HEALTH CARE STATE RANKINGS
2003

Health Care in the 50 United States

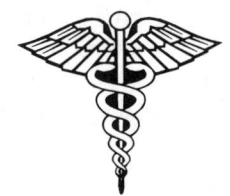

Kathleen O'Leary Morgan and Scott Morgan, Editors

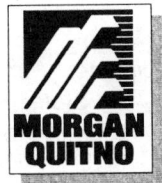

MORGAN QUITNO

Morgan Quitno Press
© Copyright 2003, All Rights Reserved

512 East 9th Street, P.O. Box 1656
Lawrence, KS 66044-8656
USA
800-457-0742 or 785-841-3534
www.statestats.com
Eleventh Edition

ISBN: 0-7401-0901-4
ISSN: 1065-1403

Health Care State Rankings 2003 sells for $54.95 ($6.00 shipping) and is only available in paper binding. For those who prefer ranking information tailored to a particular state, we also offer Health Care State Perspectives, state-specific reports for each of the 50 states. These individual guides provide information on a state's data and rank for each of the categories featured in the national Health Care State Rankings volume. Perspectives sell for $19.00 or $9.50 if ordered with Health Care State Rankings. If crime statistics are your interest, please ask about our annual Crime State Rankings ($54.95 paper). If you are interested in city and metropolitan crime data, we offer City Crime Rankings ($42.95 paper). For a general view of the states, please ask about our annual State Rankings reference book ($54.95 paper) or our monthly State Statistical Trends ($299 a year). Also available is the first edition of our Education State Rankings. This view of K-12 education at the state level is $49.95. All of our data sets are also available on CD in pdf format as well as various database formats. These sell for $100 each. Shipping and handling is $6.00 per order. For information, please visit our website at www.statestats.com.

Eleventh Edition
Printed in the United States of America
April 2003

PREFACE

As the debate rages on as to how to reel in the cost of health insurance, prescription drugs and physician and hospital services, the need for accurate and reliable health care data is more important than ever. Now in its 11th year of publication, *Health Care State Rankings* provides a solid collection of state health care information. Births and reproductive health, deaths, disease, insurance and finance, health care providers, facilities and physical fitness are compared state-by-state. Discover the answers to important health care questions, such as what percent of citizens in your state has access to primary care doctors? How many Americans do not have health insurance coverage? How much does your state spend for Medicaid? In all, more than 500 tables of state comparisons are provided, covering virtually every aspect of health care in the 50 United States.

Important Notes About *Health Care State Rankings 2003*

Health Care State Rankings 2003 presents information from government and private sector sources in one user-friendly volume. Our mission in publishing this book is to translate complicated and often convoluted health care data into easy-to-understand, meaningful state comparisons. As we revise this volume each year, we reexamine each table, update most, delete others and add new tables of interest to our readers. In this 2003 edition, our regular readers will note that a number of tables in the Finance Chapter are "repeats." The Centers For Medicare and Medicaid Services (formerly known as the Health Care Financing Administration) hopes to update its state health care expenditures numbers later this year.

We make every effort to present the data in *Health Care State Rankings 2003* as simply and straightforwardly as possible. Source information and other pertinent footnotes are clearly shown at the bottom of each page. National totals, rates and percentages are prominently displayed at the top of each table. Every other line is shaded in gray for easier reading. In addition, numerous information-finding tools are provided: a thorough table of contents, table listings at the beginning of each chapter, a roster of sources with addresses and phone numbers, a detailed index and a chapter thumb index.

For the ease of our readers, the numbers shown in *Health Care State Rankings* require no additional calculations to convert them from millions, thousands, etc. All states are ranked on a high to low basis, with any ties among the states listed alphabetically for a given ranking. Negative numbers are shown in parentheses "( )." For tables with national totals (as opposed to rates, per capitas, etc.) a separate column is included showing what percent of the national total each individual state's total represents. This column is headed by "% of USA." This percentage figure is particularly interesting when compared with a state's share of the nation's population for a particular year (provided in an appendix).

Those researchers who need information for just one state should check out our *Health Care State Perspective* series of publications. These 21-page comb bound reports feature data and ranking information for an individual state, as reported in *Health Care State Rankings 2003*. (For example *California Health Care in Perspective* features information about the state of California only.) These serve as handy, quick reference guides for those who do not want to page through the entire *Health Care State Rankings* volume searching for information for their particular state. *Health Care State Perspectives* sell for $19. When purchased with a copy of *Health Care State Rankings 2003*, these handy quick reference guides are just $9.50. For additional information, please call us toll-free at 1-800-457-0742.

Other Books From Morgan Quitno Press

In addition to *Health Care State Rankings 2003*, our company offers four other rankings reference books. The first of these, *State Rankings 2003*, is our original rankings reference book, providing a general view of the states. Statistics for categories ranging from agriculture to transportation, government finance to social welfare are featured. *Education State Rankings* is our newest state reference book, launched in the fall of 2002. This volume compares states in teachers' salaries, class sizes, graduation rates and more than 400 other categories relating to K-12 education. Our *Crime State Rankings* book provides a huge collection of user-friendly state statistics on law enforcement personnel and expenditures, corrections, juvenile crime and delinquency, arrests and offenses. For crime information that is a little closer to home, *City Crime Rankings,* compares crime in all metropolitan areas and cities of 75,000 or more population (approx. 300 cities). Numbers of crimes, crime rates and changes in crime rates over one and five years are presented for all major crime categories reported by the FBI. Final 2001 crime data are featured in the most recent 9th edition. For true data aficionados, the information in all our books also is available CD-ROM. These electronic editions provide a searchable PDF version of each book as well as the raw data in .dbf, Excel and ASCII formats.

State Statistical Trends is our popular monthly journal that examines changes in life and government for the 50 United States. Each 100-page monthly issue focuses on a different subject and provides a collection of tables, graphics and commentary showing state multi-year trends. For further information about *Trends* or any of our other publications, please call us toll-free at 1-800-457-0742 or check out our web site at www.statestats.com.

Finally, many thanks to the librarians, government and health care industry officials who help us each year. Thanks also to you, our readers. We always welcome your thoughts and suggestions, so please give us a call, send us an e-mail or drop us a note with your ideas.

- THE EDITORS

WHICH STATE IS HEALTHIEST?

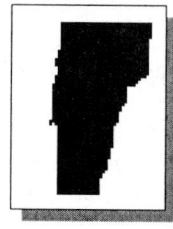

Vermont does enjoy its good health. For the third year in a row, the Green Mountain State is our Healthiest State. In our eleventh annual Healthiest State Award, Vermont's neighbor New Hampshire jumped to second followed by Nebraska in third and Iowa in fourth. Mississippi unfortunately remains consistent, bringing up the least healthy end of the rankings for the fourth year in a row. It is preceded by Louisiana in 49th, South Carolina in 48th and Alabama in 47th.

Each year we take a step back from our objective reporting of health statistics, feed some basic figures into our computer and determine which is the nation's Healthiest State. While we never claim our findings are indisputable, we do believe they provide an interesting statistical match-up of how the states are doing with regard to health care.

Methodology

The Healthiest State designation is awarded based on 21 factors chosen from the year 2003 edition of our annual reference book, *Health Care State Rankings*. These

2003 HEALTHIEST STATE AWARD

RANK	STATE	SUM	02	RANK	STATE	SUM	02
1	Vermont	18.25	1	26	Ohio	1.09	24
2	New Hampshire	17.68	4	27	Indiana	0.97	28
3	Nebraska	16.80	5	28	Michigan	(0.04)	27
4	Iowa	16.30	3	29	North Carolina	(1.38)	34
5	Minnesota	13.84	2	30	West Virginia	(1.60)	30
6	Massachusetts	13.02	9	31	Kentucky	(1.63)	33
7	Maine	12.65	11	32	Illinois	(2.85)	31
8	Hawaii	12.55	6	33	New York	(3.36)	38
9	Utah	12.39	10	34	Missouri	(3.39)	39
10	North Dakota	11.20	7	35	Maryland	(3.70)	37
11	Connecticut	10.20	8	36	Alaska	(3.84)	29
12	Washington	8.87	14	37	Tennessee	(4.67)	36
13	South Dakota	8.60	20	38	Delaware	(6.56)	43
14	California	8.30	13	39	Texas	(6.70)	42
15	Kansas	8.19	12	40	Oklahoma	(6.84)	32
16	New Jersey	7.64	15	41	Arizona	(7.41)	35
17	Rhode Island	7.34	16	42	Georgia	(8.00)	41
18	Montana	7.28	17	43	Arkansas	(8.29)	40
19	Oregon	6.99	18	44	Florida	(9.37)	44
20	Wyoming	5.88	25	45	Nevada	(12.25)	46
21	Idaho	5.29	22	46	New Mexico	(12.34)	48
22	Virginia	4.85	19	47	Alabama	(13.32)	47
23	Wisconsin	4.82	26	48	South Carolina	(13.74)	45
24	Pennsylvania	3.62	23	49	Louisiana	(16.12)	49
25	Colorado	3.49	21	50	Mississippi	(18.65)	50

factors reflect access to health care providers, affordability of health care and a generally healthy population (see box below.) All 21 factors are the same as last year. The 21 factors were divided into two groups: those that are "negative" for which a high ranking would be considered bad for a state, and those that are "positive" for which a high ranking would be considered good for a state. Rates for each of the 21 factors were processed through a formula that measures how a state compares to the national average for a given category. The positive and negative nature of each factor was taken into account as part of the formula. Once these computations were made, the factors then were weighted (factors were weighted equally.) These weighted scores were then added together to get a state's final score ("SUM" on the table above.) This way, states are assessed based on how they stack up against the national average. The end result is that the farther below the national average a state's health ranking is, the lower (and less healthy) it ranks. The farther above the national average, the higher (and healthier) a state ranks. This same methodology was used for our Dangerous State and Safest/Dangerous City Awards.

The table above shows how each state fared in the 2003 Healthiest State Award as well as its placement in 2002. Congratulations to the citizens of Vermont. We wish you continued good health!

THE EDITORS

POSITIVE (+) AND NEGATIVE (-) FACTORS CONSIDERED:
1. Births of Low Birthweight as a Percent of All Births (Table 15) -
2. Teenage Birth Rate (Table 31) -
3. Percent of Mothers Receiving Late or No Prenatal Care (Table 59) -
4. Age-Adjusted Death Rate (Table 83) -
5. Infant Mortality Rate (Table 87) -
6. Age-Adjusted Death Rate by Malignant Neoplasms (Table 154) -
7. Age-Adjusted Death Rate by Suicide (Table 175) -
8. Percent of Population Not Covered by Health Insurance (Table 234) -
9. Health Care Expenditures as a Percent of Gross State Product (Table 282) -
10. Per Capita Personal Health Expenditures (Table 285) -
11. Estimated Rate of New Cancer Cases (Table 350) -

12. AIDS Rate (Table 376) -
13. Sexually Transmitted Disease Rate (Table 412) -
14. Percent of Population Lacking Access to Primary Care (Table 439) -
15. Percent of Adults Who Are Binge Drinkers (Table 500) -
16. Percent of Adults Who Smoke (Table 501) -
17. Percent of Adults Obese (Table 505) -
18. Number of Days in Past Month When Physical Health was "Not Good" (Table 509) -
19. Beds in Community Hospitals per 100,000 Population (Table 201) +
20. Percent of Children Aged 19-35 Months Fully Immunized (Table 409) +
21. Safety Belt Usage Rate (Table 512) +

TABLE OF CONTENTS

I. Births and Reproductive Health

TABLE OF CONTENTS (continued)

TABLE OF CONTENTS (continued)

TABLE OF CONTENTS (continued)

III. Facilities

TABLE OF CONTENTS (continued)

IV. Finance

TABLE OF CONTENTS (continued)

TABLE OF CONTENTS (continued)

V. Incidence of Disease

TABLE OF CONTENTS (continued)

TABLE OF CONTENTS (continued)

VII. Physical Fitness

VIII. Appendix

IX. Sources

X. Index

I. BIRTHS AND REPRODUCTIVE HEALTH

I. BIRTHS AND REPRODUCTIVE HEALTH
(CONTINUED)

Abortions

Births in 2001

National Total = 4,025,933 Live Births*

ALPHA ORDER

RANK	STATE	BIRTHS	% of USA
24	Alabama	60,454	1.5%
47	Alaska	10,003	0.2%
14	Arizona	85,597	2.1%
34	Arkansas	37,010	0.9%
1	California	527,759	13.1%
22	Colorado	67,007	1.7%
30	Connecticut	42,648	1.1%
45	Delaware	10,749	0.3%
4	Florida	205,793	5.1%
8	Georgia	133,526	3.3%
40	Hawaii	17,072	0.4%
38	Idaho	20,688	0.5%
5	Illinois	184,064	4.6%
13	Indiana	86,459	2.1%
33	Iowa	37,619	0.9%
32	Kansas	38,869	1.0%
26	Kentucky	54,658	1.4%
23	Louisiana	65,352	1.6%
42	Maine	13,759	0.3%
19	Maryland	73,218	1.8%
15	Massachusetts	81,077	2.0%
9	Michigan	133,427	3.3%
21	Minnesota	67,562	1.7%
31	Mississippi	42,282	1.1%
18	Missouri	75,464	1.9%
44	Montana	10,970	0.3%
37	Nebraska	24,820	0.6%
35	Nevada	31,382	0.8%
41	New Hampshire	14,656	0.4%
11	New Jersey	115,795	2.9%
36	New Mexico	27,128	0.7%
3	New York	254,026	6.3%
10	North Carolina	118,185	2.9%
48	North Dakota	7,629	0.2%
6	Ohio	151,570	3.8%
27	Oklahoma	50,118	1.2%
29	Oregon	45,322	1.1%
7	Pennsylvania	143,495	3.6%
43	Rhode Island	12,713	0.3%
25	South Carolina	55,756	1.4%
46	South Dakota	10,483	0.3%
17	Tennessee	78,340	1.9%
2	Texas	365,410	9.1%
28	Utah	47,959	1.2%
49	Vermont	6,366	0.2%
12	Virginia	98,884	2.5%
16	Washington	79,570	2.0%
39	West Virginia	20,428	0.5%
20	Wisconsin	69,072	1.7%
50	Wyoming	6,115	0.2%

RANK ORDER

RANK	STATE	BIRTHS	% of USA
1	California	527,759	13.1%
2	Texas	365,410	9.1%
3	New York	254,026	6.3%
4	Florida	205,793	5.1%
5	Illinois	184,064	4.6%
6	Ohio	151,570	3.8%
7	Pennsylvania	143,495	3.6%
8	Georgia	133,526	3.3%
9	Michigan	133,427	3.3%
10	North Carolina	118,185	2.9%
11	New Jersey	115,795	2.9%
12	Virginia	98,884	2.5%
13	Indiana	86,459	2.1%
14	Arizona	85,597	2.1%
15	Massachusetts	81,077	2.0%
16	Washington	79,570	2.0%
17	Tennessee	78,340	1.9%
18	Missouri	75,464	1.9%
19	Maryland	73,218	1.8%
20	Wisconsin	69,072	1.7%
21	Minnesota	67,562	1.7%
22	Colorado	67,007	1.7%
23	Louisiana	65,352	1.6%
24	Alabama	60,454	1.5%
25	South Carolina	55,756	1.4%
26	Kentucky	54,658	1.4%
27	Oklahoma	50,118	1.2%
28	Utah	47,959	1.2%
29	Oregon	45,322	1.1%
30	Connecticut	42,648	1.1%
31	Mississippi	42,282	1.1%
32	Kansas	38,869	1.0%
33	Iowa	37,619	0.9%
34	Arkansas	37,010	0.9%
35	Nevada	31,382	0.8%
36	New Mexico	27,128	0.7%
37	Nebraska	24,820	0.6%
38	Idaho	20,688	0.5%
39	West Virginia	20,428	0.5%
40	Hawaii	17,072	0.4%
41	New Hampshire	14,656	0.4%
42	Maine	13,759	0.3%
43	Rhode Island	12,713	0.3%
44	Montana	10,970	0.3%
45	Delaware	10,749	0.3%
46	South Dakota	10,483	0.3%
47	Alaska	10,003	0.2%
48	North Dakota	7,629	0.2%
49	Vermont	6,366	0.2%
50	Wyoming	6,115	0.2%
	District of Columbia	7,625	0.2%

Source: U.S. Department of Health and Human Services, National Center for Health Statistics
"National Vital Statistics Reports" (Vol. 51, No. 2, December 18, 2002)
*Final data by state of residence.

Birth Rate in 2001

National Rate = 14.1 Live Births per 1,000 Population*

ALPHA ORDER

RANK ORDER

RANK	STATE	RATE		RANK	STATE	RATE
30	Alabama	13.7		1	Utah	21.8
6	Alaska	16.0		2	Texas	17.6
3	Arizona	17.1		3	Arizona	17.1
20	Arkansas	14.3		4	Georgia	16.5
9	California	15.5		5	Nevada	16.1
8	Colorado	15.9		6	Alaska	16.0
40	Connecticut	12.9		6	Idaho	16.0
26	Delaware	13.9		8	Colorado	15.9
37	Florida	13.2		9	California	15.5
4	Georgia	16.5		10	New Mexico	15.4
17	Hawaii	14.5		11	Mississippi	15.1
6	Idaho	16.0		11	North Carolina	15.1
13	Illinois	15.0		13	Illinois	15.0
19	Indiana	14.4		14	Louisiana	14.9
38	Iowa	13.0		15	Nebraska	14.8
17	Kansas	14.5		15	Oklahoma	14.8
31	Kentucky	13.6		17	Hawaii	14.5
14	Louisiana	14.9		17	Kansas	14.5
49	Maine	10.9		19	Indiana	14.4
26	Maryland	13.9		20	Arkansas	14.3
38	Massachusetts	13.0		21	South Carolina	14.1
35	Michigan	13.4		21	South Dakota	14.1
29	Minnesota	13.8		23	New Jersey	14.0
11	Mississippi	15.1		23	Tennessee	14.0
31	Missouri	13.6		23	Virginia	14.0
44	Montana	12.3		26	Delaware	13.9
15	Nebraska	14.8		26	Maryland	13.9
5	Nevada	16.1		26	New York	13.9
47	New Hampshire	11.9		29	Minnesota	13.8
23	New Jersey	14.0		30	Alabama	13.7
10	New Mexico	15.4		31	Kentucky	13.6
26	New York	13.9		31	Missouri	13.6
11	North Carolina	15.1		31	Washington	13.6
45	North Dakota	12.2		34	Oregon	13.5
35	Ohio	13.4		35	Michigan	13.4
15	Oklahoma	14.8		35	Ohio	13.4
34	Oregon	13.5		37	Florida	13.2
46	Pennsylvania	12.0		38	Iowa	13.0
42	Rhode Island	12.7		38	Massachusetts	13.0
21	South Carolina	14.1		40	Connecticut	12.9
21	South Dakota	14.1		40	Wisconsin	12.9
23	Tennessee	14.0		42	Rhode Island	12.7
2	Texas	17.6		42	Wyoming	12.7
1	Utah	21.8		44	Montana	12.3
50	Vermont	10.6		45	North Dakota	12.2
23	Virginia	14.0		46	Pennsylvania	12.0
31	Washington	13.6		47	New Hampshire	11.9
48	West Virginia	11.4		48	West Virginia	11.4
40	Wisconsin	12.9		49	Maine	10.9
42	Wyoming	12.7		50	Vermont	10.6
					District of Columbia	14.8

Source: U.S. Department of Health and Human Services, National Center for Health Statistics
    "National Vital Statistics Reports" (Vol. 51, No. 2, December 18, 2002). National figure revised by
    "National Vital Statistics Reports" (Vol. 51, No. 4, February 6, 2003)
*Final data by state of residence.

Births in 2000

National Total = 4,058,814 Births*

ALPHA ORDER

RANK	STATE	BIRTHS	% of USA
24	Alabama	63,299	1.6%
47	Alaska	9,974	0.2%
14	Arizona	85,273	2.1%
34	Arkansas	37,783	0.9%
1	California	531,959	13.1%
23	Colorado	65,438	1.6%
31	Connecticut	43,026	1.1%
44	Delaware	11,051	0.3%
4	Florida	204,125	5.0%
9	Georgia	132,644	3.3%
40	Hawaii	17,551	0.4%
39	Idaho	20,366	0.5%
5	Illinois	185,036	4.6%
13	Indiana	87,699	2.2%
33	Iowa	38,266	0.9%
32	Kansas	39,666	1.0%
26	Kentucky	56,029	1.4%
21	Louisiana	67,898	1.7%
42	Maine	13,603	0.3%
19	Maryland	74,316	1.8%
15	Massachusetts	81,614	2.0%
8	Michigan	136,171	3.4%
22	Minnesota	67,604	1.7%
30	Mississippi	44,075	1.1%
18	Missouri	76,463	1.9%
45	Montana	10,957	0.3%
37	Nebraska	24,646	0.6%
35	Nevada	30,829	0.8%
41	New Hampshire	14,609	0.4%
11	New Jersey	115,632	2.8%
36	New Mexico	27,223	0.7%
3	New York	258,737	6.4%
10	North Carolina	120,311	3.0%
48	North Dakota	7,676	0.2%
6	Ohio	155,472	3.8%
27	Oklahoma	49,782	1.2%
29	Oregon	45,804	1.1%
7	Pennsylvania	146,281	3.6%
43	Rhode Island	12,505	0.3%
25	South Carolina	56,114	1.4%
46	South Dakota	10,345	0.3%
17	Tennessee	79,611	2.0%
2	Texas	363,414	9.0%
28	Utah	47,353	1.2%
49	Vermont	6,500	0.2%
12	Virginia	98,938	2.4%
16	Washington	81,036	2.0%
38	West Virginia	20,865	0.5%
20	Wisconsin	69,326	1.7%
50	Wyoming	6,253	0.2%

RANK ORDER

RANK	STATE	BIRTHS	% of USA
1	California	531,959	13.1%
2	Texas	363,414	9.0%
3	New York	258,737	6.4%
4	Florida	204,125	5.0%
5	Illinois	185,036	4.6%
6	Ohio	155,472	3.8%
7	Pennsylvania	146,281	3.6%
8	Michigan	136,171	3.4%
9	Georgia	132,644	3.3%
10	North Carolina	120,311	3.0%
11	New Jersey	115,632	2.8%
12	Virginia	98,938	2.4%
13	Indiana	87,699	2.2%
14	Arizona	85,273	2.1%
15	Massachusetts	81,614	2.0%
16	Washington	81,036	2.0%
17	Tennessee	79,611	2.0%
18	Missouri	76,463	1.9%
19	Maryland	74,316	1.8%
20	Wisconsin	69,326	1.7%
21	Louisiana	67,898	1.7%
22	Minnesota	67,604	1.7%
23	Colorado	65,438	1.6%
24	Alabama	63,299	1.6%
25	South Carolina	56,114	1.4%
26	Kentucky	56,029	1.4%
27	Oklahoma	49,782	1.2%
28	Utah	47,353	1.2%
29	Oregon	45,804	1.1%
30	Mississippi	44,075	1.1%
31	Connecticut	43,026	1.1%
32	Kansas	39,666	1.0%
33	Iowa	38,266	0.9%
34	Arkansas	37,783	0.9%
35	Nevada	30,829	0.8%
36	New Mexico	27,223	0.7%
37	Nebraska	24,646	0.6%
38	West Virginia	20,865	0.5%
39	Idaho	20,366	0.5%
40	Hawaii	17,551	0.4%
41	New Hampshire	14,609	0.4%
42	Maine	13,603	0.3%
43	Rhode Island	12,505	0.3%
44	Delaware	11,051	0.3%
45	Montana	10,957	0.3%
46	South Dakota	10,345	0.3%
47	Alaska	9,974	0.2%
48	North Dakota	7,676	0.2%
49	Vermont	6,500	0.2%
50	Wyoming	6,253	0.2%
	District of Columbia	7,666	0.2%

Source: U.S. Department of Health and Human Services, National Center for Health Statistics
"National Vital Statistics Reports" (Vol. 50, No. 5, February 12, 2002)
*Final data by state of residence.

Birth Rate in 2000

National Rate = 14.4 Live Births per 1,000 Population*

ALPHA ORDER

RANK	STATE	RATE
22	Alabama	14.4
6	Alaska	16.0
3	Arizona	17.5
18	Arkansas	14.7
8	California	15.8
8	Colorado	15.8
41	Connecticut	13.0
21	Delaware	14.5
37	Florida	13.3
4	Georgia	16.7
15	Hawaii	14.9
6	Idaho	16.0
14	Illinois	15.2
18	Indiana	14.7
37	Iowa	13.3
15	Kansas	14.9
28	Kentucky	14.1
12	Louisiana	15.5
50	Maine	10.8
25	Maryland	14.2
39	Massachusetts	13.2
35	Michigan	13.7
30	Minnesota	14.0
8	Mississippi	15.8
32	Missouri	13.9
44	Montana	12.3
17	Nebraska	14.8
5	Nevada	16.4
47	New Hampshire	12.0
28	New Jersey	14.1
11	New Mexico	15.6
25	New York	14.2
12	North Carolina	15.5
45	North Dakota	12.2
34	Ohio	13.8
18	Oklahoma	14.7
35	Oregon	13.7
45	Pennsylvania	12.2
43	Rhode Island	12.6
24	South Carolina	14.3
30	South Dakota	14.0
22	Tennessee	14.4
2	Texas	17.8
1	Utah	21.9
49	Vermont	10.9
25	Virginia	14.2
32	Washington	13.9
48	West Virginia	11.6
40	Wisconsin	13.1
41	Wyoming	13.0

RANK ORDER

RANK	STATE	RATE
1	Utah	21.9
2	Texas	17.8
3	Arizona	17.5
4	Georgia	16.7
5	Nevada	16.4
6	Alaska	16.0
6	Idaho	16.0
8	California	15.8
8	Colorado	15.8
8	Mississippi	15.8
11	New Mexico	15.6
12	Louisiana	15.5
12	North Carolina	15.5
14	Illinois	15.2
15	Hawaii	14.9
15	Kansas	14.9
17	Nebraska	14.8
18	Arkansas	14.7
18	Indiana	14.7
18	Oklahoma	14.7
21	Delaware	14.5
22	Alabama	14.4
22	Tennessee	14.4
24	South Carolina	14.3
25	Maryland	14.2
25	New York	14.2
25	Virginia	14.2
28	Kentucky	14.1
28	New Jersey	14.1
30	Minnesota	14.0
30	South Dakota	14.0
32	Missouri	13.9
32	Washington	13.9
34	Ohio	13.8
35	Michigan	13.7
35	Oregon	13.7
37	Florida	13.3
37	Iowa	13.3
39	Massachusetts	13.2
40	Wisconsin	13.1
41	Connecticut	13.0
41	Wyoming	13.0
43	Rhode Island	12.6
44	Montana	12.3
45	North Dakota	12.2
45	Pennsylvania	12.2
47	New Hampshire	12.0
48	West Virginia	11.6
49	Vermont	10.9
50	Maine	10.8
	District of Columbia	14.8

Source: U.S. Department of Health and Human Services, National Center for Health Statistics
"National Vital Statistics Reports" (Vol. 50, No. 5, February 12, 2002). National figure revised by
"National Vital Statistics Reports" (Vol. 51, No. 4, February 6, 2003)
*Final data by state of residence.

Birth Rate in 1990

National Rate = 16.7 Births per 1,000 Population*

ALPHA ORDER

RANK	STATE	RATE
26	Alabama	15.7
1	Alaska	21.6
4	Arizona	18.8
29	Arkansas	15.5
3	California	20.6
20	Colorado	16.2
38	Connecticut	15.2
15	Delaware	16.7
32	Florida	15.4
9	Georgia	17.4
6	Hawaii	18.5
18	Idaho	16.3
10	Illinois	17.1
28	Indiana	15.6
48	Iowa	14.2
26	Kansas	15.7
43	Kentucky	14.8
10	Louisiana	17.1
49	Maine	14.1
13	Maryland	16.8
32	Massachusetts	15.4
16	Michigan	16.5
29	Minnesota	15.5
12	Mississippi	16.9
29	Missouri	15.5
45	Montana	14.5
32	Nebraska	15.4
8	Nevada	18.0
22	New Hampshire	15.8
22	New Jersey	15.8
7	New Mexico	18.1
16	New York	16.5
22	North Carolina	15.8
45	North Dakota	14.5
32	Ohio	15.4
39	Oklahoma	15.1
39	Oregon	15.1
45	Pennsylvania	14.5
39	Rhode Island	15.1
13	South Carolina	16.8
22	South Dakota	15.8
32	Tennessee	15.4
5	Texas	18.6
2	Utah	21.1
44	Vermont	14.7
21	Virginia	16.1
18	Washington	16.3
50	West Virginia	12.6
42	Wisconsin	14.9
32	Wyoming	15.4

RANK ORDER

RANK	STATE	RATE
1	Alaska	21.6
2	Utah	21.1
3	California	20.6
4	Arizona	18.8
5	Texas	18.6
6	Hawaii	18.5
7	New Mexico	18.1
8	Nevada	18.0
9	Georgia	17.4
10	Illinois	17.1
10	Louisiana	17.1
12	Mississippi	16.9
13	Maryland	16.8
13	South Carolina	16.8
15	Delaware	16.7
16	Michigan	16.5
16	New York	16.5
18	Idaho	16.3
18	Washington	16.3
20	Colorado	16.2
21	Virginia	16.1
22	New Hampshire	15.8
22	New Jersey	15.8
22	North Carolina	15.8
22	South Dakota	15.8
26	Alabama	15.7
26	Kansas	15.7
28	Indiana	15.6
29	Arkansas	15.5
29	Minnesota	15.5
29	Missouri	15.5
32	Florida	15.4
32	Massachusetts	15.4
32	Nebraska	15.4
32	Ohio	15.4
32	Tennessee	15.4
32	Wyoming	15.4
38	Connecticut	15.2
39	Oklahoma	15.1
39	Oregon	15.1
39	Rhode Island	15.1
42	Wisconsin	14.9
43	Kentucky	14.8
44	Vermont	14.7
45	Montana	14.5
45	North Dakota	14.5
45	Pennsylvania	14.5
48	Iowa	14.2
49	Maine	14.1
50	West Virginia	12.6
	District of Columbia	19.5

Source: U.S. Department of Health and Human Services, National Center for Health Statistics
"Monthly Vital Statistics Report" (Vol. 41, No. 9, Supplement, February 25, 1993)
*Final data by state of residence.

Birth Rate in 1980

National Rate = 15.9 Births per 1,000 Population*

ALPHA ORDER

RANK	STATE	RATE
27	Alabama	16.3
2	Alaska	23.7
11	Arizona	18.4
27	Arkansas	16.3
18	California	17.0
15	Colorado	17.2
50	Connecticut	12.5
33	Delaware	15.8
45	Florida	13.5
19	Georgia	16.9
10	Hawaii	18.8
4	Idaho	21.4
20	Illinois	16.6
30	Indiana	16.1
24	Iowa	16.4
15	Kansas	17.2
27	Kentucky	16.3
6	Louisiana	19.5
41	Maine	14.6
43	Maryland	14.2
49	Massachusetts	12.7
34	Michigan	15.7
20	Minnesota	16.6
9	Mississippi	19.0
30	Missouri	16.1
13	Montana	18.1
14	Nebraska	17.4
20	Nevada	16.6
39	New Hampshire	14.9
47	New Jersey	13.2
5	New Mexico	20.0
44	New York	13.6
42	North Carolina	14.4
11	North Dakota	18.4
34	Ohio	15.7
15	Oklahoma	17.2
24	Oregon	16.4
46	Pennsylvania	13.4
48	Rhode Island	12.9
20	South Carolina	16.6
7	South Dakota	19.2
37	Tennessee	15.1
7	Texas	19.2
1	Utah	28.6
36	Vermont	15.4
40	Virginia	14.7
24	Washington	16.4
37	West Virginia	15.1
32	Wisconsin	15.9
3	Wyoming	22.5

RANK ORDER

RANK	STATE	RATE
1	Utah	28.6
2	Alaska	23.7
3	Wyoming	22.5
4	Idaho	21.4
5	New Mexico	20.0
6	Louisiana	19.5
7	South Dakota	19.2
7	Texas	19.2
9	Mississippi	19.0
10	Hawaii	18.8
11	Arizona	18.4
11	North Dakota	18.4
13	Montana	18.1
14	Nebraska	17.4
15	Colorado	17.2
15	Kansas	17.2
15	Oklahoma	17.2
18	California	17.0
19	Georgia	16.9
20	Illinois	16.6
20	Minnesota	16.6
20	Nevada	16.6
20	South Carolina	16.6
24	Iowa	16.4
24	Oregon	16.4
24	Washington	16.4
27	Alabama	16.3
27	Arkansas	16.3
27	Kentucky	16.3
30	Indiana	16.1
30	Missouri	16.1
32	Wisconsin	15.9
33	Delaware	15.8
34	Michigan	15.7
34	Ohio	15.7
36	Vermont	15.4
37	Tennessee	15.1
37	West Virginia	15.1
39	New Hampshire	14.9
40	Virginia	14.7
41	Maine	14.6
42	North Carolina	14.4
43	Maryland	14.2
44	New York	13.6
45	Florida	13.5
46	Pennsylvania	13.4
47	New Jersey	13.2
48	Rhode Island	12.9
49	Massachusetts	12.7
50	Connecticut	12.5
	District of Columbia	14.7

*Source: U.S. Department of Health and Human Services, National Center for Health Statistics
"Vital Statistics of the United States, 1980" and "Monthly Vital Statistics Report"*
*Live births by state of residence.

Fertility Rate in 2001

National Rate = 65.3 Live Births per 1,000 Women 15 to 44 Years Old*

ALPHA ORDER

RANK	STATE	RATE
31	Alabama	62.4
5	Alaska	75.5
2	Arizona	84.0
19	Arkansas	67.5
14	California	69.5
7	Colorado	74.6
38	Connecticut	61.0
37	Delaware	61.5
21	Florida	67.0
10	Georgia	71.1
9	Hawaii	71.4
6	Idaho	75.4
14	Illinois	69.5
23	Indiana	66.1
28	Iowa	63.4
16	Kansas	68.1
32	Kentucky	62.3
20	Louisiana	67.2
49	Maine	50.0
40	Maryland	60.9
45	Massachusetts	59.1
38	Michigan	61.0
27	Minnesota	63.5
18	Mississippi	67.6
29	Missouri	63.2
36	Montana	61.8
13	Nebraska	69.7
4	Nevada	79.4
48	New Hampshire	52.0
22	New Jersey	66.3
8	New Mexico	72.8
25	New York	64.4
12	North Carolina	70.4
43	North Dakota	59.3
34	Ohio	61.9
11	Oklahoma	70.8
24	Oregon	65.3
46	Pennsylvania	57.7
44	Rhode Island	59.2
30	South Carolina	62.8
17	South Dakota	67.7
26	Tennessee	64.3
3	Texas	79.9
1	Utah	95.0
50	Vermont	47.9
40	Virginia	60.9
34	Washington	61.9
47	West Virginia	55.6
42	Wisconsin	60.2
33	Wyoming	62.0

RANK ORDER

RANK	STATE	RATE
1	Utah	95.0
2	Arizona	84.0
3	Texas	79.9
4	Nevada	79.4
5	Alaska	75.5
6	Idaho	75.4
7	Colorado	74.6
8	New Mexico	72.8
9	Hawaii	71.4
10	Georgia	71.1
11	Oklahoma	70.8
12	North Carolina	70.4
13	Nebraska	69.7
14	California	69.5
14	Illinois	69.5
16	Kansas	68.1
17	South Dakota	67.7
18	Mississippi	67.6
19	Arkansas	67.5
20	Louisiana	67.2
21	Florida	67.0
22	New Jersey	66.3
23	Indiana	66.1
24	Oregon	65.3
25	New York	64.4
26	Tennessee	64.3
27	Minnesota	63.5
28	Iowa	63.4
29	Missouri	63.2
30	South Carolina	62.8
31	Alabama	62.4
32	Kentucky	62.3
33	Wyoming	62.0
34	Ohio	61.9
34	Washington	61.9
36	Montana	61.8
37	Delaware	61.5
38	Connecticut	61.0
38	Michigan	61.0
40	Maryland	60.9
40	Virginia	60.9
42	Wisconsin	60.2
43	North Dakota	59.3
44	Rhode Island	59.2
45	Massachusetts	59.1
46	Pennsylvania	57.7
47	West Virginia	55.6
48	New Hampshire	52.0
49	Maine	50.0
50	Vermont	47.9
	District of Columbia	63.9

Source: U.S. Department of Health and Human Services, National Center for Health Statistics
"National Vital Statistics Reports" (Vol. 51, No. 2, December 18, 2002). National figure revised by
"National Vital Statistics Reports" (Vol. 51, No. 4, February 6, 2003)
*Final data by state of residence.

Births to White Women in 2001

National Total = 3,177,626 Live Births to White Women*

ALPHA ORDER

RANK	STATE	BIRTHS	% of USA
26	Alabama	40,604	1.3%
47	Alaska	6,383	0.2%
13	Arizona	75,219	2.4%
33	Arkansas	28,836	0.9%
1	California	428,238	13.5%
18	Colorado	61,056	1.9%
30	Connecticut	35,612	1.1%
45	Delaware	7,668	0.2%
4	Florida	152,207	4.8%
9	Georgia	85,648	2.7%
50	Hawaii	3,815	0.1%
38	Idaho	19,944	0.6%
5	Illinois	142,474	4.5%
12	Indiana	75,393	2.4%
31	Iowa	35,324	1.1%
32	Kansas	34,622	1.1%
22	Kentucky	48,968	1.5%
28	Louisiana	36,899	1.2%
41	Maine	13,280	0.4%
24	Maryland	45,068	1.4%
15	Massachusetts	67,786	2.1%
8	Michigan	105,235	3.3%
21	Minnesota	57,982	1.8%
36	Mississippi	22,808	0.7%
17	Missouri	62,504	2.0%
43	Montana	9,442	0.3%
37	Nebraska	22,496	0.7%
34	Nevada	26,284	0.8%
40	New Hampshire	13,954	0.4%
11	New Jersey	85,110	2.7%
35	New Mexico	22,810	0.7%
3	New York	182,191	5.7%
10	North Carolina	85,315	2.7%
46	North Dakota	6,625	0.2%
6	Ohio	125,507	3.9%
27	Oklahoma	39,218	1.2%
25	Oregon	41,284	1.3%
7	Pennsylvania	119,015	3.7%
42	Rhode Island	10,960	0.3%
29	South Carolina	35,866	1.1%
44	South Dakota	8,475	0.3%
19	Tennessee	60,216	1.9%
2	Texas	311,979	9.8%
23	Utah	45,440	1.4%
48	Vermont	6,237	0.2%
14	Virginia	70,946	2.2%
16	Washington	67,437	2.1%
39	West Virginia	19,576	0.6%
20	Wisconsin	59,383	1.9%
49	Wyoming	5,717	0.2%

RANK ORDER

RANK	STATE	BIRTHS	% of USA
1	California	428,238	13.5%
2	Texas	311,979	9.8%
3	New York	182,191	5.7%
4	Florida	152,207	4.8%
5	Illinois	142,474	4.5%
6	Ohio	125,507	3.9%
7	Pennsylvania	119,015	3.7%
8	Michigan	105,235	3.3%
9	Georgia	85,648	2.7%
10	North Carolina	85,315	2.7%
11	New Jersey	85,110	2.7%
12	Indiana	75,393	2.4%
13	Arizona	75,219	2.4%
14	Virginia	70,946	2.2%
15	Massachusetts	67,786	2.1%
16	Washington	67,437	2.1%
17	Missouri	62,504	2.0%
18	Colorado	61,056	1.9%
19	Tennessee	60,216	1.9%
20	Wisconsin	59,383	1.9%
21	Minnesota	57,982	1.8%
22	Kentucky	48,968	1.5%
23	Utah	45,440	1.4%
24	Maryland	45,068	1.4%
25	Oregon	41,284	1.3%
26	Alabama	40,604	1.3%
27	Oklahoma	39,218	1.2%
28	Louisiana	36,899	1.2%
29	South Carolina	35,866	1.1%
30	Connecticut	35,612	1.1%
31	Iowa	35,324	1.1%
32	Kansas	34,622	1.1%
33	Arkansas	28,836	0.9%
34	Nevada	26,284	0.8%
35	New Mexico	22,810	0.7%
36	Mississippi	22,808	0.7%
37	Nebraska	22,496	0.7%
38	Idaho	19,944	0.6%
39	West Virginia	19,576	0.6%
40	New Hampshire	13,954	0.4%
41	Maine	13,280	0.4%
42	Rhode Island	10,960	0.3%
43	Montana	9,442	0.3%
44	South Dakota	8,475	0.3%
45	Delaware	7,668	0.2%
46	North Dakota	6,625	0.2%
47	Alaska	6,383	0.2%
48	Vermont	6,237	0.2%
49	Wyoming	5,717	0.2%
50	Hawaii	3,815	0.1%
	District of Columbia	2,570	0.1%

Source: U.S. Department of Health and Human Services, National Center for Health Statistics
"National Vital Statistics Reports" (Vol. 51, No. 2, December 18, 2002)
*Final data by state of residence. By race of mother.

White Births as a Percent of All Births in 2001

National Percent = 78.9% of Live Births*

ALPHA ORDER

RANK	STATE	PERCENT
43	Alabama	67.2
46	Alaska	63.8
14	Arizona	87.9
34	Arkansas	77.9
30	California	81.1
9	Colorado	91.1
26	Connecticut	83.5
42	Delaware	71.3
37	Florida	74.0
45	Georgia	64.1
50	Hawaii	22.3
3	Idaho	96.4
35	Illinois	77.4
15	Indiana	87.2
7	Iowa	93.9
13	Kansas	89.1
12	Kentucky	89.6
48	Louisiana	56.5
2	Maine	96.5
47	Maryland	61.6
25	Massachusetts	83.6
32	Michigan	78.9
20	Minnesota	85.8
49	Mississippi	53.9
28	Missouri	82.8
18	Montana	86.1
11	Nebraska	90.6
24	Nevada	83.8
5	New Hampshire	95.2
38	New Jersey	73.5
23	New Mexico	84.1
40	New York	71.7
39	North Carolina	72.2
16	North Dakota	86.8
28	Ohio	82.8
33	Oklahoma	78.3
9	Oregon	91.1
27	Pennsylvania	82.9
17	Rhode Island	86.2
44	South Carolina	64.3
31	South Dakota	80.8
36	Tennessee	76.9
21	Texas	85.4
6	Utah	94.7
1	Vermont	98.0
40	Virginia	71.7
22	Washington	84.8
4	West Virginia	95.8
19	Wisconsin	86.0
8	Wyoming	93.5

RANK ORDER

RANK	STATE	PERCENT
1	Vermont	98.0
2	Maine	96.5
3	Idaho	96.4
4	West Virginia	95.8
5	New Hampshire	95.2
6	Utah	94.7
7	Iowa	93.9
8	Wyoming	93.5
9	Colorado	91.1
9	Oregon	91.1
11	Nebraska	90.6
12	Kentucky	89.6
13	Kansas	89.1
14	Arizona	87.9
15	Indiana	87.2
16	North Dakota	86.8
17	Rhode Island	86.2
18	Montana	86.1
19	Wisconsin	86.0
20	Minnesota	85.8
21	Texas	85.4
22	Washington	84.8
23	New Mexico	84.1
24	Nevada	83.8
25	Massachusetts	83.6
26	Connecticut	83.5
27	Pennsylvania	82.9
28	Missouri	82.8
28	Ohio	82.8
30	California	81.1
31	South Dakota	80.8
32	Michigan	78.9
33	Oklahoma	78.3
34	Arkansas	77.9
35	Illinois	77.4
36	Tennessee	76.9
37	Florida	74.0
38	New Jersey	73.5
39	North Carolina	72.2
40	New York	71.7
40	Virginia	71.7
42	Delaware	71.3
43	Alabama	67.2
44	South Carolina	64.3
45	Georgia	64.1
46	Alaska	63.8
47	Maryland	61.6
48	Louisiana	56.5
49	Mississippi	53.9
50	Hawaii	22.3

District of Columbia	33.7

Source: Morgan Quitno Press using data from U.S. Dept. of Health and Human Services, Nat'l Center for Health Statistics
"National Vital Statistics Reports" (Vol. 51, No. 2, December 18, 2002)
*Final data by state of residence. By race of mother.

Births to Black Women in 2001

National Total = 606,156 Live Births to Black Women*

ALPHA ORDER

RANK	STATE	BIRTHS	% of USA
15	Alabama	19,199	3.2%
41	Alaska	441	0.1%
31	Arizona	2,762	0.5%
22	Arkansas	7,435	1.2%
5	California	33,774	5.6%
29	Colorado	2,971	0.5%
24	Connecticut	5,134	0.8%
32	Delaware	2,710	0.4%
2	Florida	47,186	7.8%
3	Georgia	43,727	7.2%
39	Hawaii	527	0.1%
47	Idaho	86	0.0%
6	Illinois	33,203	5.5%
20	Indiana	9,649	1.6%
35	Iowa	1,266	0.2%
30	Kansas	2,781	0.5%
25	Kentucky	4,930	0.8%
8	Louisiana	27,058	4.5%
44	Maine	153	0.0%
9	Maryland	24,252	4.0%
21	Massachusetts	8,205	1.4%
10	Michigan	23,613	3.9%
26	Minnesota	4,767	0.8%
17	Mississippi	18,817	3.1%
19	Missouri	11,134	1.8%
49	Montana	42	0.0%
34	Nebraska	1,373	0.2%
33	Nevada	2,518	0.4%
43	New Hampshire	208	0.0%
13	New Jersey	20,583	3.4%
40	New Mexico	511	0.1%
1	New York	52,190	8.6%
7	North Carolina	28,393	4.7%
45	North Dakota	102	0.0%
11	Ohio	22,994	3.8%
27	Oklahoma	4,612	0.8%
37	Oregon	944	0.2%
14	Pennsylvania	20,238	3.3%
36	Rhode Island	1,112	0.2%
16	South Carolina	18,927	3.1%
46	South Dakota	101	0.0%
18	Tennessee	16,603	2.7%
4	Texas	40,750	6.7%
42	Utah	342	0.1%
50	Vermont	31	0.0%
12	Virginia	22,272	3.7%
28	Washington	3,334	0.6%
38	West Virginia	704	0.1%
23	Wisconsin	6,567	1.1%
48	Wyoming	65	0.0%

RANK ORDER

RANK	STATE	BIRTHS	% of USA
1	New York	52,190	8.6%
2	Florida	47,186	7.8%
3	Georgia	43,727	7.2%
4	Texas	40,750	6.7%
5	California	33,774	5.6%
6	Illinois	33,203	5.5%
7	North Carolina	28,393	4.7%
8	Louisiana	27,058	4.5%
9	Maryland	24,252	4.0%
10	Michigan	23,613	3.9%
11	Ohio	22,994	3.8%
12	Virginia	22,272	3.7%
13	New Jersey	20,583	3.4%
14	Pennsylvania	20,238	3.3%
15	Alabama	19,199	3.2%
16	South Carolina	18,927	3.1%
17	Mississippi	18,817	3.1%
18	Tennessee	16,603	2.7%
19	Missouri	11,134	1.8%
20	Indiana	9,649	1.6%
21	Massachusetts	8,205	1.4%
22	Arkansas	7,435	1.2%
23	Wisconsin	6,567	1.1%
24	Connecticut	5,134	0.8%
25	Kentucky	4,930	0.8%
26	Minnesota	4,767	0.8%
27	Oklahoma	4,612	0.8%
28	Washington	3,334	0.6%
29	Colorado	2,971	0.5%
30	Kansas	2,781	0.5%
31	Arizona	2,762	0.5%
32	Delaware	2,710	0.4%
33	Nevada	2,518	0.4%
34	Nebraska	1,373	0.2%
35	Iowa	1,266	0.2%
36	Rhode Island	1,112	0.2%
37	Oregon	944	0.2%
38	West Virginia	704	0.1%
39	Hawaii	527	0.1%
40	New Mexico	511	0.1%
41	Alaska	441	0.1%
42	Utah	342	0.1%
43	New Hampshire	208	0.0%
44	Maine	153	0.0%
45	North Dakota	102	0.0%
46	South Dakota	101	0.0%
47	Idaho	86	0.0%
48	Wyoming	65	0.0%
49	Montana	42	0.0%
50	Vermont	31	0.0%
	District of Columbia	4,860	0.8%

Source: U.S. Department of Health and Human Services, National Center for Health Statistics "National Vital Statistics Reports" (Vol. 51, No. 2, December 18, 2002)
*Final data by state of residence. By race of mother.

Black Births as a Percent of All Births in 2001

National Percent = 15.1% of Live Births*

ALPHA ORDER			RANK ORDER		
RANK	STATE	PERCENT	RANK	STATE	PERCENT
6	Alabama	31.8	1	Mississippi	44.5
33	Alaska	4.4	2	Louisiana	41.4
38	Arizona	3.2	3	South Carolina	33.9
13	Arkansas	20.1	4	Maryland	33.1
31	California	6.4	5	Georgia	32.7
33	Colorado	4.4	6	Alabama	31.8
20	Connecticut	12.0	7	Delaware	25.2
7	Delaware	25.2	8	North Carolina	24.0
9	Florida	22.9	9	Florida	22.9
5	Georgia	32.7	10	Virginia	22.5
39	Hawaii	3.1	11	Tennessee	21.2
49	Idaho	0.4	12	New York	20.5
14	Illinois	18.0	13	Arkansas	20.1
21	Indiana	11.2	14	Illinois	18.0
36	Iowa	3.4	15	New Jersey	17.8
29	Kansas	7.2	16	Michigan	17.7
26	Kentucky	9.0	17	Ohio	15.2
2	Louisiana	41.4	18	Missouri	14.8
44	Maine	1.1	19	Pennsylvania	14.1
4	Maryland	33.1	20	Connecticut	12.0
23	Massachusetts	10.1	21	Indiana	11.2
16	Michigan	17.7	21	Texas	11.2
30	Minnesota	7.1	23	Massachusetts	10.1
1	Mississippi	44.5	24	Wisconsin	9.5
18	Missouri	14.8	25	Oklahoma	9.2
49	Montana	0.4	26	Kentucky	9.0
32	Nebraska	5.5	27	Rhode Island	8.7
28	Nevada	8.0	28	Nevada	8.0
42	New Hampshire	1.4	29	Kansas	7.2
15	New Jersey	17.8	30	Minnesota	7.1
41	New Mexico	1.9	31	California	6.4
12	New York	20.5	32	Nebraska	5.5
8	North Carolina	24.0	33	Alaska	4.4
43	North Dakota	1.3	33	Colorado	4.4
17	Ohio	15.2	35	Washington	4.2
25	Oklahoma	9.2	36	Iowa	3.4
40	Oregon	2.1	36	West Virginia	3.4
19	Pennsylvania	14.1	38	Arizona	3.2
27	Rhode Island	8.7	39	Hawaii	3.1
3	South Carolina	33.9	40	Oregon	2.1
46	South Dakota	1.0	41	New Mexico	1.9
11	Tennessee	21.2	42	New Hampshire	1.4
21	Texas	11.2	43	North Dakota	1.3
47	Utah	0.7	44	Maine	1.1
48	Vermont	0.5	44	Wyoming	1.1
10	Virginia	22.5	46	South Dakota	1.0
35	Washington	4.2	47	Utah	0.7
36	West Virginia	3.4	48	Vermont	0.5
24	Wisconsin	9.5	49	Idaho	0.4
44	Wyoming	1.1	49	Montana	0.4
				District of Columbia	63.7

Source: Morgan Quitno Press using data from U.S. Dept. of Health and Human Services, Nat'l Center for Health Statistics "National Vital Statistics Reports" (Vol. 51, No. 2, December 18, 2002)
Final data by state of residence. By race of mother.

Births to Hispanic Women in 2001

National Total = 851,851 Live Births to Hispanic Women*

ALPHA ORDER

RANK	STATE	BIRTHS	% of USA
34	Alabama	2,254	0.3%
42	Alaska	652	0.1%
6	Arizona	36,183	4.2%
33	Arkansas	2,649	0.3%
1	California	261,071	30.6%
8	Colorado	19,730	2.3%
19	Connecticut	6,913	0.8%
40	Delaware	1,083	0.1%
4	Florida	49,629	5.8%
9	Georgia	15,699	1.8%
35	Hawaii	2,237	0.3%
32	Idaho	2,753	0.3%
5	Illinois	40,973	4.8%
21	Indiana	5,898	0.7%
36	Iowa	2,232	0.3%
25	Kansas	4,906	0.6%
39	Kentucky	1,509	0.2%
38	Louisiana	1,557	0.2%
47	Maine	173	0.0%
22	Maryland	5,301	0.6%
14	Massachusetts	9,444	1.1%
18	Michigan	7,335	0.9%
27	Minnesota	4,543	0.5%
41	Mississippi	719	0.1%
30	Missouri	2,981	0.3%
45	Montana	377	0.0%
31	Nebraska	2,946	0.3%
13	Nevada	10,855	1.3%
44	New Hampshire	509	0.1%
7	New Jersey	23,497	2.8%
11	New Mexico	14,126	1.7%
3	New York	54,544	6.4%
10	North Carolina	14,539	1.7%
48	North Dakota	140	0.0%
26	Ohio	4,598	0.5%
24	Oklahoma	4,942	0.6%
17	Oregon	7,902	0.9%
16	Pennsylvania	8,192	1.0%
37	Rhode Island	2,196	0.3%
29	South Carolina	2,988	0.4%
46	South Dakota	257	0.0%
28	Tennessee	3,905	0.5%
2	Texas	172,354	20.2%
20	Utah	6,543	0.8%
50	Vermont	35	0.0%
15	Virginia	9,143	1.1%
12	Washington	12,140	1.4%
49	West Virginia	83	0.0%
23	Wisconsin	5,152	0.6%
43	Wyoming	569	0.1%

RANK ORDER

RANK	STATE	BIRTHS	% of USA
1	California	261,071	30.6%
2	Texas	172,354	20.2%
3	New York	54,544	6.4%
4	Florida	49,629	5.8%
5	Illinois	40,973	4.8%
6	Arizona	36,183	4.2%
7	New Jersey	23,497	2.8%
8	Colorado	19,730	2.3%
9	Georgia	15,699	1.8%
10	North Carolina	14,539	1.7%
11	New Mexico	14,126	1.7%
12	Washington	12,140	1.4%
13	Nevada	10,855	1.3%
14	Massachusetts	9,444	1.1%
15	Virginia	9,143	1.1%
16	Pennsylvania	8,192	1.0%
17	Oregon	7,902	0.9%
18	Michigan	7,335	0.9%
19	Connecticut	6,913	0.8%
20	Utah	6,543	0.8%
21	Indiana	5,898	0.7%
22	Maryland	5,301	0.6%
23	Wisconsin	5,152	0.6%
24	Oklahoma	4,942	0.6%
25	Kansas	4,906	0.6%
26	Ohio	4,598	0.5%
27	Minnesota	4,543	0.5%
28	Tennessee	3,905	0.5%
29	South Carolina	2,988	0.4%
30	Missouri	2,981	0.3%
31	Nebraska	2,946	0.3%
32	Idaho	2,753	0.3%
33	Arkansas	2,649	0.3%
34	Alabama	2,254	0.3%
35	Hawaii	2,237	0.3%
36	Iowa	2,232	0.3%
37	Rhode Island	2,196	0.3%
38	Louisiana	1,557	0.2%
39	Kentucky	1,509	0.2%
40	Delaware	1,083	0.1%
41	Mississippi	719	0.1%
42	Alaska	652	0.1%
43	Wyoming	569	0.1%
44	New Hampshire	509	0.1%
45	Montana	377	0.0%
46	South Dakota	257	0.0%
47	Maine	173	0.0%
48	North Dakota	140	0.0%
49	West Virginia	83	0.0%
50	Vermont	35	0.0%
	District of Columbia	895	0.1%

Source: U.S. Department of Health and Human Services, National Center for Health Statistics
"National Vital Statistics Reports" (Vol. 51, No. 2, December 18, 2002)
*Final data by state of residence. By race of mother. Persons of Hispanic origin may be of any race.

Hispanic Births as a Percent of All Births in 2001

National Percent = 21.2% of Live Births*

ALPHA ORDER

RANK	STATE	PERCENT
39	Alabama	3.7
32	Alaska	6.5
4	Arizona	42.3
28	Arkansas	7.2
2	California	49.5
6	Colorado	29.4
13	Connecticut	16.2
23	Delaware	10.1
7	Florida	24.1
21	Georgia	11.8
17	Hawaii	13.1
16	Idaho	13.3
8	Illinois	22.3
30	Indiana	6.8
33	Iowa	5.9
18	Kansas	12.6
43	Kentucky	2.8
45	Louisiana	2.4
48	Maine	1.3
28	Maryland	7.2
22	Massachusetts	11.6
35	Michigan	5.5
31	Minnesota	6.7
47	Mississippi	1.7
38	Missouri	4.0
41	Montana	3.4
20	Nebraska	11.9
5	Nevada	34.6
40	New Hampshire	3.5
10	New Jersey	20.3
1	New Mexico	52.1
9	New York	21.5
19	North Carolina	12.3
46	North Dakota	1.8
42	Ohio	3.0
24	Oklahoma	9.9
11	Oregon	17.4
34	Pennsylvania	5.7
12	Rhode Island	17.3
36	South Carolina	5.4
44	South Dakota	2.5
37	Tennessee	5.0
3	Texas	47.2
15	Utah	13.6
49	Vermont	0.5
26	Virginia	9.2
14	Washington	15.3
50	West Virginia	0.4
27	Wisconsin	7.5
25	Wyoming	9.3

RANK ORDER

RANK	STATE	PERCENT
1	New Mexico	52.1
2	California	49.5
3	Texas	47.2
4	Arizona	42.3
5	Nevada	34.6
6	Colorado	29.4
7	Florida	24.1
8	Illinois	22.3
9	New York	21.5
10	New Jersey	20.3
11	Oregon	17.4
12	Rhode Island	17.3
13	Connecticut	16.2
14	Washington	15.3
15	Utah	13.6
16	Idaho	13.3
17	Hawaii	13.1
18	Kansas	12.6
19	North Carolina	12.3
20	Nebraska	11.9
21	Georgia	11.8
22	Massachusetts	11.6
23	Delaware	10.1
24	Oklahoma	9.9
25	Wyoming	9.3
26	Virginia	9.2
27	Wisconsin	7.5
28	Arkansas	7.2
28	Maryland	7.2
30	Indiana	6.8
31	Minnesota	6.7
32	Alaska	6.5
33	Iowa	5.9
34	Pennsylvania	5.7
35	Michigan	5.5
36	South Carolina	5.4
37	Tennessee	5.0
38	Missouri	4.0
39	Alabama	3.7
40	New Hampshire	3.5
41	Montana	3.4
42	Ohio	3.0
43	Kentucky	2.8
44	South Dakota	2.5
45	Louisiana	2.4
46	North Dakota	1.8
47	Mississippi	1.7
48	Maine	1.3
49	Vermont	0.5
50	West Virginia	0.4

District of Columbia   11.7

Source: Morgan Quitno Press using data from U.S. Dept. of Health and Human Services, Nat'l Center for Health Statistics "National Vital Statistics Reports" (Vol. 51, No. 2, December 18, 2002)

*Final data by state of residence. By race of mother. Persons of Hispanic origin may be of any race.

Births of Low Birthweight in 2001

National Total = 308,747 Live Births*

ALPHA ORDER

RANK	STATE	BIRTHS	% of USA
18	Alabama	5,812	1.9%
47	Alaska	566	0.2%
17	Arizona	5,957	1.9%
29	Arkansas	3,250	1.1%
1	California	33,228	10.8%
21	Colorado	5,720	1.9%
30	Connecticut	3,143	1.0%
41	Delaware	996	0.3%
4	Florida	16,776	5.4%
7	Georgia	11,750	3.8%
39	Hawaii	1,385	0.4%
40	Idaho	1,326	0.4%
5	Illinois	14,731	4.8%
16	Indiana	6,569	2.1%
34	Iowa	2,409	0.8%
32	Kansas	2,709	0.9%
25	Kentucky	4,539	1.5%
14	Louisiana	6,825	2.2%
44	Maine	830	0.3%
15	Maryland	6,580	2.1%
19	Massachusetts	5,773	1.9%
9	Michigan	10,642	3.4%
27	Minnesota	4,254	1.4%
26	Mississippi	4,505	1.5%
20	Missouri	5,741	1.9%
45	Montana	758	0.2%
38	Nebraska	1,649	0.5%
35	Nevada	2,380	0.8%
42	New Hampshire	957	0.3%
11	New Jersey	9,170	3.0%
36	New Mexico	2,145	0.7%
3	New York	19,481	6.3%
10	North Carolina	10,572	3.4%
49	North Dakota	472	0.2%
6	Ohio	12,094	3.9%
28	Oklahoma	3,908	1.3%
33	Oregon	2,512	0.8%
8	Pennsylvania	11,346	3.7%
43	Rhode Island	931	0.3%
22	South Carolina	5,340	1.7%
46	South Dakota	671	0.2%
13	Tennessee	7,212	2.3%
2	Texas	27,603	8.9%
31	Utah	3,077	1.0%
50	Vermont	377	0.1%
12	Virginia	7,761	2.5%
23	Washington	4,599	1.5%
37	West Virginia	1,730	0.6%
24	Wisconsin	4,552	1.5%
48	Wyoming	510	0.2%

RANK ORDER

RANK	STATE	BIRTHS	% of USA
1	California	33,228	10.8%
2	Texas	27,603	8.9%
3	New York	19,481	6.3%
4	Florida	16,776	5.4%
5	Illinois	14,731	4.8%
6	Ohio	12,094	3.9%
7	Georgia	11,750	3.8%
8	Pennsylvania	11,346	3.7%
9	Michigan	10,642	3.4%
10	North Carolina	10,572	3.4%
11	New Jersey	9,170	3.0%
12	Virginia	7,761	2.5%
13	Tennessee	7,212	2.3%
14	Louisiana	6,825	2.2%
15	Maryland	6,580	2.1%
16	Indiana	6,569	2.1%
17	Arizona	5,957	1.9%
18	Alabama	5,812	1.9%
19	Massachusetts	5,773	1.9%
20	Missouri	5,741	1.9%
21	Colorado	5,720	1.9%
22	South Carolina	5,340	1.7%
23	Washington	4,599	1.5%
24	Wisconsin	4,552	1.5%
25	Kentucky	4,539	1.5%
26	Mississippi	4,505	1.5%
27	Minnesota	4,254	1.4%
28	Oklahoma	3,908	1.3%
29	Arkansas	3,250	1.1%
30	Connecticut	3,143	1.0%
31	Utah	3,077	1.0%
32	Kansas	2,709	0.9%
33	Oregon	2,512	0.8%
34	Iowa	2,409	0.8%
35	Nevada	2,380	0.8%
36	New Mexico	2,145	0.7%
37	West Virginia	1,730	0.6%
38	Nebraska	1,649	0.5%
39	Hawaii	1,385	0.4%
40	Idaho	1,326	0.4%
41	Delaware	996	0.3%
42	New Hampshire	957	0.3%
43	Rhode Island	931	0.3%
44	Maine	830	0.3%
45	Montana	758	0.2%
46	South Dakota	671	0.2%
47	Alaska	566	0.2%
48	Wyoming	510	0.2%
49	North Dakota	472	0.2%
50	Vermont	377	0.1%
	District of Columbia	924	0.3%

Source: U.S. Department of Health and Human Services, National Center for Health Statistics
    "National Vital Statistics Reports" (Vol. 51, No. 2, December 18, 2002)
*Final data by state of residence. Births of less than 2,500 grams (5 pounds 8 ounces).

Births of Low Birthweight as a Percent of All Births in 2001

National Percent = 7.7% of Live Births*

ALPHA ORDER				RANK ORDER		
RANK	STATE	PERCENT		RANK	STATE	PERCENT
3	Alabama	9.6		1	Mississippi	10.7
49	Alaska	5.7		2	Louisiana	10.4
33	Arizona	7.0		3	Alabama	9.6
9	Arkansas	8.8		3	South Carolina	9.6
43	California	6.3		5	Delaware	9.3
11	Colorado	8.5		6	Tennessee	9.2
30	Connecticut	7.4		7	Maryland	9.0
5	Delaware	9.3		8	North Carolina	8.9
15	Florida	8.2		9	Arkansas	8.8
9	Georgia	8.8		9	Georgia	8.8
16	Hawaii	8.1		11	Colorado	8.5
39	Idaho	6.4		11	West Virginia	8.5
17	Illinois	8.0		13	Kentucky	8.3
26	Indiana	7.6		13	Wyoming	8.3
39	Iowa	6.4		15	Florida	8.2
33	Kansas	7.0		16	Hawaii	8.1
13	Kentucky	8.3		17	Illinois	8.0
2	Louisiana	10.4		17	Michigan	8.0
46	Maine	6.0		17	Ohio	8.0
7	Maryland	9.0		20	New Jersey	7.9
32	Massachusetts	7.2		20	New Mexico	7.9
17	Michigan	8.0		20	Pennsylvania	7.9
43	Minnesota	6.3		20	Virginia	7.9
1	Mississippi	10.7		24	Oklahoma	7.8
26	Missouri	7.6		25	New York	7.7
35	Montana	6.9		26	Indiana	7.6
36	Nebraska	6.6		26	Missouri	7.6
26	Nevada	7.6		26	Nevada	7.6
38	New Hampshire	6.5		26	Texas	7.6
20	New Jersey	7.9		30	Connecticut	7.4
20	New Mexico	7.9		31	Rhode Island	7.3
25	New York	7.7		32	Massachusetts	7.2
8	North Carolina	8.9		33	Arizona	7.0
45	North Dakota	6.2		33	Kansas	7.0
17	Ohio	8.0		35	Montana	6.9
24	Oklahoma	7.8		36	Nebraska	6.6
50	Oregon	5.5		36	Wisconsin	6.6
20	Pennsylvania	7.9		38	New Hampshire	6.5
31	Rhode Island	7.3		39	Idaho	6.4
3	South Carolina	9.6		39	Iowa	6.4
39	South Dakota	6.4		39	South Dakota	6.4
6	Tennessee	9.2		39	Utah	6.4
26	Texas	7.6		43	California	6.3
39	Utah	6.4		43	Minnesota	6.3
47	Vermont	5.9		45	North Dakota	6.2
20	Virginia	7.9		46	Maine	6.0
48	Washington	5.8		47	Vermont	5.9
11	West Virginia	8.5		48	Washington	5.8
36	Wisconsin	6.6		49	Alaska	5.7
13	Wyoming	8.3		50	Oregon	5.5
					District of Columbia	12.1

Source: U.S. Department of Health and Human Services, National Center for Health Statistics
"National Vital Statistics Reports" (Vol. 51, No. 2, December 18, 2002)
*Final data by state of residence. Births of less than 2,500 grams (5 pounds 8 ounces).

Births of Low Birthweight to White Women in 2001

National Total = 212,228 Live Births*

ALPHA ORDER

RANK	STATE	BIRTHS	% of USA
24	Alabama	3,070	1.4%
49	Alaska	333	0.2%
13	Arizona	5,010	2.4%
33	Arkansas	2,148	1.0%
1	California	24,661	11.6%
14	Colorado	5,007	2.4%
29	Connecticut	2,370	1.1%
44	Delaware	589	0.3%
4	Florida	10,386	4.9%
11	Georgia	5,771	2.7%
50	Hawaii	247	0.1%
39	Idaho	1,275	0.6%
5	Illinois	9,463	4.5%
12	Indiana	5,225	2.5%
32	Iowa	2,160	1.0%
30	Kansas	2,247	1.1%
19	Kentucky	3,828	1.8%
27	Louisiana	2,831	1.3%
41	Maine	800	0.4%
23	Maryland	3,144	1.5%
17	Massachusetts	4,574	2.2%
8	Michigan	6,971	3.3%
22	Minnesota	3,426	1.6%
36	Mississippi	1,769	0.8%
18	Missouri	4,189	2.0%
43	Montana	655	0.3%
38	Nebraska	1,409	0.7%
34	Nevada	1,852	0.9%
40	New Hampshire	898	0.4%
10	New Jersey	5,787	2.7%
35	New Mexico	1,799	0.8%
3	New York	12,151	5.7%
9	North Carolina	6,258	2.9%
47	North Dakota	405	0.2%
6	Ohio	8,811	4.2%
26	Oklahoma	2,846	1.3%
31	Oregon	2,217	1.0%
7	Pennsylvania	8,238	3.9%
42	Rhode Island	738	0.3%
28	South Carolina	2,613	1.2%
45	South Dakota	535	0.3%
15	Tennessee	4,833	2.3%
2	Texas	21,377	10.1%
25	Utah	2,902	1.4%
48	Vermont	369	0.2%
16	Virginia	4,587	2.2%
20	Washington	3,711	1.7%
37	West Virginia	1,637	0.8%
21	Wisconsin	3,485	1.6%
46	Wyoming	458	0.2%

RANK ORDER

RANK	STATE	BIRTHS	% of USA
1	California	24,661	11.6%
2	Texas	21,377	10.1%
3	New York	12,151	5.7%
4	Florida	10,386	4.9%
5	Illinois	9,463	4.5%
6	Ohio	8,811	4.2%
7	Pennsylvania	8,238	3.9%
8	Michigan	6,971	3.3%
9	North Carolina	6,258	2.9%
10	New Jersey	5,787	2.7%
11	Georgia	5,771	2.7%
12	Indiana	5,225	2.5%
13	Arizona	5,010	2.4%
14	Colorado	5,007	2.4%
15	Tennessee	4,833	2.3%
16	Virginia	4,587	2.2%
17	Massachusetts	4,574	2.2%
18	Missouri	4,189	2.0%
19	Kentucky	3,828	1.8%
20	Washington	3,711	1.7%
21	Wisconsin	3,485	1.6%
22	Minnesota	3,426	1.6%
23	Maryland	3,144	1.5%
24	Alabama	3,070	1.4%
25	Utah	2,902	1.4%
26	Oklahoma	2,846	1.3%
27	Louisiana	2,831	1.3%
28	South Carolina	2,613	1.2%
29	Connecticut	2,370	1.1%
30	Kansas	2,247	1.1%
31	Oregon	2,217	1.0%
32	Iowa	2,160	1.0%
33	Arkansas	2,148	1.0%
34	Nevada	1,852	0.9%
35	New Mexico	1,799	0.8%
36	Mississippi	1,769	0.8%
37	West Virginia	1,637	0.8%
38	Nebraska	1,409	0.7%
39	Idaho	1,275	0.6%
40	New Hampshire	898	0.4%
41	Maine	800	0.4%
42	Rhode Island	738	0.3%
43	Montana	655	0.3%
44	Delaware	589	0.3%
45	South Dakota	535	0.3%
46	Wyoming	458	0.2%
47	North Dakota	405	0.2%
48	Vermont	369	0.2%
49	Alaska	333	0.2%
50	Hawaii	247	0.1%
	District of Columbia	163	0.1%

Source: U.S. Department of Health and Human Services, National Center for Health Statistics "National Vital Statistics Reports" (Vol. 51, No. 2, December 18, 2002)
Final data by state of residence. Births of less than 2,500 grams (5 pounds 8 ounces).

Births of Low Birthweight to White Women
As a Percent of All Births to White Women in 2001
National Percent = 6.7% of Live Births to White Women*

ALPHA ORDER

RANK	STATE	PERCENT
10	Alabama	7.6
50	Alaska	5.2
25	Arizona	6.7
11	Arkansas	7.5
47	California	5.8
2	Colorado	8.2
25	Connecticut	6.7
8	Delaware	7.7
22	Florida	6.8
25	Georgia	6.7
33	Hawaii	6.5
36	Idaho	6.4
31	Illinois	6.6
15	Indiana	7.0
41	Iowa	6.1
33	Kansas	6.5
6	Kentucky	7.8
8	Louisiana	7.7
43	Maine	6.0
15	Maryland	7.0
22	Massachusetts	6.8
31	Michigan	6.6
44	Minnesota	5.9
6	Mississippi	7.8
25	Missouri	6.7
19	Montana	6.9
39	Nebraska	6.3
15	Nevada	7.0
36	New Hampshire	6.4
22	New Jersey	6.8
5	New Mexico	7.9
25	New York	6.7
12	North Carolina	7.3
41	North Dakota	6.1
15	Ohio	7.0
12	Oklahoma	7.3
49	Oregon	5.4
19	Pennsylvania	6.9
25	Rhode Island	6.7
12	South Carolina	7.3
39	South Dakota	6.3
3	Tennessee	8.0
19	Texas	6.9
36	Utah	6.4
44	Vermont	5.9
33	Virginia	6.5
48	Washington	5.5
1	West Virginia	8.4
44	Wisconsin	5.9
3	Wyoming	8.0

RANK ORDER

RANK	STATE	PERCENT
1	West Virginia	8.4
2	Colorado	8.2
3	Tennessee	8.0
3	Wyoming	8.0
5	New Mexico	7.9
6	Kentucky	7.8
6	Mississippi	7.8
8	Delaware	7.7
8	Louisiana	7.7
10	Alabama	7.6
11	Arkansas	7.5
12	North Carolina	7.3
12	Oklahoma	7.3
12	South Carolina	7.3
15	Indiana	7.0
15	Maryland	7.0
15	Nevada	7.0
15	Ohio	7.0
19	Montana	6.9
19	Pennsylvania	6.9
19	Texas	6.9
22	Florida	6.8
22	Massachusetts	6.8
22	New Jersey	6.8
25	Arizona	6.7
25	Connecticut	6.7
25	Georgia	6.7
25	Missouri	6.7
25	New York	6.7
25	Rhode Island	6.7
31	Illinois	6.6
31	Michigan	6.6
33	Hawaii	6.5
33	Kansas	6.5
33	Virginia	6.5
36	Idaho	6.4
36	New Hampshire	6.4
36	Utah	6.4
39	Nebraska	6.3
39	South Dakota	6.3
41	Iowa	6.1
41	North Dakota	6.1
43	Maine	6.0
44	Minnesota	5.9
44	Vermont	5.9
44	Wisconsin	5.9
47	California	5.8
48	Washington	5.5
49	Oregon	5.4
50	Alaska	5.2
	District of Columbia	6.3

Source: U.S. Department of Health and Human Services, National Center for Health Statistics
"National Vital Statistics Reports" (Vol. 51, No. 2, December 18, 2002)
*Final data by state of residence. Births of less than 2,500 grams (5 pounds 8 ounces).

Births of Low Birthweight to Black Women in 2001

National Total = 78,423 Live Births*

ALPHA ORDER

RANK	STATE	BIRTHS	% of USA
14	Alabama	2,687	3.4%
41	Alaska	48	0.1%
29	Arizona	378	0.5%
21	Arkansas	1,044	1.3%
6	California	3,907	5.0%
28	Colorado	415	0.5%
26	Connecticut	621	0.8%
30	Delaware	372	0.5%
2	Florida	5,878	7.5%
3	Georgia	5,624	7.2%
40	Hawaii	60	0.1%
46	Idaho	9	0.0%
5	Illinois	4,558	5.8%
20	Indiana	1,242	1.6%
34	Iowa	173	0.2%
31	Kansas	345	0.4%
24	Kentucky	660	0.8%
8	Louisiana	3,883	5.0%
44	Maine	14	0.0%
10	Maryland	3,134	4.0%
23	Massachusetts	832	1.1%
9	Michigan	3,317	4.2%
27	Minnesota	467	0.6%
15	Mississippi	2,683	3.4%
19	Missouri	1,406	1.8%
49	Montana	2	0.0%
35	Nebraska	170	0.2%
32	Nevada	326	0.4%
43	New Hampshire	29	0.0%
17	New Jersey	2,595	3.3%
39	New Mexico	67	0.1%
1	New York	5,892	7.5%
7	North Carolina	3,906	5.0%
48	North Dakota	5	0.0%
11	Ohio	3,069	3.9%
25	Oklahoma	628	0.8%
37	Oregon	95	0.1%
13	Pennsylvania	2,771	3.5%
36	Rhode Island	131	0.2%
16	South Carolina	2,647	3.4%
47	South Dakota	6	0.0%
18	Tennessee	2,252	2.9%
4	Texas	5,242	6.7%
42	Utah	37	0.0%
50	Vermont	1	0.0%
12	Virginia	2,775	3.5%
33	Washington	324	0.4%
38	West Virginia	81	0.1%
22	Wisconsin	861	1.1%
45	Wyoming	11	0.0%

RANK ORDER

RANK	STATE	BIRTHS	% of USA
1	New York	5,892	7.5%
2	Florida	5,878	7.5%
3	Georgia	5,624	7.2%
4	Texas	5,242	6.7%
5	Illinois	4,558	5.8%
6	California	3,907	5.0%
7	North Carolina	3,906	5.0%
8	Louisiana	3,883	5.0%
9	Michigan	3,317	4.2%
10	Maryland	3,134	4.0%
11	Ohio	3,069	3.9%
12	Virginia	2,775	3.5%
13	Pennsylvania	2,771	3.5%
14	Alabama	2,687	3.4%
15	Mississippi	2,683	3.4%
16	South Carolina	2,647	3.4%
17	New Jersey	2,595	3.3%
18	Tennessee	2,252	2.9%
19	Missouri	1,406	1.8%
20	Indiana	1,242	1.6%
21	Arkansas	1,044	1.3%
22	Wisconsin	861	1.1%
23	Massachusetts	832	1.1%
24	Kentucky	660	0.8%
25	Oklahoma	628	0.8%
26	Connecticut	621	0.8%
27	Minnesota	467	0.6%
28	Colorado	415	0.5%
29	Arizona	378	0.5%
30	Delaware	372	0.5%
31	Kansas	345	0.4%
32	Nevada	326	0.4%
33	Washington	324	0.4%
34	Iowa	173	0.2%
35	Nebraska	170	0.2%
36	Rhode Island	131	0.2%
37	Oregon	95	0.1%
38	West Virginia	81	0.1%
39	New Mexico	67	0.1%
40	Hawaii	60	0.1%
41	Alaska	48	0.1%
42	Utah	37	0.0%
43	New Hampshire	29	0.0%
44	Maine	14	0.0%
45	Wyoming	11	0.0%
46	Idaho	9	0.0%
47	South Dakota	6	0.0%
48	North Dakota	5	0.0%
49	Montana	2	0.0%
50	Vermont	1	0.0%
	District of Columbia	743	0.9%

Source: U.S. Department of Health and Human Services, National Center for Health Statistics
"National Vital Statistics Reports" (Vol. 51, No. 2, December 18, 2002)
*Final data by state of residence. Births of less than 2,500 grams (5 pounds 8 ounces).

Births of Low Birthweight to Black Women
As a Percent of All Births to Black Women in 2001
National Percent = 13.0% of Live Births to Black Women*

ALPHA ORDER

RANK	STATE	PERCENT
5	Alabama	14.0
38	Alaska	10.9
10	Arizona	13.7
3	Arkansas	14.1
34	California	11.6
5	Colorado	14.0
32	Connecticut	12.1
10	Delaware	13.7
28	Florida	12.5
22	Georgia	12.9
36	Hawaii	11.4
NA	Idaho**	NA
10	Illinois	13.7
22	Indiana	12.9
10	Iowa	13.7
30	Kansas	12.4
17	Kentucky	13.4
1	Louisiana	14.4
NA	Maine**	NA
22	Maryland	12.9
40	Massachusetts	10.2
3	Michigan	14.1
42	Minnesota	9.8
2	Mississippi	14.3
26	Missouri	12.6
NA	Montana**	NA
30	Nebraska	12.4
21	Nevada	13.0
8	New Hampshire	13.9
26	New Jersey	12.6
19	New Mexico	13.1
37	New York	11.3
9	North Carolina	13.8
NA	North Dakota**	NA
17	Ohio	13.4
15	Oklahoma	13.6
41	Oregon	10.1
10	Pennsylvania	13.7
33	Rhode Island	11.8
5	South Carolina	14.0
NA	South Dakota**	NA
15	Tennessee	13.6
22	Texas	12.9
39	Utah	10.8
NA	Vermont**	NA
28	Virginia	12.5
42	Washington	9.8
35	West Virginia	11.5
19	Wisconsin	13.1
NA	Wyoming**	NA

RANK ORDER

RANK	STATE	PERCENT
1	Louisiana	14.4
2	Mississippi	14.3
3	Arkansas	14.1
3	Michigan	14.1
5	Alabama	14.0
5	Colorado	14.0
5	South Carolina	14.0
8	New Hampshire	13.9
9	North Carolina	13.8
10	Arizona	13.7
10	Delaware	13.7
10	Illinois	13.7
10	Iowa	13.7
10	Pennsylvania	13.7
15	Oklahoma	13.6
15	Tennessee	13.6
17	Kentucky	13.4
17	Ohio	13.4
19	New Mexico	13.1
19	Wisconsin	13.1
21	Nevada	13.0
22	Georgia	12.9
22	Indiana	12.9
22	Maryland	12.9
22	Texas	12.9
26	Missouri	12.6
26	New Jersey	12.6
28	Florida	12.5
28	Virginia	12.5
30	Kansas	12.4
30	Nebraska	12.4
32	Connecticut	12.1
33	Rhode Island	11.8
34	California	11.6
35	West Virginia	11.5
36	Hawaii	11.4
37	New York	11.3
38	Alaska	10.9
39	Utah	10.8
40	Massachusetts	10.2
41	Oregon	10.1
42	Minnesota	9.8
42	Washington	9.8
NA	Idaho**	NA
NA	Maine**	NA
NA	Montana**	NA
NA	North Dakota**	NA
NA	South Dakota**	NA
NA	Vermont**	NA
NA	Wyoming**	NA
	District of Columbia	15.3

Source: U.S. Department of Health and Human Services, National Center for Health Statistics
"National Vital Statistics Reports" (Vol. 51, No. 2, December 18, 2002)
*Final data by state of residence. Births of less than 2,500 grams (5 pounds 8 ounces).
**Not available. Fewer than 20 births of low birthweight to black women.

Births of Low Birthweight to Hispanic Women in 2001

National Total = 55,092 Live Births*

ALPHA ORDER

RANK	STATE	BIRTHS	% of USA
36	Alabama	155	0.3%
43	Alaska	41	0.1%
6	Arizona	2,399	4.4%
35	Arkansas	157	0.3%
1	California	14,784	26.8%
7	Colorado	1,657	3.0%
16	Connecticut	565	1.0%
40	Delaware	70	0.1%
4	Florida	3,222	5.8%
11	Georgia	889	1.6%
32	Hawaii	171	0.3%
30	Idaho	187	0.3%
5	Illinois	2,689	4.9%
21	Indiana	389	0.7%
37	Iowa	139	0.3%
25	Kansas	292	0.5%
38	Kentucky	115	0.2%
39	Louisiana	103	0.2%
48	Maine	7	0.0%
22	Maryland	365	0.7%
12	Massachusetts	778	1.4%
19	Michigan	453	0.8%
27	Minnesota	280	0.5%
42	Mississippi	50	0.1%
33	Missouri	169	0.3%
44	Montana	30	0.1%
31	Nebraska	183	0.3%
14	Nevada	691	1.3%
44	New Hampshire	30	0.1%
8	New Jersey	1,647	3.0%
9	New Mexico	1,124	2.0%
3	New York	4,050	7.4%
10	North Carolina	890	1.6%
47	North Dakota	11	0.0%
23	Ohio	319	0.6%
25	Oklahoma	292	0.5%
20	Oregon	440	0.8%
13	Pennsylvania	721	1.3%
34	Rhode Island	167	0.3%
29	South Carolina	196	0.4%
46	South Dakota	21	0.0%
28	Tennessee	253	0.5%
2	Texas	11,820	21.5%
18	Utah	485	0.9%
50	Vermont	1	0.0%
17	Virginia	527	1.0%
15	Washington	636	1.2%
49	West Virginia	4	0.0%
24	Wisconsin	318	0.6%
41	Wyoming	52	0.1%

RANK ORDER

RANK	STATE	BIRTHS	% of USA
1	California	14,784	26.8%
2	Texas	11,820	21.5%
3	New York	4,050	7.4%
4	Florida	3,222	5.8%
5	Illinois	2,689	4.9%
6	Arizona	2,399	4.4%
7	Colorado	1,657	3.0%
8	New Jersey	1,647	3.0%
9	New Mexico	1,124	2.0%
10	North Carolina	890	1.6%
11	Georgia	889	1.6%
12	Massachusetts	778	1.4%
13	Pennsylvania	721	1.3%
14	Nevada	691	1.3%
15	Washington	636	1.2%
16	Connecticut	565	1.0%
17	Virginia	527	1.0%
18	Utah	485	0.9%
19	Michigan	453	0.8%
20	Oregon	440	0.8%
21	Indiana	389	0.7%
22	Maryland	365	0.7%
23	Ohio	319	0.6%
24	Wisconsin	318	0.6%
25	Kansas	292	0.5%
25	Oklahoma	292	0.5%
27	Minnesota	280	0.5%
28	Tennessee	253	0.5%
29	South Carolina	196	0.4%
30	Idaho	187	0.3%
31	Nebraska	183	0.3%
32	Hawaii	171	0.3%
33	Missouri	169	0.3%
34	Rhode Island	167	0.3%
35	Arkansas	157	0.3%
36	Alabama	155	0.3%
37	Iowa	139	0.3%
38	Kentucky	115	0.2%
39	Louisiana	103	0.2%
40	Delaware	70	0.1%
41	Wyoming	52	0.1%
42	Mississippi	50	0.1%
43	Alaska	41	0.1%
44	Montana	30	0.1%
44	New Hampshire	30	0.1%
46	South Dakota	21	0.0%
47	North Dakota	11	0.0%
48	Maine	7	0.0%
49	West Virginia	4	0.0%
50	Vermont	1	0.0%
	District of Columbia	58	0.1%

Source: U.S. Department of Health and Human Services, National Center for Health Statistics
"National Vital Statistics Reports" (Vol. 51, No. 2, December 18, 2002)
*Final data by state of residence. Births of less than 2,500 grams (5 pounds 8 ounces). Hispanic can be of any race.

Births of Low Birthweight to Hispanic Women
As a Percent of All Births to Hispanic Women in 2001
National Percent = 6.5% of Live Births to Hispanic Women*

<u>ALPHA ORDER</u>

RANK	STATE	PERCENT
17	Alabama	6.9
30	Alaska	6.3
21	Arizona	6.6
38	Arkansas	5.9
42	California	5.7
3	Colorado	8.4
5	Connecticut	8.2
26	Delaware	6.5
26	Florida	6.5
42	Georgia	5.7
10	Hawaii	7.6
20	Idaho	6.8
21	Illinois	6.6
21	Indiana	6.6
31	Iowa	6.2
37	Kansas	6.0
9	Kentucky	7.7
21	Louisiana	6.6
NA	Maine**	NA
17	Maryland	6.9
4	Massachusetts	8.3
31	Michigan	6.2
31	Minnesota	6.2
14	Mississippi	7.0
42	Missouri	5.7
7	Montana	8.0
31	Nebraska	6.2
29	Nevada	6.4
38	New Hampshire	5.9
14	New Jersey	7.0
7	New Mexico	8.0
12	New York	7.4
36	North Carolina	6.1
NA	North Dakota**	NA
14	Ohio	7.0
38	Oklahoma	5.9
45	Oregon	5.6
2	Pennsylvania	8.8
10	Rhode Island	7.6
21	South Carolina	6.6
5	South Dakota	8.2
26	Tennessee	6.5
17	Texas	6.9
12	Utah	7.4
NA	Vermont**	NA
41	Virginia	5.8
46	Washington	5.2
NA	West Virginia**	NA
31	Wisconsin	6.2
1	Wyoming	9.1

<u>RANK ORDER</u>

RANK	STATE	PERCENT
1	Wyoming	9.1
2	Pennsylvania	8.8
3	Colorado	8.4
4	Massachusetts	8.3
5	Connecticut	8.2
5	South Dakota	8.2
7	Montana	8.0
7	New Mexico	8.0
9	Kentucky	7.7
10	Hawaii	7.6
10	Rhode Island	7.6
12	New York	7.4
12	Utah	7.4
14	Mississippi	7.0
14	New Jersey	7.0
14	Ohio	7.0
17	Alabama	6.9
17	Maryland	6.9
17	Texas	6.9
20	Idaho	6.8
21	Arizona	6.6
21	Illinois	6.6
21	Indiana	6.6
21	Louisiana	6.6
21	South Carolina	6.6
26	Delaware	6.5
26	Florida	6.5
26	Tennessee	6.5
29	Nevada	6.4
30	Alaska	6.3
31	Iowa	6.2
31	Michigan	6.2
31	Minnesota	6.2
31	Nebraska	6.2
31	Wisconsin	6.2
36	North Carolina	6.1
37	Kansas	6.0
38	Arkansas	5.9
38	New Hampshire	5.9
38	Oklahoma	5.9
41	Virginia	5.8
42	California	5.7
42	Georgia	5.7
42	Missouri	5.7
45	Oregon	5.6
46	Washington	5.2
NA	Maine**	NA
NA	North Dakota**	NA
NA	Vermont**	NA
NA	West Virginia**	NA
	District of Columbia	6.5

Source: U.S. Department of Health and Human Services, National Center for Health Statistics
  "National Vital Statistics Reports" (Vol. 51, No. 2, December 18, 2002)
*Final data by state of residence. Births of less than 2,500 grams (5 pounds 8 ounces). Hispanic can be of any race.
**Not available. Fewer than 20 births of low birthweight to Hispanic women.

Births to Unmarried Women in 2001

National Total = 1,349,249 Live Births*

ALPHA ORDER

RANK	STATE	BIRTHS	% of USA
22	Alabama	20,777	1.5%
47	Alaska	3,281	0.2%
12	Arizona	33,776	2.5%
30	Arkansas	13,378	1.0%
1	California	172,764	12.8%
28	Colorado	16,732	1.2%
32	Connecticut	12,433	0.9%
43	Delaware	4,290	0.3%
4	Florida	80,221	5.9%
7	Georgia	49,834	3.7%
39	Hawaii	5,632	0.4%
40	Idaho	4,557	0.3%
5	Illinois	63,449	4.7%
13	Indiana	30,676	2.3%
35	Iowa	10,824	0.8%
34	Kansas	11,628	0.9%
27	Kentucky	17,317	1.3%
14	Louisiana	30,267	2.2%
42	Maine	4,369	0.3%
18	Maryland	25,198	1.9%
21	Massachusetts	21,641	1.6%
9	Michigan	45,742	3.4%
25	Minnesota	17,782	1.3%
24	Mississippi	19,582	1.5%
17	Missouri	26,235	1.9%
46	Montana	3,440	0.3%
37	Nebraska	6,870	0.5%
33	Nevada	11,679	0.9%
44	New Hampshire	3,542	0.3%
11	New Jersey	33,807	2.5%
31	New Mexico	12,552	0.9%
3	New York	90,746	6.7%
10	North Carolina	40,507	3.0%
48	North Dakota	2,127	0.2%
6	Ohio	53,239	3.9%
26	Oklahoma	17,637	1.3%
29	Oregon	13,764	1.0%
8	Pennsylvania	48,536	3.6%
41	Rhode Island	4,543	0.3%
20	South Carolina	22,343	1.7%
45	South Dakota	3,516	0.3%
16	Tennessee	27,974	2.1%
2	Texas	113,420	8.4%
36	Utah	8,327	0.6%
49	Vermont	1,972	0.1%
15	Virginia	29,930	2.2%
19	Washington	22,880	1.7%
38	West Virginia	6,638	0.5%
23	Wisconsin	20,686	1.5%
50	Wyoming	1,813	0.1%

RANK ORDER

RANK	STATE	BIRTHS	% of USA
1	California	172,764	12.8%
2	Texas	113,420	8.4%
3	New York	90,746	6.7%
4	Florida	80,221	5.9%
5	Illinois	63,449	4.7%
6	Ohio	53,239	3.9%
7	Georgia	49,834	3.7%
8	Pennsylvania	48,536	3.6%
9	Michigan	45,742	3.4%
10	North Carolina	40,507	3.0%
11	New Jersey	33,807	2.5%
12	Arizona	33,776	2.5%
13	Indiana	30,676	2.3%
14	Louisiana	30,267	2.2%
15	Virginia	29,930	2.2%
16	Tennessee	27,974	2.1%
17	Missouri	26,235	1.9%
18	Maryland	25,198	1.9%
19	Washington	22,880	1.7%
20	South Carolina	22,343	1.7%
21	Massachusetts	21,641	1.6%
22	Alabama	20,777	1.5%
23	Wisconsin	20,686	1.5%
24	Mississippi	19,582	1.5%
25	Minnesota	17,782	1.3%
26	Oklahoma	17,637	1.3%
27	Kentucky	17,317	1.3%
28	Colorado	16,732	1.2%
29	Oregon	13,764	1.0%
30	Arkansas	13,378	1.0%
31	New Mexico	12,552	0.9%
32	Connecticut	12,433	0.9%
33	Nevada	11,679	0.9%
34	Kansas	11,628	0.9%
35	Iowa	10,824	0.8%
36	Utah	8,327	0.6%
37	Nebraska	6,870	0.5%
38	West Virginia	6,638	0.5%
39	Hawaii	5,632	0.4%
40	Idaho	4,557	0.3%
41	Rhode Island	4,543	0.3%
42	Maine	4,369	0.3%
43	Delaware	4,290	0.3%
44	New Hampshire	3,542	0.3%
45	South Dakota	3,516	0.3%
46	Montana	3,440	0.3%
47	Alaska	3,281	0.2%
48	North Dakota	2,127	0.2%
49	Vermont	1,972	0.1%
50	Wyoming	1,813	0.1%
	District of Columbia	4,376	0.3%

Source: U.S. Department of Health and Human Services, National Center for Health Statistics
"National Vital Statistics Reports" (Vol. 51, No. 2, December 18, 2002)
*Final data by state of residence.

Births to Unmarried Women as a Percent of All Births in 2001

National Percent = 33.5% of Live Births*

ALPHA ORDER			RANK ORDER		
RANK	STATE	PERCENT	RANK	STATE	PERCENT
19	Alabama	34.4	1	Louisiana	46.3
26	Alaska	32.8	1	Mississippi	46.3
6	Arizona	39.5	1	New Mexico	46.3
10	Arkansas	36.1	4	South Carolina	40.1
27	California	32.7	5	Delaware	39.9
47	Colorado	25.0	6	Arizona	39.5
39	Connecticut	29.2	7	Florida	39.0
5	Delaware	39.9	8	Georgia	37.3
7	Florida	39.0	9	Nevada	37.2
8	Georgia	37.3	10	Arkansas	36.1
25	Hawaii	33.0	11	New York	35.7
49	Idaho	22.0	11	Rhode Island	35.7
18	Illinois	34.5	11	Tennessee	35.7
14	Indiana	35.5	14	Indiana	35.5
41	Iowa	28.8	15	Oklahoma	35.2
36	Kansas	29.9	16	Ohio	35.1
30	Kentucky	31.7	17	Missouri	34.8
1	Louisiana	46.3	18	Illinois	34.5
29	Maine	31.8	19	Alabama	34.4
19	Maryland	34.4	19	Maryland	34.4
45	Massachusetts	26.7	21	Michigan	34.3
21	Michigan	34.3	21	North Carolina	34.3
46	Minnesota	26.3	23	Pennsylvania	33.8
1	Mississippi	46.3	24	South Dakota	33.5
17	Missouri	34.8	25	Hawaii	33.0
31	Montana	31.4	26	Alaska	32.8
44	Nebraska	27.7	27	California	32.7
9	Nevada	37.2	28	West Virginia	32.5
48	New Hampshire	24.2	29	Maine	31.8
39	New Jersey	29.2	30	Kentucky	31.7
1	New Mexico	46.3	31	Montana	31.4
11	New York	35.7	32	Texas	31.0
21	North Carolina	34.3	32	Vermont	31.0
43	North Dakota	27.9	34	Oregon	30.4
16	Ohio	35.1	35	Virginia	30.3
15	Oklahoma	35.2	36	Kansas	29.9
34	Oregon	30.4	36	Wisconsin	29.9
23	Pennsylvania	33.8	38	Wyoming	29.6
11	Rhode Island	35.7	39	Connecticut	29.2
4	South Carolina	40.1	39	New Jersey	29.2
24	South Dakota	33.5	41	Iowa	28.8
11	Tennessee	35.7	41	Washington	28.8
32	Texas	31.0	43	North Dakota	27.9
50	Utah	17.4	44	Nebraska	27.7
32	Vermont	31.0	45	Massachusetts	26.7
35	Virginia	30.3	46	Minnesota	26.3
41	Washington	28.8	47	Colorado	25.0
28	West Virginia	32.5	48	New Hampshire	24.2
36	Wisconsin	29.9	49	Idaho	22.0
38	Wyoming	29.6	50	Utah	17.4
				District of Columbia	57.4

Source: U.S. Dept. of Health and Human Services, Nat'l Center for Health Statistics
   "National Vital Statistics Reports" (Vol. 51, No. 2, December 18, 2002)
*Final data by state of residence.

Births to Unmarried White Women in 2001

National Total = 879,848 Live Births*

ALPHA ORDER				RANK ORDER			
RANK	STATE	BIRTHS	% of USA	RANK	STATE	BIRTHS	% of USA
33	Alabama	7,638	0.9%	1	California	141,305	16.1%
49	Alaska	1,422	0.2%	2	Texas	86,986	9.9%
8	Arizona	27,790	3.2%	3	New York	52,619	6.0%
35	Arkansas	7,546	0.9%	4	Florida	47,056	5.3%
1	California	141,305	16.1%	5	Illinois	37,345	4.2%
19	Colorado	14,625	1.7%	6	Ohio	35,425	4.0%
31	Connecticut	8,814	1.0%	7	Pennsylvania	32,400	3.7%
44	Delaware	2,304	0.3%	8	Arizona	27,790	3.2%
4	Florida	47,056	5.3%	9	Michigan	27,719	3.2%
11	Georgia	20,554	2.3%	10	Indiana	23,146	2.6%
50	Hawaii	706	0.1%	11	Georgia	20,554	2.3%
39	Idaho	4,281	0.5%	12	North Carolina	20,513	2.3%
5	Illinois	37,345	4.2%	13	New Jersey	19,831	2.3%
10	Indiana	23,146	2.6%	14	Washington	18,519	2.1%
28	Iowa	9,589	1.1%	15	Missouri	17,345	2.0%
29	Kansas	9,306	1.1%	16	Massachusetts	15,961	1.8%
21	Kentucky	13,639	1.6%	17	Tennessee	15,608	1.8%
27	Louisiana	9,664	1.1%	18	Virginia	15,440	1.8%
40	Maine	4,196	0.5%	19	Colorado	14,625	1.7%
25	Maryland	10,381	1.2%	20	Wisconsin	14,325	1.6%
16	Massachusetts	15,961	1.8%	21	Kentucky	13,639	1.6%
9	Michigan	27,719	3.2%	22	Minnesota	13,174	1.5%
22	Minnesota	13,174	1.5%	23	Oregon	12,315	1.4%
38	Mississippi	5,111	0.6%	24	Oklahoma	11,565	1.3%
15	Missouri	17,345	2.0%	25	Maryland	10,381	1.2%
43	Montana	2,437	0.3%	26	New Mexico	9,714	1.1%
37	Nebraska	5,542	0.6%	27	Louisiana	9,664	1.1%
30	Nevada	9,078	1.0%	28	Iowa	9,589	1.1%
42	New Hampshire	3,416	0.4%	29	Kansas	9,306	1.1%
13	New Jersey	19,831	2.3%	30	Nevada	9,078	1.0%
26	New Mexico	9,714	1.1%	31	Connecticut	8,814	1.0%
3	New York	52,619	6.0%	32	South Carolina	8,617	1.0%
12	North Carolina	20,513	2.3%	33	Alabama	7,638	0.9%
48	North Dakota	1,503	0.2%	34	Utah	7,573	0.9%
6	Ohio	35,425	4.0%	35	Arkansas	7,546	0.9%
24	Oklahoma	11,565	1.3%	36	West Virginia	6,072	0.7%
23	Oregon	12,315	1.4%	37	Nebraska	5,542	0.6%
7	Pennsylvania	32,400	3.7%	38	Mississippi	5,111	0.6%
41	Rhode Island	3,532	0.4%	39	Idaho	4,281	0.5%
32	South Carolina	8,617	1.0%	40	Maine	4,196	0.5%
45	South Dakota	2,053	0.2%	41	Rhode Island	3,532	0.4%
17	Tennessee	15,608	1.8%	42	New Hampshire	3,416	0.4%
2	Texas	86,986	9.9%	43	Montana	2,437	0.3%
34	Utah	7,573	0.9%	44	Delaware	2,304	0.3%
46	Vermont	1,939	0.2%	45	South Dakota	2,053	0.2%
18	Virginia	15,440	1.8%	46	Vermont	1,939	0.2%
14	Washington	18,519	2.1%	47	Wyoming	1,592	0.2%
36	West Virginia	6,072	0.7%	48	North Dakota	1,503	0.2%
20	Wisconsin	14,325	1.6%	49	Alaska	1,422	0.2%
47	Wyoming	1,592	0.2%	50	Hawaii	706	0.1%
					District of Columbia	617	0.1%

Source: U.S. Department of Health and Human Services, National Center for Health Statistics
"National Vital Statistics Reports" (Vol. 51, No. 2, December 18, 2002)
*Final data by state of residence. By race of mother.

Births to Unmarried White Women
As a Percent of All Births to White Women in 2001
National Percent = 27.7% of Live Births*

ALPHA ORDER

RANK	STATE	PERCENT
48	Alabama	18.8
45	Alaska	22.3
2	Arizona	36.9
25	Arkansas	26.2
4	California	33.0
35	Colorado	24.0
30	Connecticut	24.8
11	Delaware	30.0
9	Florida	30.9
35	Georgia	24.0
49	Hawaii	18.5
47	Idaho	21.5
25	Illinois	26.2
10	Indiana	30.7
22	Iowa	27.1
23	Kansas	26.9
16	Kentucky	27.9
25	Louisiana	26.2
6	Maine	31.6
41	Maryland	23.0
39	Massachusetts	23.5
24	Michigan	26.3
42	Minnesota	22.7
44	Mississippi	22.4
18	Missouri	27.8
29	Montana	25.8
31	Nebraska	24.6
3	Nevada	34.5
32	New Hampshire	24.5
40	New Jersey	23.3
1	New Mexico	42.6
14	New York	28.9
35	North Carolina	24.0
42	North Dakota	22.7
15	Ohio	28.2
13	Oklahoma	29.5
12	Oregon	29.8
21	Pennsylvania	27.2
5	Rhode Island	32.2
35	South Carolina	24.0
33	South Dakota	24.2
28	Tennessee	25.9
16	Texas	27.9
50	Utah	16.7
7	Vermont	31.1
46	Virginia	21.8
20	Washington	27.5
8	West Virginia	31.0
34	Wisconsin	24.1
18	Wyoming	27.8

RANK ORDER

RANK	STATE	PERCENT
1	New Mexico	42.6
2	Arizona	36.9
3	Nevada	34.5
4	California	33.0
5	Rhode Island	32.2
6	Maine	31.6
7	Vermont	31.1
8	West Virginia	31.0
9	Florida	30.9
10	Indiana	30.7
11	Delaware	30.0
12	Oregon	29.8
13	Oklahoma	29.5
14	New York	28.9
15	Ohio	28.2
16	Kentucky	27.9
16	Texas	27.9
18	Missouri	27.8
18	Wyoming	27.8
20	Washington	27.5
21	Pennsylvania	27.2
22	Iowa	27.1
23	Kansas	26.9
24	Michigan	26.3
25	Arkansas	26.2
25	Illinois	26.2
25	Louisiana	26.2
28	Tennessee	25.9
29	Montana	25.8
30	Connecticut	24.8
31	Nebraska	24.6
32	New Hampshire	24.5
33	South Dakota	24.2
34	Wisconsin	24.1
35	Colorado	24.0
35	Georgia	24.0
35	North Carolina	24.0
35	South Carolina	24.0
39	Massachusetts	23.5
40	New Jersey	23.3
41	Maryland	23.0
42	Minnesota	22.7
42	North Dakota	22.7
44	Mississippi	22.4
45	Alaska	22.3
46	Virginia	21.8
47	Idaho	21.5
48	Alabama	18.8
49	Hawaii	18.5
50	Utah	16.7
	District of Columbia	24.0

Source: U.S. Dept. of Health and Human Services, Nat'l Center for Health Statistics
   "National Vital Statistics Reports" (Vol. 51, No. 2, December 18, 2002)
*Final data by state of residence. By race of mother.

Births to Unmarried Black Women in 2001

National Total = 414,533 Live Births*

ALPHA ORDER

RANK	STATE	BIRTHS	% of USA
17	Alabama	13,028	3.1%
40	Alaska	196	0.0%
31	Arizona	1,764	0.4%
21	Arkansas	5,642	1.4%
6	California	21,145	5.1%
33	Colorado	1,525	0.4%
25	Connecticut	3,391	0.8%
28	Delaware	1,952	0.5%
2	Florida	31,784	7.7%
3	Georgia	28,740	6.9%
42	Hawaii	110	0.0%
46	Idaho	35	0.0%
4	Illinois	25,401	6.1%
20	Indiana	7,312	1.8%
34	Iowa	942	0.2%
29	Kansas	1,947	0.5%
24	Kentucky	3,540	0.9%
7	Louisiana	20,218	4.9%
44	Maine	61	0.0%
12	Maryland	14,429	3.5%
23	Massachusetts	4,835	1.2%
10	Michigan	17,332	4.2%
27	Minnesota	2,739	0.7%
13	Mississippi	14,230	3.4%
19	Missouri	8,504	2.1%
49	Montana	26	0.0%
35	Nebraska	939	0.2%
32	Nevada	1,739	0.4%
43	New Hampshire	85	0.0%
16	New Jersey	13,357	3.2%
39	New Mexico	297	0.1%
1	New York	34,652	8.4%
8	North Carolina	18,693	4.5%
47	North Dakota	29	0.0%
9	Ohio	17,363	4.2%
26	Oklahoma	3,253	0.8%
37	Oregon	609	0.1%
11	Pennsylvania	15,480	3.7%
36	Rhode Island	757	0.2%
15	South Carolina	13,521	3.3%
45	South Dakota	44	0.0%
18	Tennessee	12,064	2.9%
5	Texas	25,159	6.1%
41	Utah	152	0.0%
50	Vermont	14	0.0%
14	Virginia	14,011	3.4%
30	Washington	1,779	0.4%
38	West Virginia	541	0.1%
22	Wisconsin	5,411	1.3%
47	Wyoming	29	0.0%

RANK ORDER

RANK	STATE	BIRTHS	% of USA
1	New York	34,652	8.4%
2	Florida	31,784	7.7%
3	Georgia	28,740	6.9%
4	Illinois	25,401	6.1%
5	Texas	25,159	6.1%
6	California	21,145	5.1%
7	Louisiana	20,218	4.9%
8	North Carolina	18,693	4.5%
9	Ohio	17,363	4.2%
10	Michigan	17,332	4.2%
11	Pennsylvania	15,480	3.7%
12	Maryland	14,429	3.5%
13	Mississippi	14,230	3.4%
14	Virginia	14,011	3.4%
15	South Carolina	13,521	3.3%
16	New Jersey	13,357	3.2%
17	Alabama	13,028	3.1%
18	Tennessee	12,064	2.9%
19	Missouri	8,504	2.1%
20	Indiana	7,312	1.8%
21	Arkansas	5,642	1.4%
22	Wisconsin	5,411	1.3%
23	Massachusetts	4,835	1.2%
24	Kentucky	3,540	0.9%
25	Connecticut	3,391	0.8%
26	Oklahoma	3,253	0.8%
27	Minnesota	2,739	0.7%
28	Delaware	1,952	0.5%
29	Kansas	1,947	0.5%
30	Washington	1,779	0.4%
31	Arizona	1,764	0.4%
32	Nevada	1,739	0.4%
33	Colorado	1,525	0.4%
34	Iowa	942	0.2%
35	Nebraska	939	0.2%
36	Rhode Island	757	0.2%
37	Oregon	609	0.1%
38	West Virginia	541	0.1%
39	New Mexico	297	0.1%
40	Alaska	196	0.0%
41	Utah	152	0.0%
42	Hawaii	110	0.0%
43	New Hampshire	85	0.0%
44	Maine	61	0.0%
45	South Dakota	44	0.0%
46	Idaho	35	0.0%
47	North Dakota	29	0.0%
47	Wyoming	29	0.0%
49	Montana	26	0.0%
50	Vermont	14	0.0%
	District of Columbia	3,727	0.9%

Source: U.S. Department of Health and Human Services, National Center for Health Statistics
"National Vital Statistics Reports" (Vol. 51, No. 2, December 18, 2002)
*Final data by state of residence. By race of mother.

Births to Unmarried Black Women
As a Percent of All Births to Black Women in 2001
National Percent = 68.4% of Live Births*

<u>ALPHA ORDER</u>

RANK	STATE	PERCENT
22	Alabama	67.9
43	Alaska	44.4
30	Arizona	63.9
6	Arkansas	75.9
32	California	62.6
40	Colorado	51.3
25	Connecticut	66.0
14	Delaware	72.0
23	Florida	67.4
27	Georgia	65.7
50	Hawaii	20.9
47	Idaho	40.7
3	Illinois	76.5
7	Indiana	75.8
11	Iowa	74.4
18	Kansas	70.0
15	Kentucky	71.8
10	Louisiana	74.7
48	Maine	39.9
35	Maryland	59.5
36	Massachusetts	58.9
12	Michigan	73.4
38	Minnesota	57.5
8	Mississippi	75.6
5	Missouri	76.4
33	Montana	61.9
20	Nebraska	68.4
19	Nevada	69.1
46	New Hampshire	40.9
28	New Jersey	64.9
37	New Mexico	58.1
24	New York	66.4
26	North Carolina	65.8
49	North Dakota	28.4
9	Ohio	75.5
17	Oklahoma	70.5
29	Oregon	64.5
3	Pennsylvania	76.5
21	Rhode Island	68.1
16	South Carolina	71.4
45	South Dakota	43.6
13	Tennessee	72.7
34	Texas	61.7
43	Utah	44.4
41	Vermont	45.2
31	Virginia	62.9
39	Washington	53.4
2	West Virginia	76.8
1	Wisconsin	82.4
42	Wyoming	44.6

<u>RANK ORDER</u>

RANK	STATE	PERCENT
1	Wisconsin	82.4
2	West Virginia	76.8
3	Illinois	76.5
3	Pennsylvania	76.5
5	Missouri	76.4
6	Arkansas	75.9
7	Indiana	75.8
8	Mississippi	75.6
9	Ohio	75.5
10	Louisiana	74.7
11	Iowa	74.4
12	Michigan	73.4
13	Tennessee	72.7
14	Delaware	72.0
15	Kentucky	71.8
16	South Carolina	71.4
17	Oklahoma	70.5
18	Kansas	70.0
19	Nevada	69.1
20	Nebraska	68.4
21	Rhode Island	68.1
22	Alabama	67.9
23	Florida	67.4
24	New York	66.4
25	Connecticut	66.0
26	North Carolina	65.8
27	Georgia	65.7
28	New Jersey	64.9
29	Oregon	64.5
30	Arizona	63.9
31	Virginia	62.9
32	California	62.6
33	Montana	61.9
34	Texas	61.7
35	Maryland	59.5
36	Massachusetts	58.9
37	New Mexico	58.1
38	Minnesota	57.5
39	Washington	53.4
40	Colorado	51.3
41	Vermont	45.2
42	Wyoming	44.6
43	Alaska	44.4
43	Utah	44.4
45	South Dakota	43.6
46	New Hampshire	40.9
47	Idaho	40.7
48	Maine	39.9
49	North Dakota	28.4
50	Hawaii	20.9
	District of Columbia	76.7

Source: U.S. Dept. of Health and Human Services, Nat'l Center for Health Statistics
"National Vital Statistics Reports" (Vol. 51, No. 2, December 18, 2002)
*Final data by state of residence. By race of mother.

Births to Unmarried Hispanic Women in 2001

National Total = 361,689 Live Births*

ALPHA ORDER

RANK	STATE	BIRTHS	% of USA
39	Alabama	557	0.2%
43	Alaska	225	0.1%
5	Arizona	18,400	5.1%
34	Arkansas	979	0.3%
1	California	108,473	30.0%
8	Colorado	7,613	2.1%
16	Connecticut	4,271	1.2%
38	Delaware	598	0.2%
4	Florida	19,315	5.3%
11	Georgia	6,162	1.7%
33	Hawaii	989	0.3%
35	Idaho	942	0.3%
6	Illinois	17,150	4.7%
20	Indiana	2,820	0.8%
36	Iowa	924	0.3%
26	Kansas	2,063	0.6%
37	Kentucky	608	0.2%
40	Louisiana	532	0.1%
47	Maine	65	0.0%
22	Maryland	2,303	0.6%
12	Massachusetts	5,756	1.6%
19	Michigan	3,071	0.8%
25	Minnesota	2,179	0.6%
41	Mississippi	290	0.1%
30	Missouri	1,261	0.3%
45	Montana	153	0.0%
32	Nebraska	1,212	0.3%
15	Nevada	4,635	1.3%
44	New Hampshire	190	0.1%
7	New Jersey	12,380	3.4%
9	New Mexico	7,375	2.0%
3	New York	32,298	8.9%
10	North Carolina	6,723	1.9%
48	North Dakota	42	0.0%
24	Ohio	2,271	0.6%
27	Oklahoma	2,035	0.6%
18	Oregon	3,256	0.9%
13	Pennsylvania	4,980	1.4%
29	Rhode Island	1,302	0.4%
31	South Carolina	1,259	0.3%
46	South Dakota	134	0.0%
28	Tennessee	1,698	0.5%
2	Texas	57,981	16.0%
21	Utah	2,539	0.7%
50	Vermont	11	0.0%
17	Virginia	3,648	1.0%
14	Washington	4,961	1.4%
49	West Virginia	30	0.0%
22	Wisconsin	2,303	0.6%
42	Wyoming	236	0.1%

RANK ORDER

RANK	STATE	BIRTHS	% of USA
1	California	108,473	30.0%
2	Texas	57,981	16.0%
3	New York	32,298	8.9%
4	Florida	19,315	5.3%
5	Arizona	18,400	5.1%
6	Illinois	17,150	4.7%
7	New Jersey	12,380	3.4%
8	Colorado	7,613	2.1%
9	New Mexico	7,375	2.0%
10	North Carolina	6,723	1.9%
11	Georgia	6,162	1.7%
12	Massachusetts	5,756	1.6%
13	Pennsylvania	4,980	1.4%
14	Washington	4,961	1.4%
15	Nevada	4,635	1.3%
16	Connecticut	4,271	1.2%
17	Virginia	3,648	1.0%
18	Oregon	3,256	0.9%
19	Michigan	3,071	0.8%
20	Indiana	2,820	0.8%
21	Utah	2,539	0.7%
22	Maryland	2,303	0.6%
22	Wisconsin	2,303	0.6%
24	Ohio	2,271	0.6%
25	Minnesota	2,179	0.6%
26	Kansas	2,063	0.6%
27	Oklahoma	2,035	0.6%
28	Tennessee	1,698	0.5%
29	Rhode Island	1,302	0.4%
30	Missouri	1,261	0.3%
31	South Carolina	1,259	0.3%
32	Nebraska	1,212	0.3%
33	Hawaii	989	0.3%
34	Arkansas	979	0.3%
35	Idaho	942	0.3%
36	Iowa	924	0.3%
37	Kentucky	608	0.2%
38	Delaware	598	0.2%
39	Alabama	557	0.2%
40	Louisiana	532	0.1%
41	Mississippi	290	0.1%
42	Wyoming	236	0.1%
43	Alaska	225	0.1%
44	New Hampshire	190	0.1%
45	Montana	153	0.0%
46	South Dakota	134	0.0%
47	Maine	65	0.0%
48	North Dakota	42	0.0%
49	West Virginia	30	0.0%
50	Vermont	11	0.0%
	District of Columbia	491	0.1%

Source: U.S. Department of Health and Human Services, National Center for Health Statistics
    "National Vital Statistics Reports" (Vol. 51, No. 2, December 18, 2002)
*Final data by state of residence. By race of mother. Persons of Hispanic origin may be of any race.

Births to Unmarried Hispanic Women
As a Percent of All Births to Hispanic Women in 2001
National Percent = 42.5% of Live Births*

RANK	STATE	PERCENT
50	Alabama	24.7
44	Alaska	34.5
10	Arizona	50.9
42	Arkansas	37.0
25	California	41.5
39	Colorado	38.6
1	Connecticut	61.8
6	Delaware	55.2
37	Florida	38.9
36	Georgia	39.3
16	Hawaii	44.2
45	Idaho	34.2
23	Illinois	41.9
13	Indiana	47.8
27	Iowa	41.4
21	Kansas	42.1
33	Kentucky	40.3
45	Louisiana	34.2
40	Maine	37.6
18	Maryland	43.4
2	Massachusetts	60.9
23	Michigan	41.9
12	Minnesota	48.0
33	Mississippi	40.3
20	Missouri	42.3
32	Montana	40.6
30	Nebraska	41.1
19	Nevada	42.7
41	New Hampshire	37.3
7	New Jersey	52.7
8	New Mexico	52.2
5	New York	59.2
14	North Carolina	46.2
49	North Dakota	30.0
11	Ohio	49.4
28	Oklahoma	41.2
28	Oregon	41.2
3	Pennsylvania	60.8
4	Rhode Island	59.3
21	South Carolina	42.1
9	South Dakota	52.1
17	Tennessee	43.5
47	Texas	33.6
38	Utah	38.8
48	Vermont	31.4
35	Virginia	39.9
31	Washington	40.9
43	West Virginia	36.1
15	Wisconsin	44.7
25	Wyoming	41.5

RANK	STATE	PERCENT
1	Connecticut	61.8
2	Massachusetts	60.9
3	Pennsylvania	60.8
4	Rhode Island	59.3
5	New York	59.2
6	Delaware	55.2
7	New Jersey	52.7
8	New Mexico	52.2
9	South Dakota	52.1
10	Arizona	50.9
11	Ohio	49.4
12	Minnesota	48.0
13	Indiana	47.8
14	North Carolina	46.2
15	Wisconsin	44.7
16	Hawaii	44.2
17	Tennessee	43.5
18	Maryland	43.4
19	Nevada	42.7
20	Missouri	42.3
21	Kansas	42.1
21	South Carolina	42.1
23	Illinois	41.9
23	Michigan	41.9
25	California	41.5
25	Wyoming	41.5
27	Iowa	41.4
28	Oklahoma	41.2
28	Oregon	41.2
30	Nebraska	41.1
31	Washington	40.9
32	Montana	40.6
33	Kentucky	40.3
33	Mississippi	40.3
35	Virginia	39.9
36	Georgia	39.3
37	Florida	38.9
38	Utah	38.8
39	Colorado	38.6
40	Maine	37.6
41	New Hampshire	37.3
42	Arkansas	37.0
43	West Virginia	36.1
44	Alaska	34.5
45	Idaho	34.2
45	Louisiana	34.2
47	Texas	33.6
48	Vermont	31.4
49	North Dakota	30.0
50	Alabama	24.7
	District of Columbia	54.9

Source: U.S. Dept. of Health and Human Services, Nat'l Center for Health Statistics
    "National Vital Statistics Reports" (Vol. 51, No. 2, December 18, 2002)
*Final data by state of residence. By race of mother. Persons of Hispanic origin may be of any race.

Births to Teenage Mothers in 2001

National Total = 445,944 Live Births*

RANK	STATE	BIRTHS	% of USA
17	Alabama	8,820	2.0%
46	Alaska	1,056	0.2%
11	Arizona	11,653	2.6%
27	Arkansas	5,941	1.3%
1	California	53,007	11.9%
23	Colorado	7,169	1.6%
36	Connecticut	3,081	0.7%
41	Delaware	1,259	0.3%
3	Florida	24,217	5.4%
6	Georgia	17,279	3.9%
40	Hawaii	1,672	0.4%
39	Idaho	2,203	0.5%
5	Illinois	19,758	4.4%
14	Indiana	10,109	2.3%
35	Iowa	3,574	0.8%
32	Kansas	4,472	1.0%
24	Kentucky	7,120	1.6%
13	Louisiana	10,373	2.3%
44	Maine	1,215	0.3%
26	Maryland	6,756	1.5%
29	Massachusetts	4,984	1.1%
10	Michigan	13,457	3.0%
28	Minnesota	5,240	1.2%
22	Mississippi	7,340	1.6%
16	Missouri	9,317	2.1%
42	Montana	1,258	0.3%
38	Nebraska	2,393	0.5%
34	Nevada	3,677	0.8%
47	New Hampshire	914	0.2%
19	New Jersey	7,693	1.7%
31	New Mexico	4,529	1.0%
4	New York	20,012	4.5%
8	North Carolina	14,336	3.2%
49	North Dakota	673	0.2%
7	Ohio	17,034	3.8%
21	Oklahoma	7,476	1.7%
30	Oregon	4,820	1.1%
9	Pennsylvania	13,567	3.0%
43	Rhode Island	1,236	0.3%
18	South Carolina	7,901	1.8%
45	South Dakota	1,148	0.3%
12	Tennessee	10,838	2.4%
2	Texas	52,782	11.8%
33	Utah	3,884	0.9%
50	Vermont	524	0.1%
15	Virginia	9,439	2.1%
20	Washington	7,517	1.7%
37	West Virginia	2,683	0.6%
25	Wisconsin	6,775	1.5%
48	Wyoming	782	0.2%

RANK	STATE	BIRTHS	% of USA
1	California	53,007	11.9%
2	Texas	52,782	11.8%
3	Florida	24,217	5.4%
4	New York	20,012	4.5%
5	Illinois	19,758	4.4%
6	Georgia	17,279	3.9%
7	Ohio	17,034	3.8%
8	North Carolina	14,336	3.2%
9	Pennsylvania	13,567	3.0%
10	Michigan	13,457	3.0%
11	Arizona	11,653	2.6%
12	Tennessee	10,838	2.4%
13	Louisiana	10,373	2.3%
14	Indiana	10,109	2.3%
15	Virginia	9,439	2.1%
16	Missouri	9,317	2.1%
17	Alabama	8,820	2.0%
18	South Carolina	7,901	1.8%
19	New Jersey	7,693	1.7%
20	Washington	7,517	1.7%
21	Oklahoma	7,476	1.7%
22	Mississippi	7,340	1.6%
23	Colorado	7,169	1.6%
24	Kentucky	7,120	1.6%
25	Wisconsin	6,775	1.5%
26	Maryland	6,756	1.5%
27	Arkansas	5,941	1.3%
28	Minnesota	5,240	1.2%
29	Massachusetts	4,984	1.1%
30	Oregon	4,820	1.1%
31	New Mexico	4,529	1.0%
32	Kansas	4,472	1.0%
33	Utah	3,884	0.9%
34	Nevada	3,677	0.8%
35	Iowa	3,574	0.8%
36	Connecticut	3,081	0.7%
37	West Virginia	2,683	0.6%
38	Nebraska	2,393	0.5%
39	Idaho	2,203	0.5%
40	Hawaii	1,672	0.4%
41	Delaware	1,259	0.3%
42	Montana	1,258	0.3%
43	Rhode Island	1,236	0.3%
44	Maine	1,215	0.3%
45	South Dakota	1,148	0.3%
46	Alaska	1,056	0.2%
47	New Hampshire	914	0.2%
48	Wyoming	782	0.2%
49	North Dakota	673	0.2%
50	Vermont	524	0.1%
	District of Columbia	981	0.2%

Source: Morgan Quitno Press using data from U.S. Dept. of Health and Human Services, Nat'l Center for Health Statistics (unpublished data)
*Live births to women 15 to 19 years old by state of residence.

Teenage Birth Rate in 2001

National Rate = 45.3 Births per 1,000 Women 15 to 19 Years Old*

ALPHA ORDER

RANK	STATE	RATE
9	Alabama	57.8
32	Alaska	37.7
3	Arizona	65.3
5	Arkansas	64.2
22	California	45.2
20	Colorado	45.7
44	Connecticut	29.4
16	Delaware	48.2
15	Florida	49.3
6	Georgia	60.9
24	Hawaii	42.5
27	Idaho	40.6
17	Illinois	47.3
18	Indiana	47.2
42	Iowa	33.0
23	Kansas	43.0
14	Kentucky	51.4
9	Louisiana	57.8
47	Maine	27.1
30	Maryland	38.2
48	Massachusetts	25.0
34	Michigan	37.2
45	Minnesota	27.9
1	Mississippi	66.7
19	Missouri	46.1
37	Montana	35.6
36	Nebraska	36.0
12	Nevada	56.4
50	New Hampshire	21.0
43	New Jersey	29.9
4	New Mexico	64.5
39	New York	34.1
13	North Carolina	55.2
46	North Dakota	27.2
25	Ohio	42.2
8	Oklahoma	58.0
26	Oregon	40.9
40	Pennsylvania	33.6
33	Rhode Island	37.4
11	South Carolina	57.4
35	South Dakota	37.1
7	Tennessee	58.4
2	Texas	66.5
30	Utah	38.2
49	Vermont	23.9
28	Virginia	39.4
38	Washington	34.9
21	West Virginia	45.5
41	Wisconsin	33.4
29	Wyoming	38.6

RANK ORDER

RANK	STATE	RATE
1	Mississippi	66.7
2	Texas	66.5
3	Arizona	65.3
4	New Mexico	64.5
5	Arkansas	64.2
6	Georgia	60.9
7	Tennessee	58.4
8	Oklahoma	58.0
9	Alabama	57.8
9	Louisiana	57.8
11	South Carolina	57.4
12	Nevada	56.4
13	North Carolina	55.2
14	Kentucky	51.4
15	Florida	49.3
16	Delaware	48.2
17	Illinois	47.3
18	Indiana	47.2
19	Missouri	46.1
20	Colorado	45.7
21	West Virginia	45.5
22	California	45.2
23	Kansas	43.0
24	Hawaii	42.5
25	Ohio	42.2
26	Oregon	40.9
27	Idaho	40.6
28	Virginia	39.4
29	Wyoming	38.6
30	Maryland	38.2
30	Utah	38.2
32	Alaska	37.7
33	Rhode Island	37.4
34	Michigan	37.2
35	South Dakota	37.1
36	Nebraska	36.0
37	Montana	35.6
38	Washington	34.9
39	New York	34.1
40	Pennsylvania	33.6
41	Wisconsin	33.4
42	Iowa	33.0
43	New Jersey	29.9
44	Connecticut	29.4
45	Minnesota	27.9
46	North Dakota	27.2
47	Maine	27.1
48	Massachusetts	25.0
49	Vermont	23.9
50	New Hampshire	21.0
	District of Columbia	74.9

Source: U.S. Department of Health and Human Services, National Center for Health Statistics
"National Vital Statistics Reports" (Vol. 51, No. 2, December 18, 2002). National figure revised by
"National Vital Statistics Reports" (Vol. 51, No. 4, February 6, 2003)
*Final data by state of residence.

Births to Teenage Mothers as a Percent of Births in 2001

National Percent = 11.1% of Live Births*

ALPHA ORDER				RANK ORDER		
RANK	STATE	PERCENT		RANK	STATE	PERCENT
6	Alabama	14.6		1	Mississippi	17.4
27	Alaska	10.6		2	New Mexico	16.7
10	Arizona	13.6		3	Arkansas	16.1
3	Arkansas	16.1		4	Louisiana	15.9
31	California	10.0		5	Oklahoma	14.9
25	Colorado	10.7		6	Alabama	14.6
47	Connecticut	7.2		7	Texas	14.4
18	Delaware	11.7		8	South Carolina	14.2
17	Florida	11.8		9	Tennessee	13.8
13	Georgia	12.9		10	Arizona	13.6
32	Hawaii	9.8		11	West Virginia	13.1
27	Idaho	10.6		12	Kentucky	13.0
25	Illinois	10.7		13	Georgia	12.9
18	Indiana	11.7		14	Wyoming	12.8
36	Iowa	9.5		15	Missouri	12.3
21	Kansas	11.5		16	North Carolina	12.1
12	Kentucky	13.0		17	Florida	11.8
4	Louisiana	15.9		18	Delaware	11.7
41	Maine	8.8		18	Indiana	11.7
40	Maryland	9.2		18	Nevada	11.7
50	Massachusetts	6.1		21	Kansas	11.5
30	Michigan	10.1		21	Montana	11.5
46	Minnesota	7.8		23	Ohio	11.2
1	Mississippi	17.4		24	South Dakota	11.0
15	Missouri	12.3		25	Colorado	10.7
21	Montana	11.5		25	Illinois	10.7
35	Nebraska	9.6		27	Alaska	10.6
18	Nevada	11.7		27	Idaho	10.6
49	New Hampshire	6.2		27	Oregon	10.6
48	New Jersey	6.6		30	Michigan	10.1
2	New Mexico	16.7		31	California	10.0
45	New York	7.9		32	Hawaii	9.8
16	North Carolina	12.1		32	Wisconsin	9.8
41	North Dakota	8.8		34	Rhode Island	9.7
23	Ohio	11.2		35	Nebraska	9.6
5	Oklahoma	14.9		36	Iowa	9.5
27	Oregon	10.6		36	Pennsylvania	9.5
36	Pennsylvania	9.5		36	Virginia	9.5
34	Rhode Island	9.7		39	Washington	9.4
8	South Carolina	14.2		40	Maryland	9.2
24	South Dakota	11.0		41	Maine	8.8
9	Tennessee	13.8		41	North Dakota	8.8
7	Texas	14.4		43	Vermont	8.2
44	Utah	8.1		44	Utah	8.1
43	Vermont	8.2		45	New York	7.9
36	Virginia	9.5		46	Minnesota	7.8
39	Washington	9.4		47	Connecticut	7.2
11	West Virginia	13.1		48	New Jersey	6.6
32	Wisconsin	9.8		49	New Hampshire	6.2
14	Wyoming	12.8		50	Massachusetts	6.1
					District of Columbia	12.9

Source: Morgan Quitno Press using data from U.S. Dept. of Health and Human Services, Nat'l Center for Health Statistics (unpublished data)

*Live births to women age 15 to 19 years old by state of residence.

Births to White Teenage Mothers in 2001

National Total = 318,563 Live Births*

ALPHA ORDER					RANK ORDER			
RANK	STATE	BIRTHS	% of USA		RANK	STATE	BIRTHS	% of USA
20	Alabama	4,870	1.5%		1	California	45,199	14.2%
48	Alaska	480	0.2%		2	Texas	44,515	14.0%
7	Arizona	9,997	3.1%		3	Florida	15,135	4.8%
25	Arkansas	4,042	1.3%		4	New York	12,674	4.0%
1	California	45,199	14.2%		5	Illinois	12,442	3.9%
15	Colorado	6,430	2.0%		6	Ohio	12,134	3.8%
37	Connecticut	2,272	0.7%		7	Arizona	9,997	3.1%
46	Delaware	689	0.2%		8	Georgia	9,458	3.0%
3	Florida	15,135	4.8%		9	Pennsylvania	9,369	2.9%
8	Georgia	9,458	3.0%		10	Michigan	8,948	2.8%
50	Hawaii	216	0.1%		11	North Carolina	8,550	2.7%
38	Idaho	2,099	0.7%		12	Indiana	8,088	2.5%
5	Illinois	12,442	3.9%		13	Tennessee	7,411	2.3%
12	Indiana	8,088	2.5%		14	Missouri	6,866	2.2%
32	Iowa	3,190	1.0%		15	Colorado	6,430	2.0%
29	Kansas	3,773	1.2%		16	Washington	6,304	2.0%
17	Kentucky	6,126	1.9%		17	Kentucky	6,126	1.9%
24	Louisiana	4,243	1.3%		18	Virginia	5,453	1.7%
40	Maine	1,158	0.4%		19	Oklahoma	5,269	1.7%
33	Maryland	2,990	0.9%		20	Alabama	4,870	1.5%
28	Massachusetts	3,794	1.2%		21	Wisconsin	4,600	1.4%
10	Michigan	8,948	2.8%		22	New Jersey	4,560	1.4%
30	Minnesota	3,750	1.2%		23	Oregon	4,402	1.4%
35	Mississippi	2,902	0.9%		24	Louisiana	4,243	1.3%
14	Missouri	6,866	2.2%		25	Arkansas	4,042	1.3%
42	Montana	916	0.3%		26	South Carolina	3,946	1.2%
39	Nebraska	1,994	0.6%		27	New Mexico	3,835	1.2%
34	Nevada	2,966	0.9%		28	Massachusetts	3,794	1.2%
43	New Hampshire	879	0.3%		29	Kansas	3,773	1.2%
22	New Jersey	4,560	1.4%		30	Minnesota	3,750	1.2%
27	New Mexico	3,835	1.2%		31	Utah	3,623	1.1%
4	New York	12,674	4.0%		32	Iowa	3,190	1.0%
11	North Carolina	8,550	2.7%		33	Maryland	2,990	0.9%
49	North Dakota	474	0.1%		34	Nevada	2,966	0.9%
6	Ohio	12,134	3.8%		35	Mississippi	2,902	0.9%
19	Oklahoma	5,269	1.7%		36	West Virginia	2,538	0.8%
23	Oregon	4,402	1.4%		37	Connecticut	2,272	0.7%
9	Pennsylvania	9,369	2.9%		38	Idaho	2,099	0.7%
41	Rhode Island	953	0.3%		39	Nebraska	1,994	0.6%
26	South Carolina	3,946	1.2%		40	Maine	1,158	0.4%
45	South Dakota	699	0.2%		41	Rhode Island	953	0.3%
13	Tennessee	7,411	2.3%		42	Montana	916	0.3%
2	Texas	44,515	14.0%		43	New Hampshire	879	0.3%
31	Utah	3,623	1.1%		44	Wyoming	709	0.2%
47	Vermont	515	0.2%		45	South Dakota	699	0.2%
18	Virginia	5,453	1.7%		46	Delaware	689	0.2%
16	Washington	6,304	2.0%		47	Vermont	515	0.2%
36	West Virginia	2,538	0.8%		48	Alaska	480	0.2%
21	Wisconsin	4,600	1.4%		49	North Dakota	474	0.1%
44	Wyoming	709	0.2%		50	Hawaii	216	0.1%
						District of Columbia	118	0.0%

Source: Morgan Quitno Press using data from U.S. Dept. of Health and Human Services, Nat'l Center for Health Statistics (unpublished data)

*Live births to women 15 to 19 years old by state of residence.

White Teenage Birth Rate in 2001

National Rate = 46.3 Births per 1,000 White Teenage Women*

ALPHA ORDER

RANK	STATE	RATE
14	Alabama	47.9
36	Alaska	32.0
3	Arizona	83.4
7	Arkansas	56.5
4	California	74.3
9	Colorado	55.6
40	Connecticut	28.6
29	Delaware	35.8
16	Florida	45.0
8	Georgia	56.3
31	Hawaii	34.5
20	Idaho	42.8
22	Illinois	42.4
20	Indiana	42.8
37	Iowa	31.1
18	Kansas	44.2
12	Kentucky	49.1
24	Louisiana	40.9
41	Maine	27.8
39	Maryland	29.4
48	Massachusetts	23.5
33	Michigan	32.8
47	Minnesota	23.8
13	Mississippi	48.3
23	Missouri	41.2
38	Montana	30.4
30	Nebraska	34.6
5	Nevada	69.9
49	New Hampshire	21.7
42	New Jersey	27.3
1	New Mexico	91.6
34	New York	32.7
11	North Carolina	49.5
50	North Dakota	20.3
28	Ohio	36.6
6	Oklahoma	57.7
17	Oregon	44.4
42	Pennsylvania	27.3
35	Rhode Island	32.4
15	South Carolina	45.9
45	South Dakota	27.0
10	Tennessee	50.9
2	Texas	85.0
27	Utah	37.4
46	Vermont	24.3
31	Virginia	34.5
25	Washington	39.3
19	West Virginia	44.1
44	Wisconsin	27.1
26	Wyoming	38.8

RANK ORDER

RANK	STATE	RATE
1	New Mexico	91.6
2	Texas	85.0
3	Arizona	83.4
4	California	74.3
5	Nevada	69.9
6	Oklahoma	57.7
7	Arkansas	56.5
8	Georgia	56.3
9	Colorado	55.6
10	Tennessee	50.9
11	North Carolina	49.5
12	Kentucky	49.1
13	Mississippi	48.3
14	Alabama	47.9
15	South Carolina	45.9
16	Florida	45.0
17	Oregon	44.4
18	Kansas	44.2
19	West Virginia	44.1
20	Idaho	42.8
20	Indiana	42.8
22	Illinois	42.4
23	Missouri	41.2
24	Louisiana	40.9
25	Washington	39.3
26	Wyoming	38.8
27	Utah	37.4
28	Ohio	36.6
29	Delaware	35.8
30	Nebraska	34.6
31	Hawaii	34.5
31	Virginia	34.5
33	Michigan	32.8
34	New York	32.7
35	Rhode Island	32.4
36	Alaska	32.0
37	Iowa	31.1
38	Montana	30.4
39	Maryland	29.4
40	Connecticut	28.6
41	Maine	27.8
42	New Jersey	27.3
42	Pennsylvania	27.3
44	Wisconsin	27.1
45	South Dakota	27.0
46	Vermont	24.3
47	Minnesota	23.8
48	Massachusetts	23.5
49	New Hampshire	21.7
50	North Dakota	20.3
	District of Columbia	19.8

Source: Morgan Quitno Press using data from U.S. Dept. of Health and Human Services, Nat'l Center for Health Statistics
(unpublished data)

*Live births to women age 15 to 19 years old by state of residence. Rates calculated using Census 2000 figures for white females ages 15 to 19 years old.

Births to White Teenage Mothers as a Percent of White Births in 2001

National Percent = 10.0% of White Live Births*

ALPHA ORDER

RANK	STATE	PERCENT
11	Alabama	12.0
41	Alaska	7.5
5	Arizona	13.3
3	Arkansas	14.0
20	California	10.6
21	Colorado	10.5
46	Connecticut	6.4
28	Delaware	9.0
24	Florida	9.9
14	Georgia	11.0
48	Hawaii	5.7
21	Idaho	10.5
31	Illinois	8.7
18	Indiana	10.7
28	Iowa	9.0
17	Kansas	10.9
8	Kentucky	12.5
12	Louisiana	11.5
31	Maine	8.7
44	Maryland	6.6
49	Massachusetts	5.6
34	Michigan	8.5
45	Minnesota	6.5
7	Mississippi	12.7
14	Missouri	11.0
25	Montana	9.7
30	Nebraska	8.9
13	Nevada	11.3
47	New Hampshire	6.3
50	New Jersey	5.4
1	New Mexico	16.8
43	New York	7.0
23	North Carolina	10.0
42	North Dakota	7.2
25	Ohio	9.7
4	Oklahoma	13.4
18	Oregon	10.7
38	Pennsylvania	7.9
31	Rhode Island	8.7
14	South Carolina	11.0
36	South Dakota	8.2
10	Tennessee	12.3
2	Texas	14.3
37	Utah	8.0
35	Vermont	8.3
39	Virginia	7.7
27	Washington	9.3
6	West Virginia	13.0
39	Wisconsin	7.7
9	Wyoming	12.4

RANK ORDER

RANK	STATE	PERCENT
1	New Mexico	16.8
2	Texas	14.3
3	Arkansas	14.0
4	Oklahoma	13.4
5	Arizona	13.3
6	West Virginia	13.0
7	Mississippi	12.7
8	Kentucky	12.5
9	Wyoming	12.4
10	Tennessee	12.3
11	Alabama	12.0
12	Louisiana	11.5
13	Nevada	11.3
14	Georgia	11.0
14	Missouri	11.0
14	South Carolina	11.0
17	Kansas	10.9
18	Indiana	10.7
18	Oregon	10.7
20	California	10.6
21	Colorado	10.5
21	Idaho	10.5
23	North Carolina	10.0
24	Florida	9.9
25	Montana	9.7
25	Ohio	9.7
27	Washington	9.3
28	Delaware	9.0
28	Iowa	9.0
30	Nebraska	8.9
31	Illinois	8.7
31	Maine	8.7
31	Rhode Island	8.7
34	Michigan	8.5
35	Vermont	8.3
36	South Dakota	8.2
37	Utah	8.0
38	Pennsylvania	7.9
39	Virginia	7.7
39	Wisconsin	7.7
41	Alaska	7.5
42	North Dakota	7.2
43	New York	7.0
44	Maryland	6.6
45	Minnesota	6.5
46	Connecticut	6.4
47	New Hampshire	6.3
48	Hawaii	5.7
49	Massachusetts	5.6
50	New Jersey	5.4
	District of Columbia	4.6

Source: Morgan Quitno Press using data from U.S. Dept. of Health and Human Services, Nat'l Center for Health Statistics (unpublished data)

*Live births to women age 15 to 19 years old by state of residence.

Births to Black Teenage Mothers in 2001

National Total = 110,843 Live Births*

ALPHA ORDER

RANK	STATE	BIRTHS	% of USA
13	Alabama	3,893	3.5%
40	Alaska	63	0.1%
30	Arizona	532	0.5%
21	Arkansas	1,824	1.6%
8	California	4,900	4.4%
31	Colorado	492	0.4%
26	Connecticut	750	0.7%
29	Delaware	556	0.5%
1	Florida	8,694	7.8%
3	Georgia	7,669	6.9%
42	Hawaii	38	0.0%
46	Idaho	14	0.0%
4	Illinois	7,120	6.4%
20	Indiana	1,954	1.8%
34	Iowa	297	0.3%
28	Kansas	558	0.5%
24	Kentucky	952	0.9%
6	Louisiana	5,990	5.4%
43	Maine	21	0.0%
16	Maryland	3,670	3.3%
25	Massachusetts	940	0.8%
11	Michigan	4,272	3.9%
27	Minnesota	732	0.7%
10	Mississippi	4,341	3.9%
19	Missouri	2,338	2.1%
48	Montana	9	0.0%
35	Nebraska	278	0.3%
32	Nevada	487	0.4%
43	New Hampshire	21	0.0%
18	New Jersey	3,005	2.7%
39	New Mexico	99	0.1%
5	New York	6,833	6.2%
7	North Carolina	5,259	4.7%
49	North Dakota	8	0.0%
9	Ohio	4,769	4.3%
23	Oklahoma	990	0.9%
37	Oregon	163	0.1%
12	Pennsylvania	4,031	3.6%
36	Rhode Island	186	0.2%
14	South Carolina	3,880	3.5%
45	South Dakota	20	0.0%
17	Tennessee	3,335	3.0%
2	Texas	7,813	7.0%
41	Utah	53	0.0%
50	Vermont	5	0.0%
15	Virginia	3,844	3.5%
33	Washington	477	0.4%
38	West Virginia	139	0.1%
22	Wisconsin	1,660	1.5%
47	Wyoming	11	0.0%

RANK ORDER

RANK	STATE	BIRTHS	% of USA
1	Florida	8,694	7.8%
2	Texas	7,813	7.0%
3	Georgia	7,669	6.9%
4	Illinois	7,120	6.4%
5	New York	6,833	6.2%
6	Louisiana	5,990	5.4%
7	North Carolina	5,259	4.7%
8	California	4,900	4.4%
9	Ohio	4,769	4.3%
10	Mississippi	4,341	3.9%
11	Michigan	4,272	3.9%
12	Pennsylvania	4,031	3.6%
13	Alabama	3,893	3.5%
14	South Carolina	3,880	3.5%
15	Virginia	3,844	3.5%
16	Maryland	3,670	3.3%
17	Tennessee	3,335	3.0%
18	New Jersey	3,005	2.7%
19	Missouri	2,338	2.1%
20	Indiana	1,954	1.8%
21	Arkansas	1,824	1.6%
22	Wisconsin	1,660	1.5%
23	Oklahoma	990	0.9%
24	Kentucky	952	0.9%
25	Massachusetts	940	0.8%
26	Connecticut	750	0.7%
27	Minnesota	732	0.7%
28	Kansas	558	0.5%
29	Delaware	556	0.5%
30	Arizona	532	0.5%
31	Colorado	492	0.4%
32	Nevada	487	0.4%
33	Washington	477	0.4%
34	Iowa	297	0.3%
35	Nebraska	278	0.3%
36	Rhode Island	186	0.2%
37	Oregon	163	0.1%
38	West Virginia	139	0.1%
39	New Mexico	99	0.1%
40	Alaska	63	0.1%
41	Utah	53	0.0%
42	Hawaii	38	0.0%
43	Maine	21	0.0%
43	New Hampshire	21	0.0%
45	South Dakota	20	0.0%
46	Idaho	14	0.0%
47	Wyoming	11	0.0%
48	Montana	9	0.0%
49	North Dakota	8	0.0%
50	Vermont	5	0.0%
	District of Columbia	858	0.8%

Source: Morgan Quitno Press using data from U.S. Dept. of Health and Human Services, Nat'l Center for Health Statistics
    (unpublished data)
*Live births to women 15 to 19 years old by state of residence.

Black Teenage Birth Rate in 2001

National Rate = 76.6 Births per 1,000 Black Teenage Women*

ALPHA ORDER			RANK ORDER		
RANK	STATE	RATE	RANK	STATE	RATE
31	Alabama	73.1	1	Wisconsin	119.2
27	Alaska	76.9	2	South Dakota	112.4
16	Arizona	84.6	3	Iowa	108.6
9	Arkansas	90.4	4	Minnesota	98.1
45	California	57.7	5	Nevada	97.2
23	Colorado	79.3	6	Indiana	91.5
44	Connecticut	60.0	7	Ohio	91.1
12	Delaware	85.5	8	Illinois	90.6
22	Florida	82.0	9	Arkansas	90.4
25	Georgia	77.1	10	Nebraska	88.9
35	Hawaii	69.5	11	Missouri	87.5
42	Idaho	64.2	12	Delaware	85.5
8	Illinois	90.6	12	Rhode Island	85.5
6	Indiana	91.5	14	Kansas	84.7
3	Iowa	108.6	14	Louisiana	84.7
14	Kansas	84.7	16	Arizona	84.6
28	Kentucky	76.8	17	Tennessee	84.2
14	Louisiana	84.7	18	Mississippi	84.1
41	Maine	64.4	18	Montana	84.1
39	Maryland	65.1	20	Pennsylvania	83.8
38	Massachusetts	68.3	21	Oklahoma	83.5
24	Michigan	78.0	22	Florida	82.0
4	Minnesota	98.1	23	Colorado	79.3
18	Mississippi	84.1	24	Michigan	78.0
11	Missouri	87.5	25	Georgia	77.1
18	Montana	84.1	26	Texas	77.0
10	Nebraska	88.9	27	Alaska	76.9
5	Nevada	97.2	28	Kentucky	76.8
48	New Hampshire	52.6	29	Oregon	76.1
35	New Jersey	69.5	30	North Carolina	75.5
34	New Mexico	71.7	31	Alabama	73.1
47	New York	57.3	32	South Carolina	72.8
30	North Carolina	75.5	33	Wyoming	72.4
49	North Dakota	45.5	34	New Mexico	71.7
7	Ohio	91.1	35	Hawaii	69.5
21	Oklahoma	83.5	35	New Jersey	69.5
29	Oregon	76.1	37	Virginia	68.5
20	Pennsylvania	83.8	38	Massachusetts	68.3
12	Rhode Island	85.5	39	Maryland	65.1
32	South Carolina	72.8	40	Washington	64.5
2	South Dakota	112.4	41	Maine	64.4
17	Tennessee	84.2	42	Idaho	64.2
26	Texas	77.0	43	West Virginia	62.9
46	Utah	57.5	44	Connecticut	60.0
50	Vermont	30.3	45	California	57.7
37	Virginia	68.5	46	Utah	57.5
40	Washington	64.5	47	New York	57.3
43	West Virginia	62.9	48	New Hampshire	52.6
1	Wisconsin	119.2	49	North Dakota	45.5
33	Wyoming	72.4	50	Vermont	30.3
				District of Columbia	72.1

Source: Morgan Quitno Press using data from U.S. Dept. of Health and Human Services, Nat'l Center for Health Statistics
   (unpublished data)
*Live births to women age 15 to 19 years old by state of residence. Rates calculated using Census 2000 figures for black females ages 15 to 19 years old.

Births to Black Teenage Mothers as a Percent of Black Births in 2001

National Percent = 18.3% of Black Live Births*

ALPHA ORDER   RANK ORDER

RANK	STATE	PERCENT	RANK	STATE	PERCENT
13	Alabama	20.3	1	Wisconsin	25.3
43	Alaska	14.3	2	Arkansas	24.5
22	Arizona	19.3	3	Iowa	23.5
2	Arkansas	24.5	4	Mississippi	23.1
42	California	14.5	5	Louisiana	22.1
34	Colorado	16.6	6	Oklahoma	21.5
40	Connecticut	14.6	7	Illinois	21.4
11	Delaware	20.5	7	Montana	21.4
27	Florida	18.4	9	Missouri	21.0
29	Georgia	17.5	10	Ohio	20.7
50	Hawaii	7.2	11	Delaware	20.5
35	Idaho	16.3	11	South Carolina	20.5
7	Illinois	21.4	13	Alabama	20.3
13	Indiana	20.3	13	Indiana	20.3
3	Iowa	23.5	15	Nebraska	20.2
16	Kansas	20.1	16	Kansas	20.1
22	Kentucky	19.3	16	Tennessee	20.1
5	Louisiana	22.1	18	Pennsylvania	19.9
45	Maine	13.7	19	South Dakota	19.8
39	Maryland	15.1	20	West Virginia	19.7
47	Massachusetts	11.5	21	New Mexico	19.4
28	Michigan	18.1	22	Arizona	19.3
38	Minnesota	15.4	22	Kentucky	19.3
4	Mississippi	23.1	22	Nevada	19.3
9	Missouri	21.0	25	Texas	19.2
7	Montana	21.4	26	North Carolina	18.5
15	Nebraska	20.2	27	Florida	18.4
22	Nevada	19.3	28	Michigan	18.1
48	New Hampshire	10.1	29	Georgia	17.5
40	New Jersey	14.6	30	Oregon	17.3
21	New Mexico	19.4	30	Virginia	17.3
46	New York	13.1	32	Wyoming	16.9
26	North Carolina	18.5	33	Rhode Island	16.7
49	North Dakota	7.8	34	Colorado	16.6
10	Ohio	20.7	35	Idaho	16.3
6	Oklahoma	21.5	36	Vermont	16.1
30	Oregon	17.3	37	Utah	15.5
18	Pennsylvania	19.9	38	Minnesota	15.4
33	Rhode Island	16.7	39	Maryland	15.1
11	South Carolina	20.5	40	Connecticut	14.6
19	South Dakota	19.8	40	New Jersey	14.6
16	Tennessee	20.1	42	California	14.5
25	Texas	19.2	43	Alaska	14.3
37	Utah	15.5	43	Washington	14.3
36	Vermont	16.1	45	Maine	13.7
30	Virginia	17.3	46	New York	13.1
43	Washington	14.3	47	Massachusetts	11.5
20	West Virginia	19.7	48	New Hampshire	10.1
1	Wisconsin	25.3	49	North Dakota	7.8
32	Wyoming	16.9	50	Hawaii	7.2
				District of Columbia	17.7

Source: Morgan Quitno Press using data from U.S. Dept. of Health and Human Services, Nat'l Center for Health Statistics (unpublished data)
*Live births to women 15 to 19 years old by state of residence.

Births to Teenage Mothers in 1990

National Total = 521,826 Live Births*

ALPHA ORDER

RANK	STATE	BIRTHS	% of USA
15	Alabama	11,252	2.2%
47	Alaska	1,142	0.2%
19	Arizona	9,612	1.8%
27	Arkansas	7,011	1.3%
1	California	69,712	13.4%
28	Colorado	5,975	1.1%
33	Connecticut	4,038	0.8%
44	Delaware	1,277	0.2%
3	Florida	27,017	5.2%
8	Georgia	18,369	3.5%
39	Hawaii	2,122	0.4%
40	Idaho	2,009	0.4%
5	Illinois	24,967	4.8%
12	Indiana	12,335	2.4%
34	Iowa	3,989	0.8%
31	Kansas	4,722	0.9%
20	Kentucky	9,349	1.8%
13	Louisiana	12,270	2.4%
41	Maine	1,857	0.4%
23	Maryland	8,143	1.6%
26	Massachusetts	7,266	1.4%
7	Michigan	20,312	3.9%
29	Minnesota	5,342	1.0%
21	Mississippi	8,909	1.7%
16	Missouri	11,227	2.2%
43	Montana	1,331	0.3%
38	Nebraska	2,352	0.5%
37	Nevada	2,663	0.5%
45	New Hampshire	1,258	0.2%
17	New Jersey	10,068	1.9%
32	New Mexico	4,367	0.8%
4	New York	26,608	5.1%
10	North Carolina	16,506	3.2%
49	North Dakota	793	0.2%
6	Ohio	22,690	4.3%
24	Oklahoma	7,590	1.5%
30	Oregon	5,084	1.0%
9	Pennsylvania	18,216	3.5%
42	Rhode Island	1,564	0.3%
18	South Carolina	9,721	1.9%
46	South Dakota	1,172	0.2%
11	Tennessee	12,928	2.5%
2	Texas	48,302	9.3%
36	Utah	3,707	0.7%
50	Vermont	702	0.1%
14	Virginia	11,353	2.2%
22	Washington	8,397	1.6%
35	West Virginia	3,976	0.8%
25	Wisconsin	7,281	1.4%
48	Wyoming	943	0.2%

RANK ORDER

RANK	STATE	BIRTHS	% of USA
1	California	69,712	13.4%
2	Texas	48,302	9.3%
3	Florida	27,017	5.2%
4	New York	26,608	5.1%
5	Illinois	24,967	4.8%
6	Ohio	22,690	4.3%
7	Michigan	20,312	3.9%
8	Georgia	18,369	3.5%
9	Pennsylvania	18,216	3.5%
10	North Carolina	16,506	3.2%
11	Tennessee	12,928	2.5%
12	Indiana	12,335	2.4%
13	Louisiana	12,270	2.4%
14	Virginia	11,353	2.2%
15	Alabama	11,252	2.2%
16	Missouri	11,227	2.2%
17	New Jersey	10,068	1.9%
18	South Carolina	9,721	1.9%
19	Arizona	9,612	1.8%
20	Kentucky	9,349	1.8%
21	Mississippi	8,909	1.7%
22	Washington	8,397	1.6%
23	Maryland	8,143	1.6%
24	Oklahoma	7,590	1.5%
25	Wisconsin	7,281	1.4%
26	Massachusetts	7,266	1.4%
27	Arkansas	7,011	1.3%
28	Colorado	5,975	1.1%
29	Minnesota	5,342	1.0%
30	Oregon	5,084	1.0%
31	Kansas	4,722	0.9%
32	New Mexico	4,367	0.8%
33	Connecticut	4,038	0.8%
34	Iowa	3,989	0.8%
35	West Virginia	3,976	0.8%
36	Utah	3,707	0.7%
37	Nevada	2,663	0.5%
38	Nebraska	2,352	0.5%
39	Hawaii	2,122	0.4%
40	Idaho	2,009	0.4%
41	Maine	1,857	0.4%
42	Rhode Island	1,564	0.3%
43	Montana	1,331	0.3%
44	Delaware	1,277	0.2%
45	New Hampshire	1,258	0.2%
46	South Dakota	1,172	0.2%
47	Alaska	1,142	0.2%
48	Wyoming	943	0.2%
49	North Dakota	793	0.2%
50	Vermont	702	0.1%
	District of Columbia	2,030	0.4%

Source: U.S. Department of Health and Human Services, Centers for Disease Control and Prevention
"Surveillance for Pregnancy and Birth Rates Among Teenagers" (MMWR, Vol. 42, No. SS-6, 12/17/93)
*Women aged 15 to 19 years old.

Teenage Birth Rate in 1990

National Rate = 59.9 Live Births per 1,000 Teenage Women*

ALPHA ORDER				RANK ORDER		
RANK	**STATE**	**RATE**		**RANK**	**STATE**	**RATE**
11	Alabama	71.0		1	Mississippi	81.0
17	Alaska	65.3		2	Arkansas	80.1
4	Arizona	75.5		3	New Mexico	78.2
2	Arkansas	80.1		4	Arizona	75.5
12	California	70.6		4	Georgia	75.5
28	Colorado	54.5		6	Texas	75.3
45	Connecticut	38.8		7	Louisiana	74.2
28	Delaware	54.5		8	Nevada	73.3
13	Florida	69.1		9	Tennessee	72.3
4	Georgia	75.5		10	South Carolina	71.3
20	Hawaii	61.2		11	Alabama	71.0
33	Idaho	50.6		12	California	70.6
18	Illinois	62.9		13	Florida	69.1
22	Indiana	58.6		14	Kentucky	67.6
43	Iowa	40.5		14	North Carolina	67.6
26	Kansas	56.1		16	Oklahoma	66.8
14	Kentucky	67.6		17	Alaska	65.3
7	Louisiana	74.2		18	Illinois	62.9
40	Maine	43.0		19	Missouri	62.8
30	Maryland	53.2		20	Hawaii	61.2
48	Massachusetts	35.1		21	Michigan	59.0
21	Michigan	59.0		22	Indiana	58.6
46	Minnesota	36.3		23	Ohio	57.9
1	Mississippi	81.0		24	West Virginia	57.3
19	Missouri	62.8		25	Wyoming	56.3
35	Montana	48.4		26	Kansas	56.1
42	Nebraska	42.3		27	Oregon	54.6
8	Nevada	73.3		28	Colorado	54.5
50	New Hampshire	33.0		28	Delaware	54.5
43	New Jersey	40.5		30	Maryland	53.2
3	New Mexico	78.2		31	Washington	53.1
39	New York	43.6		32	Virginia	52.9
14	North Carolina	67.6		33	Idaho	50.6
47	North Dakota	35.4		34	Utah	48.5
23	Ohio	57.9		35	Montana	48.4
16	Oklahoma	66.8		36	South Dakota	46.8
27	Oregon	54.6		37	Pennsylvania	44.9
37	Pennsylvania	44.9		38	Rhode Island	43.9
38	Rhode Island	43.9		39	New York	43.6
10	South Carolina	71.3		40	Maine	43.0
36	South Dakota	46.8		41	Wisconsin	42.6
9	Tennessee	72.3		42	Nebraska	42.3
6	Texas	75.3		43	Iowa	40.5
34	Utah	48.5		43	New Jersey	40.5
49	Vermont	34.0		45	Connecticut	38.8
32	Virginia	52.9		46	Minnesota	36.3
31	Washington	53.1		47	North Dakota	35.4
24	West Virginia	57.3		48	Massachusetts	35.1
41	Wisconsin	42.6		49	Vermont	34.0
25	Wyoming	56.3		50	New Hampshire	33.0
					District of Columbia	93.1

Source: U.S. Department of Health and Human Services, Centers for Disease Control and Prevention
    "Surveillance for Pregnancy and Birth Rates Among Teenagers" (MMWR, Vol. 42, No. SS-6, 12/17/93)
*Women aged 15 to 19 years old.

Percent Change in Teenage Birth Rate: 1990 to 2001

National Percent Change = 24.4% Decrease*

ALPHA ORDER

RANK	STATE	PERCENT CHANGE
12	Alabama	(18.6)
50	Alaska	(42.3)
4	Arizona	(13.5)
18	Arkansas	(19.9)
46	California	(36.0)
7	Colorado	(16.1)
30	Connecticut	(24.2)
1	Delaware	(11.6)
40	Florida	(28.7)
14	Georgia	(19.3)
43	Hawaii	(30.6)
17	Idaho	(19.8)
31	Illinois	(24.8)
15	Indiana	(19.5)
11	Iowa	(18.5)
28	Kansas	(23.4)
29	Kentucky	(24.0)
24	Louisiana	(22.1)
49	Maine	(37.0)
39	Maryland	(28.2)
41	Massachusetts	(28.8)
48	Michigan	(36.9)
25	Minnesota	(23.1)
9	Mississippi	(17.7)
37	Missouri	(26.6)
36	Montana	(26.4)
6	Nebraska	(14.9)
25	Nevada	(23.1)
47	New Hampshire	(36.4)
35	New Jersey	(26.2)
8	New Mexico	(17.5)
23	New York	(21.8)
10	North Carolina	(18.3)
27	North Dakota	(23.2)
38	Ohio	(27.1)
3	Oklahoma	(13.2)
32	Oregon	(25.1)
33	Pennsylvania	(25.2)
5	Rhode Island	(14.8)
15	South Carolina	(19.5)
20	South Dakota	(20.7)
13	Tennessee	(19.2)
2	Texas	(11.7)
21	Utah	(21.2)
42	Vermont	(29.7)
34	Virginia	(25.5)
45	Washington	(34.3)
19	West Virginia	(20.6)
22	Wisconsin	(21.6)
44	Wyoming	(31.4)

RANK ORDER

RANK	STATE	PERCENT CHANGE
1	Delaware	(11.6)
2	Texas	(11.7)
3	Oklahoma	(13.2)
4	Arizona	(13.5)
5	Rhode Island	(14.8)
6	Nebraska	(14.9)
7	Colorado	(16.1)
8	New Mexico	(17.5)
9	Mississippi	(17.7)
10	North Carolina	(18.3)
11	Iowa	(18.5)
12	Alabama	(18.6)
13	Tennessee	(19.2)
14	Georgia	(19.3)
15	Indiana	(19.5)
15	South Carolina	(19.5)
17	Idaho	(19.8)
18	Arkansas	(19.9)
19	West Virginia	(20.6)
20	South Dakota	(20.7)
21	Utah	(21.2)
22	Wisconsin	(21.6)
23	New York	(21.8)
24	Louisiana	(22.1)
25	Minnesota	(23.1)
25	Nevada	(23.1)
27	North Dakota	(23.2)
28	Kansas	(23.4)
29	Kentucky	(24.0)
30	Connecticut	(24.2)
31	Illinois	(24.8)
32	Oregon	(25.1)
33	Pennsylvania	(25.2)
34	Virginia	(25.5)
35	New Jersey	(26.2)
36	Montana	(26.4)
37	Missouri	(26.6)
38	Ohio	(27.1)
39	Maryland	(28.2)
40	Florida	(28.7)
41	Massachusetts	(28.8)
42	Vermont	(29.7)
43	Hawaii	(30.6)
44	Wyoming	(31.4)
45	Washington	(34.3)
46	California	(36.0)
47	New Hampshire	(36.4)
48	Michigan	(36.9)
49	Maine	(37.0)
50	Alaska	(42.3)
	District of Columbia	(19.5)

Source: Morgan Quitno Press using data from U.S. Department of Health and Human Services
"National Vital Statistics Reports" (Vol. 51, No. 2, December 18, 2002) and
"Surveillance for Pregnancy and Birth Rates Among Teenagers" (MMWR, Vol. 42, No. SS-6, 12/17/93)
*Women aged 15 to 19 years old.

Births to Teenage Mothers in 1980

National Total = 562,330 Live Births*

ALPHA ORDER

RANK	STATE	BIRTHS	% of USA
15	Alabama	13,096	2.3%
49	Alaska	1,123	0.2%
25	Arizona	8,235	1.5%
26	Arkansas	8,060	1.4%
1	California	56,138	10.0%
29	Colorado	6,592	1.2%
36	Connecticut	4,408	0.8%
45	Delaware	1,572	0.3%
6	Florida	24,042	4.3%
9	Georgia	19,137	3.4%
40	Hawaii	2,085	0.4%
38	Idaho	2,645	0.5%
3	Illinois	29,798	5.3%
12	Indiana	15,331	2.7%
31	Iowa	5,962	1.1%
30	Kansas	6,090	1.1%
16	Kentucky	12,559	2.2%
10	Louisiana	16,504	2.9%
39	Maine	2,522	0.4%
23	Maryland	8,885	1.6%
27	Massachusetts	7,765	1.4%
8	Michigan	20,401	3.6%
28	Minnesota	7,048	1.3%
19	Mississippi	11,079	2.0%
14	Missouri	13,312	2.4%
43	Montana	1,761	0.3%
37	Nebraska	3,313	0.6%
41	Nevada	2,048	0.4%
47	New Hampshire	1,475	0.3%
18	New Jersey	11,904	2.1%
34	New Mexico	4,758	0.8%
4	New York	28,206	5.0%
11	North Carolina	16,192	2.9%
48	North Dakota	1,304	0.2%
5	Ohio	26,567	4.7%
21	Oklahoma	10,206	1.8%
33	Oregon	5,731	1.0%
7	Pennsylvania	22,029	3.9%
46	Rhode Island	1,502	0.3%
20	South Carolina	10,282	1.8%
42	South Dakota	1,797	0.3%
13	Tennessee	13,792	2.5%
2	Texas	50,125	8.9%
35	Utah	4,594	0.8%
50	Vermont	1,024	0.2%
17	Virginia	12,138	2.2%
24	Washington	8,495	1.5%
32	West Virginia	5,911	1.1%
22	Wisconsin	9,220	1.6%
44	Wyoming	1,634	0.3%

RANK ORDER

RANK	STATE	BIRTHS	% of USA
1	California	56,138	10.0%
2	Texas	50,125	8.9%
3	Illinois	29,798	5.3%
4	New York	28,206	5.0%
5	Ohio	26,567	4.7%
6	Florida	24,042	4.3%
7	Pennsylvania	22,029	3.9%
8	Michigan	20,401	3.6%
9	Georgia	19,137	3.4%
10	Louisiana	16,504	2.9%
11	North Carolina	16,192	2.9%
12	Indiana	15,331	2.7%
13	Tennessee	13,792	2.5%
14	Missouri	13,312	2.4%
15	Alabama	13,096	2.3%
16	Kentucky	12,559	2.2%
17	Virginia	12,138	2.2%
18	New Jersey	11,904	2.1%
19	Mississippi	11,079	2.0%
20	South Carolina	10,282	1.8%
21	Oklahoma	10,206	1.8%
22	Wisconsin	9,220	1.6%
23	Maryland	8,885	1.6%
24	Washington	8,495	1.5%
25	Arizona	8,235	1.5%
26	Arkansas	8,060	1.4%
27	Massachusetts	7,765	1.4%
28	Minnesota	7,048	1.3%
29	Colorado	6,592	1.2%
30	Kansas	6,090	1.1%
31	Iowa	5,962	1.1%
32	West Virginia	5,911	1.1%
33	Oregon	5,731	1.0%
34	New Mexico	4,758	0.8%
35	Utah	4,594	0.8%
36	Connecticut	4,408	0.8%
37	Nebraska	3,313	0.6%
38	Idaho	2,645	0.5%
39	Maine	2,522	0.4%
40	Hawaii	2,085	0.4%
41	Nevada	2,048	0.4%
42	South Dakota	1,797	0.3%
43	Montana	1,761	0.3%
44	Wyoming	1,634	0.3%
45	Delaware	1,572	0.3%
46	Rhode Island	1,502	0.3%
47	New Hampshire	1,475	0.3%
48	North Dakota	1,304	0.2%
49	Alaska	1,123	0.2%
50	Vermont	1,024	0.2%
	District of Columbia	1,933	0.3%

Source: U.S. Department of Health and Human Services, National Center for Health Statistics
    "Vital Statistics of the United States, 1980" (Vol. I-Natality, issued 1984)
*Births to women age 15 to 19 years old.

Teenage Birth Rate in 1980

National Rate = 53.0 Live Births per 1,000 Teenage Women*

ALPHA ORDER			RANK ORDER		
RANK	STATE	RATE	RANK	STATE	RATE
10	Alabama	68.3	1	Mississippi	83.7
15	Alaska	64.4	2	Wyoming	78.7
12	Arizona	65.5	3	Louisiana	76.0
5	Arkansas	74.5	4	Oklahoma	74.6
25	California	53.3	5	Arkansas	74.5
31	Colorado	49.9	6	Texas	74.3
49	Connecticut	30.5	7	Kentucky	72.3
28	Delaware	51.2	8	Georgia	71.9
18	Florida	58.5	9	New Mexico	71.8
8	Georgia	71.9	10	Alabama	68.3
30	Hawaii	50.7	11	West Virginia	67.8
17	Idaho	59.5	12	Arizona	65.5
24	Illinois	55.8	13	Utah	65.2
21	Indiana	57.5	14	South Carolina	64.8
39	Iowa	43.0	15	Alaska	64.4
23	Kansas	56.8	16	Tennessee	64.1
7	Kentucky	72.3	17	Idaho	59.5
3	Louisiana	76.0	18	Florida	58.5
34	Maine	47.4	18	Nevada	58.5
38	Maryland	43.4	20	Missouri	57.8
50	Massachusetts	28.1	21	Indiana	57.5
37	Michigan	45.0	21	North Carolina	57.5
44	Minnesota	35.4	23	Kansas	56.8
1	Mississippi	83.7	24	Illinois	55.8
20	Missouri	57.8	25	California	53.3
32	Montana	48.5	26	South Dakota	52.6
36	Nebraska	45.1	27	Ohio	52.5
18	Nevada	58.5	28	Delaware	51.2
47	New Hampshire	33.6	29	Oregon	50.9
45	New Jersey	35.2	30	Hawaii	50.7
9	New Mexico	71.8	31	Colorado	49.9
46	New York	34.8	32	Montana	48.5
21	North Carolina	57.5	33	Virginia	48.3
40	North Dakota	41.7	34	Maine	47.4
27	Ohio	52.5	35	Washington	46.7
4	Oklahoma	74.6	36	Nebraska	45.1
29	Oregon	50.9	37	Michigan	45.0
41	Pennsylvania	40.5	38	Maryland	43.4
48	Rhode Island	33.0	39	Iowa	43.0
14	South Carolina	64.8	40	North Dakota	41.7
26	South Dakota	52.6	41	Pennsylvania	40.5
16	Tennessee	64.1	42	Vermont	39.5
6	Texas	74.3	42	Wisconsin	39.5
13	Utah	65.2	44	Minnesota	35.4
42	Vermont	39.5	45	New Jersey	35.2
33	Virginia	48.3	46	New York	34.8
35	Washington	46.7	47	New Hampshire	33.6
11	West Virginia	67.8	48	Rhode Island	33.0
42	Wisconsin	39.5	49	Connecticut	30.5
2	Wyoming	78.7	50	Massachusetts	28.1
				District of Columbia	62.4

Source: U.S. Department of Health and Human Services, Centers for Disease Control and Prevention
"Surveillance for Pregnancy and Birth Rates Among Teenagers" (MMWR, Vol. 42, No. SS-6, 12/17/93)
*Women aged 15 to 19 years old.

Percent Change in Teenage Birth Rate: 1980 to 2001

National Percent Change = 14.5% Decrease*

ALPHA ORDER

RANK	STATE	PERCENT CHANGE
20	Alabama	(15.4)
48	Alaska	(41.5)
2	Arizona	(0.3)
15	Arkansas	(13.8)
17	California	(15.2)
8	Colorado	(8.4)
4	Connecticut	(3.6)
7	Delaware	(5.9)
22	Florida	(15.7)
19	Georgia	(15.3)
23	Hawaii	(16.2)
42	Idaho	(31.8)
17	Illinois	(15.2)
26	Indiana	(17.9)
35	Iowa	(23.3)
37	Kansas	(24.3)
40	Kentucky	(28.9)
36	Louisiana	(23.9)
49	Maine	(42.8)
14	Maryland	(12.0)
12	Massachusetts	(11.0)
25	Michigan	(17.3)
33	Minnesota	(21.2)
32	Mississippi	(20.3)
30	Missouri	(20.2)
39	Montana	(26.6)
30	Nebraska	(20.2)
4	Nevada	(3.6)
45	New Hampshire	(37.5)
16	New Jersey	(15.1)
10	New Mexico	(10.2)
3	New York	(2.0)
6	North Carolina	(4.0)
44	North Dakota	(34.8)
28	Ohio	(19.6)
34	Oklahoma	(22.3)
28	Oregon	(19.6)
24	Pennsylvania	(17.0)
1	Rhode Island	13.3
13	South Carolina	(11.4)
41	South Dakota	(29.5)
9	Tennessee	(8.9)
11	Texas	(10.5)
47	Utah	(41.4)
46	Vermont	(39.5)
27	Virginia	(18.4)
38	Washington	(25.3)
43	West Virginia	(32.9)
20	Wisconsin	(15.4)
50	Wyoming	(51.0)

RANK ORDER

RANK	STATE	PERCENT CHANGE
1	Rhode Island	13.3
2	Arizona	(0.3)
3	New York	(2.0)
4	Connecticut	(3.6)
4	Nevada	(3.6)
6	North Carolina	(4.0)
7	Delaware	(5.9)
8	Colorado	(8.4)
9	Tennessee	(8.9)
10	New Mexico	(10.2)
11	Texas	(10.5)
12	Massachusetts	(11.0)
13	South Carolina	(11.4)
14	Maryland	(12.0)
15	Arkansas	(13.8)
16	New Jersey	(15.1)
17	California	(15.2)
17	Illinois	(15.2)
19	Georgia	(15.3)
20	Alabama	(15.4)
20	Wisconsin	(15.4)
22	Florida	(15.7)
23	Hawaii	(16.2)
24	Pennsylvania	(17.0)
25	Michigan	(17.3)
26	Indiana	(17.9)
27	Virginia	(18.4)
28	Ohio	(19.6)
28	Oregon	(19.6)
30	Missouri	(20.2)
30	Nebraska	(20.2)
32	Mississippi	(20.3)
33	Minnesota	(21.2)
34	Oklahoma	(22.3)
35	Iowa	(23.3)
36	Louisiana	(23.9)
37	Kansas	(24.3)
38	Washington	(25.3)
39	Montana	(26.6)
40	Kentucky	(28.9)
41	South Dakota	(29.5)
42	Idaho	(31.8)
43	West Virginia	(32.9)
44	North Dakota	(34.8)
45	New Hampshire	(37.5)
46	Vermont	(39.5)
47	Utah	(41.4)
48	Alaska	(41.5)
49	Maine	(42.8)
50	Wyoming	(51.0)

District of Columbia   20.0

*Source: Morgan Quitno Press using data from U.S. Department of Health and Human Services
"National Vital Statistics Reports" (Vol. 51, No. 2, December 18, 2002) and
"Surveillance for Pregnancy and Birth Rates Among Teenagers" (MMWR, Vol. 42, No. SS-6, 12/17/93)*
*Women aged 15 to 19 years old.

Pregnancy Rate for 15 to 19 Year Old Women in 1999

National Rate = 68.1 Births and Abortions per 1,000 Women 15-19 Years Old*

ALPHA ORDER

RANK	STATE	RATE
9	Alabama	80.2
NA	Alaska**	NA
7	Arizona	81.7
8	Arkansas	80.7
NA	California**	NA
28	Colorado	56.1
25	Connecticut	60.5
3	Delaware	85.5
NA	Florida**	NA
2	Georgia	87.4
18	Hawaii	68.7
36	Idaho	47.9
14	Illinois	74.1
24	Indiana	62.6
37	Iowa	47.6
15	Kansas	73.7
21	Kentucky	63.9
13	Louisiana	75.6
43	Maine	43.0
30	Maryland	55.2
35	Massachusetts	52.0
31	Michigan	54.4
40	Minnesota	44.0
12	Mississippi	79.7
27	Missouri	56.8
32	Montana	53.3
34	Nebraska	52.4
5	Nevada	82.4
NA	New Hampshire**	NA
26	New Jersey	59.4
4	New Mexico	82.6
11	New York	79.8
6	North Carolina	82.2
45	North Dakota	39.5
22	Ohio	63.8
NA	Oklahoma**	NA
17	Oregon	72.1
33	Pennsylvania	52.8
19	Rhode Island	66.5
16	South Carolina	72.3
41	South Dakota	43.5
9	Tennessee	80.2
1	Texas	88.1
38	Utah	46.3
42	Vermont	43.1
23	Virginia	63.1
20	Washington	65.6
29	West Virginia	56.0
39	Wisconsin	46.1
44	Wyoming	41.8

RANK ORDER

RANK	STATE	RATE
1	Texas	88.1
2	Georgia	87.4
3	Delaware	85.5
4	New Mexico	82.6
5	Nevada	82.4
6	North Carolina	82.2
7	Arizona	81.7
8	Arkansas	80.7
9	Alabama	80.2
9	Tennessee	80.2
11	New York	79.8
12	Mississippi	79.7
13	Louisiana	75.6
14	Illinois	74.1
15	Kansas	73.7
16	South Carolina	72.3
17	Oregon	72.1
18	Hawaii	68.7
19	Rhode Island	66.5
20	Washington	65.6
21	Kentucky	63.9
22	Ohio	63.8
23	Virginia	63.1
24	Indiana	62.6
25	Connecticut	60.5
26	New Jersey	59.4
27	Missouri	56.8
28	Colorado	56.1
29	West Virginia	56.0
30	Maryland	55.2
31	Michigan	54.4
32	Montana	53.3
33	Pennsylvania	52.8
34	Nebraska	52.4
35	Massachusetts	52.0
36	Idaho	47.9
37	Iowa	47.6
38	Utah	46.3
39	Wisconsin	46.1
40	Minnesota	44.0
41	South Dakota	43.5
42	Vermont	43.1
43	Maine	43.0
44	Wyoming	41.8
45	North Dakota	39.5
NA	Alaska**	NA
NA	California**	NA
NA	Florida**	NA
NA	New Hampshire**	NA
NA	Oklahoma**	NA

District of Columbia   192.8

Source: Morgan Quitno Press using data from US Dept of Health & Human Serv's, Centers for Disease Control-Prevention "Abortion Surveillance-United States, 1999" (Morbidity Mortality Weekly Report, Vol. 51, No. SS-9, 11/29/02)
The sum of live births and legal induced abortions per 1,000 women aged 15-19 years old. Births by state of residence, abortions by state of occurrence. Miscarriages are not included in these rates. National rate includes only states reporting abortions and births.
***Not available.*

Percent Change in Pregnancy Rate for 15 to 19 Year Old Women: 1997 to 1999

National Percent Change = 4.5% Decrease*

ALPHA ORDER				RANK ORDER		
RANK	STATE	PERCENT CHANGE		RANK	STATE	PERCENT CHANGE
13	Alabama	(3.5)		1	New Jersey	7.4
NA	Alaska**	NA		2	Idaho	1.5
8	Arizona	(2.4)		3	Maryland	0.4
26	Arkansas	(5.8)		4	Kansas	(0.1)
NA	California**	NA		5	Hawaii	(1.4)
40	Colorado	(11.4)		6	Mississippi	(1.7)
35	Connecticut	(8.5)		6	Nebraska	(1.7)
43	Delaware	(20.8)		8	Arizona	(2.4)
NA	Florida**	NA		9	New Mexico	(2.7)
22	Georgia	(5.0)		9	North Dakota	(2.7)
5	Hawaii	(1.4)		11	Pennsylvania	(2.9)
2	Idaho	1.5		12	Louisiana	(3.4)
NA	Illinois**	NA		13	Alabama	(3.5)
25	Indiana	(5.3)		13	Oregon	(3.5)
NA	Iowa**	NA		13	Tennessee	(3.5)
4	Kansas	(0.1)		16	South Carolina	(3.6)
34	Kentucky	(7.9)		17	New York	(3.7)
12	Louisiana	(3.4)		18	Texas	(3.8)
32	Maine	(6.9)		19	North Carolina	(4.0)
3	Maryland	0.4		19	Virginia	(4.0)
36	Massachusetts	(8.6)		21	West Virginia	(4.6)
38	Michigan	(9.0)		22	Georgia	(5.0)
31	Minnesota	(6.6)		23	Utah	(5.1)
6	Mississippi	(1.7)		23	Wisconsin	(5.1)
29	Missouri	(6.4)		25	Indiana	(5.3)
27	Montana	(6.0)		26	Arkansas	(5.8)
6	Nebraska	(1.7)		27	Montana	(6.0)
38	Nevada	(9.0)		28	Wyoming	(6.1)
NA	New Hampshire**	NA		29	Missouri	(6.4)
1	New Jersey	7.4		29	Washington	(6.4)
9	New Mexico	(2.7)		31	Minnesota	(6.6)
17	New York	(3.7)		32	Maine	(6.9)
19	North Carolina	(4.0)		33	Ohio	(7.1)
9	North Dakota	(2.7)		34	Kentucky	(7.9)
33	Ohio	(7.1)		35	Connecticut	(8.5)
NA	Oklahoma**	NA		36	Massachusetts	(8.6)
13	Oregon	(3.5)		36	South Dakota	(8.6)
11	Pennsylvania	(2.9)		38	Michigan	(9.0)
42	Rhode Island	(13.5)		38	Nevada	(9.0)
16	South Carolina	(3.6)		40	Colorado	(11.4)
36	South Dakota	(8.6)		41	Vermont	(11.7)
13	Tennessee	(3.5)		42	Rhode Island	(13.5)
18	Texas	(3.8)		43	Delaware	(20.8)
23	Utah	(5.1)		NA	Alaska**	NA
41	Vermont	(11.7)		NA	California**	NA
19	Virginia	(4.0)		NA	Florida**	NA
29	Washington	(6.4)		NA	Illinois**	NA
21	West Virginia	(4.6)		NA	Iowa**	NA
23	Wisconsin	(5.1)		NA	New Hampshire**	NA
28	Wyoming	(6.1)		NA	Oklahoma**	NA

District of Columbia (9.0)

Source: Morgan Quitno Press using data from US Dept of Health & Human Serv's, Centers for Disease Control-Prevention
"Abortion Surveillance-United States, 1999" (Morbidity Mortality Weekly Report, Vol. 51, No. SS-9, 11/29/02)
*The sum of live births and legal induced abortions per 1,000 women aged 15-19 years old. Births by state of residence, abortions by state of occurrence. Miscarriages are not included in these rates. National rate includes only states reporting abortions and births.
**Not available.

Births to Women 35 to 54 Years Old in 2001

National Total = 549,619 Live Births*

ALPHA ORDER

RANK	STATE	BIRTHS	% of USA
27	Alabama	5,338	1.0%
44	Alaska	1,414	0.3%
17	Arizona	9,525	1.7%
38	Arkansas	2,680	0.5%
1	California	86,016	15.7%
18	Colorado	9,437	1.7%
20	Connecticut	9,138	1.7%
45	Delaware	1,412	0.3%
4	Florida	29,241	5.3%
12	Georgia	15,312	2.8%
36	Hawaii	2,866	0.5%
41	Idaho	1,955	0.4%
5	Illinois	26,516	4.8%
21	Indiana	8,627	1.6%
31	Iowa	4,120	0.7%
29	Kansas	4,292	0.8%
28	Kentucky	5,005	0.9%
24	Louisiana	5,928	1.1%
42	Maine	1,909	0.3%
13	Maryland	13,380	2.4%
8	Massachusetts	17,983	3.3%
10	Michigan	17,169	3.1%
16	Minnesota	10,319	1.9%
34	Mississippi	3,188	0.6%
22	Missouri	8,239	1.5%
46	Montana	1,320	0.2%
35	Nebraska	2,943	0.5%
33	Nevada	3,795	0.7%
39	New Hampshire	2,628	0.5%
6	New Jersey	24,014	4.4%
37	New Mexico	2,850	0.5%
2	New York	48,127	8.8%
14	North Carolina	13,165	2.4%
49	North Dakota	848	0.2%
9	Ohio	17,877	3.3%
32	Oklahoma	3,986	0.7%
25	Oregon	5,683	1.0%
7	Pennsylvania	21,827	4.0%
40	Rhode Island	2,124	0.4%
26	South Carolina	5,633	1.0%
47	South Dakota	1,142	0.2%
23	Tennessee	7,275	1.3%
3	Texas	38,010	6.9%
30	Utah	4,226	0.8%
48	Vermont	1,066	0.2%
11	Virginia	15,626	2.8%
15	Washington	11,548	2.1%
43	West Virginia	1,686	0.3%
19	Wisconsin	9,289	1.7%
50	Wyoming	525	0.1%

RANK ORDER

RANK	STATE	BIRTHS	% of USA
1	California	86,016	15.7%
2	New York	48,127	8.8%
3	Texas	38,010	6.9%
4	Florida	29,241	5.3%
5	Illinois	26,516	4.8%
6	New Jersey	24,014	4.4%
7	Pennsylvania	21,827	4.0%
8	Massachusetts	17,983	3.3%
9	Ohio	17,877	3.3%
10	Michigan	17,169	3.1%
11	Virginia	15,626	2.8%
12	Georgia	15,312	2.8%
13	Maryland	13,380	2.4%
14	North Carolina	13,165	2.4%
15	Washington	11,548	2.1%
16	Minnesota	10,319	1.9%
17	Arizona	9,525	1.7%
18	Colorado	9,437	1.7%
19	Wisconsin	9,289	1.7%
20	Connecticut	9,138	1.7%
21	Indiana	8,627	1.6%
22	Missouri	8,239	1.5%
23	Tennessee	7,275	1.3%
24	Louisiana	5,928	1.1%
25	Oregon	5,683	1.0%
26	South Carolina	5,633	1.0%
27	Alabama	5,338	1.0%
28	Kentucky	5,005	0.9%
29	Kansas	4,292	0.8%
30	Utah	4,226	0.8%
31	Iowa	4,120	0.7%
32	Oklahoma	3,986	0.7%
33	Nevada	3,795	0.7%
34	Mississippi	3,188	0.6%
35	Nebraska	2,943	0.5%
36	Hawaii	2,866	0.5%
37	New Mexico	2,850	0.5%
38	Arkansas	2,680	0.5%
39	New Hampshire	2,628	0.5%
40	Rhode Island	2,124	0.4%
41	Idaho	1,955	0.4%
42	Maine	1,909	0.3%
43	West Virginia	1,686	0.3%
44	Alaska	1,414	0.3%
45	Delaware	1,412	0.3%
46	Montana	1,320	0.2%
47	South Dakota	1,142	0.2%
48	Vermont	1,066	0.2%
49	North Dakota	848	0.2%
50	Wyoming	525	0.1%
	District of Columbia	1,397	0.3%

Source: Morgan Quitno Press using data from U.S. Dept of Health & Human Services, National Center for Health Statistics
    (unpublished data)
*By state of residence.

Births to Women 35 to 54 Years Old as a Percent of All Births in 2001

National Percent = 13.7% of Live Births*

ALPHA ORDER

RANK	STATE	PERCENT
44	Alabama	8.8
17	Alaska	14.1
29	Arizona	11.1
50	Arkansas	7.2
10	California	16.3
17	Colorado	14.1
2	Connecticut	21.4
21	Delaware	13.1
16	Florida	14.2
28	Georgia	11.5
7	Hawaii	16.8
40	Idaho	9.4
15	Illinois	14.4
39	Indiana	10.0
32	Iowa	11.0
32	Kansas	11.0
42	Kentucky	9.2
43	Louisiana	9.1
19	Maine	13.9
5	Maryland	18.3
1	Massachusetts	22.2
22	Michigan	12.9
12	Minnesota	15.3
49	Mississippi	7.5
34	Missouri	10.9
25	Montana	12.0
26	Nebraska	11.9
24	Nevada	12.1
6	New Hampshire	17.9
3	New Jersey	20.7
36	New Mexico	10.5
4	New York	18.9
29	North Carolina	11.1
29	North Dakota	11.1
27	Ohio	11.8
48	Oklahoma	8.0
23	Oregon	12.5
13	Pennsylvania	15.2
8	Rhode Island	16.7
38	South Carolina	10.1
34	South Dakota	10.9
41	Tennessee	9.3
37	Texas	10.4
44	Utah	8.8
8	Vermont	16.7
11	Virginia	15.8
14	Washington	14.5
47	West Virginia	8.3
20	Wisconsin	13.4
46	Wyoming	8.6

RANK ORDER

RANK	STATE	PERCENT
1	Massachusetts	22.2
2	Connecticut	21.4
3	New Jersey	20.7
4	New York	18.9
5	Maryland	18.3
6	New Hampshire	17.9
7	Hawaii	16.8
8	Rhode Island	16.7
8	Vermont	16.7
10	California	16.3
11	Virginia	15.8
12	Minnesota	15.3
13	Pennsylvania	15.2
14	Washington	14.5
15	Illinois	14.4
16	Florida	14.2
17	Alaska	14.1
17	Colorado	14.1
19	Maine	13.9
20	Wisconsin	13.4
21	Delaware	13.1
22	Michigan	12.9
23	Oregon	12.5
24	Nevada	12.1
25	Montana	12.0
26	Nebraska	11.9
27	Ohio	11.8
28	Georgia	11.5
29	Arizona	11.1
29	North Carolina	11.1
29	North Dakota	11.1
32	Iowa	11.0
32	Kansas	11.0
34	Missouri	10.9
34	South Dakota	10.9
36	New Mexico	10.5
37	Texas	10.4
38	South Carolina	10.1
39	Indiana	10.0
40	Idaho	9.4
41	Tennessee	9.3
42	Kentucky	9.2
43	Louisiana	9.1
44	Alabama	8.8
44	Utah	8.8
46	Wyoming	8.6
47	West Virginia	8.3
48	Oklahoma	8.0
49	Mississippi	7.5
50	Arkansas	7.2

| | District of Columbia | 18.3 |

Source: Morgan Quitno Press using data from U.S. Dept of Health & Human Services, National Center for Health Statistics
     (unpublished data)
*By state of residence.

Births by Vaginal Delivery in 2001

National Total = 3,043,605 Live Births*

RANK	STATE	BIRTHS	% of USA
24	Alabama	43,769	1.4%
45	Alaska	8,112	0.3%
13	Arizona	68,478	2.2%
34	Arkansas	26,795	0.9%
1	California	395,291	13.0%
21	Colorado	53,874	1.8%
30	Connecticut	32,285	1.1%
47	Delaware	8,008	0.3%
4	Florida	151,464	5.0%
9	Georgia	101,079	3.3%
40	Hawaii	13,641	0.4%
38	Idaho	16,819	0.6%
5	Illinois	143,018	4.7%
14	Indiana	66,314	2.2%
33	Iowa	28,929	1.0%
32	Kansas	29,618	1.0%
26	Kentucky	40,338	1.3%
23	Louisiana	45,812	1.5%
42	Maine	10,443	0.3%
20	Maryland	54,621	1.8%
16	Massachusetts	60,483	2.0%
8	Michigan	102,205	3.4%
22	Minnesota	53,306	1.8%
31	Mississippi	29,724	1.0%
18	Missouri	57,428	1.9%
44	Montana	8,600	0.3%
37	Nebraska	18,838	0.6%
35	Nevada	23,944	0.8%
41	New Hampshire	11,285	0.4%
11	New Jersey	82,330	2.7%
36	New Mexico	22,082	0.7%
3	New York	188,233	6.2%
10	North Carolina	88,757	2.9%
48	North Dakota	6,019	0.2%
6	Ohio	118,679	3.9%
28	Oklahoma	37,137	1.2%
29	Oregon	35,804	1.2%
7	Pennsylvania	110,491	3.6%
43	Rhode Island	9,649	0.3%
25	South Carolina	41,036	1.3%
46	South Dakota	8,072	0.3%
17	Tennessee	57,815	1.9%
2	Texas	269,307	8.8%
27	Utah	39,710	1.3%
49	Vermont	5,233	0.2%
12	Virginia	74,559	2.4%
15	Washington	61,587	2.0%
39	West Virginia	14,994	0.5%
19	Wisconsin	55,879	1.8%
50	Wyoming	4,886	0.2%

RANK	STATE	BIRTHS	% of USA
1	California	395,291	13.0%
2	Texas	269,307	8.8%
3	New York	188,233	6.2%
4	Florida	151,464	5.0%
5	Illinois	143,018	4.7%
6	Ohio	118,679	3.9%
7	Pennsylvania	110,491	3.6%
8	Michigan	102,205	3.4%
9	Georgia	101,079	3.3%
10	North Carolina	88,757	2.9%
11	New Jersey	82,330	2.7%
12	Virginia	74,559	2.4%
13	Arizona	68,478	2.2%
14	Indiana	66,314	2.2%
15	Washington	61,587	2.0%
16	Massachusetts	60,483	2.0%
17	Tennessee	57,815	1.9%
18	Missouri	57,428	1.9%
19	Wisconsin	55,879	1.8%
20	Maryland	54,621	1.8%
21	Colorado	53,874	1.8%
22	Minnesota	53,306	1.8%
23	Louisiana	45,812	1.5%
24	Alabama	43,769	1.4%
25	South Carolina	41,036	1.3%
26	Kentucky	40,338	1.3%
27	Utah	39,710	1.3%
28	Oklahoma	37,137	1.2%
29	Oregon	35,804	1.2%
30	Connecticut	32,285	1.1%
31	Mississippi	29,724	1.0%
32	Kansas	29,618	1.0%
33	Iowa	28,929	1.0%
34	Arkansas	26,795	0.9%
35	Nevada	23,944	0.8%
36	New Mexico	22,082	0.7%
37	Nebraska	18,838	0.6%
38	Idaho	16,819	0.6%
39	West Virginia	14,994	0.5%
40	Hawaii	13,641	0.4%
41	New Hampshire	11,285	0.4%
42	Maine	10,443	0.3%
43	Rhode Island	9,649	0.3%
44	Montana	8,600	0.3%
45	Alaska	8,112	0.3%
46	South Dakota	8,072	0.3%
47	Delaware	8,008	0.3%
48	North Dakota	6,019	0.2%
49	Vermont	5,233	0.2%
50	Wyoming	4,886	0.2%
	District of Columbia	5,719	0.2%

Source: Morgan Quitno Press using data from U.S. Dept of Health & Human Services, National Center for Health Statistics "National Vital Statistics Reports" (Vol. 51, No. 2, December 18, 2002)

*By state of residence.

Percent of Births by Vaginal Delivery in 2001

National Percent = 75.6% of Live Births*

ALPHA ORDER

RANK	STATE	PERCENT
46	Alabama	72.4
5	Alaska	81.1
8	Arizona	80.0
46	Arkansas	72.4
34	California	74.9
7	Colorado	80.4
30	Connecticut	75.7
37	Delaware	74.5
43	Florida	73.6
30	Georgia	75.7
9	Hawaii	79.9
4	Idaho	81.3
16	Illinois	77.7
22	Indiana	76.7
21	Iowa	76.9
25	Kansas	76.2
40	Kentucky	73.8
50	Louisiana	70.1
27	Maine	75.9
35	Maryland	74.6
35	Massachusetts	74.6
23	Michigan	76.6
12	Minnesota	78.9
49	Mississippi	70.3
26	Missouri	76.1
14	Montana	78.4
27	Nebraska	75.9
24	Nevada	76.3
18	New Hampshire	77.0
48	New Jersey	71.1
3	New Mexico	81.4
38	New York	74.1
33	North Carolina	75.1
12	North Dakota	78.9
15	Ohio	78.3
38	Oklahoma	74.1
11	Oregon	79.0
18	Pennsylvania	77.0
27	Rhode Island	75.9
43	South Carolina	73.6
18	South Dakota	77.0
40	Tennessee	73.8
42	Texas	73.7
1	Utah	82.8
2	Vermont	82.2
32	Virginia	75.4
17	Washington	77.4
45	West Virginia	73.4
6	Wisconsin	80.9
9	Wyoming	79.9

RANK ORDER

RANK	STATE	PERCENT
1	Utah	82.8
2	Vermont	82.2
3	New Mexico	81.4
4	Idaho	81.3
5	Alaska	81.1
6	Wisconsin	80.9
7	Colorado	80.4
8	Arizona	80.0
9	Hawaii	79.9
9	Wyoming	79.9
11	Oregon	79.0
12	Minnesota	78.9
12	North Dakota	78.9
14	Montana	78.4
15	Ohio	78.3
16	Illinois	77.7
17	Washington	77.4
18	New Hampshire	77.0
18	Pennsylvania	77.0
18	South Dakota	77.0
21	Iowa	76.9
22	Indiana	76.7
23	Michigan	76.6
24	Nevada	76.3
25	Kansas	76.2
26	Missouri	76.1
27	Maine	75.9
27	Nebraska	75.9
27	Rhode Island	75.9
30	Connecticut	75.7
30	Georgia	75.7
32	Virginia	75.4
33	North Carolina	75.1
34	California	74.9
35	Maryland	74.6
35	Massachusetts	74.6
37	Delaware	74.5
38	New York	74.1
38	Oklahoma	74.1
40	Kentucky	73.8
40	Tennessee	73.8
42	Texas	73.7
43	Florida	73.6
43	South Carolina	73.6
45	West Virginia	73.4
46	Alabama	72.4
46	Arkansas	72.4
48	New Jersey	71.1
49	Mississippi	70.3
50	Louisiana	70.1

District of Columbia	75.0

Source: Morgan Quitno Press using data from U.S. Dept of Health & Human Services, National Center for Health Statistics "National Vital Statistics Reports" (Vol. 51, No. 2, December 18, 2002)
By state of residence.

Births by Cesarean Delivery in 2001

National Total = 982,328 Live Cesarean Births*

ALPHA ORDER

RANK	STATE	BIRTHS	% of USA
21	Alabama	16,685	1.7%
47	Alaska	1,891	0.2%
20	Arizona	17,119	1.7%
30	Arkansas	10,215	1.0%
1	California	132,468	13.5%
26	Colorado	13,133	1.3%
29	Connecticut	10,363	1.1%
44	Delaware	2,741	0.3%
4	Florida	54,329	5.5%
9	Georgia	32,447	3.3%
40	Hawaii	3,431	0.3%
39	Idaho	3,869	0.4%
5	Illinois	41,046	4.2%
15	Indiana	20,145	2.1%
33	Iowa	8,690	0.9%
32	Kansas	9,251	0.9%
23	Kentucky	14,320	1.5%
16	Louisiana	19,540	2.0%
42	Maine	3,316	0.3%
17	Maryland	18,597	1.9%
13	Massachusetts	20,594	2.1%
10	Michigan	31,222	3.2%
24	Minnesota	14,256	1.5%
28	Mississippi	12,558	1.3%
18	Missouri	18,036	1.8%
46	Montana	2,370	0.2%
36	Nebraska	5,982	0.6%
35	Nevada	7,438	0.8%
41	New Hampshire	3,371	0.3%
6	New Jersey	33,465	3.4%
38	New Mexico	5,046	0.5%
3	New York	65,793	6.7%
11	North Carolina	29,428	3.0%
48	North Dakota	1,610	0.2%
8	Ohio	32,891	3.3%
27	Oklahoma	12,981	1.3%
31	Oregon	9,518	1.0%
7	Pennsylvania	33,004	3.4%
43	Rhode Island	3,064	0.3%
22	South Carolina	14,720	1.5%
45	South Dakota	2,411	0.2%
14	Tennessee	20,525	2.1%
2	Texas	96,103	9.8%
34	Utah	8,249	0.8%
50	Vermont	1,133	0.1%
12	Virginia	24,325	2.5%
19	Washington	17,983	1.8%
37	West Virginia	5,434	0.6%
25	Wisconsin	13,193	1.3%
49	Wyoming	1,229	0.1%

RANK ORDER

RANK	STATE	BIRTHS	% of USA
1	California	132,468	13.5%
2	Texas	96,103	9.8%
3	New York	65,793	6.7%
4	Florida	54,329	5.5%
5	Illinois	41,046	4.2%
6	New Jersey	33,465	3.4%
7	Pennsylvania	33,004	3.4%
8	Ohio	32,891	3.3%
9	Georgia	32,447	3.3%
10	Michigan	31,222	3.2%
11	North Carolina	29,428	3.0%
12	Virginia	24,325	2.5%
13	Massachusetts	20,594	2.1%
14	Tennessee	20,525	2.1%
15	Indiana	20,145	2.1%
16	Louisiana	19,540	2.0%
17	Maryland	18,597	1.9%
18	Missouri	18,036	1.8%
19	Washington	17,983	1.8%
20	Arizona	17,119	1.7%
21	Alabama	16,685	1.7%
22	South Carolina	14,720	1.5%
23	Kentucky	14,320	1.5%
24	Minnesota	14,256	1.5%
25	Wisconsin	13,193	1.3%
26	Colorado	13,133	1.3%
27	Oklahoma	12,981	1.3%
28	Mississippi	12,558	1.3%
29	Connecticut	10,363	1.1%
30	Arkansas	10,215	1.0%
31	Oregon	9,518	1.0%
32	Kansas	9,251	0.9%
33	Iowa	8,690	0.9%
34	Utah	8,249	0.8%
35	Nevada	7,438	0.8%
36	Nebraska	5,982	0.6%
37	West Virginia	5,434	0.6%
38	New Mexico	5,046	0.5%
39	Idaho	3,869	0.4%
40	Hawaii	3,431	0.3%
41	New Hampshire	3,371	0.3%
42	Maine	3,316	0.3%
43	Rhode Island	3,064	0.3%
44	Delaware	2,741	0.3%
45	South Dakota	2,411	0.2%
46	Montana	2,370	0.2%
47	Alaska	1,891	0.2%
48	North Dakota	1,610	0.2%
49	Wyoming	1,229	0.1%
50	Vermont	1,133	0.1%
	District of Columbia	1,906	0.2%

Source: Morgan Quitno Press using data from U.S. Dept of Health & Human Services, National Center for Health Statistics
"National Vital Statistics Reports" (Vol. 51, No. 2, December 18, 2002)
*By state of residence.

Percent of Births by Cesarean Delivery in 2001

National Percent = 24.4% of Live Births*

ALPHA ORDER

RANK	STATE	PERCENT
4	Alabama	27.6
46	Alaska	18.9
43	Arizona	20.0
4	Arkansas	27.6
17	California	25.1
44	Colorado	19.6
20	Connecticut	24.3
14	Delaware	25.5
7	Florida	26.4
20	Georgia	24.3
41	Hawaii	20.1
47	Idaho	18.7
35	Illinois	22.3
29	Indiana	23.3
30	Iowa	23.1
26	Kansas	23.8
10	Kentucky	26.2
1	Louisiana	29.9
22	Maine	24.1
15	Maryland	25.4
15	Massachusetts	25.4
28	Michigan	23.4
38	Minnesota	21.1
2	Mississippi	29.7
25	Missouri	23.9
37	Montana	21.6
22	Nebraska	24.1
27	Nevada	23.7
31	New Hampshire	23.0
3	New Jersey	28.9
48	New Mexico	18.6
12	New York	25.9
18	North Carolina	24.9
38	North Dakota	21.1
36	Ohio	21.7
12	Oklahoma	25.9
40	Oregon	21.0
31	Pennsylvania	23.0
22	Rhode Island	24.1
7	South Carolina	26.4
31	South Dakota	23.0
10	Tennessee	26.2
9	Texas	26.3
50	Utah	17.2
49	Vermont	17.8
19	Virginia	24.6
34	Washington	22.6
6	West Virginia	26.6
45	Wisconsin	19.1
41	Wyoming	20.1

RANK ORDER

RANK	STATE	PERCENT
1	Louisiana	29.9
2	Mississippi	29.7
3	New Jersey	28.9
4	Alabama	27.6
4	Arkansas	27.6
6	West Virginia	26.6
7	Florida	26.4
7	South Carolina	26.4
9	Texas	26.3
10	Kentucky	26.2
10	Tennessee	26.2
12	New York	25.9
12	Oklahoma	25.9
14	Delaware	25.5
15	Maryland	25.4
15	Massachusetts	25.4
17	California	25.1
18	North Carolina	24.9
19	Virginia	24.6
20	Connecticut	24.3
20	Georgia	24.3
22	Maine	24.1
22	Nebraska	24.1
22	Rhode Island	24.1
25	Missouri	23.9
26	Kansas	23.8
27	Nevada	23.7
28	Michigan	23.4
29	Indiana	23.3
30	Iowa	23.1
31	New Hampshire	23.0
31	Pennsylvania	23.0
31	South Dakota	23.0
34	Washington	22.6
35	Illinois	22.3
36	Ohio	21.7
37	Montana	21.6
38	Minnesota	21.1
38	North Dakota	21.1
40	Oregon	21.0
41	Hawaii	20.1
41	Wyoming	20.1
43	Arizona	20.0
44	Colorado	19.6
45	Wisconsin	19.1
46	Alaska	18.9
47	Idaho	18.7
48	New Mexico	18.6
49	Vermont	17.8
50	Utah	17.2
	District of Columbia	25.0

Source: U.S. Department of Health and Human Services, National Center for Health Statistics
    "National Vital Statistics Reports" (Vol. 51, No. 2, December 18, 2002)
*Final data by state of residence.

Percent Change in Rate of Cesarean Births: 1995 to 2001

National Percent Change = 17.3% Increase*

ALPHA ORDER			RANK ORDER		
RANK	STATE	PERCENT CHANGE	RANK	STATE	PERCENT CHANGE
34	Alabama	15.5	1	Washington	31.4
45	Alaska	12.5	2	Rhode Island	29.6
18	Arizona	19.0	3	Massachusetts	28.9
43	Arkansas	12.7	4	Kansas	28.6
15	California	19.5	5	Colorado	28.1
5	Colorado	28.1	6	Oregon	24.3
8	Connecticut	22.7	7	Minnesota	23.4
11	Delaware	21.4	8	Connecticut	22.7
19	Florida	18.9	9	Iowa	22.2
27	Georgia	16.8	10	Wisconsin	21.7
13	Hawaii	20.4	11	Delaware	21.4
40	Idaho	14.0	12	Maryland	21.0
27	Illinois	16.8	13	Hawaii	20.4
22	Indiana	18.3	14	Tennessee	19.6
9	Iowa	22.2	15	California	19.5
4	Kansas	28.6	16	Nebraska	19.3
26	Kentucky	17.0	17	New Hampshire	19.2
24	Louisiana	17.7	18	Arizona	19.0
32	Maine	15.9	19	Florida	18.9
12	Maryland	21.0	19	Missouri	18.9
3	Massachusetts	28.9	21	Pennsylvania	18.6
29	Michigan	16.4	22	Indiana	18.3
7	Minnesota	23.4	23	Nevada	17.9
47	Mississippi	11.2	24	Louisiana	17.7
19	Missouri	18.9	25	North Carolina	17.5
42	Montana	13.7	26	Kentucky	17.0
16	Nebraska	19.3	27	Georgia	16.8
23	Nevada	17.9	27	Illinois	16.8
17	New Hampshire	19.2	29	Michigan	16.4
30	New Jersey	16.1	30	New Jersey	16.1
46	New Mexico	12.0	30	Oklahoma	16.1
44	New York	12.6	32	Maine	15.9
25	North Carolina	17.5	33	South Carolina	15.8
36	North Dakota	14.7	34	Alabama	15.5
38	Ohio	14.2	35	South Dakota	15.0
30	Oklahoma	16.1	36	North Dakota	14.7
6	Oregon	24.3	37	Virginia	14.4
21	Pennsylvania	18.6	38	Ohio	14.2
2	Rhode Island	29.6	39	Vermont	14.1
33	South Carolina	15.8	40	Idaho	14.0
35	South Dakota	15.0	41	Texas	13.9
14	Tennessee	19.6	42	Montana	13.7
41	Texas	13.9	43	Arkansas	12.7
49	Utah	8.9	44	New York	12.6
39	Vermont	14.1	45	Alaska	12.5
37	Virginia	14.4	46	New Mexico	12.0
1	Washington	31.4	47	Mississippi	11.2
48	West Virginia	9.0	48	West Virginia	9.0
10	Wisconsin	21.7	49	Utah	8.9
50	Wyoming	8.1	50	Wyoming	8.1
				District of Columbia	17.9

Source: Morgan Quitno Press using data from U.S. Dept of Health & Human Services, National Center for Health Statistics "National Vital Statistics Reports" (Vol. 51, No. 2, December 18, 2002) and unpublished data.

*By state of residence.

Percent of Vaginal Births After a Cesarean (VBAC) in 2001

National Percent = 16.4% of Live Births to Women Who Have Had a Cesarean*

ALPHA ORDER

RANK	STATE	PERCENT
44	Alabama	11.8
5	Alaska	24.5
30	Arizona	16.7
42	Arkansas	12.7
47	California	10.9
8	Colorado	23.5
23	Connecticut	18.8
28	Delaware	17.0
45	Florida	11.1
37	Georgia	14.7
20	Hawaii	19.3
3	Idaho	26.3
13	Illinois	21.4
32	Indiana	16.6
27	Iowa	17.7
34	Kansas	15.8
43	Kentucky	12.4
50	Louisiana	8.2
39	Maine	13.9
18	Maryland	20.3
19	Massachusetts	19.5
30	Michigan	16.7
17	Minnesota	20.5
49	Mississippi	8.6
21	Missouri	19.1
22	Montana	18.9
35	Nebraska	15.5
36	Nevada	15.4
11	New Hampshire	22.2
14	New Jersey	21.3
4	New Mexico	24.7
12	New York	22.1
29	North Carolina	16.9
7	North Dakota	23.7
5	Ohio	24.5
45	Oklahoma	11.1
16	Oregon	21.0
9	Pennsylvania	23.3
25	Rhode Island	18.7
40	South Carolina	13.6
23	South Dakota	18.8
38	Tennessee	14.4
48	Texas	10.6
2	Utah	29.1
1	Vermont	40.0
33	Virginia	16.4
26	Washington	18.6
41	West Virginia	13.4
10	Wisconsin	23.0
15	Wyoming	21.2

RANK ORDER

RANK	STATE	PERCENT
1	Vermont	40.0
2	Utah	29.1
3	Idaho	26.3
4	New Mexico	24.7
5	Alaska	24.5
5	Ohio	24.5
7	North Dakota	23.7
8	Colorado	23.5
9	Pennsylvania	23.3
10	Wisconsin	23.0
11	New Hampshire	22.2
12	New York	22.1
13	Illinois	21.4
14	New Jersey	21.3
15	Wyoming	21.2
16	Oregon	21.0
17	Minnesota	20.5
18	Maryland	20.3
19	Massachusetts	19.5
20	Hawaii	19.3
21	Missouri	19.1
22	Montana	18.9
23	Connecticut	18.8
23	South Dakota	18.8
25	Rhode Island	18.7
26	Washington	18.6
27	Iowa	17.7
28	Delaware	17.0
29	North Carolina	16.9
30	Arizona	16.7
30	Michigan	16.7
32	Indiana	16.6
33	Virginia	16.4
34	Kansas	15.8
35	Nebraska	15.5
36	Nevada	15.4
37	Georgia	14.7
38	Tennessee	14.4
39	Maine	13.9
40	South Carolina	13.6
41	West Virginia	13.4
42	Arkansas	12.7
43	Kentucky	12.4
44	Alabama	11.8
45	Florida	11.1
45	Oklahoma	11.1
47	California	10.9
48	Texas	10.6
49	Mississippi	8.6
50	Louisiana	8.2
	District of Columbia	14.0

Source: U.S. Department of Health and Human Services, National Center for Health Statistics
"National Vital Statistics Reports" (Vol. 51, No. 2, December 18, 2002)
*Vaginal births after a cesarean delivery as a percent of all births to women with a previous cesarean delivery giving birth in 2001.

Percent of Mothers Beginning Prenatal Care in First Trimester in 2001

National Percent = 83.4% of Mothers*

ALPHA ORDER

RANK	STATE	PERCENT
34	Alabama	82.4
38	Alaska	80.5
48	Arizona	76.7
41	Arkansas	79.8
16	California	85.4
41	Colorado	79.8
5	Connecticut	88.7
10	Delaware	87.2
23	Florida	84.1
14	Georgia	86.2
22	Hawaii	84.2
35	Idaho	81.8
24	Illinois	84.0
37	Indiana	80.6
6	Iowa	88.4
11	Kansas	86.9
12	Kentucky	86.7
27	Louisiana	83.2
7	Maine	88.2
26	Maryland	83.7
3	Massachusetts	89.7
19	Michigan	84.5
19	Minnesota	84.5
32	Mississippi	82.7
8	Missouri	87.7
33	Montana	82.6
27	Nebraska	83.2
49	Nevada	75.7
2	New Hampshire	90.6
41	New Jersey	79.8
50	New Mexico	69.0
38	New York	80.5
21	North Carolina	84.4
15	North Dakota	85.8
9	Ohio	87.3
47	Oklahoma	77.4
36	Oregon	81.5
17	Pennsylvania	85.2
1	Rhode Island	91.4
45	South Carolina	79.2
46	South Dakota	78.3
31	Tennessee	82.8
40	Texas	80.3
44	Utah	79.3
4	Vermont	89.3
18	Virginia	85.1
27	Washington	83.2
13	West Virginia	86.3
25	Wisconsin	83.8
30	Wyoming	82.9

RANK ORDER

RANK	STATE	PERCENT
1	Rhode Island	91.4
2	New Hampshire	90.6
3	Massachusetts	89.7
4	Vermont	89.3
5	Connecticut	88.7
6	Iowa	88.4
7	Maine	88.2
8	Missouri	87.7
9	Ohio	87.3
10	Delaware	87.2
11	Kansas	86.9
12	Kentucky	86.7
13	West Virginia	86.3
14	Georgia	86.2
15	North Dakota	85.8
16	California	85.4
17	Pennsylvania	85.2
18	Virginia	85.1
19	Michigan	84.5
19	Minnesota	84.5
21	North Carolina	84.4
22	Hawaii	84.2
23	Florida	84.1
24	Illinois	84.0
25	Wisconsin	83.8
26	Maryland	83.7
27	Louisiana	83.2
27	Nebraska	83.2
27	Washington	83.2
30	Wyoming	82.9
31	Tennessee	82.8
32	Mississippi	82.7
33	Montana	82.6
34	Alabama	82.4
35	Idaho	81.8
36	Oregon	81.5
37	Indiana	80.6
38	Alaska	80.5
38	New York	80.5
40	Texas	80.3
41	Arkansas	79.8
41	Colorado	79.8
41	New Jersey	79.8
44	Utah	79.3
45	South Carolina	79.2
46	South Dakota	78.3
47	Oklahoma	77.4
48	Arizona	76.7
49	Nevada	75.7
50	New Mexico	69.0
	District of Columbia	74.4

Source: U.S. Department of Health and Human Services, National Center for Health Statistics
"National Vital Statistics Reports" (Vol. 51, No. 2, December 18, 2002)
*Final data by state of residence.

Percent of White Mothers Beginning Prenatal Care in First Trimester in 2001

National Percent = 85.2% of White Mothers*

ALPHA ORDER

RANK	STATE	PERCENT
21	Alabama	87.4
34	Alaska	84.2
48	Arizona	77.4
39	Arkansas	82.4
30	California	85.4
46	Colorado	80.2
5	Connecticut	89.7
10	Delaware	88.9
25	Florida	87.0
10	Georgia	88.9
13	Hawaii	88.5
42	Idaho	82.0
27	Illinois	86.5
41	Indiana	82.1
10	Iowa	88.9
19	Kansas	87.6
20	Kentucky	87.5
4	Louisiana	90.4
15	Maine	88.3
18	Maryland	87.7
2	Massachusetts	91.3
16	Michigan	87.8
24	Minnesota	87.1
6	Mississippi	89.3
8	Missouri	89.2
31	Montana	85.3
32	Nebraska	84.5
49	Nevada	76.3
3	New Hampshire	91.0
38	New Jersey	83.3
50	New Mexico	70.3
35	New York	83.9
23	North Carolina	87.3
14	North Dakota	88.4
9	Ohio	89.1
47	Oklahoma	79.5
43	Oregon	81.8
21	Pennsylvania	87.4
1	Rhode Island	92.4
33	South Carolina	84.3
40	South Dakota	82.2
29	Tennessee	85.7
44	Texas	80.5
45	Utah	80.3
6	Vermont	89.3
16	Virginia	87.8
36	Washington	83.8
26	West Virginia	86.8
28	Wisconsin	86.2
37	Wyoming	83.4

RANK ORDER

RANK	STATE	PERCENT
1	Rhode Island	92.4
2	Massachusetts	91.3
3	New Hampshire	91.0
4	Louisiana	90.4
5	Connecticut	89.7
6	Mississippi	89.3
6	Vermont	89.3
8	Missouri	89.2
9	Ohio	89.1
10	Delaware	88.9
10	Georgia	88.9
10	Iowa	88.9
13	Hawaii	88.5
14	North Dakota	88.4
15	Maine	88.3
16	Michigan	87.8
16	Virginia	87.8
18	Maryland	87.7
19	Kansas	87.6
20	Kentucky	87.5
21	Alabama	87.4
21	Pennsylvania	87.4
23	North Carolina	87.3
24	Minnesota	87.1
25	Florida	87.0
26	West Virginia	86.8
27	Illinois	86.5
28	Wisconsin	86.2
29	Tennessee	85.7
30	California	85.4
31	Montana	85.3
32	Nebraska	84.5
33	South Carolina	84.3
34	Alaska	84.2
35	New York	83.9
36	Washington	83.8
37	Wyoming	83.4
38	New Jersey	83.3
39	Arkansas	82.4
40	South Dakota	82.2
41	Indiana	82.1
42	Idaho	82.0
43	Oregon	81.8
44	Texas	80.5
45	Utah	80.3
46	Colorado	80.2
47	Oklahoma	79.5
48	Arizona	77.4
49	Nevada	76.3
50	New Mexico	70.3
	District of Columbia	84.2

Source: U.S. Department of Health and Human Services, National Center for Health Statistics
"National Vital Statistics Reports" (Vol. 51, No. 2, December 18, 2002)
*Final data by state of residence.

Percent of Black Mothers Beginning Prenatal Care in First Trimester in 2001

National Percent = 74.5% of Black Mothers*

ALPHA ORDER			RANK ORDER		
RANK	STATE	PERCENT	RANK	STATE	PERCENT
36	Alabama	71.7	1	Hawaii	92.0
6	Alaska	82.3	2	Rhode Island	84.5
28	Arizona	75.8	3	Wyoming	83.1
38	Arkansas	69.9	4	Montana	82.9
5	California	82.5	5	California	82.5
34	Colorado	72.7	6	Alaska	82.3
7	Connecticut	81.9	7	Connecticut	81.9
8	Delaware	81.5	8	Delaware	81.5
29	Florida	75.1	9	Idaho	81.0
10	Georgia	80.6	10	Georgia	80.6
1	Hawaii	92.0	11	Maine	79.7
9	Idaho	81.0	12	Kansas	79.5
32	Illinois	72.9	12	Massachusetts	79.5
43	Indiana	68.9	12	New Hampshire	79.5
16	Iowa	79.0	15	Kentucky	79.3
12	Kansas	79.5	16	Iowa	79.0
15	Kentucky	79.3	17	Missouri	78.7
31	Louisiana	73.4	18	North Dakota	78.4
11	Maine	79.7	19	Vermont	77.4
24	Maryland	76.5	20	Ohio	77.2
12	Massachusetts	79.5	21	Texas	77.0
41	Michigan	69.3	21	Washington	77.0
46	Minnesota	66.5	23	Oregon	76.6
30	Mississippi	74.9	24	Maryland	76.5
17	Missouri	78.7	24	Virginia	76.5
4	Montana	82.9	26	West Virginia	76.2
44	Nebraska	68.0	27	North Carolina	75.9
45	Nevada	67.6	28	Arizona	75.8
12	New Hampshire	79.5	29	Florida	75.1
48	New Jersey	63.4	30	Mississippi	74.9
47	New Mexico	65.8	31	Louisiana	73.4
37	New York	70.3	32	Illinois	72.9
27	North Carolina	75.9	32	Pennsylvania	72.9
18	North Dakota	78.4	34	Colorado	72.7
20	Ohio	77.2	35	Tennessee	72.2
42	Oklahoma	69.2	36	Alabama	71.7
23	Oregon	76.6	37	New York	70.3
32	Pennsylvania	72.9	38	Arkansas	69.9
2	Rhode Island	84.5	39	Wisconsin	69.6
40	South Carolina	69.5	40	South Carolina	69.5
50	South Dakota	59.0	41	Michigan	69.3
35	Tennessee	72.2	42	Oklahoma	69.2
21	Texas	77.0	43	Indiana	68.9
49	Utah	61.7	44	Nebraska	68.0
19	Vermont	77.4	45	Nevada	67.6
24	Virginia	76.5	46	Minnesota	66.5
21	Washington	77.0	47	New Mexico	65.8
26	West Virginia	76.2	48	New Jersey	63.4
39	Wisconsin	69.6	49	Utah	61.7
3	Wyoming	83.1	50	South Dakota	59.0
				District of Columbia	68.7

Source: U.S. Department of Health and Human Services, National Center for Health Statistics
"National Vital Statistics Reports" (Vol. 51, No. 2, December 18, 2002)
*Final data by state of residence.

Percent of Hispanic Mothers Beginning Prenatal Care in First Trimester in 2001

National Percent = 75.7% of Hispanic Mothers*

ALPHA ORDER

RANK	STATE	PERCENT
50	Alabama	52.3
5	Alaska	82.2
38	Arizona	66.7
35	Arkansas	67.4
4	California	82.4
42	Colorado	65.1
11	Connecticut	78.5
23	Delaware	73.0
7	Florida	81.7
17	Georgia	76.5
3	Hawaii	83.3
33	Idaho	69.5
16	Illinois	76.8
45	Indiana	63.2
18	Iowa	74.7
28	Kansas	71.0
35	Kentucky	67.4
2	Louisiana	84.0
14	Maine	77.5
24	Maryland	72.6
8	Massachusetts	81.6
26	Michigan	71.2
46	Minnesota	62.8
26	Mississippi	71.2
13	Missouri	78.0
10	Montana	79.8
34	Nebraska	68.3
46	Nevada	62.8
9	New Hampshire	81.2
35	New Jersey	67.4
40	New Mexico	66.3
20	New York	73.2
29	North Carolina	69.9
12	North Dakota	78.1
15	Ohio	77.3
41	Oklahoma	65.4
29	Oregon	69.9
20	Pennsylvania	73.2
1	Rhode Island	87.5
43	South Carolina	63.9
39	South Dakota	66.5
49	Tennessee	57.1
19	Texas	74.2
48	Utah	60.8
6	Vermont	81.8
31	Virginia	69.8
22	Washington	73.1
44	West Virginia	63.4
31	Wisconsin	69.8
25	Wyoming	71.6

RANK ORDER

RANK	STATE	PERCENT
1	Rhode Island	87.5
2	Louisiana	84.0
3	Hawaii	83.3
4	California	82.4
5	Alaska	82.2
6	Vermont	81.8
7	Florida	81.7
8	Massachusetts	81.6
9	New Hampshire	81.2
10	Montana	79.8
11	Connecticut	78.5
12	North Dakota	78.1
13	Missouri	78.0
14	Maine	77.5
15	Ohio	77.3
16	Illinois	76.8
17	Georgia	76.5
18	Iowa	74.7
19	Texas	74.2
20	New York	73.2
20	Pennsylvania	73.2
22	Washington	73.1
23	Delaware	73.0
24	Maryland	72.6
25	Wyoming	71.6
26	Michigan	71.2
26	Mississippi	71.2
28	Kansas	71.0
29	North Carolina	69.9
29	Oregon	69.9
31	Virginia	69.8
31	Wisconsin	69.8
33	Idaho	69.5
34	Nebraska	68.3
35	Arkansas	67.4
35	Kentucky	67.4
35	New Jersey	67.4
38	Arizona	66.7
39	South Dakota	66.5
40	New Mexico	66.3
41	Oklahoma	65.4
42	Colorado	65.1
43	South Carolina	63.9
44	West Virginia	63.4
45	Indiana	63.2
46	Minnesota	62.8
46	Nevada	62.8
48	Utah	60.8
49	Tennessee	57.1
50	Alabama	52.3

| | District of Columbia | 70.9 |

Source: U.S. Department of Health and Human Services, National Center for Health Statistics
"National Vital Statistics Reports" (Vol. 51, No. 2, December 18, 2002)
*Final data by state of residence. Persons of Hispanic origin may be of any race.

Percent of Mothers Receiving Late or No Prenatal Care in 2001

National Percent = 3.7% of Mothers*

ALPHA ORDER

RANK	STATE	PERCENT
16	Alabama	3.9
11	Alaska	4.5
3	Arizona	6.3
10	Arkansas	4.6
37	California	2.9
8	Colorado	4.7
47	Connecticut	1.9
28	Delaware	3.3
25	Florida	3.4
35	Georgia	3.0
17	Hawaii	3.8
18	Idaho	3.7
28	Illinois	3.3
18	Indiana	3.7
43	Iowa	2.3
38	Kansas	2.7
38	Kentucky	2.7
22	Louisiana	3.6
46	Maine	2.0
18	Maryland	3.7
45	Massachusetts	2.1
22	Michigan	3.6
38	Minnesota	2.7
28	Mississippi	3.3
41	Missouri	2.6
32	Montana	3.1
32	Nebraska	3.1
2	Nevada	7.4
49	New Hampshire	1.7
5	New Jersey	5.3
1	New Mexico	7.7
6	New York	5.2
32	North Carolina	3.1
42	North Dakota	2.4
25	Ohio	3.4
4	Oklahoma	5.4
18	Oregon	3.7
28	Pennsylvania	3.3
50	Rhode Island	1.1
12	South Carolina	4.4
13	South Dakota	4.1
13	Tennessee	4.1
7	Texas	4.9
8	Utah	4.7
48	Vermont	1.8
22	Virginia	3.6
35	Washington	3.0
44	West Virginia	2.2
25	Wisconsin	3.4
15	Wyoming	4.0

RANK ORDER

RANK	STATE	PERCENT
1	New Mexico	7.7
2	Nevada	7.4
3	Arizona	6.3
4	Oklahoma	5.4
5	New Jersey	5.3
6	New York	5.2
7	Texas	4.9
8	Colorado	4.7
8	Utah	4.7
10	Arkansas	4.6
11	Alaska	4.5
12	South Carolina	4.4
13	South Dakota	4.1
13	Tennessee	4.1
15	Wyoming	4.0
16	Alabama	3.9
17	Hawaii	3.8
18	Idaho	3.7
18	Indiana	3.7
18	Maryland	3.7
18	Oregon	3.7
22	Louisiana	3.6
22	Michigan	3.6
22	Virginia	3.6
25	Florida	3.4
25	Ohio	3.4
25	Wisconsin	3.4
28	Delaware	3.3
28	Illinois	3.3
28	Mississippi	3.3
28	Pennsylvania	3.3
32	Montana	3.1
32	Nebraska	3.1
32	North Carolina	3.1
35	Georgia	3.0
35	Washington	3.0
37	California	2.9
38	Kansas	2.7
38	Kentucky	2.7
38	Minnesota	2.7
41	Missouri	2.6
42	North Dakota	2.4
43	Iowa	2.3
44	West Virginia	2.2
45	Massachusetts	2.1
46	Maine	2.0
47	Connecticut	1.9
48	Vermont	1.8
49	New Hampshire	1.7
50	Rhode Island	1.1

| | District of Columbia | 7.9 |

Source: U.S. Department of Health and Human Services, National Center for Health Statistics
   "National Vital Statistics Reports" (Vol. 51, No. 2, December 18, 2002)
*Final data by state of residence. "Late" means care begun in third trimester.

Percent of White Mothers Receiving Late or No Prenatal Care in 2001

National Percent = 3.2% of White Mothers*

ALPHA ORDER

RANK	STATE	PERCENT
19	Alabama	2.9
14	Alaska	3.3
3	Arizona	6.2
9	Arkansas	3.9
17	California	3.0
6	Colorado	4.6
45	Connecticut	1.7
22	Delaware	2.7
26	Florida	2.6
34	Georgia	2.4
22	Hawaii	2.7
12	Idaho	3.7
34	Illinois	2.4
14	Indiana	3.3
37	Iowa	2.1
30	Kansas	2.5
30	Kentucky	2.5
45	Louisiana	1.7
41	Maine	2.0
30	Maryland	2.5
45	Massachusetts	1.7
30	Michigan	2.5
41	Minnesota	2.0
43	Mississippi	1.8
37	Missouri	2.1
37	Montana	2.1
22	Nebraska	2.7
1	Nevada	7.3
49	New Hampshire	1.5
9	New Jersey	3.9
2	New Mexico	7.1
8	New York	4.0
34	North Carolina	2.4
48	North Dakota	1.6
26	Ohio	2.6
5	Oklahoma	4.7
13	Oregon	3.6
26	Pennsylvania	2.6
50	Rhode Island	0.9
16	South Carolina	3.2
26	South Dakota	2.6
17	Tennessee	3.0
4	Texas	4.9
7	Utah	4.3
43	Vermont	1.8
20	Virginia	2.8
20	Washington	2.8
37	West Virginia	2.1
22	Wisconsin	2.7
11	Wyoming	3.8

RANK ORDER

RANK	STATE	PERCENT
1	Nevada	7.3
2	New Mexico	7.1
3	Arizona	6.2
4	Texas	4.9
5	Oklahoma	4.7
6	Colorado	4.6
7	Utah	4.3
8	New York	4.0
9	Arkansas	3.9
9	New Jersey	3.9
11	Wyoming	3.8
12	Idaho	3.7
13	Oregon	3.6
14	Alaska	3.3
14	Indiana	3.3
16	South Carolina	3.2
17	California	3.0
17	Tennessee	3.0
19	Alabama	2.9
20	Virginia	2.8
20	Washington	2.8
22	Delaware	2.7
22	Hawaii	2.7
22	Nebraska	2.7
22	Wisconsin	2.7
26	Florida	2.6
26	Ohio	2.6
26	Pennsylvania	2.6
26	South Dakota	2.6
30	Kansas	2.5
30	Kentucky	2.5
30	Maryland	2.5
30	Michigan	2.5
34	Georgia	2.4
34	Illinois	2.4
34	North Carolina	2.4
37	Iowa	2.1
37	Missouri	2.1
37	Montana	2.1
37	West Virginia	2.1
41	Maine	2.0
41	Minnesota	2.0
43	Mississippi	1.8
43	Vermont	1.8
45	Connecticut	1.7
45	Louisiana	1.7
45	Massachusetts	1.7
48	North Dakota	1.6
49	New Hampshire	1.5
50	Rhode Island	0.9
	District of Columbia	3.7

Source: U.S. Department of Health and Human Services, National Center for Health Statistics
     "National Vital Statistics Reports" (Vol. 51, No. 2, December 18, 2002)
*Final data by state of residence. "Late" means care begun in third trimester.

Percent of Black Mothers Receiving Late or No Prenatal Care in 2001

National Percent = 6.5% of Black Mothers*

RANK	STATE	PERCENT
19	Alabama	6.2
NA	Alaska**	NA
22	Arizona	5.9
12	Arkansas	7.4
38	California	3.6
17	Colorado	7.0
39	Connecticut	3.3
28	Delaware	5.3
25	Florida	5.7
35	Georgia	4.2
NA	Hawaii**	NA
NA	Idaho**	NA
12	Illinois	7.4
14	Indiana	7.3
23	Iowa	5.8
30	Kansas	5.2
33	Kentucky	4.8
19	Louisiana	6.2
NA	Maine**	NA
19	Maryland	6.2
28	Massachusetts	5.3
6	Michigan	8.9
16	Minnesota	7.2
32	Mississippi	5.1
25	Missouri	5.7
NA	Montana**	NA
11	Nebraska	7.6
3	Nevada	10.2
NA	New Hampshire**	NA
2	New Jersey	11.6
4	New Mexico	9.4
5	New York	9.0
30	North Carolina	5.2
NA	North Dakota**	NA
9	Ohio	8.0
7	Oklahoma	8.2
37	Oregon	3.8
14	Pennsylvania	7.3
40	Rhode Island	2.8
18	South Carolina	6.8
NA	South Dakota**	NA
10	Tennessee	7.9
25	Texas	5.7
1	Utah	15.0
NA	Vermont**	NA
23	Virginia	5.8
34	Washington	4.7
36	West Virginia	4.1
8	Wisconsin	8.1
NA	Wyoming**	NA

RANK	STATE	PERCENT
1	Utah	15.0
2	New Jersey	11.6
3	Nevada	10.2
4	New Mexico	9.4
5	New York	9.0
6	Michigan	8.9
7	Oklahoma	8.2
8	Wisconsin	8.1
9	Ohio	8.0
10	Tennessee	7.9
11	Nebraska	7.6
12	Arkansas	7.4
12	Illinois	7.4
14	Indiana	7.3
14	Pennsylvania	7.3
16	Minnesota	7.2
17	Colorado	7.0
18	South Carolina	6.8
19	Alabama	6.2
19	Louisiana	6.2
19	Maryland	6.2
22	Arizona	5.9
23	Iowa	5.8
23	Virginia	5.8
25	Florida	5.7
25	Missouri	5.7
25	Texas	5.7
28	Delaware	5.3
28	Massachusetts	5.3
30	Kansas	5.2
30	North Carolina	5.2
32	Mississippi	5.1
33	Kentucky	4.8
34	Washington	4.7
35	Georgia	4.2
36	West Virginia	4.1
37	Oregon	3.8
38	California	3.6
39	Connecticut	3.3
40	Rhode Island	2.8
NA	Alaska**	NA
NA	Hawaii**	NA
NA	Idaho**	NA
NA	Maine**	NA
NA	Montana**	NA
NA	New Hampshire**	NA
NA	North Dakota**	NA
NA	South Dakota**	NA
NA	Vermont**	NA
NA	Wyoming**	NA
	District of Columbia	10.1

Source: U.S. Department of Health and Human Services, National Center for Health Statistics
"National Vital Statistics Reports" (Vol. 51, No. 2, December 18, 2002)
*Final data by state of residence. "Late" means care begun in third trimester.
**Insufficient data.

Percent of Hispanic Mothers Receiving Late or No Prenatal Care in 2001

National Percent = 5.9% of Hispanic Mothers*

ALPHA ORDER

RANK	STATE	PERCENT
1	Alabama	19.4
40	Alaska	3.8
4	Arizona	10.1
10	Arkansas	8.5
42	California	3.6
9	Colorado	8.8
40	Connecticut	3.8
29	Delaware	5.7
36	Florida	4.3
24	Georgia	6.2
43	Hawaii	3.2
18	Idaho	7.1
37	Illinois	4.1
13	Indiana	7.9
35	Iowa	4.7
16	Kansas	7.2
7	Kentucky	9.4
44	Louisiana	3.0
NA	Maine**	NA
28	Maryland	5.8
39	Massachusetts	3.9
31	Michigan	5.5
15	Minnesota	7.3
16	Mississippi	7.2
34	Missouri	4.8
26	Montana	5.9
26	Nebraska	5.9
3	Nevada	12.4
38	New Hampshire	4.0
12	New Jersey	8.0
10	New Mexico	8.5
18	New York	7.1
21	North Carolina	6.7
NA	North Dakota**	NA
22	Ohio	6.3
6	Oklahoma	9.5
24	Oregon	6.2
30	Pennsylvania	5.6
45	Rhode Island	1.4
8	South Carolina	9.1
NA	South Dakota**	NA
2	Tennessee	14.7
20	Texas	6.9
5	Utah	9.6
NA	Vermont**	NA
13	Virginia	7.9
33	Washington	5.3
NA	West Virginia**	NA
22	Wisconsin	6.3
31	Wyoming	5.5

RANK ORDER

RANK	STATE	PERCENT
1	Alabama	19.4
2	Tennessee	14.7
3	Nevada	12.4
4	Arizona	10.1
5	Utah	9.6
6	Oklahoma	9.5
7	Kentucky	9.4
8	South Carolina	9.1
9	Colorado	8.8
10	Arkansas	8.5
10	New Mexico	8.5
12	New Jersey	8.0
13	Indiana	7.9
13	Virginia	7.9
15	Minnesota	7.3
16	Kansas	7.2
16	Mississippi	7.2
18	Idaho	7.1
18	New York	7.1
20	Texas	6.9
21	North Carolina	6.7
22	Ohio	6.3
22	Wisconsin	6.3
24	Georgia	6.2
24	Oregon	6.2
26	Montana	5.9
26	Nebraska	5.9
28	Maryland	5.8
29	Delaware	5.7
30	Pennsylvania	5.6
31	Michigan	5.5
31	Wyoming	5.5
33	Washington	5.3
34	Missouri	4.8
35	Iowa	4.7
36	Florida	4.3
37	Illinois	4.1
38	New Hampshire	4.0
39	Massachusetts	3.9
40	Alaska	3.8
40	Connecticut	3.8
42	California	3.6
43	Hawaii	3.2
44	Louisiana	3.0
45	Rhode Island	1.4
NA	Maine**	NA
NA	North Dakota**	NA
NA	South Dakota**	NA
NA	Vermont**	NA
NA	West Virginia**	NA

District of Columbia 5.9

Source: U.S. Department of Health and Human Services, National Center for Health Statistics
    "National Vital Statistics Reports" (Vol. 51, No. 2, December 18, 2002)
*Final data by state of residence. "Late" means care begun in third trimester.
**Insufficient data.

Reported Legal Abortions in 1999

Reporting States' Total = 861,789 Abortions*

ALPHA ORDER

RANK	STATE	ABORTIONS	% of USA
17	Alabama	13,273	1.5%
NA	Alaska**	NA	NA
24	Arizona	10,765	1.2%
29	Arkansas	5,755	0.7%
NA	California**	NA	NA
33	Colorado	5,017	0.6%
18	Connecticut	12,958	1.5%
31	Delaware	5,161	0.6%
2	Florida	83,971	9.7%
8	Georgia	33,095	3.8%
36	Hawaii	4,404	0.5%
44	Idaho	867	0.1%
4	Illinois	45,924	5.3%
20	Indiana	12,109	1.4%
27	Iowa	6,106	0.7%
19	Kansas	12,395	1.4%
30	Kentucky	5,469	0.6%
21	Louisiana	12,008	1.4%
41	Maine	2,427	0.3%
22	Maryland	11,164	1.3%
11	Massachusetts	26,852	3.1%
12	Michigan	26,207	3.0%
15	Minnesota	14,342	1.7%
37	Mississippi	3,878	0.4%
25	Missouri	8,113	0.9%
39	Montana	2,499	0.3%
35	Nebraska	4,565	0.5%
28	Nevada	5,807	0.7%
NA	New Hampshire**	NA	NA
6	New Jersey	35,126	4.1%
32	New Mexico	5,098	0.6%
1	New York	137,234	15.9%
9	North Carolina	32,081	3.7%
43	North Dakota	1,345	0.2%
5	Ohio	37,041	4.3%
NA	Oklahoma**	NA	NA
16	Oregon	14,145	1.6%
7	Pennsylvania	34,494	4.0%
34	Rhode Island	5,004	0.6%
26	South Carolina	7,687	0.9%
45	South Dakota	740	0.1%
14	Tennessee	16,924	2.0%
3	Texas	80,739	9.4%
38	Utah	3,381	0.4%
42	Vermont	1,748	0.2%
10	Virginia	27,354	3.2%
13	Washington	25,523	3.0%
40	West Virginia	2,498	0.3%
23	Wisconsin	11,013	1.3%
46	Wyoming	110	0.0%

RANK ORDER

RANK	STATE	ABORTIONS	% of USA
1	New York	137,234	15.9%
2	Florida	83,971	9.7%
3	Texas	80,739	9.4%
4	Illinois	45,924	5.3%
5	Ohio	37,041	4.3%
6	New Jersey	35,126	4.1%
7	Pennsylvania	34,494	4.0%
8	Georgia	33,095	3.8%
9	North Carolina	32,081	3.7%
10	Virginia	27,354	3.2%
11	Massachusetts	26,852	3.1%
12	Michigan	26,207	3.0%
13	Washington	25,523	3.0%
14	Tennessee	16,924	2.0%
15	Minnesota	14,342	1.7%
16	Oregon	14,145	1.6%
17	Alabama	13,273	1.5%
18	Connecticut	12,958	1.5%
19	Kansas	12,395	1.4%
20	Indiana	12,109	1.4%
21	Louisiana	12,008	1.4%
22	Maryland	11,164	1.3%
23	Wisconsin	11,013	1.3%
24	Arizona	10,765	1.2%
25	Missouri	8,113	0.9%
26	South Carolina	7,687	0.9%
27	Iowa	6,106	0.7%
28	Nevada	5,807	0.7%
29	Arkansas	5,755	0.7%
30	Kentucky	5,469	0.6%
31	Delaware	5,161	0.6%
32	New Mexico	5,098	0.6%
33	Colorado	5,017	0.6%
34	Rhode Island	5,004	0.6%
35	Nebraska	4,565	0.5%
36	Hawaii	4,404	0.5%
37	Mississippi	3,878	0.4%
38	Utah	3,381	0.4%
39	Montana	2,499	0.3%
40	West Virginia	2,498	0.3%
41	Maine	2,427	0.3%
42	Vermont	1,748	0.2%
43	North Dakota	1,345	0.2%
44	Idaho	867	0.1%
45	South Dakota	740	0.1%
46	Wyoming	110	0.0%
NA	Alaska**	NA	NA
NA	California**	NA	NA
NA	New Hampshire**	NA	NA
NA	Oklahoma**	NA	NA
	District of Columbia	7,373	0.9%

Source: U.S. Department of Health and Human Services, Centers for Disease Control and Prevention
   "Abortion Surveillance-United States, 1999" (Morbidity Mortality Weekly Report, Vol. 51, No. SS-9, 11/29/02)
*By state of occurrence. Total is for reporting states only.
**Not reported.

Reported Legal Abortions per 1,000 Live Births in 1999

Reporting States' Ratio = 256 Abortions per 1,000 Live Births*

ALPHA ORDER

RANK	STATE	RATIO
23	Alabama	214
NA	Alaska**	NA
37	Arizona	133
33	Arkansas	157
NA	California**	NA
42	Colorado	81
10	Connecticut	299
2	Delaware	483
3	Florida	426
14	Georgia	261
15	Hawaii	258
45	Idaho	44
16	Illinois	252
35	Indiana	141
31	Iowa	163
7	Kansas	320
40	Kentucky	101
28	Louisiana	179
29	Maine	178
34	Maryland	155
5	Massachusetts	332
25	Michigan	196
22	Minnesota	217
41	Mississippi	91
39	Missouri	108
19	Montana	232
26	Nebraska	191
24	Nevada	198
NA	New Hampshire**	NA
9	New Jersey	308
27	New Mexico	187
1	New York	537
12	North Carolina	282
30	North Dakota	176
17	Ohio	243
NA	Oklahoma**	NA
8	Oregon	313
18	Pennsylvania	237
4	Rhode Island	405
36	South Carolina	140
44	South Dakota	70
21	Tennessee	218
20	Texas	231
43	Utah	73
13	Vermont	266
11	Virginia	287
6	Washington	321
38	West Virginia	121
32	Wisconsin	161
46	Wyoming	18

RANK ORDER

RANK	STATE	RATIO
1	New York	537
2	Delaware	483
3	Florida	426
4	Rhode Island	405
5	Massachusetts	332
6	Washington	321
7	Kansas	320
8	Oregon	313
9	New Jersey	308
10	Connecticut	299
11	Virginia	287
12	North Carolina	282
13	Vermont	266
14	Georgia	261
15	Hawaii	258
16	Illinois	252
17	Ohio	243
18	Pennsylvania	237
19	Montana	232
20	Texas	231
21	Tennessee	218
22	Minnesota	217
23	Alabama	214
24	Nevada	198
25	Michigan	196
26	Nebraska	191
27	New Mexico	187
28	Louisiana	179
29	Maine	178
30	North Dakota	176
31	Iowa	163
32	Wisconsin	161
33	Arkansas	157
34	Maryland	155
35	Indiana	141
36	South Carolina	140
37	Arizona	133
38	West Virginia	121
39	Missouri	108
40	Kentucky	101
41	Mississippi	91
42	Colorado	81
43	Utah	73
44	South Dakota	70
45	Idaho	44
46	Wyoming	18
NA	Alaska**	NA
NA	California**	NA
NA	New Hampshire**	NA
NA	Oklahoma**	NA

| | District of Columbia | 980 |

Source: U.S. Department of Health and Human Services, Centers for Disease Control and Prevention
    "Abortion Surveillance-United States, 1999" (Morbidity Mortality Weekly Report, Vol. 51, No. SS-9, 11/29/02)
*By state of occurrence. National figure is for reporting states only.
**Not reported.

Reported Legal Abortions per 1,000 Women Ages 15 to 44 in 1999

Reporting States' Rate = 17 Abortions per 1,000 Women Ages 15 to 44*

ALPHA ORDER

RANK	STATE	RATE
19	Alabama	14
NA	Alaska**	NA
29	Arizona	11
29	Arkansas	11
NA	California**	NA
41	Colorado	6
9	Connecticut	19
2	Delaware	30
3	Florida	28
12	Georgia	18
12	Hawaii	18
45	Idaho	3
15	Illinois	17
34	Indiana	9
31	Iowa	10
5	Kansas	22
41	Kentucky	6
27	Louisiana	12
34	Maine	9
34	Maryland	9
9	Massachusetts	19
27	Michigan	12
19	Minnesota	14
41	Mississippi	6
38	Missouri	7
19	Montana	14
25	Nebraska	13
17	Nevada	15
NA	New Hampshire**	NA
6	New Jersey	20
19	New Mexico	14
1	New York	34
9	North Carolina	19
31	North Dakota	10
17	Ohio	15
NA	Oklahoma**	NA
6	Oregon	20
19	Pennsylvania	14
4	Rhode Island	23
34	South Carolina	9
44	South Dakota	5
19	Tennessee	14
12	Texas	18
38	Utah	7
25	Vermont	13
15	Virginia	17
6	Washington	20
38	West Virginia	7
31	Wisconsin	10
46	Wyoming	1

RANK ORDER

RANK	STATE	RATE
1	New York	34
2	Delaware	30
3	Florida	28
4	Rhode Island	23
5	Kansas	22
6	New Jersey	20
6	Oregon	20
6	Washington	20
9	Connecticut	19
9	Massachusetts	19
9	North Carolina	19
12	Georgia	18
12	Hawaii	18
12	Texas	18
15	Illinois	17
15	Virginia	17
17	Nevada	15
17	Ohio	15
19	Alabama	14
19	Minnesota	14
19	Montana	14
19	New Mexico	14
19	Pennsylvania	14
19	Tennessee	14
25	Nebraska	13
25	Vermont	13
27	Louisiana	12
27	Michigan	12
29	Arizona	11
29	Arkansas	11
31	Iowa	10
31	North Dakota	10
31	Wisconsin	10
34	Indiana	9
34	Maine	9
34	Maryland	9
34	South Carolina	9
38	Missouri	7
38	Utah	7
38	West Virginia	7
41	Colorado	6
41	Kentucky	6
41	Mississippi	6
44	South Dakota	5
45	Idaho	3
46	Wyoming	1
NA	Alaska**	NA
NA	California**	NA
NA	New Hampshire**	NA
NA	Oklahoma**	NA
	District of Columbia	59

Source: U.S. Department of Health and Human Services, Centers for Disease Control and Prevention
   "Abortion Surveillance-United States, 1999" (Morbidity Mortality Weekly Report, Vol. 51, No. SS-9, 11/29/02)
*By state of occurrence. National figure is for reporting states only.
**Not reported.

Percent of Legal Abortions Obtained by Out-Of-State Residents in 1999

Reporting States' Percent = 8.8% of Abortions*

ALPHA ORDER

RANK	STATE	PERCENT	RANK	STATE	PERCENT
9	Alabama	17.4	1	Kansas	48.6
NA	Alaska**	NA	2	Delaware	34.8
41	Arizona	1.0	3	North Dakota	34.2
15	Arkansas	13.1	4	Rhode Island	22.0
NA	California**	NA	5	Kentucky	20.2
11	Colorado	15.0	6	Tennessee	18.8
35	Connecticut	3.4	7	South Dakota	18.6
2	Delaware	34.8	8	Nebraska	18.4
NA	Florida**	NA	9	Alabama	17.4
18	Georgia	9.5	10	Vermont	16.8
42	Hawaii	0.5	11	Colorado	15.0
36	Idaho	3.2	12	Montana	14.6
20	Illinois	9.4	13	North Carolina	14.3
34	Indiana	3.6	14	West Virginia	13.3
NA	Iowa**	NA	15	Arkansas	13.1
1	Kansas	48.6	16	Oregon	12.6
5	Kentucky	20.2	17	Nevada	10.4
NA	Louisiana**	NA	18	Georgia	9.5
38	Maine	3.0	18	Missouri	9.5
32	Maryland	4.1	20	Illinois	9.4
25	Massachusetts	6.1	21	Minnesota	8.9
37	Michigan	3.1	22	Ohio	7.8
21	Minnesota	8.9	23	Utah	6.7
29	Mississippi	4.7	24	Virginia	6.3
18	Missouri	9.5	25	Massachusetts	6.1
12	Montana	14.6	26	New Jersey	6.0
8	Nebraska	18.4	27	South Carolina	5.6
17	Nevada	10.4	28	New Mexico	5.0
NA	New Hampshire**	NA	29	Mississippi	4.7
26	New Jersey	6.0	29	Pennsylvania	4.7
28	New Mexico	5.0	31	Washington	4.3
NA	New York**	NA	32	Maryland	4.1
13	North Carolina	14.3	33	Texas	3.7
3	North Dakota	34.2	34	Indiana	3.6
22	Ohio	7.8	35	Connecticut	3.4
NA	Oklahoma**	NA	36	Idaho	3.2
16	Oregon	12.6	37	Michigan	3.1
29	Pennsylvania	4.7	38	Maine	3.0
4	Rhode Island	22.0	39	Wisconsin	2.8
27	South Carolina	5.6	40	Wyoming	1.8
7	South Dakota	18.6	41	Arizona	1.0
6	Tennessee	18.8	42	Hawaii	0.5
33	Texas	3.7	NA	Alaska**	NA
23	Utah	6.7	NA	California**	NA
10	Vermont	16.8	NA	Florida**	NA
24	Virginia	6.3	NA	Iowa**	NA
31	Washington	4.3	NA	Louisiana**	NA
14	West Virginia	13.3	NA	New Hampshire**	NA
39	Wisconsin	2.8	NA	New York**	NA
40	Wyoming	1.8	NA	Oklahoma**	NA

District of Columbia 54.9

Source: U.S. Department of Health and Human Services, Centers for Disease Control and Prevention
"Abortion Surveillance-United States, 1999" (Morbidity Mortality Weekly Report, Vol. 51, No. SS-9, 11/29/02)
By state of occurrence. National figure is for reporting states only.
**Not reported.*

Percent of Reported Legal Abortions Obtained by White Women in 1999

Reporting States' Percent = 54.6% of Abortions*

ALPHA ORDER

RANK ORDER

RANK	STATE	PERCENT		RANK	STATE	PERCENT
28	Alabama	48.5		1	Vermont	96.7
NA	Alaska**	NA		2	Idaho	93.5
NA	Arizona**	NA		3	Maine	90.9
19	Arkansas	59.8		4	West Virginia	87.7
NA	California**	NA		5	North Dakota	87.0
13	Colorado	75.9		6	Montana	86.9
NA	Connecticut**	NA		7	Oregon	84.7
23	Delaware	55.2		8	New Mexico	84.4
NA	Florida**	NA		9	South Dakota	80.9
30	Georgia	42.5		10	Iowa	80.6
36	Hawaii	25.1		11	Utah	79.1
2	Idaho	93.5		12	Rhode Island	78.0
NA	Illinois**	NA		13	Colorado	75.9
21	Indiana	59.1		14	Kansas	72.8
10	Iowa	80.6		15	Kentucky	71.8
14	Kansas	72.8		16	Texas	71.0
15	Kentucky	71.8		17	Wisconsin	69.7
32	Louisiana	41.0		18	Minnesota	67.0
3	Maine	90.9		19	Arkansas	59.8
34	Maryland	34.6		19	Ohio	59.8
NA	Massachusetts**	NA		21	Indiana	59.1
NA	Michigan**	NA		22	Missouri	58.5
18	Minnesota	67.0		23	Delaware	55.2
35	Mississippi	27.3		24	South Carolina	55.1
22	Missouri	58.5		25	Tennessee	54.0
6	Montana	86.9		26	Pennsylvania	53.9
NA	Nebraska**	NA		27	Virginia	49.7
NA	Nevada**	NA		28	Alabama	48.5
NA	New Hampshire**	NA		29	North Carolina	47.7
33	New Jersey	35.1		30	Georgia	42.5
8	New Mexico	84.4		31	New York**	42.2
31	New York**	42.2		32	Louisiana	41.0
29	North Carolina	47.7		33	New Jersey	35.1
5	North Dakota	87.0		34	Maryland	34.6
19	Ohio	59.8		35	Mississippi	27.3
NA	Oklahoma**	NA		36	Hawaii	25.1
7	Oregon	84.7		NA	Alaska**	NA
26	Pennsylvania	53.9		NA	Arizona**	NA
12	Rhode Island	78.0		NA	California**	NA
24	South Carolina	55.1		NA	Connecticut**	NA
9	South Dakota	80.9		NA	Florida**	NA
25	Tennessee	54.0		NA	Illinois**	NA
16	Texas	71.0		NA	Massachusetts**	NA
11	Utah	79.1		NA	Michigan**	NA
1	Vermont	96.7		NA	Nebraska**	NA
27	Virginia	49.7		NA	Nevada**	NA
NA	Washington**	NA		NA	New Hampshire**	NA
4	West Virginia	87.7		NA	Oklahoma**	NA
17	Wisconsin	69.7		NA	Washington**	NA
NA	Wyoming**	NA		NA	Wyoming**	NA
					District of Columbia	8.7

Source: U.S. Department of Health and Human Services, Centers for Disease Control and Prevention
   "Abortion Surveillance-United States, 1999" (Morbidity Mortality Weekly Report, Vol. 51, No. SS-9, 11/29/02)
*By state of occurrence. Includes those of Hispanic ethnicity. National percent is for reporting states only.
**Not reported. New York's number is for New York City only.

Percent of Reported Legal Abortions Obtained by Black Women in 1999

Reporting States' Percent = 36.2% of Abortions*

ALPHA ORDER

RANK	STATE	PERCENT
5	Alabama	49.8
NA	Alaska**	NA
NA	Arizona**	NA
15	Arkansas	36.9
NA	California**	NA
27	Colorado	4.8
NA	Connecticut**	NA
12	Delaware	41.2
NA	Florida**	NA
3	Georgia	54.2
29	Hawaii	3.0
33	Idaho	1.2
NA	Illinois**	NA
17	Indiana	27.4
25	Iowa	6.3
20	Kansas	21.5
19	Kentucky	21.6
4	Louisiana	51.4
35	Maine	1.0
2	Maryland	56.3
NA	Massachusetts**	NA
NA	Michigan**	NA
22	Minnesota	16.9
1	Mississippi	71.0
14	Missouri	37.0
36	Montana	0.4
NA	Nebraska**	NA
NA	Nevada**	NA
NA	New Hampshire**	NA
7	New Jersey	44.4
29	New Mexico	3.0
6	New York**	48.2
11	North Carolina	42.4
32	North Dakota	2.2
16	Ohio	34.2
NA	Oklahoma**	NA
26	Oregon	5.7
9	Pennsylvania	42.6
23	Rhode Island	14.5
9	South Carolina	42.6
28	South Dakota	3.9
8	Tennessee	42.7
21	Texas	20.3
31	Utah	2.7
34	Vermont	1.1
13	Virginia	39.5
NA	Washington**	NA
24	West Virginia	10.5
18	Wisconsin	23.9
NA	Wyoming**	NA

RANK ORDER

RANK	STATE	PERCENT
1	Mississippi	71.0
2	Maryland	56.3
3	Georgia	54.2
4	Louisiana	51.4
5	Alabama	49.8
6	New York**	48.2
7	New Jersey	44.4
8	Tennessee	42.7
9	Pennsylvania	42.6
9	South Carolina	42.6
11	North Carolina	42.4
12	Delaware	41.2
13	Virginia	39.5
14	Missouri	37.0
15	Arkansas	36.9
16	Ohio	34.2
17	Indiana	27.4
18	Wisconsin	23.9
19	Kentucky	21.6
20	Kansas	21.5
21	Texas	20.3
22	Minnesota	16.9
23	Rhode Island	14.5
24	West Virginia	10.5
25	Iowa	6.3
26	Oregon	5.7
27	Colorado	4.8
28	South Dakota	3.9
29	Hawaii	3.0
29	New Mexico	3.0
31	Utah	2.7
32	North Dakota	2.2
33	Idaho	1.2
34	Vermont	1.1
35	Maine	1.0
36	Montana	0.4
NA	Alaska**	NA
NA	Arizona**	NA
NA	California**	NA
NA	Connecticut**	NA
NA	Florida**	NA
NA	Illinois**	NA
NA	Massachusetts**	NA
NA	Michigan**	NA
NA	Nebraska**	NA
NA	Nevada**	NA
NA	New Hampshire**	NA
NA	Oklahoma**	NA
NA	Washington**	NA
NA	Wyoming**	NA

District of Columbia	80.0

Source: U.S. Department of Health and Human Services, Centers for Disease Control and Prevention
"Abortion Surveillance-United States, 1999" (Morbidity Mortality Weekly Report, Vol. 51, No. SS-9, 11/29/02)
*By state of occurrence. National percent is for reporting states only.
**Not reported. New York's number is for New York City only.

Percent of Reported Legal Abortions Obtained by Hispanic Women in 1999

Reporting States' Percent = 16.8%*

ALPHA ORDER				RANK ORDER		
RANK	STATE	PERCENT		RANK	STATE	PERCENT
21	Alabama	1.6		1	New Mexico	46.4
NA	Alaska**	NA		2	Texas	34.1
NA	Arizona**	NA		3	New York**	32.1
19	Arkansas	1.9		4	New Jersey	17.2
NA	California**	NA		5	Utah	13.7
6	Colorado	11.5		6	Colorado	11.5
NA	Connecticut**	NA		7	Idaho	9.5
11	Delaware	5.5		8	Oregon	8.6
NA	Florida**	NA		9	Kansas	6.5
14	Georgia	3.4		10	Wisconsin	5.9
NA	Hawaii**	NA		11	Delaware	5.5
7	Idaho	9.5		12	Minnesota	4.3
NA	Illinois**	NA		13	Pennsylvania	4.1
NA	Indiana**	NA		14	Georgia	3.4
NA	Iowa**	NA		14	South Dakota	3.4
9	Kansas	6.5		16	South Carolina	2.5
25	Kentucky	0.2		17	Ohio	2.2
NA	Louisiana**	NA		18	Missouri	2.0
23	Maine	0.7		19	Arkansas	1.9
NA	Maryland**	NA		20	Tennessee	1.8
NA	Massachusetts**	NA		21	Alabama	1.6
NA	Michigan**	NA		22	Vermont	1.1
12	Minnesota	4.3		23	Maine	0.7
24	Mississippi	0.4		24	Mississippi	0.4
18	Missouri	2.0		25	Kentucky	0.2
NA	Montana**	NA		NA	Alaska**	NA
NA	Nebraska**	NA		NA	Arizona**	NA
NA	Nevada**	NA		NA	California**	NA
NA	New Hampshire**	NA		NA	Connecticut**	NA
4	New Jersey	17.2		NA	Florida**	NA
1	New Mexico	46.4		NA	Hawaii**	NA
3	New York**	32.1		NA	Illinois**	NA
NA	North Carolina**	NA		NA	Indiana**	NA
NA	North Dakota**	NA		NA	Iowa**	NA
17	Ohio	2.2		NA	Louisiana**	NA
NA	Oklahoma**	NA		NA	Maryland**	NA
8	Oregon	8.6		NA	Massachusetts**	NA
13	Pennsylvania	4.1		NA	Michigan**	NA
NA	Rhode Island**	NA		NA	Montana**	NA
16	South Carolina	2.5		NA	Nebraska**	NA
14	South Dakota	3.4		NA	Nevada**	NA
20	Tennessee	1.8		NA	New Hampshire**	NA
2	Texas	34.1		NA	North Carolina**	NA
5	Utah	13.7		NA	North Dakota**	NA
22	Vermont	1.1		NA	Oklahoma**	NA
NA	Virginia**	NA		NA	Rhode Island**	NA
NA	Washington**	NA		NA	Virginia**	NA
NA	West Virginia**	NA		NA	Washington**	NA
10	Wisconsin	5.9		NA	West Virginia**	NA
NA	Wyoming**	NA		NA	Wyoming**	NA
					District of Columbia	7.2

Source: U.S. Department of Health and Human Services, Centers for Disease Control and Prevention
"Abortion Surveillance-United States, 1999" (Morbidity Mortality Weekly Report, Vol. 51, No. SS-9, 11/29/02)
*By state of occurrence. National percent is for reporting states only. Hispanic can be of any race.
**Not reported. New York's number is for New York City only.

Percent of Reported Legal Abortions Obtained by Married Women in 1999

Reporting States' Percent = 18.6% of Abortions*

ALPHA ORDER			RANK ORDER		
RANK	STATE	PERCENT	RANK	STATE	PERCENT
33	Alabama	15.5	1	Utah	27.0
NA	Alaska**	NA	2	Massachusetts	26.1
NA	Arizona**	NA	3	Idaho	25.1
23	Arkansas	17.4	4	Oregon	22.7
NA	California**	NA	5	Iowa	22.2
7	Colorado	21.9	5	Nevada	22.2
NA	Connecticut**	NA	7	Colorado	21.9
30	Delaware	16.2	8	North Carolina	21.1
NA	Florida**	NA	9	Texas	20.9
19	Georgia	18.5	10	Missouri	20.5
13	Hawaii	19.5	11	Kansas	19.9
3	Idaho	25.1	11	Vermont	19.9
32	Illinois	15.9	13	Hawaii	19.5
37	Indiana	14.2	14	Minnesota	19.3
5	Iowa	22.2	15	South Dakota	19.1
11	Kansas	19.9	16	North Dakota	18.7
34	Kentucky	15.1	16	West Virginia	18.7
NA	Louisiana**	NA	16	Wisconsin	18.7
NA	Maine**	NA	19	Georgia	18.5
27	Maryland	16.8	20	Tennessee	18.0
2	Massachusetts	26.1	21	New York	17.9
34	Michigan	15.1	22	New Jersey	17.8
14	Minnesota	19.3	23	Arkansas	17.4
36	Mississippi	14.4	24	South Carolina	17.2
10	Missouri	20.5	24	Virginia	17.2
NA	Montana**	NA	26	Ohio	16.9
NA	Nebraska**	NA	27	Maryland	16.8
5	Nevada	22.2	27	Rhode Island	16.8
NA	New Hampshire**	NA	29	Pennsylvania	16.6
22	New Jersey	17.8	30	Delaware	16.2
30	New Mexico	16.2	30	New Mexico	16.2
21	New York	17.9	32	Illinois	15.9
8	North Carolina	21.1	33	Alabama	15.5
16	North Dakota	18.7	34	Kentucky	15.1
26	Ohio	16.9	34	Michigan	15.1
NA	Oklahoma**	NA	36	Mississippi	14.4
4	Oregon	22.7	37	Indiana	14.2
29	Pennsylvania	16.6	NA	Alaska**	NA
27	Rhode Island	16.8	NA	Arizona**	NA
24	South Carolina	17.2	NA	California**	NA
15	South Dakota	19.1	NA	Connecticut**	NA
20	Tennessee	18.0	NA	Florida**	NA
9	Texas	20.9	NA	Louisiana**	NA
1	Utah	27.0	NA	Maine**	NA
11	Vermont	19.9	NA	Montana**	NA
24	Virginia	17.2	NA	Nebraska**	NA
NA	Washington**	NA	NA	New Hampshire**	NA
16	West Virginia	18.7	NA	Oklahoma**	NA
16	Wisconsin	18.7	NA	Washington**	NA
NA	Wyoming**	NA	NA	Wyoming**	NA
				District of Columbia**	NA

Source: U.S. Department of Health and Human Services, Centers for Disease Control and Prevention
   "Abortion Surveillance-United States, 1999" (Morbidity Mortality Weekly Report, Vol. 51, No. SS-9, 11/29/02)
*By state of occurrence. National percent is for reporting states only.
**Not reported. New York's number is for New York City only.

Percent of Reported Legal Abortions Obtained by Unmarried Women in 1999

Reporting States' Percent = 78.1% of Abortions*

ALPHA ORDER			RANK ORDER		
RANK	STATE	PERCENT	RANK	STATE	PERCENT
2	Alabama	83.9	1	Mississippi	85.4
NA	Alaska**	NA	2	Alabama	83.9
NA	Arizona**	NA	2	Michigan	83.9
16	Arkansas	80.2	4	Delaware	83.8
NA	California**	NA	5	Kentucky	83.4
24	Colorado	77.1	5	Pennsylvania	83.4
NA	Connecticut**	NA	7	South Carolina	82.7
4	Delaware	83.8	8	New Mexico	82.1
NA	Florida**	NA	9	New Jersey	81.8
10	Georgia	81.5	10	Georgia	81.5
16	Hawaii	80.2	11	West Virginia	81.0
28	Idaho	74.7	11	Wisconsin	81.0
22	Illinois	79.1	13	South Dakota	80.9
34	Indiana	71.9	14	North Dakota	80.7
26	Iowa	75.6	14	Tennessee	80.7
18	Kansas	79.9	16	Arkansas	80.2
5	Kentucky	83.4	16	Hawaii	80.2
NA	Louisiana**	NA	18	Kansas	79.9
NA	Maine**	NA	19	Maryland	79.5
19	Maryland	79.5	20	Ohio	79.4
37	Massachusetts	65.7	21	New York	79.3
2	Michigan	83.9	22	Illinois	79.1
31	Minnesota	73.8	23	Missouri	78.1
1	Mississippi	85.4	24	Colorado	77.1
23	Missouri	78.1	25	Texas	75.8
NA	Montana**	NA	26	Iowa	75.6
NA	Nebraska**	NA	27	Oregon	75.4
29	Nevada	74.2	28	Idaho	74.7
NA	New Hampshire**	NA	29	Nevada	74.2
9	New Jersey	81.8	29	North Carolina	74.2
8	New Mexico	82.1	31	Minnesota	73.8
21	New York	79.3	32	Vermont	73.6
29	North Carolina	74.2	33	Utah	72.5
14	North Dakota	80.7	34	Indiana	71.9
20	Ohio	79.4	35	Rhode Island	71.6
NA	Oklahoma**	NA	36	Virginia	71.0
27	Oregon	75.4	37	Massachusetts	65.7
5	Pennsylvania	83.4	NA	Alaska**	NA
35	Rhode Island	71.6	NA	Arizona**	NA
7	South Carolina	82.7	NA	California**	NA
13	South Dakota	80.9	NA	Connecticut**	NA
14	Tennessee	80.7	NA	Florida**	NA
25	Texas	75.8	NA	Louisiana**	NA
33	Utah	72.5	NA	Maine**	NA
32	Vermont	73.6	NA	Montana**	NA
36	Virginia	71.0	NA	Nebraska**	NA
NA	Washington**	NA	NA	New Hampshire**	NA
11	West Virginia	81.0	NA	Oklahoma**	NA
11	Wisconsin	81.0	NA	Washington**	NA
NA	Wyoming**	NA	NA	Wyoming**	NA
				District of Columbia**	NA

Source: U.S. Department of Health and Human Services, Centers for Disease Control and Prevention
   "Abortion Surveillance-United States, 1999" (Morbidity Mortality Weekly Report, Vol. 51, No. SS-9, 11/29/02)
*By state of occurrence. National percent is for reporting states only.
**Not reported. New York's number is for New York City only.

Reported Legal Abortions Obtained by Teenagers in 1999

Reporting States' Total = 148,068 Abortions Obtained by Teenagers*

ALPHA ORDER

RANK	STATE	ABORTIONS	% of USA
16	Alabama	2,740	1.9%
NA	Alaska**	NA	NA
23	Arizona	2,060	1.4%
27	Arkansas	1,190	0.8%
NA	California**	NA	NA
28	Colorado	1,160	0.8%
15	Connecticut	2,762	1.9%
36	Delaware	795	0.5%
NA	Florida**	NA	NA
7	Georgia	6,193	4.2%
33	Hawaii	1,000	0.7%
43	Idaho	231	0.2%
3	Illinois	9,607	6.5%
19	Indiana	2,398	1.6%
26	Iowa	1,310	0.9%
17	Kansas	2,733	1.8%
31	Kentucky	1,065	0.7%
20	Louisiana	2,337	1.6%
39	Maine	583	0.4%
21	Maryland	2,145	1.4%
12	Massachusetts	4,472	3.0%
10	Michigan	4,994	3.4%
18	Minnesota	2,576	1.7%
35	Mississippi	807	0.5%
25	Missouri	1,446	1.0%
37	Montana	646	0.4%
32	Nebraska	1,026	0.7%
29	Nevada	1,078	0.7%
NA	New Hampshire**	NA	NA
6	New Jersey	6,705	4.5%
30	New Mexico	1,068	0.7%
1	New York	24,832	16.8%
8	North Carolina	5,751	3.9%
42	North Dakota	300	0.2%
4	Ohio	7,276	4.9%
NA	Oklahoma**	NA	NA
14	Oregon	3,026	2.0%
5	Pennsylvania	6,715	4.5%
34	Rhode Island	904	0.6%
24	South Carolina	1,598	1.1%
44	South Dakota	184	0.1%
13	Tennessee	3,275	2.2%
2	Texas	13,902	9.4%
37	Utah	646	0.4%
41	Vermont	372	0.3%
11	Virginia	4,749	3.2%
9	Washington	5,369	3.6%
40	West Virginia	510	0.3%
22	Wisconsin	2,094	1.4%
45	Wyoming	28	0.0%

RANK ORDER

RANK	STATE	ABORTIONS	% of USA
1	New York	24,832	16.8%
2	Texas	13,902	9.4%
3	Illinois	9,607	6.5%
4	Ohio	7,276	4.9%
5	Pennsylvania	6,715	4.5%
6	New Jersey	6,705	4.5%
7	Georgia	6,193	4.2%
8	North Carolina	5,751	3.9%
9	Washington	5,369	3.6%
10	Michigan	4,994	3.4%
11	Virginia	4,749	3.2%
12	Massachusetts	4,472	3.0%
13	Tennessee	3,275	2.2%
14	Oregon	3,026	2.0%
15	Connecticut	2,762	1.9%
16	Alabama	2,740	1.9%
17	Kansas	2,733	1.8%
18	Minnesota	2,576	1.7%
19	Indiana	2,398	1.6%
20	Louisiana	2,337	1.6%
21	Maryland	2,145	1.4%
22	Wisconsin	2,094	1.4%
23	Arizona	2,060	1.4%
24	South Carolina	1,598	1.1%
25	Missouri	1,446	1.0%
26	Iowa	1,310	0.9%
27	Arkansas	1,190	0.8%
28	Colorado	1,160	0.8%
29	Nevada	1,078	0.7%
30	New Mexico	1,068	0.7%
31	Kentucky	1,065	0.7%
32	Nebraska	1,026	0.7%
33	Hawaii	1,000	0.7%
34	Rhode Island	904	0.6%
35	Mississippi	807	0.5%
36	Delaware	795	0.5%
37	Montana	646	0.4%
37	Utah	646	0.4%
39	Maine	583	0.4%
40	West Virginia	510	0.3%
41	Vermont	372	0.3%
42	North Dakota	300	0.2%
43	Idaho	231	0.2%
44	South Dakota	184	0.1%
45	Wyoming	28	0.0%
NA	Alaska**	NA	NA
NA	California**	NA	NA
NA	Florida**	NA	NA
NA	New Hampshire**	NA	NA
NA	Oklahoma**	NA	NA
	District of Columbia	1,410	1.0%

Source: U.S. Department of Health and Human Services, Centers for Disease Control and Prevention
"Abortion Surveillance-United States, 1999" (Morbidity Mortality Weekly Report, Vol. 51, No. SS-9, 11/29/02)
*Nineteen years old and younger by state of occurrence. National total is for reporting states only.
**Not reported.

Percent of Reported Legal Abortions Obtained by Teenagers in 1999

Reporting States' Percent = 19.1% of Abortions*

RANK	STATE	PERCENT	% of USA
21	Alabama	20.7	0.0%
NA	Alaska**	NA	0.0%
31	Arizona	19.2	0.0%
21	Arkansas	20.7	0.0%
NA	California**	NA	0.0%
7	Colorado	23.1	0.0%
14	Connecticut	21.3	0.0%
6	Delaware	23.7	0.0%
NA	Florida**	NA	0.0%
36	Georgia	18.7	0.0%
8	Hawaii	22.7	0.0%
1	Idaho	26.6	0.0%
17	Illinois	21.0	0.0%
24	Indiana	19.8	0.0%
12	Iowa	21.5	0.0%
11	Kansas	22.0	0.0%
26	Kentucky	19.5	0.0%
26	Louisiana	19.5	0.0%
5	Maine	24.0	0.0%
31	Maryland	19.2	0.0%
45	Massachusetts	16.7	0.0%
35	Michigan	19.0	0.0%
40	Minnesota	18.0	0.0%
19	Mississippi	20.8	0.0%
41	Missouri	17.9	0.0%
2	Montana	25.9	0.0%
9	Nebraska	22.5	0.0%
37	Nevada	18.6	0.0%
NA	New Hampshire**	NA	0.0%
34	New Jersey	19.1	0.0%
17	New Mexico	21.0	0.0%
38	New York	18.1	0.0%
41	North Carolina	17.9	0.0%
10	North Dakota	22.3	0.0%
25	Ohio	19.7	0.0%
NA	Oklahoma**	NA	0.0%
13	Oregon	21.4	0.0%
26	Pennsylvania	19.5	0.0%
38	Rhode Island	18.1	0.0%
19	South Carolina	20.8	0.0%
4	South Dakota	24.9	0.0%
30	Tennessee	19.3	0.0%
44	Texas	17.3	0.0%
31	Utah	19.2	0.0%
14	Vermont	21.3	0.0%
43	Virginia	17.4	0.0%
16	Washington	21.1	0.0%
23	West Virginia	20.4	0.0%
26	Wisconsin	19.5	0.0%
3	Wyoming	25.4	0.0%

RANK	STATE	PERCENT	% of USA
1	Idaho	26.6	0.0%
2	Montana	25.9	0.0%
3	Wyoming	25.4	0.0%
4	South Dakota	24.9	0.0%
5	Maine	24.0	0.0%
6	Delaware	23.7	0.0%
7	Colorado	23.1	0.0%
8	Hawaii	22.7	0.0%
9	Nebraska	22.5	0.0%
10	North Dakota	22.3	0.0%
11	Kansas	22.0	0.0%
12	Iowa	21.5	0.0%
13	Oregon	21.4	0.0%
14	Connecticut	21.3	0.0%
14	Vermont	21.3	0.0%
16	Washington	21.1	0.0%
17	Illinois	21.0	0.0%
17	New Mexico	21.0	0.0%
19	Mississippi	20.8	0.0%
19	South Carolina	20.8	0.0%
21	Alabama	20.7	0.0%
21	Arkansas	20.7	0.0%
23	West Virginia	20.4	0.0%
24	Indiana	19.8	0.0%
25	Ohio	19.7	0.0%
26	Kentucky	19.5	0.0%
26	Louisiana	19.5	0.0%
26	Pennsylvania	19.5	0.0%
26	Wisconsin	19.5	0.0%
30	Tennessee	19.3	0.0%
31	Arizona	19.2	0.0%
31	Maryland	19.2	0.0%
31	Utah	19.2	0.0%
34	New Jersey	19.1	0.0%
35	Michigan	19.0	0.0%
36	Georgia	18.7	0.0%
37	Nevada	18.6	0.0%
38	New York	18.1	0.0%
38	Rhode Island	18.1	0.0%
40	Minnesota	18.0	0.0%
41	Missouri	17.9	0.0%
41	North Carolina	17.9	0.0%
43	Virginia	17.4	0.0%
44	Texas	17.3	0.0%
45	Massachusetts	16.7	0.0%
NA	Alaska**	NA	0.0%
NA	California**	NA	0.0%
NA	Florida**	NA	0.0%
NA	New Hampshire**	NA	0.0%
NA	Oklahoma**	NA	0.0%
	District of Columbia	19.1	0.0%

Source: U.S. Department of Health and Human Services, Centers for Disease Control and Prevention
   "Abortion Surveillance-United States, 1999" (Morbidity Mortality Weekly Report, Vol. 51, No. SS-9, 11/29/02)
*Nineteen years old and younger by state of occurrence. National total is for reporting states only.
**Not reported.

Reported Legal Abortions Obtained by Teenagers 17 Years and Younger in 1999

Reporting States' Total = 53,436 Abortions*

ALPHA ORDER

RANK	STATE	ABORTIONS	% of USA
16	Alabama	1,045	2.0%
NA	Alaska**	NA	NA
21	Arizona	792	1.5%
29	Arkansas	449	0.8%
NA	California**	NA	NA
24	Colorado	516	1.0%
12	Connecticut	1,269	2.4%
32	Delaware	316	0.6%
NA	Florida**	NA	NA
5	Georgia	2,527	4.7%
30	Hawaii	430	0.8%
41	Idaho	74	0.1%
NA	Illinois**	NA	NA
20	Indiana	798	1.5%
26	Iowa	488	0.9%
15	Kansas	1,085	2.0%
NA	Kentucky**	NA	NA
19	Louisiana	849	1.6%
36	Maine	236	0.4%
18	Maryland	909	1.7%
11	Massachusetts	1,595	3.0%
9	Michigan	1,849	3.5%
17	Minnesota	919	1.7%
33	Mississippi	289	0.5%
25	Missouri	499	0.9%
35	Montana	278	0.5%
31	Nebraska	380	0.7%
27	Nevada	481	0.9%
NA	New Hampshire**	NA	NA
4	New Jersey	2,742	5.1%
28	New Mexico	462	0.9%
1	New York	10,603	19.8%
8	North Carolina	2,120	4.0%
40	North Dakota	101	0.2%
3	Ohio	2,801	5.2%
NA	Oklahoma**	NA	NA
13	Oregon	1,194	2.2%
6	Pennsylvania	2,412	4.5%
34	Rhode Island	283	0.5%
23	South Carolina	682	1.3%
42	South Dakota	61	0.1%
14	Tennessee	1,177	2.2%
2	Texas	4,973	9.3%
37	Utah	226	0.4%
39	Vermont	155	0.3%
10	Virginia	1,679	3.1%
7	Washington	2,146	4.0%
38	West Virginia	200	0.4%
22	Wisconsin	755	1.4%
43	Wyoming	11	0.0%

RANK ORDER

RANK	STATE	ABORTIONS	% of USA
1	New York	10,603	19.8%
2	Texas	4,973	9.3%
3	Ohio	2,801	5.2%
4	New Jersey	2,742	5.1%
5	Georgia	2,527	4.7%
6	Pennsylvania	2,412	4.5%
7	Washington	2,146	4.0%
8	North Carolina	2,120	4.0%
9	Michigan	1,849	3.5%
10	Virginia	1,679	3.1%
11	Massachusetts	1,595	3.0%
12	Connecticut	1,269	2.4%
13	Oregon	1,194	2.2%
14	Tennessee	1,177	2.2%
15	Kansas	1,085	2.0%
16	Alabama	1,045	2.0%
17	Minnesota	919	1.7%
18	Maryland	909	1.7%
19	Louisiana	849	1.6%
20	Indiana	798	1.5%
21	Arizona	792	1.5%
22	Wisconsin	755	1.4%
23	South Carolina	682	1.3%
24	Colorado	516	1.0%
25	Missouri	499	0.9%
26	Iowa	488	0.9%
27	Nevada	481	0.9%
28	New Mexico	462	0.9%
29	Arkansas	449	0.8%
30	Hawaii	430	0.8%
31	Nebraska	380	0.7%
32	Delaware	316	0.6%
33	Mississippi	289	0.5%
34	Rhode Island	283	0.5%
35	Montana	278	0.5%
36	Maine	236	0.4%
37	Utah	226	0.4%
38	West Virginia	200	0.4%
39	Vermont	155	0.3%
40	North Dakota	101	0.2%
41	Idaho	74	0.1%
42	South Dakota	61	0.1%
43	Wyoming	11	0.0%
NA	Alaska**	NA	NA
NA	California**	NA	NA
NA	Florida**	NA	NA
NA	Illinois**	NA	NA
NA	Kentucky**	NA	NA
NA	New Hampshire**	NA	NA
NA	Oklahoma**	NA	NA
	District of Columbia	580	1.1%

Source: U.S. Department of Health and Human Services, Centers for Disease Control and Prevention
   "Abortion Surveillance-United States, 1999" (Morbidity Mortality Weekly Report, Vol. 51, No. SS-9, 11/29/02)
*By state of occurrence. National total is for reporting states only.
**Not reported.

Percent of Reported Legal Abortions Obtained
By Teenagers 17 Years and Younger in 1999
Reporting States' Percent = 7.4% of Abortions*

ALPHA ORDER

RANK	STATE	PERCENT
21	Alabama	7.9
NA	Alaska**	NA
29	Arizona	7.4
22	Arkansas	7.8
NA	California**	NA
2	Colorado	10.3
4	Connecticut	9.8
7	Delaware	9.4
NA	Florida**	NA
25	Georgia	7.6
4	Hawaii	9.8
12	Idaho	8.5
NA	Illinois**	NA
36	Indiana	6.6
19	Iowa	8.0
11	Kansas	8.8
NA	Kentucky**	NA
30	Louisiana	7.1
6	Maine	9.7
18	Maryland	8.1
42	Massachusetts	5.9
30	Michigan	7.1
38	Minnesota	6.4
27	Mississippi	7.5
39	Missouri	6.2
1	Montana	11.1
15	Nebraska	8.3
15	Nevada	8.3
NA	New Hampshire**	NA
22	New Jersey	7.8
8	New Mexico	9.1
24	New York	7.7
36	North Carolina	6.6
27	North Dakota	7.5
25	Ohio	7.6
NA	Oklahoma**	NA
13	Oregon	8.4
33	Pennsylvania	7.0
43	Rhode Island	5.7
9	South Carolina	8.9
17	South Dakota	8.2
33	Tennessee	7.0
39	Texas	6.2
35	Utah	6.7
9	Vermont	8.9
41	Virginia	6.1
13	Washington	8.4
19	West Virginia	8.0
30	Wisconsin	7.1
3	Wyoming	10.0

RANK ORDER

RANK	STATE	PERCENT
1	Montana	11.1
2	Colorado	10.3
3	Wyoming	10.0
4	Connecticut	9.8
4	Hawaii	9.8
6	Maine	9.7
7	Delaware	9.4
8	New Mexico	9.1
9	South Carolina	8.9
9	Vermont	8.9
11	Kansas	8.8
12	Idaho	8.5
13	Oregon	8.4
13	Washington	8.4
15	Nebraska	8.3
15	Nevada	8.3
17	South Dakota	8.2
18	Maryland	8.1
19	Iowa	8.0
19	West Virginia	8.0
21	Alabama	7.9
22	Arkansas	7.8
22	New Jersey	7.8
24	New York	7.7
25	Georgia	7.6
25	Ohio	7.6
27	Mississippi	7.5
27	North Dakota	7.5
29	Arizona	7.4
30	Louisiana	7.1
30	Michigan	7.1
30	Wisconsin	7.1
33	Pennsylvania	7.0
33	Tennessee	7.0
35	Utah	6.7
36	Indiana	6.6
36	North Carolina	6.6
38	Minnesota	6.4
39	Missouri	6.2
39	Texas	6.2
41	Virginia	6.1
42	Massachusetts	5.9
43	Rhode Island	5.7
NA	Alaska**	NA
NA	California**	NA
NA	Florida**	NA
NA	Illinois**	NA
NA	Kentucky**	NA
NA	New Hampshire**	NA
NA	Oklahoma**	NA

District of Columbia 7.9

Source: Morgan Quitno Press using data from US Dept of Health & Human Serv's, Centers for Disease Control-Prevention
"Abortion Surveillance-United States, 1999" (Morbidity Mortality Weekly Report, Vol. 51, No. SS-9, 11/29/02)
*By state of occurrence. National percent is for reporting states only.
**Not reported.

Percent of Teenage Abortions Obtained
By Teenagers 17 Years and Younger in 1999
Reporting States' Percent = 36.1% of Teenage Abortions*

ALPHA ORDER

RANK ORDER

RANK	STATE	PERCENT
22	Alabama	38.1
NA	Alaska**	NA
20	Arizona	38.4
23	Arkansas	37.8
NA	California**	NA
3	Colorado	44.4
1	Connecticut	46.0
15	Delaware	39.8
NA	Florida**	NA
12	Georgia	40.8
5	Hawaii	43.0
42	Idaho	32.1
NA	Illinois**	NA
40	Indiana	33.3
24	Iowa	37.3
16	Kansas	39.7
NA	Kentucky**	NA
28	Louisiana	36.3
13	Maine	40.4
9	Maryland	42.3
35	Massachusetts	35.6
25	Michigan	37.1
32	Minnesota	35.7
32	Mississippi	35.7
38	Missouri	34.5
5	Montana	43.0
26	Nebraska	36.9
2	Nevada	44.6
NA	New Hampshire**	NA
11	New Jersey	40.9
4	New Mexico	43.3
7	New York	42.7
26	North Carolina	36.9
39	North Dakota	33.6
20	Ohio	38.4
NA	Oklahoma**	NA
17	Oregon	39.4
30	Pennsylvania	36.0
43	Rhode Island	31.4
7	South Carolina	42.7
41	South Dakota	33.2
30	Tennessee	36.0
32	Texas	35.7
37	Utah	35.0
10	Vermont	41.7
36	Virginia	35.2
14	Washington	40.0
18	West Virginia	39.2
29	Wisconsin	36.1
18	Wyoming	39.2

RANK	STATE	PERCENT
1	Connecticut	46.0
2	Nevada	44.6
3	Colorado	44.4
4	New Mexico	43.3
5	Hawaii	43.0
5	Montana	43.0
7	New York	42.7
7	South Carolina	42.7
9	Maryland	42.3
10	Vermont	41.7
11	New Jersey	40.9
12	Georgia	40.8
13	Maine	40.4
14	Washington	40.0
15	Delaware	39.8
16	Kansas	39.7
17	Oregon	39.4
18	West Virginia	39.2
18	Wyoming	39.2
20	Arizona	38.4
20	Ohio	38.4
22	Alabama	38.1
23	Arkansas	37.8
24	Iowa	37.3
25	Michigan	37.1
26	Nebraska	36.9
26	North Carolina	36.9
28	Louisiana	36.3
29	Wisconsin	36.1
30	Pennsylvania	36.0
30	Tennessee	36.0
32	Minnesota	35.7
32	Mississippi	35.7
32	Texas	35.7
35	Massachusetts	35.6
36	Virginia	35.2
37	Utah	35.0
38	Missouri	34.5
39	North Dakota	33.6
40	Indiana	33.3
41	South Dakota	33.2
42	Idaho	32.1
43	Rhode Island	31.4
NA	Alaska**	NA
NA	California**	NA
NA	Florida**	NA
NA	Illinois**	NA
NA	Kentucky**	NA
NA	New Hampshire**	NA
NA	Oklahoma**	NA

District of Columbia 41.1

Source: Morgan Quitno Press using data from US Dept of Health & Human Serv's, Centers for Disease Control-Prevention
    "Abortion Surveillance-United States, 1999" (Morbidity Mortality Weekly Report, Vol. 51, No. SS-9, 11/29/02)
*By state of occurrence. National percent is for reporting states only.
**Not reported.

Reported Legal Abortions Performed at 12 Weeks or Less of Gestation in 1999

Reporting States' Total = 577,961 Abortions*

<u>ALPHA ORDER</u>

RANK	STATE	ABORTIONS	% of USA
14	Alabama	11,745	2.0%
NA	Alaska**	NA	NA
21	Arizona	8,942	1.5%
26	Arkansas	4,822	0.8%
NA	California**	NA	NA
30	Colorado	4,258	0.7%
13	Connecticut	11,757	2.0%
34	Delaware	2,989	0.5%
NA	Florida**	NA	NA
7	Georgia	27,389	4.7%
31	Hawaii	3,758	0.7%
40	Idaho	830	0.1%
NA	Illinois**	NA	NA
15	Indiana	11,623	2.0%
24	Iowa	5,539	1.0%
18	Kansas	10,419	1.8%
28	Kentucky	4,471	0.8%
19	Louisiana	9,743	1.7%
35	Maine	2,397	0.4%
17	Maryland	10,592	1.8%
NA	Massachusetts**	NA	NA
9	Michigan	22,755	3.9%
12	Minnesota	12,920	2.2%
32	Mississippi	3,438	0.6%
23	Missouri	7,447	1.3%
37	Montana	2,050	0.4%
NA	Nebraska**	NA	NA
25	Nevada	5,091	0.9%
NA	New Hampshire**	NA	NA
5	New Jersey	28,170	4.9%
29	New Mexico	4,401	0.8%
1	New York***	88,263	15.3%
6	North Carolina	27,992	4.8%
39	North Dakota	1,204	0.2%
3	Ohio	31,433	5.4%
NA	Oklahoma**	NA	NA
16	Oregon	11,579	2.0%
4	Pennsylvania	29,904	5.2%
27	Rhode Island	4,536	0.8%
22	South Carolina	7,590	1.3%
41	South Dakota	718	0.1%
11	Tennessee	16,172	2.8%
2	Texas	70,448	12.2%
33	Utah	3,109	0.5%
38	Vermont	1,677	0.3%
8	Virginia	26,274	4.5%
10	Washington	21,771	3.8%
36	West Virginia	2,174	0.4%
20	Wisconsin	9,142	1.6%
42	Wyoming	106	0.0%

<u>RANK ORDER</u>

RANK	STATE	ABORTIONS	% of USA
1	New York***	88,263	15.3%
2	Texas	70,448	12.2%
3	Ohio	31,433	5.4%
4	Pennsylvania	29,904	5.2%
5	New Jersey	28,170	4.9%
6	North Carolina	27,992	4.8%
7	Georgia	27,389	4.7%
8	Virginia	26,274	4.5%
9	Michigan	22,755	3.9%
10	Washington	21,771	3.8%
11	Tennessee	16,172	2.8%
12	Minnesota	12,920	2.2%
13	Connecticut	11,757	2.0%
14	Alabama	11,745	2.0%
15	Indiana	11,623	2.0%
16	Oregon	11,579	2.0%
17	Maryland	10,592	1.8%
18	Kansas	10,419	1.8%
19	Louisiana	9,743	1.7%
20	Wisconsin	9,142	1.6%
21	Arizona	8,942	1.5%
22	South Carolina	7,590	1.3%
23	Missouri	7,447	1.3%
24	Iowa	5,539	1.0%
25	Nevada	5,091	0.9%
26	Arkansas	4,822	0.8%
27	Rhode Island	4,536	0.8%
28	Kentucky	4,471	0.8%
29	New Mexico	4,401	0.8%
30	Colorado	4,258	0.7%
31	Hawaii	3,758	0.7%
32	Mississippi	3,438	0.6%
33	Utah	3,109	0.5%
34	Delaware	2,989	0.5%
35	Maine	2,397	0.4%
36	West Virginia	2,174	0.4%
37	Montana	2,050	0.4%
38	Vermont	1,677	0.3%
39	North Dakota	1,204	0.2%
40	Idaho	830	0.1%
41	South Dakota	718	0.1%
42	Wyoming	106	0.0%
NA	Alaska**	NA	NA
NA	California**	NA	NA
NA	Florida**	NA	NA
NA	Illinois**	NA	NA
NA	Massachusetts**	NA	NA
NA	Nebraska**	NA	NA
NA	New Hampshire**	NA	NA
NA	Oklahoma**	NA	NA
	District of Columbia	6,323	1.1%

Source: Morgan Quitno Press using data from US Dept of Health & Human Serv's, Centers for Disease Control-Prevention "Abortion Surveillance-United States, 1999" (Morbidity Mortality Weekly Report, Vol. 51, No. SS-9, 11/29/02)
*By state of occurrence. National total is for reporting states only.
**Not reported.
***New York figure is for New York City only.

Percent of Reported Legal Abortions Performed
At 12 Weeks or less of Gestation in 1999
Reporting States' Percent = 87.2% of Abortions*

ALPHA ORDER

RANK	STATE	PERCENT
20	Alabama	88.4
NA	Alaska**	NA
36	Arizona	83.1
35	Arkansas	83.8
NA	California**	NA
32	Colorado	84.9
13	Connecticut	90.8
18	Delaware	88.9
NA	Florida**	NA
37	Georgia	82.7
30	Hawaii	85.3
8	Idaho	95.7
NA	Illinois**	NA
5	Indiana	96.0
14	Iowa	90.7
34	Kansas	84.0
40	Kentucky	81.7
41	Louisiana	81.1
1	Maine	98.7
10	Maryland	94.9
NA	Massachusetts**	NA
25	Michigan	86.8
16	Minnesota	90.0
19	Mississippi	88.6
12	Missouri	91.8
38	Montana	82.0
NA	Nebraska**	NA
21	Nevada	87.7
NA	New Hampshire**	NA
42	New Jersey	80.2
27	New Mexico	86.3
28	New York***	86.2
22	North Carolina	87.3
17	North Dakota	89.4
32	Ohio	84.9
NA	Oklahoma**	NA
39	Oregon	81.8
26	Pennsylvania	86.7
14	Rhode Island	90.7
1	South Carolina	98.7
3	South Dakota	97.0
9	Tennessee	95.6
22	Texas	87.3
11	Utah	92.0
5	Vermont	96.0
5	Virginia	96.0
30	Washington	85.3
24	West Virginia	87.0
29	Wisconsin	85.4
4	Wyoming	96.4

RANK ORDER

RANK	STATE	PERCENT
1	Maine	98.7
1	South Carolina	98.7
3	South Dakota	97.0
4	Wyoming	96.4
5	Indiana	96.0
5	Vermont	96.0
5	Virginia	96.0
8	Idaho	95.7
9	Tennessee	95.6
10	Maryland	94.9
11	Utah	92.0
12	Missouri	91.8
13	Connecticut	90.8
14	Iowa	90.7
14	Rhode Island	90.7
16	Minnesota	90.0
17	North Dakota	89.4
18	Delaware	88.9
19	Mississippi	88.6
20	Alabama	88.4
21	Nevada	87.7
22	North Carolina	87.3
22	Texas	87.3
24	West Virginia	87.0
25	Michigan	86.8
26	Pennsylvania	86.7
27	New Mexico	86.3
28	New York***	86.2
29	Wisconsin	85.4
30	Hawaii	85.3
30	Washington	85.3
32	Colorado	84.9
32	Ohio	84.9
34	Kansas	84.0
35	Arkansas	83.8
36	Arizona	83.1
37	Georgia	82.7
38	Montana	82.0
39	Oregon	81.8
40	Kentucky	81.7
41	Louisiana	81.1
42	New Jersey	80.2
NA	Alaska**	NA
NA	California**	NA
NA	Florida**	NA
NA	Illinois**	NA
NA	Massachusetts**	NA
NA	Nebraska**	NA
NA	New Hampshire**	NA
NA	Oklahoma**	NA

District of Columbia 85.7

Source: Morgan Quitno Press using data from US Dept of Health & Human Serv's, Centers for Disease Control-Prevention "Abortion Surveillance-United States, 1999" (Morbidity Mortality Weekly Report, Vol. 51, No. SS-9, 11/29/02)
By state of occurrence. National percent is for reporting states only.
**Not reported.*
***New York figure is for New York City only.*

Reported Legal Abortions Performed At or After 21 Weeks of Gestation in 1999

Reporting States' Total = 9,643 Abortions*

ALPHA ORDER					RANK ORDER			
RANK	STATE		ABORTIONS	% of USA	RANK	STATE	ABORTIONS	% of USA
23	Alabama		32	0.3%	1	New York***	2,316	24.0%
NA	Alaska**		NA	NA	2	Georgia	1,105	11.5%
34	Arizona		4	0.0%	3	Texas	979	10.2%
21	Arkansas		44	0.5%	4	New Jersey	812	8.4%
NA	California**		NA	NA	5	Ohio	682	7.1%
12	Colorado		178	1.8%	6	Kansas	665	6.9%
31	Connecticut		7	0.1%	7	Washington	548	5.7%
33	Delaware		5	0.1%	8	Pennsylvania	526	5.5%
NA	Florida**		NA	NA	9	Louisiana	335	3.5%
2	Georgia		1,105	11.5%	10	Oregon	325	3.4%
20	Hawaii		48	0.5%	11	Michigan	245	2.5%
31	Idaho		7	0.1%	12	Colorado	178	1.8%
NA	Illinois**		NA	NA	13	Wisconsin	171	1.8%
38	Indiana		0	0.0%	14	Minnesota	100	1.0%
22	Iowa		38	0.4%	15	Kentucky	89	0.9%
6	Kansas		665	6.9%	16	North Carolina	74	0.8%
15	Kentucky		89	0.9%	17	Nevada	59	0.6%
9	Louisiana		335	3.5%	18	Virginia	58	0.6%
36	Maine		2	0.0%	19	Montana	50	0.5%
25	Maryland		22	0.2%	20	Hawaii	48	0.5%
NA	Massachusetts**		NA	NA	21	Arkansas	44	0.5%
11	Michigan		245	2.5%	22	Iowa	38	0.4%
14	Minnesota		100	1.0%	23	Alabama	32	0.3%
28	Mississippi		17	0.2%	24	Missouri	30	0.3%
24	Missouri		30	0.3%	25	Maryland	22	0.2%
19	Montana		50	0.5%	26	New Mexico	21	0.2%
NA	Nebraska**		NA	NA	26	Tennessee	21	0.2%
17	Nevada		59	0.6%	28	Mississippi	17	0.2%
NA	New Hampshire**		NA	NA	29	Rhode Island	12	0.1%
4	New Jersey		812	8.4%	30	South Carolina	10	0.1%
26	New Mexico		21	0.2%	31	Connecticut	7	0.1%
1	New York***		2,316	24.0%	31	Idaho	7	0.1%
16	North Carolina		74	0.8%	33	Delaware	5	0.1%
38	North Dakota		0	0.0%	34	Arizona	4	0.0%
5	Ohio		682	7.1%	34	Vermont	4	0.0%
NA	Oklahoma**		NA	NA	36	Maine	2	0.0%
10	Oregon		325	3.4%	36	West Virginia	2	0.0%
8	Pennsylvania		526	5.5%	38	Indiana	0	0.0%
29	Rhode Island		12	0.1%	38	North Dakota	0	0.0%
30	South Carolina		10	0.1%	38	South Dakota	0	0.0%
38	South Dakota		0	0.0%	38	Utah	0	0.0%
26	Tennessee		21	0.2%	38	Wyoming	0	0.0%
3	Texas		979	10.2%	NA	Alaska**	NA	NA
38	Utah		0	0.0%	NA	California**	NA	NA
34	Vermont		4	0.0%	NA	Florida**	NA	NA
18	Virginia		58	0.6%	NA	Illinois**	NA	NA
7	Washington		548	5.7%	NA	Massachusetts**	NA	NA
36	West Virginia		2	0.0%	NA	Nebraska**	NA	NA
13	Wisconsin		171	1.8%	NA	New Hampshire**	NA	NA
38	Wyoming		0	0.0%	NA	Oklahoma**	NA	NA
					District of Columbia		0	0.0%

Source: Morgan Quitno Press using data from US Dept of Health & Human Serv's, Centers for Disease Control-Prevention "Abortion Surveillance-United States, 1999" (Morbidity Mortality Weekly Report, Vol. 51, No. SS-9, 11/29/02)

*By state of occurrence. National total is for reporting states only.

**Not reported.

***New York figure is for New York City only.

Percent of Reported Legal Abortions Performed At or After 21 Weeks of Gestation in 1999
Reporting States' Percent = 1.5% of Abortions*

ALPHA ORDER

RANK	STATE	PERCENT
25	Alabama	0.2
NA	Alaska**	NA
37	Arizona	0.0
18	Arkansas	0.8
NA	California**	NA
2	Colorado	3.5
31	Connecticut	0.1
31	Delaware	0.1
NA	Florida**	NA
3	Georgia	3.3
15	Hawaii	1.1
18	Idaho	0.8
NA	Illinois**	NA
37	Indiana	0.0
21	Iowa	0.6
1	Kansas	5.4
11	Kentucky	1.6
4	Louisiana	2.8
31	Maine	0.1
25	Maryland	0.2
NA	Massachusetts**	NA
17	Michigan	0.9
20	Minnesota	0.7
22	Mississippi	0.4
22	Missouri	0.4
9	Montana	2.0
NA	Nebraska**	NA
16	Nevada	1.0
NA	New Hampshire**	NA
5	New Jersey	2.3
22	New Mexico	0.4
5	New York***	2.3
25	North Carolina	0.2
37	North Dakota	0.0
10	Ohio	1.8
NA	Oklahoma**	NA
5	Oregon	2.3
13	Pennsylvania	1.5
25	Rhode Island	0.2
31	South Carolina	0.1
37	South Dakota	0.0
31	Tennessee	0.1
14	Texas	1.2
37	Utah	0.0
25	Vermont	0.2
25	Virginia	0.2
8	Washington	2.1
31	West Virginia	0.1
11	Wisconsin	1.6
37	Wyoming	0.0

RANK ORDER

RANK	STATE	PERCENT
1	Kansas	5.4
2	Colorado	3.5
3	Georgia	3.3
4	Louisiana	2.8
5	New Jersey	2.3
5	New York***	2.3
5	Oregon	2.3
8	Washington	2.1
9	Montana	2.0
10	Ohio	1.8
11	Kentucky	1.6
11	Wisconsin	1.6
13	Pennsylvania	1.5
14	Texas	1.2
15	Hawaii	1.1
16	Nevada	1.0
17	Michigan	0.9
18	Arkansas	0.8
18	Idaho	0.8
20	Minnesota	0.7
21	Iowa	0.6
22	Mississippi	0.4
22	Missouri	0.4
22	New Mexico	0.4
25	Alabama	0.2
25	Maryland	0.2
25	North Carolina	0.2
25	Rhode Island	0.2
25	Vermont	0.2
25	Virginia	0.2
31	Connecticut	0.1
31	Delaware	0.1
31	Maine	0.1
31	South Carolina	0.1
31	Tennessee	0.1
31	West Virginia	0.1
37	Arizona	0.0
37	Indiana	0.0
37	North Dakota	0.0
37	South Dakota	0.0
37	Utah	0.0
37	Wyoming	0.0
NA	Alaska**	NA
NA	California**	NA
NA	Florida**	NA
NA	Illinois**	NA
NA	Massachusetts**	NA
NA	Nebraska**	NA
NA	New Hampshire**	NA
NA	Oklahoma**	NA

District of Columbia — 0.0

Source: Morgan Quitno Press using data from US Dept of Health & Human Serv's, Centers for Disease Control-Prevention "Abortion Surveillance-United States, 1999" (Morbidity Mortality Weekly Report, Vol. 51, No. SS-9, 11/29/02)
*By state of occurrence. National percent is for reporting states only.
**Not reported.
***New York figure is for New York City only.

II. DEATHS

II. DEATHS (Continued)

Deaths in 2000

National Total = 2,403,351 Deaths*

RANK	STATE	DEATHS	% of USA
18	Alabama	45,062	1.9%
50	Alaska	2,914	0.1%
22	Arizona	40,500	1.7%
30	Arkansas	28,217	1.2%
1	California	229,551	9.6%
32	Colorado	27,288	1.1%
27	Connecticut	30,129	1.3%
46	Delaware	6,875	0.3%
2	Florida	164,395	6.8%
11	Georgia	63,870	2.7%
43	Hawaii	8,290	0.3%
42	Idaho	9,563	0.4%
7	Illinois	106,634	4.4%
14	Indiana	55,469	2.3%
31	Iowa	28,060	1.2%
33	Kansas	24,717	1.0%
23	Kentucky	39,504	1.6%
21	Louisiana	41,138	1.7%
39	Maine	12,354	0.5%
20	Maryland	43,753	1.8%
12	Massachusetts	56,681	2.4%
8	Michigan	86,953	3.6%
24	Minnesota	37,690	1.6%
29	Mississippi	28,654	1.2%
16	Missouri	54,865	2.3%
44	Montana	8,096	0.3%
36	Nebraska	14,992	0.6%
35	Nevada	15,261	0.6%
41	New Hampshire	9,697	0.4%
9	New Jersey	74,800	3.1%
37	New Mexico	13,425	0.6%
3	New York	158,203	6.6%
10	North Carolina	71,935	3.0%
47	North Dakota	5,856	0.2%
6	Ohio	108,125	4.5%
26	Oklahoma	35,079	1.5%
28	Oregon	29,552	1.2%
5	Pennsylvania	130,813	5.4%
40	Rhode Island	10,027	0.4%
25	South Carolina	36,948	1.5%
45	South Dakota	7,021	0.3%
15	Tennessee	55,246	2.3%
4	Texas	149,939	6.2%
38	Utah	12,364	0.5%
48	Vermont	5,127	0.2%
13	Virginia	56,282	2.3%
19	Washington	43,941	1.8%
34	West Virginia	21,114	0.9%
17	Wisconsin	46,461	1.9%
49	Wyoming	3,920	0.2%

RANK	STATE	DEATHS	% of USA
1	California	229,551	9.6%
2	Florida	164,395	6.8%
3	New York	158,203	6.6%
4	Texas	149,939	6.2%
5	Pennsylvania	130,813	5.4%
6	Ohio	108,125	4.5%
7	Illinois	106,634	4.4%
8	Michigan	86,953	3.6%
9	New Jersey	74,800	3.1%
10	North Carolina	71,935	3.0%
11	Georgia	63,870	2.7%
12	Massachusetts	56,681	2.4%
13	Virginia	56,282	2.3%
14	Indiana	55,469	2.3%
15	Tennessee	55,246	2.3%
16	Missouri	54,865	2.3%
17	Wisconsin	46,461	1.9%
18	Alabama	45,062	1.9%
19	Washington	43,941	1.8%
20	Maryland	43,753	1.8%
21	Louisiana	41,138	1.7%
22	Arizona	40,500	1.7%
23	Kentucky	39,504	1.6%
24	Minnesota	37,690	1.6%
25	South Carolina	36,948	1.5%
26	Oklahoma	35,079	1.5%
27	Connecticut	30,129	1.3%
28	Oregon	29,552	1.2%
29	Mississippi	28,654	1.2%
30	Arkansas	28,217	1.2%
31	Iowa	28,060	1.2%
32	Colorado	27,288	1.1%
33	Kansas	24,717	1.0%
34	West Virginia	21,114	0.9%
35	Nevada	15,261	0.6%
36	Nebraska	14,992	0.6%
37	New Mexico	13,425	0.6%
38	Utah	12,364	0.5%
39	Maine	12,354	0.5%
40	Rhode Island	10,027	0.4%
41	New Hampshire	9,697	0.4%
42	Idaho	9,563	0.4%
43	Hawaii	8,290	0.3%
44	Montana	8,096	0.3%
45	South Dakota	7,021	0.3%
46	Delaware	6,875	0.3%
47	North Dakota	5,856	0.2%
48	Vermont	5,127	0.2%
49	Wyoming	3,920	0.2%
50	Alaska	2,914	0.1%
	District of Columbia	6,001	0.2%

Source: U.S. Department of Health and Human Services, National Center for Health Statistics "National Vital Statistics Reports" (Vol. 50, No. 15, September 16, 2002)
Final data by state of residence.

Death Rate in 2000

National Rate = 873.1 Deaths per 100,000 Population*

ALPHA ORDER

RANK	STATE	RATE
7	Alabama	1,027.0
50	Alaska	468.4
35	Arizona	829.5
2	Arkansas	1,095.2
47	California	682.5
48	Colorado	659.7
22	Connecticut	913.8
26	Delaware	902.0
4	Florida	1,072.2
39	Georgia	804.1
46	Hawaii	703.0
44	Idaho	751.1
31	Illinois	875.1
20	Indiana	928.1
13	Iowa	975.2
21	Kansas	927.2
11	Kentucky	991.2
17	Louisiana	940.3
12	Maine	981.6
34	Maryland	838.4
23	Massachusetts	913.6
30	Michigan	876.7
41	Minnesota	780.7
6	Mississippi	1,028.1
10	Missouri	997.1
24	Montana	911.8
27	Nebraska	897.5
37	Nevada	811.6
40	New Hampshire	797.5
25	New Jersey	911.7
42	New Mexico	768.1
32	New York	865.5
19	North Carolina	928.5
18	North Dakota	930.6
14	Ohio	959.4
5	Oklahoma	1,037.8
28	Oregon	884.5
3	Pennsylvania	1,091.5
8	Rhode Island	1,006.6
16	South Carolina	941.5
15	South Dakota	952.3
9	Tennessee	998.4
45	Texas	735.4
49	Utah	571.2
33	Vermont	857.6
38	Virginia	807.4
43	Washington	756.2
1	West Virginia	1,171.5
29	Wisconsin	877.4
36	Wyoming	815.1

RANK ORDER

RANK	STATE	RATE
1	West Virginia	1,171.5
2	Arkansas	1,095.2
3	Pennsylvania	1,091.5
4	Florida	1,072.2
5	Oklahoma	1,037.8
6	Mississippi	1,028.1
7	Alabama	1,027.0
8	Rhode Island	1,006.6
9	Tennessee	998.4
10	Missouri	997.1
11	Kentucky	991.2
12	Maine	981.6
13	Iowa	975.2
14	Ohio	959.4
15	South Dakota	952.3
16	South Carolina	941.5
17	Louisiana	940.3
18	North Dakota	930.6
19	North Carolina	928.5
20	Indiana	928.1
21	Kansas	927.2
22	Connecticut	913.8
23	Massachusetts	913.6
24	Montana	911.8
25	New Jersey	911.7
26	Delaware	902.0
27	Nebraska	897.5
28	Oregon	884.5
29	Wisconsin	877.4
30	Michigan	876.7
31	Illinois	875.1
32	New York	865.5
33	Vermont	857.6
34	Maryland	838.4
35	Arizona	829.5
36	Wyoming	815.1
37	Nevada	811.6
38	Virginia	807.4
39	Georgia	804.1
40	New Hampshire	797.5
41	Minnesota	780.7
42	New Mexico	768.1
43	Washington	756.2
44	Idaho	751.1
45	Texas	735.4
46	Hawaii	703.0
47	California	682.5
48	Colorado	659.7
49	Utah	571.2
50	Alaska	468.4

| | District of Columbia | 1,157.7 |

Source: U.S. Department of Health and Human Services, National Center for Health Statistics
   "National Vital Statistics Reports" (Vol. 50, No. 15, September 16, 2002)
*Final data by state of residence. Not age-adjusted.

Age-Adjusted Death Rate in 2000

National Rate = 872.0 Deaths per 100,000 Population*

ALPHA ORDER			RANK ORDER		
RANK	STATE	RATE	RANK	STATE	RATE
4	Alabama	1,013.3	1	Mississippi	1,074.1
24	Alaska	861.4	2	Louisiana	1,020.1
29	Arizona	844.0	3	Tennessee	1,019.9
8	Arkansas	1,001.7	4	Alabama	1,013.3
49	California	765.7	5	West Virginia	1,012.5
45	Colorado	788.4	6	Kentucky	1,004.8
44	Connecticut	797.5	7	Georgia	1,002.5
16	Delaware	920.2	8	Arkansas	1,001.7
34	Florida	828.8	9	South Carolina	994.6
7	Georgia	1,002.5	10	Oklahoma	986.8
50	Hawaii	666.7	11	North Carolina	963.9
39	Idaho	811.7	12	Nevada	951.4
23	Illinois	876.9	13	Indiana	936.4
13	Indiana	936.4	14	Missouri	928.1
42	Iowa	802.4	15	Ohio	922.5
28	Kansas	851.9	16	Delaware	920.2
6	Kentucky	1,004.8	17	Maryland	911.6
2	Louisiana	1,020.1	18	Pennsylvania	903.6
22	Maine	887.4	19	Virginia	899.9
17	Maryland	911.6	20	Texas	895.8
37	Massachusetts	818.1	21	Michigan	892.7
21	Michigan	892.7	22	Maine	887.4
48	Minnesota	766.0	23	Illinois	876.9
1	Mississippi	1,074.1	24	Alaska	861.4
14	Missouri	928.1	25	Wyoming	860.4
30	Montana	843.1	26	Vermont	854.3
43	Nebraska	798.4	27	New Jersey	853.1
12	Nevada	951.4	28	Kansas	851.9
31	New Hampshire	837.1	29	Arizona	844.0
27	New Jersey	853.1	30	Montana	843.1
32	New Mexico	836.1	31	New Hampshire	837.1
40	New York	808.6	32	New Mexico	836.1
11	North Carolina	963.9	33	Oregon	834.3
47	North Dakota	766.4	34	Florida	828.8
15	Ohio	922.5	35	Rhode Island	827.2
10	Oklahoma	986.8	36	Wisconsin	826.6
33	Oregon	834.3	37	Massachusetts	818.1
18	Pennsylvania	903.6	38	South Dakota	813.2
35	Rhode Island	827.2	39	Idaho	811.7
9	South Carolina	994.6	40	New York	808.6
38	South Dakota	813.2	41	Washington	806.6
3	Tennessee	1,019.9	42	Iowa	802.4
20	Texas	895.8	43	Nebraska	798.4
46	Utah	786.1	44	Connecticut	797.5
26	Vermont	854.3	45	Colorado	788.4
19	Virginia	899.9	46	Utah	786.1
41	Washington	806.6	47	North Dakota	766.4
5	West Virginia	1,012.5	48	Minnesota	766.0
36	Wisconsin	826.6	49	California	765.7
25	Wyoming	860.4	50	Hawaii	666.7
				District of Columbia	1,043.3

Source: U.S. Department of Health and Human Services, National Center for Health Statistics
   "National Vital Statistics Reports" (Vol. 50, No. 15, September 16, 2002)
*Final data by state of residence. Age-adjusted rates eliminate the distorting effects of the aging of the population.
Rates based on the year 2000 standard population.

Death Rate in 1990

National Rate = 863 Deaths per 100,000 Population*

ALPHA ORDER

RANK	STATE	RATE
7	Alabama	974
50	Alaska	398
37	Arizona	784
2	Arkansas	1,048
44	California	719
47	Colorado	655
32	Connecticut	840
27	Delaware	864
3	Florida	1,038
35	Georgia	799
48	Hawaii	611
42	Idaho	740
19	Illinois	900
21	Indiana	894
8	Iowa	968
20	Kansas	899
11	Kentucky	951
22	Louisiana	890
18	Maine	905
34	Maryland	803
24	Massachusetts	884
31	Michigan	847
36	Minnesota	795
6	Mississippi	976
5	Missouri	984
29	Montana	859
14	Nebraska	936
38	Nevada	775
40	New Hampshire	765
16	New Jersey	910
46	New Mexico	701
13	New York	938
27	North Carolina	864
22	North Dakota	890
15	Ohio	911
9	Oklahoma	966
24	Oregon	884
4	Pennsylvania	1,026
10	Rhode Island	954
30	South Carolina	852
17	South Dakota	909
12	Tennessee	949
43	Texas	738
49	Utah	533
33	Vermont	817
38	Virginia	775
41	Washington	762
1	West Virginia	1,080
26	Wisconsin	874
45	Wyoming	706

RANK ORDER

RANK	STATE	RATE
1	West Virginia	1,080
2	Arkansas	1,048
3	Florida	1,038
4	Pennsylvania	1,026
5	Missouri	984
6	Mississippi	976
7	Alabama	974
8	Iowa	968
9	Oklahoma	966
10	Rhode Island	954
11	Kentucky	951
12	Tennessee	949
13	New York	938
14	Nebraska	936
15	Ohio	911
16	New Jersey	910
17	South Dakota	909
18	Maine	905
19	Illinois	900
20	Kansas	899
21	Indiana	894
22	Louisiana	890
22	North Dakota	890
24	Massachusetts	884
24	Oregon	884
26	Wisconsin	874
27	Delaware	864
27	North Carolina	864
29	Montana	859
30	South Carolina	852
31	Michigan	847
32	Connecticut	840
33	Vermont	817
34	Maryland	803
35	Georgia	799
36	Minnesota	795
37	Arizona	784
38	Nevada	775
38	Virginia	775
40	New Hampshire	765
41	Washington	762
42	Idaho	740
43	Texas	738
44	California	719
45	Wyoming	706
46	New Mexico	701
47	Colorado	655
48	Hawaii	611
49	Utah	533
50	Alaska	398
	District of Columbia	1,200

Source: U.S. Department of Health and Human Services, National Center for Health Statistics
    "Monthly Vital Statistics Report" (Vol. 41, No. 7(S), January 7, 1993)
*Final data by state of residence. Not age adjusted.

Death Rate in 1980

National Rate = 877 Deaths per 100,000 Population*

ALPHA ORDER

RANK	STATE	RATE
18	Alabama	912
50	Alaska	425
40	Arizona	784
4	Arkansas	994
39	California	786
47	Colorado	654
23	Connecticut	877
27	Delaware	847
1	Florida	1,072
35	Georgia	809
49	Hawaii	515
44	Idaho	715
20	Illinois	899
25	Indiana	862
14	Iowa	930
14	Kansas	930
16	Kentucky	922
28	Louisiana	846
8	Maine	960
36	Maryland	806
9	Massachusetts	959
34	Michigan	811
33	Minnesota	817
11	Mississippi	937
3	Missouri	1,008
28	Montana	846
17	Nebraska	920
43	Nevada	735
30	New Hampshire	830
12	New Jersey	936
45	New Mexico	696
6	New York	984
32	North Carolina	823
26	North Dakota	856
19	Ohio	911
13	Oklahoma	932
31	Oregon	827
2	Pennsylvania	1,041
6	Rhode Island	984
37	South Carolina	805
10	South Dakota	947
22	Tennessee	887
42	Texas	758
48	Utah	554
21	Vermont	895
38	Virginia	794
41	Washington	773
5	West Virginia	987
24	Wisconsin	867
46	Wyoming	684

RANK ORDER

RANK	STATE	RATE
1	Florida	1,072
2	Pennsylvania	1,041
3	Missouri	1,008
4	Arkansas	994
5	West Virginia	987
6	New York	984
6	Rhode Island	984
8	Maine	960
9	Massachusetts	959
10	South Dakota	947
11	Mississippi	937
12	New Jersey	936
13	Oklahoma	932
14	Iowa	930
14	Kansas	930
16	Kentucky	922
17	Nebraska	920
18	Alabama	912
19	Ohio	911
20	Illinois	899
21	Vermont	895
22	Tennessee	887
23	Connecticut	877
24	Wisconsin	867
25	Indiana	862
26	North Dakota	856
27	Delaware	847
28	Louisiana	846
28	Montana	846
30	New Hampshire	830
31	Oregon	827
32	North Carolina	823
33	Minnesota	817
34	Michigan	811
35	Georgia	809
36	Maryland	806
37	South Carolina	805
38	Virginia	794
39	California	786
40	Arizona	784
41	Washington	773
42	Texas	758
43	Nevada	735
44	Idaho	715
45	New Mexico	696
46	Wyoming	684
47	Colorado	654
48	Utah	554
49	Hawaii	515
50	Alaska	425
	District of Columbia	1,109

Source: U.S. Department of Health and Human Services, National Center for Health Statistics
"Vital Statistics of the United States 1980" and "Monthly Vital Statistics Report"
*Final data by state of residence. Not age adjusted.

Infant Deaths in 2000

National Total = 28,035 Infant Deaths*

ALPHA ORDER

RANK	STATE	DEATHS	% of USA
16	Alabama	596	2.1%
44	Alaska	68	0.2%
17	Arizona	573	2.0%
29	Arkansas	316	1.1%
1	California	2,894	10.3%
25	Colorado	404	1.4%
30	Connecticut	282	1.0%
41	Delaware	102	0.4%
5	Florida	1,425	5.1%
7	Georgia	1,126	4.0%
40	Hawaii	142	0.5%
39	Idaho	153	0.5%
4	Illinois	1,568	5.6%
13	Indiana	685	2.4%
34	Iowa	247	0.9%
31	Kansas	268	1.0%
26	Kentucky	401	1.4%
15	Louisiana	608	2.2%
46	Maine	66	0.2%
18	Maryland	562	2.0%
28	Massachusetts	376	1.3%
8	Michigan	1,119	4.0%
27	Minnesota	378	1.3%
21	Mississippi	470	1.7%
19	Missouri	547	2.0%
45	Montana	67	0.2%
36	Nebraska	180	0.6%
35	Nevada	201	0.7%
42	New Hampshire	84	0.3%
11	New Jersey	733	2.6%
36	New Mexico	180	0.6%
3	New York	1,656	5.9%
10	North Carolina	1,038	3.7%
47	North Dakota	62	0.2%
6	Ohio	1,187	4.2%
23	Oklahoma	425	1.5%
32	Oregon	255	0.9%
9	Pennsylvania	1,039	3.7%
43	Rhode Island	79	0.3%
20	South Carolina	488	1.7%
48	South Dakota	57	0.2%
12	Tennessee	724	2.6%
2	Texas	2,065	7.4%
33	Utah	248	0.9%
50	Vermont	39	0.1%
14	Virginia	682	2.4%
24	Washington	421	1.5%
38	West Virginia	158	0.6%
22	Wisconsin	457	1.6%
49	Wyoming	42	0.1%

RANK ORDER

RANK	STATE	DEATHS	% of USA
1	California	2,894	10.3%
2	Texas	2,065	7.4%
3	New York	1,656	5.9%
4	Illinois	1,568	5.6%
5	Florida	1,425	5.1%
6	Ohio	1,187	4.2%
7	Georgia	1,126	4.0%
8	Michigan	1,119	4.0%
9	Pennsylvania	1,039	3.7%
10	North Carolina	1,038	3.7%
11	New Jersey	733	2.6%
12	Tennessee	724	2.6%
13	Indiana	685	2.4%
14	Virginia	682	2.4%
15	Louisiana	608	2.2%
16	Alabama	596	2.1%
17	Arizona	573	2.0%
18	Maryland	562	2.0%
19	Missouri	547	2.0%
20	South Carolina	488	1.7%
21	Mississippi	470	1.7%
22	Wisconsin	457	1.6%
23	Oklahoma	425	1.5%
24	Washington	421	1.5%
25	Colorado	404	1.4%
26	Kentucky	401	1.4%
27	Minnesota	378	1.3%
28	Massachusetts	376	1.3%
29	Arkansas	316	1.1%
30	Connecticut	282	1.0%
31	Kansas	268	1.0%
32	Oregon	255	0.9%
33	Utah	248	0.9%
34	Iowa	247	0.9%
35	Nevada	201	0.7%
36	Nebraska	180	0.6%
36	New Mexico	180	0.6%
38	West Virginia	158	0.6%
39	Idaho	153	0.5%
40	Hawaii	142	0.5%
41	Delaware	102	0.4%
42	New Hampshire	84	0.3%
43	Rhode Island	79	0.3%
44	Alaska	68	0.2%
45	Montana	67	0.2%
46	Maine	66	0.2%
47	North Dakota	62	0.2%
48	South Dakota	57	0.2%
49	Wyoming	42	0.1%
50	Vermont	39	0.1%
	District of Columbia	92	0.3%

Source: U.S. Department of Health and Human Services, National Center for Health Statistics
    "National Vital Statistics Reports" (Vol. 50, No. 15, September 16, 2002)
*Final data. Deaths under 1 year old by state of residence.

Infant Mortality Rate in 2000

National Rate = 6.9 Infant Deaths per 1,000 Live Births*

ALPHA ORDER

RANK ORDER

RANK	STATE	RATE		RANK	STATE	RATE
2	Alabama	9.4		1	Mississippi	10.7
26	Alaska	6.8		2	Alabama	9.4
28	Arizona	6.7		3	Delaware	9.2
11	Arkansas	8.4		4	Tennessee	9.1
46	California	5.4		5	Louisiana	9.0
38	Colorado	6.2		6	South Carolina	8.7
30	Connecticut	6.6		7	North Carolina	8.6
3	Delaware	9.2		8	Georgia	8.5
24	Florida	7.0		8	Illinois	8.5
8	Georgia	8.5		8	Oklahoma	8.5
13	Hawaii	8.1		11	Arkansas	8.4
19	Idaho	7.5		12	Michigan	8.2
8	Illinois	8.5		13	Hawaii	8.1
15	Indiana	7.8		13	North Dakota	8.1
33	Iowa	6.5		15	Indiana	7.8
26	Kansas	6.8		16	Maryland	7.6
21	Kentucky	7.2		16	Ohio	7.6
5	Louisiana	9.0		16	West Virginia	7.6
49	Maine	4.9		19	Idaho	7.5
16	Maryland	7.6		20	Nebraska	7.3
50	Massachusetts	4.6		21	Kentucky	7.2
12	Michigan	8.2		21	Missouri	7.2
43	Minnesota	5.6		23	Pennsylvania	7.1
1	Mississippi	10.7		24	Florida	7.0
21	Missouri	7.2		25	Virginia	6.9
39	Montana	6.1		26	Alaska	6.8
20	Nebraska	7.3		26	Kansas	6.8
33	Nevada	6.5		28	Arizona	6.7
41	New Hampshire	5.7		28	Wyoming	6.7
36	New Jersey	6.3		30	Connecticut	6.6
30	New Mexico	6.6		30	New Mexico	6.6
35	New York	6.4		30	Wisconsin	6.6
7	North Carolina	8.6		33	Iowa	6.5
13	North Dakota	8.1		33	Nevada	6.5
16	Ohio	7.6		35	New York	6.4
8	Oklahoma	8.5		36	New Jersey	6.3
43	Oregon	5.6		36	Rhode Island	6.3
23	Pennsylvania	7.1		38	Colorado	6.2
36	Rhode Island	6.3		39	Montana	6.1
6	South Carolina	8.7		40	Vermont	6.0
45	South Dakota	5.5		41	New Hampshire	5.7
4	Tennessee	9.1		41	Texas	5.7
41	Texas	5.7		43	Minnesota	5.6
47	Utah	5.2		43	Oregon	5.6
40	Vermont	6.0		45	South Dakota	5.5
25	Virginia	6.9		46	California	5.4
47	Washington	5.2		47	Utah	5.2
16	West Virginia	7.6		47	Washington	5.2
30	Wisconsin	6.6		49	Maine	4.9
28	Wyoming	6.7		50	Massachusetts	4.6

District of Columbia		12.0

Source: U.S. Department of Health and Human Services, National Center for Health Statistics
   "National Vital Statistics Reports" (Vol. 50, No. 15, September 16, 2002)
*Final data. Deaths under 1 year old by state of residence.

Infant Mortality Rate in 1990

National Rate = 9.2 Infant Deaths per 1,000 Live Births*

ALPHA ORDER

RANK	STATE	RATE
5	Alabama	10.8
9	Alaska	10.5
27	Arizona	8.8
22	Arkansas	9.2
41	California	7.9
27	Colorado	8.8
41	Connecticut	7.9
12	Delaware	10.1
16	Florida	9.6
1	Georgia	12.4
48	Hawaii	6.7
29	Idaho	8.7
5	Illinois	10.8
16	Indiana	9.6
37	Iowa	8.1
32	Kansas	8.4
31	Kentucky	8.5
4	Louisiana	11.1
50	Maine	6.2
16	Maryland	9.6
47	Massachusetts	7.0
7	Michigan	10.7
45	Minnesota	7.3
2	Mississippi	12.1
21	Missouri	9.4
24	Montana	9.0
34	Nebraska	8.3
32	Nevada	8.4
46	New Hampshire	7.1
24	New Jersey	9.0
24	New Mexico	9.0
16	New York	9.6
8	North Carolina	10.6
40	North Dakota	8.0
15	Ohio	9.8
22	Oklahoma	9.2
34	Oregon	8.3
16	Pennsylvania	9.6
37	Rhode Island	8.1
3	South Carolina	11.7
12	South Dakota	10.1
10	Tennessee	10.3
37	Texas	8.1
44	Utah	7.5
49	Vermont	6.4
11	Virginia	10.2
43	Washington	7.8
14	West Virginia	9.9
36	Wisconsin	8.2
30	Wyoming	8.6

RANK ORDER

RANK	STATE	RATE
1	Georgia	12.4
2	Mississippi	12.1
3	South Carolina	11.7
4	Louisiana	11.1
5	Alabama	10.8
5	Illinois	10.8
7	Michigan	10.7
8	North Carolina	10.6
9	Alaska	10.5
10	Tennessee	10.3
11	Virginia	10.2
12	Delaware	10.1
12	South Dakota	10.1
14	West Virginia	9.9
15	Ohio	9.8
16	Florida	9.6
16	Indiana	9.6
16	Maryland	9.6
16	New York	9.6
16	Pennsylvania	9.6
21	Missouri	9.4
22	Arkansas	9.2
22	Oklahoma	9.2
24	Montana	9.0
24	New Jersey	9.0
24	New Mexico	9.0
27	Arizona	8.8
27	Colorado	8.8
29	Idaho	8.7
30	Wyoming	8.6
31	Kentucky	8.5
32	Kansas	8.4
32	Nevada	8.4
34	Nebraska	8.3
34	Oregon	8.3
36	Wisconsin	8.2
37	Iowa	8.1
37	Rhode Island	8.1
37	Texas	8.1
40	North Dakota	8.0
41	California	7.9
41	Connecticut	7.9
43	Washington	7.8
44	Utah	7.5
45	Minnesota	7.3
46	New Hampshire	7.1
47	Massachusetts	7.0
48	Hawaii	6.7
49	Vermont	6.4
50	Maine	6.2

District of Columbia	20.7

Source: U.S. Department of Health and Human Services, National Center for Health Statistics
"Monthly Vital Statistics Report" (Vol. 41, No. 7(S), January 7, 1993)
*Final data by state of residence. Infant deaths are those under 1 year old.

Infant Mortality Rate in 1980

National Rate = 12.6 Infant Deaths per 1,000 Live Births*

ALPHA ORDER

RANK	STATE	RATE
3	Alabama	15.2
24	Alaska	12.3
21	Arizona	12.4
17	Arkansas	12.7
35	California	11.1
46	Colorado	10.1
34	Connecticut	11.2
10	Delaware	13.9
5	Florida	14.6
6	Georgia	14.5
44	Hawaii	10.3
38	Idaho	10.7
4	Illinois	14.8
28	Indiana	11.9
29	Iowa	11.8
42	Kansas	10.4
14	Kentucky	12.9
8	Louisiana	14.3
50	Maine	9.2
9	Maryland	14.1
41	Massachusetts	10.5
15	Michigan	12.8
47	Minnesota	10.0
1	Mississippi	17.0
21	Missouri	12.4
21	Montana	12.4
32	Nebraska	11.5
38	Nevada	10.7
48	New Hampshire	9.9
19	New Jersey	12.5
32	New Mexico	11.5
19	New York	12.5
6	North Carolina	14.5
27	North Dakota	12.1
15	Ohio	12.8
17	Oklahoma	12.7
25	Oregon	12.2
13	Pennsylvania	13.2
36	Rhode Island	11.0
2	South Carolina	15.6
37	South Dakota	10.9
12	Tennessee	13.5
25	Texas	12.2
42	Utah	10.4
38	Vermont	10.7
11	Virginia	13.6
29	Washington	11.8
29	West Virginia	11.8
44	Wisconsin	10.3
49	Wyoming	9.8

RANK ORDER

RANK	STATE	RATE
1	Mississippi	17.0
2	South Carolina	15.6
3	Alabama	15.2
4	Illinois	14.8
5	Florida	14.6
6	Georgia	14.5
6	North Carolina	14.5
8	Louisiana	14.3
9	Maryland	14.1
10	Delaware	13.9
11	Virginia	13.6
12	Tennessee	13.5
13	Pennsylvania	13.2
14	Kentucky	12.9
15	Michigan	12.8
15	Ohio	12.8
17	Arkansas	12.7
17	Oklahoma	12.7
19	New Jersey	12.5
19	New York	12.5
21	Arizona	12.4
21	Missouri	12.4
21	Montana	12.4
24	Alaska	12.3
25	Oregon	12.2
25	Texas	12.2
27	North Dakota	12.1
28	Indiana	11.9
29	Iowa	11.8
29	Washington	11.8
29	West Virginia	11.8
32	Nebraska	11.5
32	New Mexico	11.5
34	Connecticut	11.2
35	California	11.1
36	Rhode Island	11.0
37	South Dakota	10.9
38	Idaho	10.7
38	Nevada	10.7
38	Vermont	10.7
41	Massachusetts	10.5
42	Kansas	10.4
42	Utah	10.4
44	Hawaii	10.3
44	Wisconsin	10.3
46	Colorado	10.1
47	Minnesota	10.0
48	New Hampshire	9.9
49	Wyoming	9.8
50	Maine	9.2
	District of Columbia	25.0

*Source: U.S. Department of Health and Human Services, National Center for Health Statistics
"Monthly Vital Statistics Report"*
Final data by state of residence. Deaths under 1 year old, exclusive of fetal deaths.

Percent Change in Infant Mortality Rate: 1990 to 2000

National Percent Change = 25.0% Decrease*

ALPHA ORDER

RANK	STATE	PERCENT CHANGE
10	Alabama	(13.0)
49	Alaska	(35.2)
32	Arizona	(23.9)
5	Arkansas	(8.7)
42	California	(31.6)
37	Colorado	(29.5)
13	Connecticut	(16.5)
6	Delaware	(8.9)
36	Florida	(27.1)
41	Georgia	(31.5)
1	Hawaii	20.9
11	Idaho	(13.8)
23	Illinois	(21.3)
14	Indiana	(18.8)
20	Iowa	(19.8)
17	Kansas	(19.0)
12	Kentucky	(15.3)
15	Louisiana	(18.9)
22	Maine	(21.0)
21	Maryland	(20.8)
48	Massachusetts	(34.3)
30	Michigan	(23.4)
29	Minnesota	(23.3)
7	Mississippi	(11.6)
30	Missouri	(23.4)
43	Montana	(32.2)
9	Nebraska	(12.0)
27	Nevada	(22.6)
19	New Hampshire	(19.7)
39	New Jersey	(30.0)
35	New Mexico	(26.7)
46	New York	(33.3)
15	North Carolina	(18.9)
2	North Dakota	1.3
26	Ohio	(22.4)
4	Oklahoma	(7.6)
45	Oregon	(32.5)
34	Pennsylvania	(26.0)
25	Rhode Island	(22.2)
33	South Carolina	(25.6)
50	South Dakota	(45.5)
8	Tennessee	(11.7)
38	Texas	(29.6)
40	Utah	(30.7)
3	Vermont	(6.3)
44	Virginia	(32.4)
46	Washington	(33.3)
28	West Virginia	(23.2)
18	Wisconsin	(19.5)
24	Wyoming	(22.1)

RANK ORDER

RANK	STATE	PERCENT CHANGE
1	Hawaii	20.9
2	North Dakota	1.3
3	Vermont	(6.3)
4	Oklahoma	(7.6)
5	Arkansas	(8.7)
6	Delaware	(8.9)
7	Mississippi	(11.6)
8	Tennessee	(11.7)
9	Nebraska	(12.0)
10	Alabama	(13.0)
11	Idaho	(13.8)
12	Kentucky	(15.3)
13	Connecticut	(16.5)
14	Indiana	(18.8)
15	Louisiana	(18.9)
15	North Carolina	(18.9)
17	Kansas	(19.0)
18	Wisconsin	(19.5)
19	New Hampshire	(19.7)
20	Iowa	(19.8)
21	Maryland	(20.8)
22	Maine	(21.0)
23	Illinois	(21.3)
24	Wyoming	(22.1)
25	Rhode Island	(22.2)
26	Ohio	(22.4)
27	Nevada	(22.6)
28	West Virginia	(23.2)
29	Minnesota	(23.3)
30	Michigan	(23.4)
30	Missouri	(23.4)
32	Arizona	(23.9)
33	South Carolina	(25.6)
34	Pennsylvania	(26.0)
35	New Mexico	(26.7)
36	Florida	(27.1)
37	Colorado	(29.5)
38	Texas	(29.6)
39	New Jersey	(30.0)
40	Utah	(30.7)
41	Georgia	(31.5)
42	California	(31.6)
43	Montana	(32.2)
44	Virginia	(32.4)
45	Oregon	(32.5)
46	New York	(33.3)
46	Washington	(33.3)
48	Massachusetts	(34.3)
49	Alaska	(35.2)
50	South Dakota	(45.5)

District of Columbia   (42.0)

Source: Morgan Quitno Press using data from US Dept of Health & Human Services, National Center for Health Statistics
"Monthly Vital Statistics Report" (Vol. 41, No. 7(S), January 7, 1993) and "National Vital Statistics Reports"
(Vol. 50, No. 15, September 16, 2002)
*By state of residence. Infant deaths are those under 1 year old.

Percent Change in Infant Mortality Rate: 1980 to 2000

National Percent Change = 45.2% Decrease*

ALPHA ORDER

RANK	STATE	PERCENT CHANGE	RANK	STATE	PERCENT CHANGE
17	Alabama	(38.2)	1	Hawaii	(21.4)
33	Alaska	(44.7)	2	Idaho	(29.9)
35	Arizona	(46.0)	3	Wyoming	(31.6)
8	Arkansas	(33.9)	4	Tennessee	(32.6)
45	California	(51.4)	5	North Dakota	(33.1)
18	Colorado	(38.6)	5	Oklahoma	(33.1)
22	Connecticut	(41.1)	7	Delaware	(33.8)
7	Delaware	(33.8)	8	Arkansas	(33.9)
46	Florida	(52.1)	9	Indiana	(34.5)
23	Georgia	(41.4)	10	Kansas	(34.6)
1	Hawaii	(21.4)	11	West Virginia	(35.6)
2	Idaho	(29.9)	12	Michigan	(35.9)
26	Illinois	(42.6)	12	Wisconsin	(35.9)
9	Indiana	(34.5)	14	Nebraska	(36.5)
34	Iowa	(44.9)	15	Louisiana	(37.1)
10	Kansas	(34.6)	15	Mississippi	(37.1)
31	Kentucky	(44.2)	17	Alabama	(38.2)
15	Louisiana	(37.1)	18	Colorado	(38.6)
38	Maine	(46.7)	19	Nevada	(39.3)
36	Maryland	(46.1)	20	Ohio	(40.6)
50	Massachusetts	(56.2)	21	North Carolina	(40.7)
12	Michigan	(35.9)	22	Connecticut	(41.1)
30	Minnesota	(44.0)	23	Georgia	(41.4)
15	Mississippi	(37.1)	24	Missouri	(41.9)
24	Missouri	(41.9)	25	New Hampshire	(42.4)
44	Montana	(50.8)	26	Illinois	(42.6)
14	Nebraska	(36.5)	26	New Mexico	(42.6)
19	Nevada	(39.3)	28	Rhode Island	(42.7)
25	New Hampshire	(42.4)	29	Vermont	(43.9)
42	New Jersey	(49.6)	30	Minnesota	(44.0)
26	New Mexico	(42.6)	31	Kentucky	(44.2)
39	New York	(48.8)	31	South Carolina	(44.2)
21	North Carolina	(40.7)	33	Alaska	(44.7)
5	North Dakota	(33.1)	34	Iowa	(44.9)
20	Ohio	(40.6)	35	Arizona	(46.0)
5	Oklahoma	(33.1)	36	Maryland	(46.1)
48	Oregon	(54.1)	37	Pennsylvania	(46.2)
37	Pennsylvania	(46.2)	38	Maine	(46.7)
28	Rhode Island	(42.7)	39	New York	(48.8)
31	South Carolina	(44.2)	40	Virginia	(49.3)
41	South Dakota	(49.5)	41	South Dakota	(49.5)
4	Tennessee	(32.6)	42	New Jersey	(49.6)
47	Texas	(53.3)	43	Utah	(50.0)
43	Utah	(50.0)	44	Montana	(50.8)
29	Vermont	(43.9)	45	California	(51.4)
40	Virginia	(49.3)	46	Florida	(52.1)
49	Washington	(55.9)	47	Texas	(53.3)
11	West Virginia	(35.6)	48	Oregon	(54.1)
12	Wisconsin	(35.9)	49	Washington	(55.9)
3	Wyoming	(31.6)	50	Massachusetts	(56.2)
				District of Columbia	(52.0)

Source: Morgan Quitno Press using data from US Dept of Health & Human Services, National Center for Health Statistics
"National Vital Statistics Reports" (Vol. 50, No. 15, September 16, 2002)
"Vital Statistics of the United States, 1980" (Vol. I-Natality, issued 1984) and unpublished data
*Final data by state of residence. Infant deaths are those occurring under 1 year, exclusive of fetal deaths.

White Infant Deaths in 2000

National Total = 18,144 Deaths*

ALPHA ORDER

RANK	STATE	DEATHS	% of USA
23	Alabama	276	1.5%
48	Alaska	37	0.2%
12	Arizona	460	2.5%
31	Arkansas	204	1.1%
1	California	2,180	12.0%
19	Colorado	332	1.8%
32	Connecticut	201	1.1%
42	Delaware	63	0.3%
5	Florida	815	4.5%
11	Georgia	497	2.7%
50	Hawaii	26	0.1%
37	Idaho	147	0.8%
4	Illinois	938	5.2%
10	Indiana	529	2.9%
30	Iowa	217	1.2%
27	Kansas	226	1.2%
18	Kentucky	334	1.8%
28	Louisiana	224	1.2%
42	Maine	63	0.3%
29	Maryland	219	1.2%
23	Massachusetts	276	1.5%
8	Michigan	646	3.6%
22	Minnesota	283	1.6%
34	Mississippi	159	0.9%
16	Missouri	373	2.1%
44	Montana	52	0.3%
39	Nebraska	143	0.8%
35	Nevada	157	0.9%
40	New Hampshire	78	0.4%
13	New Jersey	422	2.3%
38	New Mexico	144	0.8%
3	New York	992	5.5%
9	North Carolina	546	3.0%
45	North Dakota	50	0.3%
6	Ohio	813	4.5%
21	Oklahoma	308	1.7%
25	Oregon	230	1.3%
7	Pennsylvania	700	3.9%
41	Rhode Island	64	0.4%
33	South Carolina	192	1.1%
49	South Dakota	36	0.2%
14	Tennessee	414	2.3%
2	Texas	1,568	8.6%
26	Utah	228	1.3%
46	Vermont	39	0.2%
15	Virginia	383	2.1%
17	Washington	339	1.9%
36	West Virginia	148	0.8%
20	Wisconsin	328	1.8%
47	Wyoming	38	0.2%

RANK ORDER

RANK	STATE	DEATHS	% of USA
1	California	2,180	12.0%
2	Texas	1,568	8.6%
3	New York	992	5.5%
4	Illinois	938	5.2%
5	Florida	815	4.5%
6	Ohio	813	4.5%
7	Pennsylvania	700	3.9%
8	Michigan	646	3.6%
9	North Carolina	546	3.0%
10	Indiana	529	2.9%
11	Georgia	497	2.7%
12	Arizona	460	2.5%
13	New Jersey	422	2.3%
14	Tennessee	414	2.3%
15	Virginia	383	2.1%
16	Missouri	373	2.1%
17	Washington	339	1.9%
18	Kentucky	334	1.8%
19	Colorado	332	1.8%
20	Wisconsin	328	1.8%
21	Oklahoma	308	1.7%
22	Minnesota	283	1.6%
23	Alabama	276	1.5%
23	Massachusetts	276	1.5%
25	Oregon	230	1.3%
26	Utah	228	1.3%
27	Kansas	226	1.2%
28	Louisiana	224	1.2%
29	Maryland	219	1.2%
30	Iowa	217	1.2%
31	Arkansas	204	1.1%
32	Connecticut	201	1.1%
33	South Carolina	192	1.1%
34	Mississippi	159	0.9%
35	Nevada	157	0.9%
36	West Virginia	148	0.8%
37	Idaho	147	0.8%
38	New Mexico	144	0.8%
39	Nebraska	143	0.8%
40	New Hampshire	78	0.4%
41	Rhode Island	64	0.4%
42	Delaware	63	0.3%
42	Maine	63	0.3%
44	Montana	52	0.3%
45	North Dakota	50	0.3%
46	Vermont	39	0.2%
47	Wyoming	38	0.2%
48	Alaska	37	0.2%
49	South Dakota	36	0.2%
50	Hawaii	26	0.1%
	District of Columbia	7	0.0%

Source: U.S. Department of Health and Human Services, National Center for Health Statistics
   "National Vital Statistics Reports" (Vol. 50, No. 15, September 16, 2002)
*Final data. Deaths of infants under 1 year old, exclusive of fetal deaths. Based on race of the mother.

White Infant Mortality Rate in 2000

National Rate = 5.7 White Infant Deaths per 1,000 White Live Births*

ALPHA ORDER

RANK	STATE	RATE
11	Alabama	6.6
29	Alaska	5.8
20	Arizona	6.2
6	Arkansas	7.0
41	California	5.1
31	Colorado	5.6
31	Connecticut	5.6
1	Delaware	7.9
37	Florida	5.4
25	Georgia	5.9
13	Hawaii	6.5
3	Idaho	7.5
11	Illinois	6.6
7	Indiana	6.9
22	Iowa	6.0
15	Kansas	6.4
10	Kentucky	6.7
25	Louisiana	5.9
46	Maine	4.8
46	Maryland	4.8
50	Massachusetts	4.0
22	Michigan	6.0
46	Minnesota	4.8
8	Mississippi	6.8
25	Missouri	5.9
33	Montana	5.5
15	Nebraska	6.4
22	Nevada	6.0
33	New Hampshire	5.5
44	New Jersey	5.0
17	New Mexico	6.3
37	New York	5.4
17	North Carolina	6.3
3	North Dakota	7.5
17	Ohio	6.3
1	Oklahoma	7.9
33	Oregon	5.5
29	Pennsylvania	5.8
25	Rhode Island	5.9
37	South Carolina	5.4
49	South Dakota	4.3
8	Tennessee	6.8
41	Texas	5.1
41	Utah	5.1
21	Vermont	6.1
37	Virginia	5.4
45	Washington	4.9
5	West Virginia	7.4
33	Wisconsin	5.5
13	Wyoming	6.5

RANK ORDER

RANK	STATE	RATE
1	Delaware	7.9
1	Oklahoma	7.9
3	Idaho	7.5
3	North Dakota	7.5
5	West Virginia	7.4
6	Arkansas	7.0
7	Indiana	6.9
8	Mississippi	6.8
8	Tennessee	6.8
10	Kentucky	6.7
11	Alabama	6.6
11	Illinois	6.6
13	Hawaii	6.5
13	Wyoming	6.5
15	Kansas	6.4
15	Nebraska	6.4
17	New Mexico	6.3
17	North Carolina	6.3
17	Ohio	6.3
20	Arizona	6.2
21	Vermont	6.1
22	Iowa	6.0
22	Michigan	6.0
22	Nevada	6.0
25	Georgia	5.9
25	Louisiana	5.9
25	Missouri	5.9
25	Rhode Island	5.9
29	Alaska	5.8
29	Pennsylvania	5.8
31	Colorado	5.6
31	Connecticut	5.6
33	Montana	5.5
33	New Hampshire	5.5
33	Oregon	5.5
33	Wisconsin	5.5
37	Florida	5.4
37	New York	5.4
37	South Carolina	5.4
37	Virginia	5.4
41	California	5.1
41	Texas	5.1
41	Utah	5.1
44	New Jersey	5.0
45	Washington	4.9
46	Maine	4.8
46	Maryland	4.8
46	Minnesota	4.8
49	South Dakota	4.3
50	Massachusetts	4.0

District of Columbia**   NA

Source: U.S. Department of Health and Human Services, National Center for Health Statistics
   "National Vital Statistics Reports" (Vol. 50, No. 15, September 16, 2002)
*Final data. Deaths of infants under 1 year old, exclusive of fetal deaths. Based on race of the mother.
**Not available, fewer than 20 white infant deaths.

Black Infant Deaths in 2000

National Total = 8,771 Deaths*

ALPHA ORDER

RANK	STATE	DEATHS	% of USA
13	Alabama	315	3.6%
41	Alaska	6	0.1%
29	Arizona	49	0.6%
22	Arkansas	109	1.2%
7	California	453	5.2%
28	Colorado	59	0.7%
25	Connecticut	76	0.9%
30	Delaware	39	0.4%
3	Florida	595	6.8%
1	Georgia	614	7.0%
39	Hawaii	8	0.1%
48	Idaho	0	0.0%
4	Illinois	587	6.7%
20	Indiana	150	1.7%
35	Iowa	26	0.3%
31	Kansas	35	0.4%
26	Kentucky	65	0.7%
9	Louisiana	377	4.3%
44	Maine	2	0.0%
11	Maryland	328	3.7%
24	Massachusetts	80	0.9%
8	Michigan	443	5.1%
26	Minnesota	65	0.7%
14	Mississippi	305	3.5%
19	Missouri	169	1.9%
45	Montana	1	0.0%
34	Nebraska	28	0.3%
33	Nevada	30	0.3%
43	New Hampshire	5	0.1%
17	New Jersey	288	3.3%
39	New Mexico	8	0.1%
2	New York	600	6.8%
6	North Carolina	461	5.3%
45	North Dakota	1	0.0%
10	Ohio	366	4.2%
23	Oklahoma	81	0.9%
36	Oregon	16	0.2%
12	Pennsylvania	324	3.7%
37	Rhode Island	14	0.2%
16	South Carolina	293	3.3%
48	South Dakota	0	0.0%
14	Tennessee	305	3.5%
5	Texas	471	5.4%
41	Utah	6	0.1%
48	Vermont	0	0.0%
18	Virginia	279	3.2%
32	Washington	33	0.4%
38	West Virginia	10	0.1%
21	Wisconsin	112	1.3%
45	Wyoming	1	0.0%

RANK ORDER

RANK	STATE	DEATHS	% of USA
1	Georgia	614	7.0%
2	New York	600	6.8%
3	Florida	595	6.8%
4	Illinois	587	6.7%
5	Texas	471	5.4%
6	North Carolina	461	5.3%
7	California	453	5.2%
8	Michigan	443	5.1%
9	Louisiana	377	4.3%
10	Ohio	366	4.2%
11	Maryland	328	3.7%
12	Pennsylvania	324	3.7%
13	Alabama	315	3.6%
14	Mississippi	305	3.5%
14	Tennessee	305	3.5%
16	South Carolina	293	3.3%
17	New Jersey	288	3.3%
18	Virginia	279	3.2%
19	Missouri	169	1.9%
20	Indiana	150	1.7%
21	Wisconsin	112	1.3%
22	Arkansas	109	1.2%
23	Oklahoma	81	0.9%
24	Massachusetts	80	0.9%
25	Connecticut	76	0.9%
26	Kentucky	65	0.7%
26	Minnesota	65	0.7%
28	Colorado	59	0.7%
29	Arizona	49	0.6%
30	Delaware	39	0.4%
31	Kansas	35	0.4%
32	Washington	33	0.4%
33	Nevada	30	0.3%
34	Nebraska	28	0.3%
35	Iowa	26	0.3%
36	Oregon	16	0.2%
37	Rhode Island	14	0.2%
38	West Virginia	10	0.1%
39	Hawaii	8	0.1%
39	New Mexico	8	0.1%
41	Alaska	6	0.1%
41	Utah	6	0.1%
43	New Hampshire	5	0.1%
44	Maine	2	0.0%
45	Montana	1	0.0%
45	North Dakota	1	0.0%
45	Wyoming	1	0.0%
48	Idaho	0	0.0%
48	South Dakota	0	0.0%
48	Vermont	0	0.0%
	District of Columbia	83	0.9%

Source: U.S. Department of Health and Human Services, National Center for Health Statistics
  "National Vital Statistics Reports" (Vol. 50, No. 15, September 16, 2002)
*Final data. Deaths of infants under 1 year old, exclusive of fetal deaths. Based on race of the mother.

Black Infant Mortality Rate in 2000

National Rate = 14.1 Black Infant Deaths per 1,000 Black Live Births*

ALPHA ORDER

RANK	STATE	RATE
13	Alabama	15.4
NA	Alaska**	NA
6	Arizona	17.6
22	Arkansas	13.7
26	California	12.9
3	Colorado	19.5
20	Connecticut	14.4
16	Delaware	14.8
29	Florida	12.6
21	Georgia	13.9
NA	Hawaii**	NA
NA	Idaho**	NA
8	Illinois	17.1
10	Indiana	15.8
1	Iowa	21.1
31	Kansas	12.2
27	Kentucky	12.7
24	Louisiana	13.3
NA	Maine**	NA
25	Maryland	13.2
34	Massachusetts	9.9
4	Michigan	18.2
19	Minnesota	14.6
15	Mississippi	15.3
18	Missouri	14.7
NA	Montana**	NA
2	Nebraska	20.3
27	Nevada	12.7
NA	New Hampshire**	NA
23	New Jersey	13.6
NA	New Mexico**	NA
33	New York	10.9
11	North Carolina	15.7
NA	North Dakota**	NA
13	Ohio	15.4
9	Oklahoma	16.9
NA	Oregon**	NA
11	Pennsylvania	15.7
NA	Rhode Island**	NA
16	South Carolina	14.8
NA	South Dakota**	NA
5	Tennessee	18.0
32	Texas	11.4
NA	Utah**	NA
NA	Vermont**	NA
30	Virginia	12.4
35	Washington	9.4
NA	West Virginia**	NA
7	Wisconsin	17.2
NA	Wyoming**	NA

RANK ORDER

RANK	STATE	RATE
1	Iowa	21.1
2	Nebraska	20.3
3	Colorado	19.5
4	Michigan	18.2
5	Tennessee	18.0
6	Arizona	17.6
7	Wisconsin	17.2
8	Illinois	17.1
9	Oklahoma	16.9
10	Indiana	15.8
11	North Carolina	15.7
11	Pennsylvania	15.7
13	Alabama	15.4
13	Ohio	15.4
15	Mississippi	15.3
16	Delaware	14.8
16	South Carolina	14.8
18	Missouri	14.7
19	Minnesota	14.6
20	Connecticut	14.4
21	Georgia	13.9
22	Arkansas	13.7
23	New Jersey	13.6
24	Louisiana	13.3
25	Maryland	13.2
26	California	12.9
27	Kentucky	12.7
27	Nevada	12.7
29	Florida	12.6
30	Virginia	12.4
31	Kansas	12.2
32	Texas	11.4
33	New York	10.9
34	Massachusetts	9.9
35	Washington	9.4
NA	Alaska**	NA
NA	Hawaii**	NA
NA	Idaho**	NA
NA	Maine**	NA
NA	Montana**	NA
NA	New Hampshire**	NA
NA	New Mexico**	NA
NA	North Dakota**	NA
NA	Oregon**	NA
NA	Rhode Island**	NA
NA	South Dakota**	NA
NA	Utah**	NA
NA	Vermont**	NA
NA	West Virginia**	NA
NA	Wyoming**	NA

District of Columbia	16.1

Source: U.S. Department of Health and Human Services, National Center for Health Statistics
    "National Vital Statistics Reports" (Vol. 50, No. 15, September 16, 2002)
*Final data. Deaths of infants under 1 year old, exclusive of fetal deaths. Based on race of the mother.
**Not available, fewer than 20 black infant deaths.

Percent Change in White Infant Mortality Rate: 1990 to 2000

National Percent Change = 26.0% Decrease*

RANK	STATE	PERCENT CHANGE
16	Alabama	(20.5)
40	Alaska	(31.8)
26	Arizona	(24.4)
6	Arkansas	(12.5)
43	California	(32.9)
44	Colorado	(33.3)
10	Connecticut	(15.2)
2	Delaware	8.2
36	Florida	(28.9)
46	Georgia	(35.2)
1	Hawaii	27.5
7	Idaho	(13.8)
8	Illinois	(14.3)
17	Indiana	(22.5)
20	Iowa	(23.1)
13	Kansas	(16.9)
12	Kentucky	(16.3)
14	Louisiana	(19.2)
18	Maine	(22.6)
31	Maryland	(26.2)
49	Massachusetts	(40.3)
24	Michigan	(24.1)
35	Minnesota	(28.4)
15	Mississippi	(20.0)
26	Missouri	(24.4)
48	Montana	(36.0)
5	Nebraska	(11.1)
29	Nevada	(25.9)
22	New Hampshire	(23.6)
32	New Jersey	(26.5)
42	New Mexico	(32.3)
38	New York	(29.9)
24	North Carolina	(24.1)
3	North Dakota	(5.1)
21	Ohio	(23.2)
11	Oklahoma	(16.0)
41	Oregon	(32.1)
28	Pennsylvania	(25.6)
36	Rhode Island	(28.9)
45	South Carolina	(34.9)
50	South Dakota	(50.0)
9	Tennessee	(15.0)
34	Texas	(28.2)
39	Utah	(31.1)
4	Vermont	(6.2)
33	Virginia	(28.0)
47	Washington	(35.5)
19	West Virginia	(22.9)
22	Wisconsin	(23.6)
30	Wyoming	(26.1)

RANK	STATE	PERCENT CHANGE
1	Hawaii	27.5
2	Delaware	8.2
3	North Dakota	(5.1)
4	Vermont	(6.2)
5	Nebraska	(11.1)
6	Arkansas	(12.5)
7	Idaho	(13.8)
8	Illinois	(14.3)
9	Tennessee	(15.0)
10	Connecticut	(15.2)
11	Oklahoma	(16.0)
12	Kentucky	(16.3)
13	Kansas	(16.9)
14	Louisiana	(19.2)
15	Mississippi	(20.0)
16	Alabama	(20.5)
17	Indiana	(22.5)
18	Maine	(22.6)
19	West Virginia	(22.9)
20	Iowa	(23.1)
21	Ohio	(23.2)
22	New Hampshire	(23.6)
22	Wisconsin	(23.6)
24	Michigan	(24.1)
24	North Carolina	(24.1)
26	Arizona	(24.4)
26	Missouri	(24.4)
28	Pennsylvania	(25.6)
29	Nevada	(25.9)
30	Wyoming	(26.1)
31	Maryland	(26.2)
32	New Jersey	(26.5)
33	Virginia	(28.0)
34	Texas	(28.2)
35	Minnesota	(28.4)
36	Florida	(28.9)
36	Rhode Island	(28.9)
38	New York	(29.9)
39	Utah	(31.1)
40	Alaska	(31.8)
41	Oregon	(32.1)
42	New Mexico	(32.3)
43	California	(32.9)
44	Colorado	(33.3)
45	South Carolina	(34.9)
46	Georgia	(35.2)
47	Washington	(35.5)
48	Montana	(36.0)
49	Massachusetts	(40.3)
50	South Dakota	(50.0)

District of Columbia**   NA

Source: Morgan Quitno Press using data from US Dept of Health & Human Services, National Center for Health Statistics
"National Vital Statistics Reports" (Vol. 50, No. 15, September 16, 2002) and "Vital Statistics of the United States"
*Final data. Deaths of infants under 1 year old, exclusive of fetal deaths. Based on race of the mother.
**Not available, fewer than 20 white infant deaths.

Percent Change in Black Infant Mortality Rate: 1990 to 2000

National Percent Change = 17.1% Decrease*

ALPHA ORDER

RANK	STATE	RCENT CHANGE
11	Alabama	(3.1)
NA	Alaska**	NA
5	Arizona	5.4
8	Arkansas	0.7
16	California	(9.2)
3	Colorado	18.2
17	Connecticut	(10.0)
31	Delaware	(23.7)
29	Florida	(22.2)
30	Georgia	(22.8)
NA	Hawaii**	NA
NA	Idaho**	NA
26	Illinois	(20.5)
9	Indiana	(1.2)
4	Iowa	17.2
27	Kansas	(20.8)
15	Kentucky	(6.6)
25	Louisiana	(19.4)
NA	Maine**	NA
24	Maryland	(19.0)
12	Massachusetts	(4.8)
18	Michigan	(13.3)
32	Minnesota	(25.9)
13	Mississippi	(5.0)
21	Missouri	(16.0)
NA	Montana**	NA
2	Nebraska	20.8
7	Nevada	1.6
NA	New Hampshire**	NA
28	New Jersey	(21.4)
NA	New Mexico**	NA
35	New York	(37.0)
10	North Carolina	(1.9)
NA	North Dakota**	NA
20	Ohio	(15.8)
1	Oklahoma	28.0
NA	Oregon**	NA
22	Pennsylvania	(16.5)
NA	Rhode Island**	NA
19	South Carolina	(13.5)
NA	South Dakota**	NA
6	Tennessee	2.9
23	Texas	(18.0)
NA	Utah**	NA
NA	Vermont**	NA
33	Virginia	(34.0)
34	Washington	(35.2)
NA	West Virginia**	NA
13	Wisconsin	(5.0)
NA	Wyoming**	NA

RANK ORDER

RANK	STATE	PERCENT CHANGE
1	Oklahoma	28.0
2	Nebraska	20.8
3	Colorado	18.2
4	Iowa	17.2
5	Arizona	5.4
6	Tennessee	2.9
7	Nevada	1.6
8	Arkansas	0.7
9	Indiana	(1.2)
10	North Carolina	(1.9)
11	Alabama	(3.1)
12	Massachusetts	(4.8)
13	Mississippi	(5.0)
13	Wisconsin	(5.0)
15	Kentucky	(6.6)
16	California	(9.2)
17	Connecticut	(10.0)
18	Michigan	(13.3)
19	South Carolina	(13.5)
20	Ohio	(15.8)
21	Missouri	(16.0)
22	Pennsylvania	(16.5)
23	Texas	(18.0)
24	Maryland	(19.0)
25	Louisiana	(19.4)
26	Illinois	(20.5)
27	Kansas	(20.8)
28	New Jersey	(21.4)
29	Florida	(22.2)
30	Georgia	(22.8)
31	Delaware	(23.7)
32	Minnesota	(25.9)
33	Virginia	(34.0)
34	Washington	(35.2)
35	New York	(37.0)
NA	Alaska**	NA
NA	Hawaii**	NA
NA	Idaho**	NA
NA	Maine**	NA
NA	Montana**	NA
NA	New Hampshire**	NA
NA	New Mexico**	NA
NA	North Dakota**	NA
NA	Oregon**	NA
NA	Rhode Island**	NA
NA	South Dakota**	NA
NA	Utah**	NA
NA	Vermont**	NA
NA	West Virginia**	NA
NA	Wyoming**	NA

District of Columbia (34.0)

Source: Morgan Quitno Press using data from US Dept of Health & Human Services, National Center for Health Statistics "National Vital Statistics Reports" (Vol. 50, No. 15, September 16, 2002) and "Vital Statistics of the United States"
*Final data. Deaths of infants under 1 year old, exclusive of fetal deaths. Based on race of the mother.
**Not available, fewer than 20 black infant deaths.

Neonatal Deaths in 2000

National Total = 18,776 Deaths*

ALPHA ORDER

RANK	STATE	DEATHS	% of USA
17	Alabama	369	2.0%
47	Alaska	35	0.2%
18	Arizona	367	2.0%
30	Arkansas	183	1.0%
1	California	1,960	10.4%
24	Colorado	281	1.5%
29	Connecticut	214	1.1%
41	Delaware	71	0.4%
5	Florida	925	4.9%
8	Georgia	758	4.0%
38	Hawaii	107	0.6%
37	Idaho	109	0.6%
4	Illinois	1,072	5.7%
14	Indiana	464	2.5%
34	Iowa	162	0.9%
31	Kansas	176	0.9%
26	Kentucky	256	1.4%
16	Louisiana	394	2.1%
44	Maine	47	0.3%
15	Maryland	416	2.2%
23	Massachusetts	288	1.5%
7	Michigan	781	4.2%
27	Minnesota	252	1.3%
22	Mississippi	289	1.5%
19	Missouri	362	1.9%
45	Montana	44	0.2%
36	Nebraska	120	0.6%
35	Nevada	126	0.7%
43	New Hampshire	59	0.3%
11	New Jersey	500	2.7%
40	New Mexico	101	0.5%
3	New York	1,178	6.3%
9	North Carolina	747	4.0%
46	North Dakota	41	0.2%
6	Ohio	826	4.4%
25	Oklahoma	259	1.4%
33	Oregon	165	0.9%
10	Pennsylvania	729	3.9%
42	Rhode Island	62	0.3%
20	South Carolina	341	1.8%
48	South Dakota	32	0.2%
13	Tennessee	472	2.5%
2	Texas	1,225	6.5%
32	Utah	166	0.9%
50	Vermont	25	0.1%
12	Virginia	473	2.5%
28	Washington	245	1.3%
39	West Virginia	103	0.5%
21	Wisconsin	302	1.6%
49	Wyoming	29	0.2%

RANK ORDER

RANK	STATE	DEATHS	% of USA
1	California	1,960	10.4%
2	Texas	1,225	6.5%
3	New York	1,178	6.3%
4	Illinois	1,072	5.7%
5	Florida	925	4.9%
6	Ohio	826	4.4%
7	Michigan	781	4.2%
8	Georgia	758	4.0%
9	North Carolina	747	4.0%
10	Pennsylvania	729	3.9%
11	New Jersey	500	2.7%
12	Virginia	473	2.5%
13	Tennessee	472	2.5%
14	Indiana	464	2.5%
15	Maryland	416	2.2%
16	Louisiana	394	2.1%
17	Alabama	369	2.0%
18	Arizona	367	2.0%
19	Missouri	362	1.9%
20	South Carolina	341	1.8%
21	Wisconsin	302	1.6%
22	Mississippi	289	1.5%
23	Massachusetts	288	1.5%
24	Colorado	281	1.5%
25	Oklahoma	259	1.4%
26	Kentucky	256	1.4%
27	Minnesota	252	1.3%
28	Washington	245	1.3%
29	Connecticut	214	1.1%
30	Arkansas	183	1.0%
31	Kansas	176	0.9%
32	Utah	166	0.9%
33	Oregon	165	0.9%
34	Iowa	162	0.9%
35	Nevada	126	0.7%
36	Nebraska	120	0.6%
37	Idaho	109	0.6%
38	Hawaii	107	0.6%
39	West Virginia	103	0.5%
40	New Mexico	101	0.5%
41	Delaware	71	0.4%
42	Rhode Island	62	0.3%
43	New Hampshire	59	0.3%
44	Maine	47	0.3%
45	Montana	44	0.2%
46	North Dakota	41	0.2%
47	Alaska	35	0.2%
48	South Dakota	32	0.2%
49	Wyoming	29	0.2%
50	Vermont	25	0.1%
	District of Columbia	68	0.4%

Source: U.S. Department of Health and Human Services, National Center for Health Statistics
"National Vital Statistics Reports" (Vol. 50, No. 15, September 16, 2002)
*Final data. Deaths of infants under 28 days, exclusive of fetal deaths.

Neonatal Death Rate in 2000

National Rate = 4.6 Deaths per 1,000 Live Births*

ALPHA ORDER

RANK	STATE	RATE
7	Alabama	5.8
44	Alaska	3.5
32	Arizona	4.3
23	Arkansas	4.8
40	California	3.7
32	Colorado	4.3
18	Connecticut	5.0
2	Delaware	6.4
29	Florida	4.5
10	Georgia	5.7
4	Hawaii	6.1
13	Idaho	5.4
7	Illinois	5.8
14	Indiana	5.3
35	Iowa	4.2
30	Kansas	4.4
26	Kentucky	4.6
7	Louisiana	5.8
44	Maine	3.5
12	Maryland	5.6
44	Massachusetts	3.5
10	Michigan	5.7
40	Minnesota	3.7
1	Mississippi	6.6
25	Missouri	4.7
37	Montana	4.0
21	Nebraska	4.9
36	Nevada	4.1
37	New Hampshire	4.0
32	New Jersey	4.3
40	New Mexico	3.7
26	New York	4.6
3	North Carolina	6.2
14	North Dakota	5.3
14	Ohio	5.3
17	Oklahoma	5.2
43	Oregon	3.6
18	Pennsylvania	5.0
18	Rhode Island	5.0
4	South Carolina	6.1
49	South Dakota	3.1
6	Tennessee	5.9
48	Texas	3.4
44	Utah	3.5
39	Vermont	3.8
23	Virginia	4.8
50	Washington	3.0
21	West Virginia	4.9
30	Wisconsin	4.4
26	Wyoming	4.6

RANK ORDER

RANK	STATE	RATE
1	Mississippi	6.6
2	Delaware	6.4
3	North Carolina	6.2
4	Hawaii	6.1
4	South Carolina	6.1
6	Tennessee	5.9
7	Alabama	5.8
7	Illinois	5.8
7	Louisiana	5.8
10	Georgia	5.7
10	Michigan	5.7
12	Maryland	5.6
13	Idaho	5.4
14	Indiana	5.3
14	North Dakota	5.3
14	Ohio	5.3
17	Oklahoma	5.2
18	Connecticut	5.0
18	Pennsylvania	5.0
18	Rhode Island	5.0
21	Nebraska	4.9
21	West Virginia	4.9
23	Arkansas	4.8
23	Virginia	4.8
25	Missouri	4.7
26	Kentucky	4.6
26	New York	4.6
26	Wyoming	4.6
29	Florida	4.5
30	Kansas	4.4
30	Wisconsin	4.4
32	Arizona	4.3
32	Colorado	4.3
32	New Jersey	4.3
35	Iowa	4.2
36	Nevada	4.1
37	Montana	4.0
37	New Hampshire	4.0
39	Vermont	3.8
40	California	3.7
40	Minnesota	3.7
40	New Mexico	3.7
43	Oregon	3.6
44	Alaska	3.5
44	Maine	3.5
44	Massachusetts	3.5
44	Utah	3.5
48	Texas	3.4
49	South Dakota	3.1
50	Washington	3.0
	District of Columbia	8.9

Source: U.S. Department of Health and Human Services, National Center for Health Statistics
    "National Vital Statistics Reports" (Vol. 50, No. 15, September 16, 2002)
*Final data. Deaths of infants under 28 days, exclusive of fetal deaths.

White Neonatal Deaths in 2000

National Total = 12,201 Deaths*

ALPHA ORDER

RANK	STATE	DEATHS	% of USA
24	Alabama	168	1.4%
50	Alaska	21	0.2%
12	Arizona	299	2.5%
33	Arkansas	109	0.9%
1	California	1,492	12.2%
17	Colorado	230	1.9%
26	Connecticut	157	1.3%
43	Delaware	43	0.4%
6	Florida	529	4.3%
11	Georgia	333	2.7%
49	Hawaii	22	0.2%
34	Idaho	105	0.9%
4	Illinois	669	5.5%
10	Indiana	373	3.1%
31	Iowa	141	1.2%
29	Kansas	144	1.2%
20	Kentucky	209	1.7%
29	Louisiana	144	1.2%
42	Maine	46	0.4%
25	Maryland	163	1.3%
19	Massachusetts	211	1.7%
8	Michigan	451	3.7%
23	Minnesota	189	1.5%
38	Mississippi	91	0.7%
16	Missouri	245	2.0%
45	Montana	32	0.3%
36	Nebraska	97	0.8%
34	Nevada	105	0.9%
40	New Hampshire	55	0.5%
13	New Jersey	297	2.4%
39	New Mexico	84	0.7%
3	New York	701	5.7%
9	North Carolina	397	3.3%
44	North Dakota	33	0.3%
5	Ohio	566	4.6%
22	Oklahoma	192	1.6%
27	Oregon	150	1.2%
7	Pennsylvania	507	4.2%
41	Rhode Island	48	0.4%
32	South Carolina	135	1.1%
48	South Dakota	24	0.2%
15	Tennessee	266	2.2%
2	Texas	933	7.6%
27	Utah	150	1.2%
47	Vermont	25	0.2%
14	Virginia	268	2.2%
21	Washington	199	1.6%
37	West Virginia	95	0.8%
18	Wisconsin	224	1.8%
46	Wyoming	27	0.2%

RANK ORDER

RANK	STATE	DEATHS	% of USA
1	California	1,492	12.2%
2	Texas	933	7.6%
3	New York	701	5.7%
4	Illinois	669	5.5%
5	Ohio	566	4.6%
6	Florida	529	4.3%
7	Pennsylvania	507	4.2%
8	Michigan	451	3.7%
9	North Carolina	397	3.3%
10	Indiana	373	3.1%
11	Georgia	333	2.7%
12	Arizona	299	2.5%
13	New Jersey	297	2.4%
14	Virginia	268	2.2%
15	Tennessee	266	2.2%
16	Missouri	245	2.0%
17	Colorado	230	1.9%
18	Wisconsin	224	1.8%
19	Massachusetts	211	1.7%
20	Kentucky	209	1.7%
21	Washington	199	1.6%
22	Oklahoma	192	1.6%
23	Minnesota	189	1.5%
24	Alabama	168	1.4%
25	Maryland	163	1.3%
26	Connecticut	157	1.3%
27	Oregon	150	1.2%
27	Utah	150	1.2%
29	Kansas	144	1.2%
29	Louisiana	144	1.2%
31	Iowa	141	1.2%
32	South Carolina	135	1.1%
33	Arkansas	109	0.9%
34	Idaho	105	0.9%
34	Nevada	105	0.9%
36	Nebraska	97	0.8%
37	West Virginia	95	0.8%
38	Mississippi	91	0.7%
39	New Mexico	84	0.7%
40	New Hampshire	55	0.5%
41	Rhode Island	48	0.4%
42	Maine	46	0.4%
43	Delaware	43	0.4%
44	North Dakota	33	0.3%
45	Montana	32	0.3%
46	Wyoming	27	0.2%
47	Vermont	25	0.2%
48	South Dakota	24	0.2%
49	Hawaii	22	0.2%
50	Alaska	21	0.2%
	District of Columbia	7	0.1%

Source: U.S. Department of Health and Human Services, National Center for Health Statistics
"National Vital Statistics Reports" (Vol. 50, No. 15, September 16, 2002)
*Final data. Deaths of infants under 28 days, exclusive of fetal deaths. Based on race of the mother.

White Neonatal Death Rate in 2000

National Rate = 3.8 White Neonatal Deaths per 1,000 White Live Births*

ALPHA ORDER			RANK ORDER		
RANK	STATE	RATE	RANK	STATE	RATE
20	Alabama	4.0	1	Hawaii	5.5
44	Alaska	3.3	2	Delaware	5.4
20	Arizona	4.0	3	Idaho	5.3
34	Arkansas	3.7	4	Oklahoma	5.0
39	California	3.5	5	Indiana	4.9
23	Colorado	3.9	5	North Dakota	4.9
11	Connecticut	4.4	7	West Virginia	4.8
2	Delaware	5.4	8	Illinois	4.7
39	Florida	3.5	9	North Carolina	4.6
23	Georgia	3.9	9	Wyoming	4.6
1	Hawaii	5.5	11	Connecticut	4.4
3	Idaho	5.3	11	Nebraska	4.4
8	Illinois	4.7	11	Ohio	4.4
5	Indiana	4.9	11	Rhode Island	4.4
23	Iowa	3.9	15	Tennessee	4.3
19	Kansas	4.1	16	Kentucky	4.2
16	Kentucky	4.2	16	Michigan	4.2
30	Louisiana	3.8	16	Pennsylvania	4.2
39	Maine	3.5	19	Kansas	4.1
37	Maryland	3.6	20	Alabama	4.0
47	Massachusetts	3.1	20	Arizona	4.0
16	Michigan	4.2	20	Nevada	4.0
46	Minnesota	3.2	23	Colorado	3.9
23	Mississippi	3.9	23	Georgia	3.9
23	Missouri	3.9	23	Iowa	3.9
43	Montana	3.4	23	Mississippi	3.9
11	Nebraska	4.4	23	Missouri	3.9
20	Nevada	4.0	23	New Hampshire	3.9
23	New Hampshire	3.9	23	Vermont	3.9
39	New Jersey	3.5	30	Louisiana	3.8
34	New Mexico	3.7	30	New York	3.8
30	New York	3.8	30	South Carolina	3.8
9	North Carolina	4.6	30	Virginia	3.8
5	North Dakota	4.9	34	Arkansas	3.7
11	Ohio	4.4	34	New Mexico	3.7
4	Oklahoma	5.0	34	Wisconsin	3.7
37	Oregon	3.6	37	Maryland	3.6
16	Pennsylvania	4.2	37	Oregon	3.6
11	Rhode Island	4.4	39	California	3.5
30	South Carolina	3.8	39	Florida	3.5
50	South Dakota	2.8	39	Maine	3.5
15	Tennessee	4.3	39	New Jersey	3.5
48	Texas	3.0	43	Montana	3.4
44	Utah	3.3	44	Alaska	3.3
23	Vermont	3.9	44	Utah	3.3
30	Virginia	3.8	46	Minnesota	3.2
49	Washington	2.9	47	Massachusetts	3.1
7	West Virginia	4.8	48	Texas	3.0
34	Wisconsin	3.7	49	Washington	2.9
9	Wyoming	4.6	50	South Dakota	2.8
				District of Columbia**	NA

Source: U.S. Department of Health and Human Services, National Center for Health Statistics
   "National Vital Statistics Reports" (Vol. 50, No. 15, September 16, 2002)
*Final data. Deaths of infants under 28 days, exclusive of fetal deaths. Based on race of the mother.
**Not available. Fewer than 20 white neonatal deaths.

Black Neonatal Deaths in 2000

National Total = 5,843 Deaths*

ALPHA ORDER

RANK ORDER

RANK	STATE	DEATHS	% of USA
15	Alabama	201	3.4%
43	Alaska	2	0.0%
30	Arizona	27	0.5%
21	Arkansas	73	1.2%
7	California	290	5.0%
28	Colorado	43	0.7%
24	Connecticut	52	0.9%
29	Delaware	28	0.5%
3	Florida	384	6.6%
2	Georgia	415	7.1%
39	Hawaii	7	0.1%
46	Idaho	0	0.0%
4	Illinois	371	6.3%
20	Indiana	88	1.5%
33	Iowa	17	0.3%
31	Kansas	26	0.4%
25	Kentucky	46	0.8%
10	Louisiana	245	4.2%
46	Maine	0	0.0%
11	Maryland	244	4.2%
23	Massachusetts	62	1.1%
6	Michigan	313	5.4%
27	Minnesota	44	0.8%
16	Mississippi	195	3.3%
19	Missouri	114	2.0%
44	Montana	1	0.0%
32	Nebraska	19	0.3%
35	Nevada	13	0.2%
42	New Hampshire	3	0.1%
17	New Jersey	189	3.2%
40	New Mexico	6	0.1%
1	New York	430	7.4%
5	North Carolina	328	5.6%
44	North Dakota	1	0.0%
9	Ohio	253	4.3%
25	Oklahoma	46	0.8%
37	Oregon	11	0.2%
12	Pennsylvania	214	3.7%
35	Rhode Island	13	0.2%
13	South Carolina	204	3.5%
46	South Dakota	0	0.0%
14	Tennessee	203	3.5%
8	Texas	275	4.7%
41	Utah	5	0.1%
46	Vermont	0	0.0%
17	Virginia	189	3.2%
34	Washington	16	0.3%
38	West Virginia	8	0.1%
22	Wisconsin	68	1.2%
46	Wyoming	0	0.0%

RANK	STATE	DEATHS	% of USA
1	New York	430	7.4%
2	Georgia	415	7.1%
3	Florida	384	6.6%
4	Illinois	371	6.3%
5	North Carolina	328	5.6%
6	Michigan	313	5.4%
7	California	290	5.0%
8	Texas	275	4.7%
9	Ohio	253	4.3%
10	Louisiana	245	4.2%
11	Maryland	244	4.2%
12	Pennsylvania	214	3.7%
13	South Carolina	204	3.5%
14	Tennessee	203	3.5%
15	Alabama	201	3.4%
16	Mississippi	195	3.3%
17	New Jersey	189	3.2%
17	Virginia	189	3.2%
19	Missouri	114	2.0%
20	Indiana	88	1.5%
21	Arkansas	73	1.2%
22	Wisconsin	68	1.2%
23	Massachusetts	62	1.1%
24	Connecticut	52	0.9%
25	Kentucky	46	0.8%
25	Oklahoma	46	0.8%
27	Minnesota	44	0.8%
28	Colorado	43	0.7%
29	Delaware	28	0.5%
30	Arizona	27	0.5%
31	Kansas	26	0.4%
32	Nebraska	19	0.3%
33	Iowa	17	0.3%
34	Washington	16	0.3%
35	Nevada	13	0.2%
35	Rhode Island	13	0.2%
37	Oregon	11	0.2%
38	West Virginia	8	0.1%
39	Hawaii	7	0.1%
40	New Mexico	6	0.1%
41	Utah	5	0.1%
42	New Hampshire	3	0.1%
43	Alaska	2	0.0%
44	Montana	1	0.0%
44	North Dakota	1	0.0%
46	Idaho	0	0.0%
46	Maine	0	0.0%
46	South Dakota	0	0.0%
46	Vermont	0	0.0%
46	Wyoming	0	0.0%
	District of Columbia	61	1.0%

Source: U.S. Department of Health and Human Services, National Center for Health Statistics
"National Vital Statistics Reports" (Vol. 50, No. 15, September 16, 2002)
*Final data. Deaths of infants under 28 days, exclusive of fetal deaths. Based on race of the mother.

Black Neonatal Death Rate in 2000

National Rate = 9.4 Black Neonatal Deaths per 1,000 Black Live Births*

ALPHA ORDER

RANK	STATE	RATE
14	Alabama	9.8
NA	Alaska**	NA
17	Arizona	9.7
20	Arkansas	9.2
27	California	8.3
1	Colorado	14.2
11	Connecticut	9.9
7	Delaware	10.6
28	Florida	8.1
19	Georgia	9.4
NA	Hawaii**	NA
NA	Idaho**	NA
5	Illinois	10.8
20	Indiana	9.2
NA	Iowa**	NA
22	Kansas	9.1
23	Kentucky	9.0
25	Louisiana	8.6
NA	Maine**	NA
14	Maryland	9.8
30	Massachusetts	7.7
2	Michigan	12.9
11	Minnesota	9.9
14	Mississippi	9.8
11	Missouri	9.9
NA	Montana**	NA
NA	Nebraska**	NA
NA	Nevada**	NA
NA	New Hampshire**	NA
24	New Jersey	8.9
NA	New Mexico**	NA
29	New York	7.8
4	North Carolina	11.2
NA	North Dakota**	NA
6	Ohio	10.7
18	Oklahoma	9.6
NA	Oregon**	NA
9	Pennsylvania	10.3
NA	Rhode Island**	NA
9	South Carolina	10.3
NA	South Dakota**	NA
3	Tennessee	12.0
31	Texas	6.7
NA	Utah**	NA
NA	Vermont**	NA
26	Virginia	8.4
NA	Washington**	NA
NA	West Virginia**	NA
8	Wisconsin	10.5
NA	Wyoming**	NA

RANK ORDER

RANK	STATE	RATE
1	Colorado	14.2
2	Michigan	12.9
3	Tennessee	12.0
4	North Carolina	11.2
5	Illinois	10.8
6	Ohio	10.7
7	Delaware	10.6
8	Wisconsin	10.5
9	Pennsylvania	10.3
9	South Carolina	10.3
11	Connecticut	9.9
11	Minnesota	9.9
11	Missouri	9.9
14	Alabama	9.8
14	Maryland	9.8
14	Mississippi	9.8
17	Arizona	9.7
18	Oklahoma	9.6
19	Georgia	9.4
20	Arkansas	9.2
20	Indiana	9.2
22	Kansas	9.1
23	Kentucky	9.0
24	New Jersey	8.9
25	Louisiana	8.6
26	Virginia	8.4
27	California	8.3
28	Florida	8.1
29	New York	7.8
30	Massachusetts	7.7
31	Texas	6.7
NA	Alaska**	NA
NA	Hawaii**	NA
NA	Idaho**	NA
NA	Iowa**	NA
NA	Maine**	NA
NA	Montana**	NA
NA	Nebraska**	NA
NA	Nevada**	NA
NA	New Hampshire**	NA
NA	New Mexico**	NA
NA	North Dakota**	NA
NA	Oregon**	NA
NA	Rhode Island**	NA
NA	South Dakota**	NA
NA	Utah**	NA
NA	Vermont**	NA
NA	Washington**	NA
NA	West Virginia**	NA
NA	Wyoming**	NA

District of Columbia 11.8

Source: U.S. Department of Health and Human Services, National Center for Health Statistics
   "National Vital Statistics Reports" (Vol. 50, No. 15, September 16, 2002)
*Final data. Deaths of infants under 28 days, exclusive of fetal deaths. Based on race of the mother.
**Not available. Fewer than 20 black neonatal deaths.

Deaths by AIDS in 2000

National Total = 14,478 Deaths*

ALPHA ORDER

ALPHA ORDER | | | | RANK ORDER | | | |

RANK	STATE	DEATHS	% of USA	RANK	STATE	DEATHS	% of USA
18	Alabama	203	1.4%	1	New York	2,233	15.4%
44	Alaska	11	0.1%	2	Florida	1,801	12.4%
22	Arizona	158	1.1%	3	California	1,467	10.1%
29	Arkansas	74	0.5%	4	Texas	1,083	7.5%
3	California	1,467	10.1%	5	New Jersey	830	5.7%
26	Colorado	91	0.6%	6	Georgia	744	5.1%
19	Connecticut	201	1.4%	7	Maryland	553	3.8%
31	Delaware	68	0.5%	8	Pennsylvania	501	3.5%
2	Florida	1,801	12.4%	9	Illinois	479	3.3%
6	Georgia	744	5.1%	10	North Carolina	465	3.2%
36	Hawaii	27	0.2%	11	Louisiana	386	2.7%
45	Idaho	10	0.1%	12	Tennessee	288	2.0%
9	Illinois	479	3.3%	12	Virginia	288	2.0%
24	Indiana	118	0.8%	14	South Carolina	261	1.8%
39	Iowa	23	0.2%	15	Ohio	250	1.7%
36	Kansas	27	0.2%	16	Michigan	247	1.7%
32	Kentucky	64	0.4%	17	Massachusetts	224	1.5%
11	Louisiana	386	2.7%	18	Alabama	203	1.4%
42	Maine	17	0.1%	19	Connecticut	201	1.4%
7	Maryland	553	3.8%	20	Missouri	163	1.1%
17	Massachusetts	224	1.5%	21	Mississippi	160	1.1%
16	Michigan	247	1.7%	22	Arizona	158	1.1%
30	Minnesota	71	0.5%	23	Washington	127	0.9%
21	Mississippi	160	1.1%	24	Indiana	118	0.8%
20	Missouri	163	1.1%	25	Oklahoma	110	0.8%
46	Montana	8	0.1%	26	Colorado	91	0.6%
38	Nebraska	25	0.2%	27	Nevada	89	0.6%
27	Nevada	89	0.6%	28	Wisconsin	75	0.5%
41	New Hampshire	18	0.1%	29	Arkansas	74	0.5%
5	New Jersey	830	5.7%	30	Minnesota	71	0.5%
35	New Mexico	31	0.2%	31	Delaware	68	0.5%
1	New York	2,233	15.4%	32	Kentucky	64	0.4%
10	North Carolina	465	3.2%	33	Oregon	60	0.4%
47	North Dakota	5	0.0%	34	Rhode Island	38	0.3%
15	Ohio	250	1.7%	35	New Mexico	31	0.2%
25	Oklahoma	110	0.8%	36	Hawaii	27	0.2%
33	Oregon	60	0.4%	36	Kansas	27	0.2%
8	Pennsylvania	501	3.5%	38	Nebraska	25	0.2%
34	Rhode Island	38	0.3%	39	Iowa	23	0.2%
14	South Carolina	261	1.8%	40	Utah	22	0.2%
49	South Dakota	4	0.0%	41	New Hampshire	18	0.1%
12	Tennessee	288	2.0%	42	Maine	17	0.1%
4	Texas	1,083	7.5%	43	West Virginia	16	0.1%
40	Utah	22	0.2%	44	Alaska	11	0.1%
47	Vermont	5	0.0%	45	Idaho	10	0.1%
12	Virginia	288	2.0%	46	Montana	8	0.1%
23	Washington	127	0.9%	47	North Dakota	5	0.0%
43	West Virginia	16	0.1%	47	Vermont	5	0.0%
28	Wisconsin	75	0.5%	49	South Dakota	4	0.0%
50	Wyoming	3	0.0%	50	Wyoming	3	0.0%
					District of Columbia	256	1.8%

Source: U.S. Department of Health and Human Services, National Center for Health Statistics
   "National Vital Statistics Reports" (Vol. 50, No. 15, September 16, 2002)
*AIDS is Acquired Immunodeficiency Syndrome. It is a specific group of diseases or conditions which are indicative
of severe immunosuppression related to infection with the Human Immunodeficiency Virus (HIV).

Death Rate by AIDS in 2000

National Rate = 5.3 Deaths per 100,000 Population*

ALPHA ORDER				RANK ORDER		
RANK	STATE	RATE		RANK	STATE	RATE
15	Alabama	4.6		1	New York	12.2
NA	Alaska**	NA		2	Florida	11.7
23	Arizona	3.2		3	Maryland	10.6
25	Arkansas	2.9		4	New Jersey	10.1
16	California	4.4		5	Georgia	9.4
28	Colorado	2.2		6	Delaware	8.9
9	Connecticut	6.1		7	Louisiana	8.8
6	Delaware	8.9		8	South Carolina	6.7
2	Florida	11.7		9	Connecticut	6.1
5	Georgia	9.4		10	North Carolina	6.0
27	Hawaii	2.3		11	Mississippi	5.7
NA	Idaho**	NA		12	Texas	5.3
19	Illinois	3.9		13	Tennessee	5.2
31	Indiana	2.0		14	Nevada	4.7
40	Iowa	0.8		15	Alabama	4.6
38	Kansas	1.0		16	California	4.4
34	Kentucky	1.6		17	Pennsylvania	4.2
7	Louisiana	8.8		18	Virginia	4.1
NA	Maine**	NA		19	Illinois	3.9
3	Maryland	10.6		20	Rhode Island	3.8
21	Massachusetts	3.6		21	Massachusetts	3.6
26	Michigan	2.5		22	Oklahoma	3.3
35	Minnesota	1.5		23	Arizona	3.2
11	Mississippi	5.7		24	Missouri	3.0
24	Missouri	3.0		25	Arkansas	2.9
NA	Montana**	NA		26	Michigan	2.5
35	Nebraska	1.5		27	Hawaii	2.3
14	Nevada	4.7		28	Colorado	2.2
NA	New Hampshire**	NA		28	Ohio	2.2
4	New Jersey	10.1		28	Washington	2.2
32	New Mexico	1.8		31	Indiana	2.0
1	New York	12.2		32	New Mexico	1.8
10	North Carolina	6.0		32	Oregon	1.8
NA	North Dakota**	NA		34	Kentucky	1.6
28	Ohio	2.2		35	Minnesota	1.5
22	Oklahoma	3.3		35	Nebraska	1.5
32	Oregon	1.8		37	Wisconsin	1.4
17	Pennsylvania	4.2		38	Kansas	1.0
20	Rhode Island	3.8		38	Utah	1.0
8	South Carolina	6.7		40	Iowa	0.8
NA	South Dakota**	NA		NA	Alaska**	NA
13	Tennessee	5.2		NA	Idaho**	NA
12	Texas	5.3		NA	Maine**	NA
38	Utah	1.0		NA	Montana**	NA
NA	Vermont**	NA		NA	New Hampshire**	NA
18	Virginia	4.1		NA	North Dakota**	NA
28	Washington	2.2		NA	South Dakota**	NA
NA	West Virginia**	NA		NA	Vermont**	NA
37	Wisconsin	1.4		NA	West Virginia**	NA
NA	Wyoming**	NA		NA	Wyoming**	NA
					District of Columbia	49.4

Source: U.S. Department of Health and Human Services, National Center for Health Statistics
    "National Vital Statistics Reports" (Vol. 50, No. 15, September 16, 2002)
*AIDS is Acquired Immunodeficiency Syndrome. It is a specific group of diseases or conditions which are indicative
of severe immunosuppression related to infection with the Human Immunodeficiency Virus (HIV). Not age-adjusted.
**Insufficient data to determine a reliable rate.

Age-Adjusted Death Rate by AIDS in 2000

National Rate = 5.3 Deaths per 100,000 Population*

ALPHA ORDER

ALPHA ORDER

RANK ORDER

RANK	STATE	RATE
15	Alabama	4.6
NA	Alaska**	NA
22	Arizona	3.4
24	Arkansas	3.0
16	California	4.4
29	Colorado	2.1
11	Connecticut	5.9
7	Delaware	8.6
1	Florida	12.1
6	Georgia	9.1
27	Hawaii	2.2
NA	Idaho**	NA
18	Illinois	3.9
31	Indiana	2.0
40	Iowa	0.8
39	Kansas	1.0
34	Kentucky	1.6
5	Louisiana	9.2
NA	Maine**	NA
3	Maryland	10.0
21	Massachusetts	3.5
26	Michigan	2.5
35	Minnesota	1.5
9	Mississippi	6.0
24	Missouri	3.0
NA	Montana**	NA
35	Nebraska	1.5
14	Nevada	4.7
NA	New Hampshire**	NA
4	New Jersey	9.8
32	New Mexico	1.8
2	New York	12.0
9	North Carolina	6.0
NA	North Dakota**	NA
27	Ohio	2.2
22	Oklahoma	3.4
32	Oregon	1.8
17	Pennsylvania	4.2
20	Rhode Island	3.7
8	South Carolina	6.5
NA	South Dakota**	NA
13	Tennessee	5.1
12	Texas	5.4
38	Utah	1.3
NA	Vermont**	NA
18	Virginia	3.9
29	Washington	2.1
NA	West Virginia**	NA
37	Wisconsin	1.4
NA	Wyoming**	NA

RANK	STATE	RATE
1	Florida	12.1
2	New York	12.0
3	Maryland	10.0
4	New Jersey	9.8
5	Louisiana	9.2
6	Georgia	9.1
7	Delaware	8.6
8	South Carolina	6.5
9	Mississippi	6.0
9	North Carolina	6.0
11	Connecticut	5.9
12	Texas	5.4
13	Tennessee	5.1
14	Nevada	4.7
15	Alabama	4.6
16	California	4.4
17	Pennsylvania	4.2
18	Illinois	3.9
18	Virginia	3.9
20	Rhode Island	3.7
21	Massachusetts	3.5
22	Arizona	3.4
22	Oklahoma	3.4
24	Arkansas	3.0
24	Missouri	3.0
26	Michigan	2.5
27	Hawaii	2.2
27	Ohio	2.2
29	Colorado	2.1
29	Washington	2.1
31	Indiana	2.0
32	New Mexico	1.8
32	Oregon	1.8
34	Kentucky	1.6
35	Minnesota	1.5
35	Nebraska	1.5
37	Wisconsin	1.4
38	Utah	1.3
39	Kansas	1.0
40	Iowa	0.8
NA	Alaska**	NA
NA	Idaho**	NA
NA	Maine**	NA
NA	Montana**	NA
NA	New Hampshire**	NA
NA	North Dakota**	NA
NA	South Dakota**	NA
NA	Vermont**	NA
NA	West Virginia**	NA
NA	Wyoming**	NA

District of Columbia   45.6

Source: U.S. Department of Health and Human Services, National Center for Health Statistics
    "National Vital Statistics Reports" (Vol. 50, No. 15, September 16, 2002)
*AIDS is Acquired Immunodeficiency Syndrome. It is a specific group of diseases or conditions which are indicative of severe immunosuppression related to infection with the Human Immunodeficiency Virus (HIV). Age-adjusted rates based on the year 2000 standard population.
**Insufficient data to determine a reliable rate.

Estimated Deaths by Cancer in 2003

National Estimated Total = 556,500 Deaths

RANK	STATE	DEATHS	% of USA
20	Alabama	9,800	1.8%
50	Alaska	700	0.1%
21	Arizona	9,700	1.7%
32	Arkansas	6,100	1.1%
1	California	52,200	9.4%
30	Colorado	6,300	1.1%
28	Connecticut	6,900	1.2%
45	Delaware	1,700	0.3%
2	Florida	40,100	7.2%
11	Georgia	13,900	2.5%
43	Hawaii	2,000	0.4%
42	Idaho	2,300	0.4%
7	Illinois	25,000	4.5%
14	Indiana	13,000	2.3%
29	Iowa	6,400	1.2%
33	Kansas	5,200	0.9%
23	Kentucky	9,200	1.7%
22	Louisiana	9,400	1.7%
38	Maine	3,000	0.5%
19	Maryland	10,200	1.8%
13	Massachusetts	13,600	2.4%
8	Michigan	19,800	3.6%
24	Minnesota	9,100	1.6%
31	Mississippi	6,200	1.1%
16	Missouri	12,300	2.2%
44	Montana	1,900	0.3%
36	Nebraska	3,400	0.6%
35	Nevada	4,300	0.8%
40	New Hampshire	2,500	0.4%
9	New Jersey	17,600	3.2%
37	New Mexico	3,100	0.6%
3	New York	35,800	6.4%
10	North Carolina	16,500	3.0%
47	North Dakota	1,300	0.2%
6	Ohio	25,200	4.5%
26	Oklahoma	7,400	1.3%
27	Oregon	7,200	1.3%
5	Pennsylvania	29,600	5.3%
41	Rhode Island	2,400	0.4%
25	South Carolina	8,600	1.5%
46	South Dakota	1,600	0.3%
15	Tennessee	12,700	2.3%
4	Texas	34,800	6.3%
39	Utah	2,600	0.5%
47	Vermont	1,300	0.2%
12	Virginia	13,700	2.5%
17	Washington	11,200	2.0%
34	West Virginia	4,700	0.8%
18	Wisconsin	10,800	1.9%
49	Wyoming	900	0.2%

RANK	STATE	DEATHS	% of USA
1	California	52,200	9.4%
2	Florida	40,100	7.2%
3	New York	35,800	6.4%
4	Texas	34,800	6.3%
5	Pennsylvania	29,600	5.3%
6	Ohio	25,200	4.5%
7	Illinois	25,000	4.5%
8	Michigan	19,800	3.6%
9	New Jersey	17,600	3.2%
10	North Carolina	16,500	3.0%
11	Georgia	13,900	2.5%
12	Virginia	13,700	2.5%
13	Massachusetts	13,600	2.4%
14	Indiana	13,000	2.3%
15	Tennessee	12,700	2.3%
16	Missouri	12,300	2.2%
17	Washington	11,200	2.0%
18	Wisconsin	10,800	1.9%
19	Maryland	10,200	1.8%
20	Alabama	9,800	1.8%
21	Arizona	9,700	1.7%
22	Louisiana	9,400	1.7%
23	Kentucky	9,200	1.7%
24	Minnesota	9,100	1.6%
25	South Carolina	8,600	1.5%
26	Oklahoma	7,400	1.3%
27	Oregon	7,200	1.3%
28	Connecticut	6,900	1.2%
29	Iowa	6,400	1.2%
30	Colorado	6,300	1.1%
31	Mississippi	6,200	1.1%
32	Arkansas	6,100	1.1%
33	Kansas	5,200	0.9%
34	West Virginia	4,700	0.8%
35	Nevada	4,300	0.8%
36	Nebraska	3,400	0.6%
37	New Mexico	3,100	0.6%
38	Maine	3,000	0.5%
39	Utah	2,600	0.5%
40	New Hampshire	2,500	0.4%
41	Rhode Island	2,400	0.4%
42	Idaho	2,300	0.4%
43	Hawaii	2,000	0.4%
44	Montana	1,900	0.3%
45	Delaware	1,700	0.3%
46	South Dakota	1,600	0.3%
47	North Dakota	1,300	0.2%
47	Vermont	1,300	0.2%
49	Wyoming	900	0.2%
50	Alaska	700	0.1%
	District of Columbia	1,100	0.2%

Source: American Cancer Society
"Cancer Facts & Figures 2003" (Copyright 2003, Reprinted with permission from the American Cancer Society)

Estimated Death Rate by Cancer in 2003

National Estimated Rate = 193.0 Deaths per 100,000 Population*

ALPHA ORDER

RANK	STATE	RATE
10	Alabama	218.4
50	Alaska	108.7
41	Arizona	177.8
5	Arkansas	225.1
47	California	148.7
48	Colorado	139.8
26	Connecticut	199.4
18	Delaware	210.6
3	Florida	239.9
44	Georgia	162.4
45	Hawaii	160.7
42	Idaho	171.5
28	Illinois	198.4
16	Indiana	211.1
11	Iowa	217.9
34	Kansas	191.5
6	Kentucky	224.8
20	Louisiana	209.7
4	Maine	231.8
36	Maryland	186.9
15	Massachusetts	211.6
31	Michigan	197.0
39	Minnesota	181.3
13	Mississippi	215.9
12	Missouri	216.8
22	Montana	208.9
32	Nebraska	196.6
30	Nevada	197.8
33	New Hampshire	196.1
24	New Jersey	204.9
43	New Mexico	167.1
36	New York	186.9
29	North Carolina	198.3
23	North Dakota	205.0
8	Ohio	220.6
14	Oklahoma	211.8
25	Oregon	204.5
2	Pennsylvania	240.0
7	Rhode Island	224.4
21	South Carolina	209.4
19	South Dakota	210.2
9	Tennessee	219.1
46	Texas	159.8
49	Utah	112.3
17	Vermont	210.8
35	Virginia	187.8
38	Washington	184.5
1	West Virginia	260.8
27	Wisconsin	198.5
40	Wyoming	180.5

RANK ORDER

RANK	STATE	RATE
1	West Virginia	260.8
2	Pennsylvania	240.0
3	Florida	239.9
4	Maine	231.8
5	Arkansas	225.1
6	Kentucky	224.8
7	Rhode Island	224.4
8	Ohio	220.6
9	Tennessee	219.1
10	Alabama	218.4
11	Iowa	217.9
12	Missouri	216.8
13	Mississippi	215.9
14	Oklahoma	211.8
15	Massachusetts	211.6
16	Indiana	211.1
17	Vermont	210.8
18	Delaware	210.6
19	South Dakota	210.2
20	Louisiana	209.7
21	South Carolina	209.4
22	Montana	208.9
23	North Dakota	205.0
24	New Jersey	204.9
25	Oregon	204.5
26	Connecticut	199.4
27	Wisconsin	198.5
28	Illinois	198.4
29	North Carolina	198.3
30	Nevada	197.8
31	Michigan	197.0
32	Nebraska	196.6
33	New Hampshire	196.1
34	Kansas	191.5
35	Virginia	187.8
36	Maryland	186.9
36	New York	186.9
38	Washington	184.5
39	Minnesota	181.3
40	Wyoming	180.5
41	Arizona	177.8
42	Idaho	171.5
43	New Mexico	167.1
44	Georgia	162.4
45	Hawaii	160.7
46	Texas	159.8
47	California	148.7
48	Colorado	139.8
49	Utah	112.3
50	Alaska	108.7

District of Columbia	192.7

Source: Morgan Quitno Press using data from American Cancer Society
   "Cancer Facts & Figures 2003" (Copyright 2003, Reprinted with permission from the American Cancer Society)
*Rates calculated using 2002 Census resident population estimates. Not age-adjusted.

Age-Adjusted Death Rate by Cancer for Males in 1999

National Rate = 259.1 Deaths per 100,000 Male Population*

ALPHA ORDER

RANK	STATE	RATE
4	Alabama	298.0
43	Alaska	229.2
45	Arizona	229.0
6	Arkansas	291.0
46	California	224.5
48	Colorado	215.5
34	Connecticut	244.9
7	Delaware	290.4
30	Florida	249.6
10	Georgia	284.8
49	Hawaii	198.5
44	Idaho	229.1
21	Illinois	268.3
15	Indiana	278.3
35	Iowa	244.8
36	Kansas	243.3
3	Kentucky	304.3
2	Louisiana	314.7
12	Maine	280.4
14	Maryland	278.5
23	Massachusetts	267.9
28	Michigan	259.5
40	Minnesota	239.0
1	Mississippi	315.4
19	Missouri	270.7
37	Montana	242.0
41	Nebraska	237.5
26	Nevada	263.1
20	New Hampshire	270.2
25	New Jersey	265.7
47	New Mexico	219.0
32	New York	248.1
11	North Carolina	283.7
42	North Dakota	236.8
17	Ohio	275.3
23	Oklahoma	267.9
33	Oregon	245.5
18	Pennsylvania	271.8
13	Rhode Island	279.3
9	South Carolina	286.9
31	South Dakota	249.1
5	Tennessee	296.7
27	Texas	260.9
50	Utah	188.3
22	Vermont	268.1
16	Virginia	277.3
39	Washington	239.2
8	West Virginia	289.1
29	Wisconsin	252.0
38	Wyoming	240.6

RANK ORDER

RANK	STATE	RATE
1	Mississippi	315.4
2	Louisiana	314.7
3	Kentucky	304.3
4	Alabama	298.0
5	Tennessee	296.7
6	Arkansas	291.0
7	Delaware	290.4
8	West Virginia	289.1
9	South Carolina	286.9
10	Georgia	284.8
11	North Carolina	283.7
12	Maine	280.4
13	Rhode Island	279.3
14	Maryland	278.5
15	Indiana	278.3
16	Virginia	277.3
17	Ohio	275.3
18	Pennsylvania	271.8
19	Missouri	270.7
20	New Hampshire	270.2
21	Illinois	268.3
22	Vermont	268.1
23	Massachusetts	267.9
23	Oklahoma	267.9
25	New Jersey	265.7
26	Nevada	263.1
27	Texas	260.9
28	Michigan	259.5
29	Wisconsin	252.0
30	Florida	249.6
31	South Dakota	249.1
32	New York	248.1
33	Oregon	245.5
34	Connecticut	244.9
35	Iowa	244.8
36	Kansas	243.3
37	Montana	242.0
38	Wyoming	240.6
39	Washington	239.2
40	Minnesota	239.0
41	Nebraska	237.5
42	North Dakota	236.8
43	Alaska	229.2
44	Idaho	229.1
45	Arizona	229.0
46	California	224.5
47	New Mexico	219.0
48	Colorado	215.5
49	Hawaii	198.5
50	Utah	188.3
	District of Columbia	322.7

Source: American Cancer Society
"Cancer Facts & Figures 2003" (Copyright 2003, Reprinted with permission from the American Cancer Society)
*For 1995 to 1999. Age-adjusted to the 2000 U.S. standard population.

Age-Adjusted Death Rate by Cancer for Females in 1999

National Rate = 171.4 Deaths per 100,000 Female Population*

ALPHA ORDER

RANK	STATE	RATE
30	Alabama	169.6
23	Alaska	173.1
44	Arizona	157.0
24	Arkansas	172.0
39	California	161.7
48	Colorado	148.8
27	Connecticut	171.0
1	Delaware	197.8
35	Florida	165.6
33	Georgia	167.3
49	Hawaii	130.9
47	Idaho	154.1
15	Illinois	177.9
12	Indiana	180.9
40	Iowa	160.4
41	Kansas	160.0
10	Kentucky	183.6
4	Louisiana	187.5
2	Maine	189.4
8	Maryland	184.9
13	Massachusetts	179.7
22	Michigan	173.8
38	Minnesota	162.3
25	Mississippi	171.6
17	Missouri	176.6
37	Montana	163.8
43	Nebraska	157.2
3	Nevada	187.6
5	New Hampshire	187.0
6	New Jersey	186.2
46	New Mexico	156.3
20	New York	174.2
32	North Carolina	167.9
45	North Dakota	156.8
11	Ohio	182.9
31	Oklahoma	169.1
21	Oregon	174.1
14	Pennsylvania	179.0
9	Rhode Island	184.1
29	South Carolina	170.4
42	South Dakota	158.4
18	Tennessee	175.7
36	Texas	165.0
50	Utah	128.8
15	Vermont	177.9
19	Virginia	175.6
26	Washington	171.1
7	West Virginia	186.0
34	Wisconsin	166.2
27	Wyoming	171.0

RANK ORDER

RANK	STATE	RATE
1	Delaware	197.8
2	Maine	189.4
3	Nevada	187.6
4	Louisiana	187.5
5	New Hampshire	187.0
6	New Jersey	186.2
7	West Virginia	186.0
8	Maryland	184.9
9	Rhode Island	184.1
10	Kentucky	183.6
11	Ohio	182.9
12	Indiana	180.9
13	Massachusetts	179.7
14	Pennsylvania	179.0
15	Illinois	177.9
15	Vermont	177.9
17	Missouri	176.6
18	Tennessee	175.7
19	Virginia	175.6
20	New York	174.2
21	Oregon	174.1
22	Michigan	173.8
23	Alaska	173.1
24	Arkansas	172.0
25	Mississippi	171.6
26	Washington	171.1
27	Connecticut	171.0
27	Wyoming	171.0
29	South Carolina	170.4
30	Alabama	169.6
31	Oklahoma	169.1
32	North Carolina	167.9
33	Georgia	167.3
34	Wisconsin	166.2
35	Florida	165.6
36	Texas	165.0
37	Montana	163.8
38	Minnesota	162.3
39	California	161.7
40	Iowa	160.4
41	Kansas	160.0
42	South Dakota	158.4
43	Nebraska	157.2
44	Arizona	157.0
45	North Dakota	156.8
46	New Mexico	156.3
47	Idaho	154.1
48	Colorado	148.8
49	Hawaii	130.9
50	Utah	128.8
	District of Columbia	199.1

Source: American Cancer Society

"Cancer Facts & Figures 2003" (Copyright 2003, Reprinted with permission from the American Cancer Society)
For 1995 to 1999. Age-adjusted to the 2000 U.S. standard population.

Estimated Deaths by Female Breast Cancer in 2003

National Estimated Total = 39,800 Deaths

ALPHA ORDER

RANK	STATE	DEATHS	% of USA
22	Alabama	600	1.5%
43	Alaska	100	0.3%
18	Arizona	700	1.8%
31	Arkansas	400	1.0%
1	California	4,000	10.1%
26	Colorado	500	1.3%
26	Connecticut	500	1.3%
43	Delaware	100	0.3%
4	Florida	2,500	6.3%
11	Georgia	1,000	2.5%
43	Hawaii	100	0.3%
36	Idaho	200	0.5%
6	Illinois	1,900	4.8%
13	Indiana	900	2.3%
31	Iowa	400	1.0%
31	Kansas	400	1.0%
22	Kentucky	600	1.5%
18	Louisiana	700	1.8%
36	Maine	200	0.5%
16	Maryland	800	2.0%
13	Massachusetts	900	2.3%
8	Michigan	1,400	3.5%
22	Minnesota	600	1.5%
26	Mississippi	500	1.3%
16	Missouri	800	2.0%
43	Montana	100	0.3%
36	Nebraska	200	0.5%
34	Nevada	300	0.8%
36	New Hampshire	200	0.5%
8	New Jersey	1,400	3.5%
36	New Mexico	200	0.5%
2	New York	2,800	7.0%
10	North Carolina	1,100	2.8%
43	North Dakota	100	0.3%
6	Ohio	1,900	4.8%
26	Oklahoma	500	1.3%
26	Oregon	500	1.3%
5	Pennsylvania	2,100	5.3%
36	Rhode Island	200	0.5%
22	South Carolina	600	1.5%
43	South Dakota	100	0.3%
13	Tennessee	900	2.3%
3	Texas	2,600	6.5%
36	Utah	200	0.5%
43	Vermont	100	0.3%
11	Virginia	1,000	2.5%
18	Washington	700	1.8%
34	West Virginia	300	0.8%
18	Wisconsin	700	1.8%
43	Wyoming	100	0.3%

RANK ORDER

RANK	STATE	DEATHS	% of USA
1	California	4,000	10.1%
2	New York	2,800	7.0%
3	Texas	2,600	6.5%
4	Florida	2,500	6.3%
5	Pennsylvania	2,100	5.3%
6	Illinois	1,900	4.8%
6	Ohio	1,900	4.8%
8	Michigan	1,400	3.5%
8	New Jersey	1,400	3.5%
10	North Carolina	1,100	2.8%
11	Georgia	1,000	2.5%
11	Virginia	1,000	2.5%
13	Indiana	900	2.3%
13	Massachusetts	900	2.3%
13	Tennessee	900	2.3%
16	Maryland	800	2.0%
16	Missouri	800	2.0%
18	Arizona	700	1.8%
18	Louisiana	700	1.8%
18	Washington	700	1.8%
18	Wisconsin	700	1.8%
22	Alabama	600	1.5%
22	Kentucky	600	1.5%
22	Minnesota	600	1.5%
22	South Carolina	600	1.5%
26	Colorado	500	1.3%
26	Connecticut	500	1.3%
26	Mississippi	500	1.3%
26	Oklahoma	500	1.3%
26	Oregon	500	1.3%
31	Arkansas	400	1.0%
31	Iowa	400	1.0%
31	Kansas	400	1.0%
34	Nevada	300	0.8%
34	West Virginia	300	0.8%
36	Idaho	200	0.5%
36	Maine	200	0.5%
36	Nebraska	200	0.5%
36	New Hampshire	200	0.5%
36	New Mexico	200	0.5%
36	Rhode Island	200	0.5%
36	Utah	200	0.5%
43	Alaska	100	0.3%
43	Delaware	100	0.3%
43	Hawaii	100	0.3%
43	Montana	100	0.3%
43	North Dakota	100	0.3%
43	South Dakota	100	0.3%
43	Vermont	100	0.3%
43	Wyoming	100	0.3%
	District of Columbia	100	0.3%

Age-Adjusted Death Rate by Female Breast Cancer in 1999

National Rate = 28.8 Deaths per Female Population*

ALPHA ORDER

RANK	STATE	RATE
40	Alabama	26.7
47	Alaska	24.8
45	Arizona	25.8
40	Arkansas	26.7
36	California	27.1
48	Colorado	24.6
11	Connecticut	29.7
1	Delaware	32.6
32	Florida	27.4
23	Georgia	28.3
50	Hawaii	20.4
40	Idaho	26.7
5	Illinois	31.0
15	Indiana	29.2
31	Iowa	27.5
44	Kansas	26.5
24	Kentucky	28.1
8	Louisiana	30.8
16	Maine	28.8
4	Maryland	31.4
10	Massachusetts	30.4
13	Michigan	29.5
26	Minnesota	27.8
20	Mississippi	28.5
22	Missouri	28.4
43	Montana	26.6
36	Nebraska	27.1
25	Nevada	27.9
11	New Hampshire	29.7
2	New Jersey	32.2
34	New Mexico	27.2
3	New York	31.5
17	North Carolina	28.7
34	North Dakota	27.2
9	Ohio	30.7
28	Oklahoma	27.7
28	Oregon	27.7
7	Pennsylvania	30.9
5	Rhode Island	31.0
18	South Carolina	28.6
46	South Dakota	25.2
20	Tennessee	28.5
39	Texas	26.8
49	Utah	24.5
18	Vermont	28.6
13	Virginia	29.5
36	Washington	27.1
30	West Virginia	27.6
26	Wisconsin	27.8
33	Wyoming	27.3

RANK ORDER

RANK	STATE	RATE
1	Delaware	32.6
2	New Jersey	32.2
3	New York	31.5
4	Maryland	31.4
5	Illinois	31.0
5	Rhode Island	31.0
7	Pennsylvania	30.9
8	Louisiana	30.8
9	Ohio	30.7
10	Massachusetts	30.4
11	Connecticut	29.7
11	New Hampshire	29.7
13	Michigan	29.5
13	Virginia	29.5
15	Indiana	29.2
16	Maine	28.8
17	North Carolina	28.7
18	South Carolina	28.6
18	Vermont	28.6
20	Mississippi	28.5
20	Tennessee	28.5
22	Missouri	28.4
23	Georgia	28.3
24	Kentucky	28.1
25	Nevada	27.9
26	Minnesota	27.8
26	Wisconsin	27.8
28	Oklahoma	27.7
28	Oregon	27.7
30	West Virginia	27.6
31	Iowa	27.5
32	Florida	27.4
33	Wyoming	27.3
34	New Mexico	27.2
34	North Dakota	27.2
36	California	27.1
36	Nebraska	27.1
36	Washington	27.1
39	Texas	26.8
40	Alabama	26.7
40	Arkansas	26.7
40	Idaho	26.7
43	Montana	26.6
44	Kansas	26.5
45	Arizona	25.8
46	South Dakota	25.2
47	Alaska	24.8
48	Colorado	24.6
49	Utah	24.5
50	Hawaii	20.4
	District of Columbia	39.1

Source: American Cancer Society
"Cancer Facts & Figures 2003" (Copyright 2003, Reprinted with permission from the American Cancer Society)
*For 1995 to 1999. Age-adjusted to the 2000 U.S. standard population.

Estimated Deaths by Colon and Rectum Cancer in 2003

National Estimated Total = 57,100 Deaths

ALPHA ORDER

RANK	STATE	DEATHS	% of USA
22	Alabama	900	1.6%
48	Alaska	100	0.2%
19	Arizona	1,000	1.8%
30	Arkansas	600	1.1%
1	California	5,000	8.8%
30	Colorado	600	1.1%
28	Connecticut	700	1.2%
42	Delaware	200	0.4%
3	Florida	3,900	6.8%
13	Georgia	1,300	2.3%
42	Hawaii	200	0.4%
42	Idaho	200	0.4%
7	Illinois	2,600	4.6%
13	Indiana	1,300	2.3%
26	Iowa	800	1.4%
33	Kansas	500	0.9%
22	Kentucky	900	1.6%
19	Louisiana	1,000	1.8%
37	Maine	300	0.5%
17	Maryland	1,100	1.9%
11	Massachusetts	1,400	2.5%
8	Michigan	2,000	3.5%
22	Minnesota	900	1.6%
30	Mississippi	600	1.1%
13	Missouri	1,300	2.3%
42	Montana	200	0.4%
36	Nebraska	400	0.7%
33	Nevada	500	0.9%
37	New Hampshire	300	0.5%
9	New Jersey	1,900	3.3%
37	New Mexico	300	0.5%
2	New York	4,000	7.0%
10	North Carolina	1,600	2.8%
48	North Dakota	100	0.2%
6	Ohio	2,700	4.7%
26	Oklahoma	800	1.4%
28	Oregon	700	1.2%
5	Pennsylvania	3,300	5.8%
37	Rhode Island	300	0.5%
22	South Carolina	900	1.6%
42	South Dakota	200	0.4%
16	Tennessee	1,200	2.1%
4	Texas	3,600	6.3%
37	Utah	300	0.5%
42	Vermont	200	0.4%
11	Virginia	1,400	2.5%
19	Washington	1,000	1.8%
33	West Virginia	500	0.9%
17	Wisconsin	1,100	1.9%
48	Wyoming	100	0.2%

RANK ORDER

RANK	STATE	DEATHS	% of USA
1	California	5,000	8.8%
2	New York	4,000	7.0%
3	Florida	3,900	6.8%
4	Texas	3,600	6.3%
5	Pennsylvania	3,300	5.8%
6	Ohio	2,700	4.7%
7	Illinois	2,600	4.6%
8	Michigan	2,000	3.5%
9	New Jersey	1,900	3.3%
10	North Carolina	1,600	2.8%
11	Massachusetts	1,400	2.5%
11	Virginia	1,400	2.5%
13	Georgia	1,300	2.3%
13	Indiana	1,300	2.3%
13	Missouri	1,300	2.3%
16	Tennessee	1,200	2.1%
17	Maryland	1,100	1.9%
17	Wisconsin	1,100	1.9%
19	Arizona	1,000	1.8%
19	Louisiana	1,000	1.8%
19	Washington	1,000	1.8%
22	Alabama	900	1.6%
22	Kentucky	900	1.6%
22	Minnesota	900	1.6%
22	South Carolina	900	1.6%
26	Iowa	800	1.4%
26	Oklahoma	800	1.4%
28	Connecticut	700	1.2%
28	Oregon	700	1.2%
30	Arkansas	600	1.1%
30	Colorado	600	1.1%
30	Mississippi	600	1.1%
33	Kansas	500	0.9%
33	Nevada	500	0.9%
33	West Virginia	500	0.9%
36	Nebraska	400	0.7%
37	Maine	300	0.5%
37	New Hampshire	300	0.5%
37	New Mexico	300	0.5%
37	Rhode Island	300	0.5%
37	Utah	300	0.5%
42	Delaware	200	0.4%
42	Hawaii	200	0.4%
42	Idaho	200	0.4%
42	Montana	200	0.4%
42	South Dakota	200	0.4%
42	Vermont	200	0.4%
48	Alaska	100	0.2%
48	North Dakota	100	0.2%
48	Wyoming	100	0.2%
	District of Columbia	100	0.2%

Source: American Cancer Society
"Cancer Facts & Figures 2003" (Copyright 2003, Reprinted with permission from the American Cancer Society)

Estimated Death Rate by Colon and Rectum Cancer in 2003

National Estimated Rate = 19.8 Deaths per 100,000 Population*

ALPHA ORDER

RANK	STATE	RATE
31	Alabama	20.1
45	Alaska	15.5
38	Arizona	18.3
17	Arkansas	22.1
48	California	14.2
49	Colorado	13.3
28	Connecticut	20.2
7	Delaware	24.8
10	Florida	23.3
46	Georgia	15.2
43	Hawaii	16.1
47	Idaho	14.9
27	Illinois	20.6
23	Indiana	21.1
4	Iowa	27.2
37	Kansas	18.4
19	Kentucky	22.0
16	Louisiana	22.3
11	Maine	23.2
28	Maryland	20.2
22	Massachusetts	21.8
33	Michigan	19.9
39	Minnesota	17.9
24	Mississippi	20.9
14	Missouri	22.9
19	Montana	22.0
12	Nebraska	23.1
13	Nevada	23.0
9	New Hampshire	23.5
17	New Jersey	22.1
42	New Mexico	16.2
24	New York	20.9
35	North Carolina	19.2
44	North Dakota	15.8
8	Ohio	23.6
14	Oklahoma	22.9
33	Oregon	19.9
5	Pennsylvania	26.8
2	Rhode Island	28.0
21	South Carolina	21.9
6	South Dakota	26.3
26	Tennessee	20.7
40	Texas	16.5
50	Utah	13.0
1	Vermont	32.4
35	Virginia	19.2
40	Washington	16.5
3	West Virginia	27.7
28	Wisconsin	20.2
31	Wyoming	20.1

RANK ORDER

RANK	STATE	RATE
1	Vermont	32.4
2	Rhode Island	28.0
3	West Virginia	27.7
4	Iowa	27.2
5	Pennsylvania	26.8
6	South Dakota	26.3
7	Delaware	24.8
8	Ohio	23.6
9	New Hampshire	23.5
10	Florida	23.3
11	Maine	23.2
12	Nebraska	23.1
13	Nevada	23.0
14	Missouri	22.9
14	Oklahoma	22.9
16	Louisiana	22.3
17	Arkansas	22.1
17	New Jersey	22.1
19	Kentucky	22.0
19	Montana	22.0
21	South Carolina	21.9
22	Massachusetts	21.8
23	Indiana	21.1
24	Mississippi	20.9
24	New York	20.9
26	Tennessee	20.7
27	Illinois	20.6
28	Connecticut	20.2
28	Maryland	20.2
28	Wisconsin	20.2
31	Alabama	20.1
31	Wyoming	20.1
33	Michigan	19.9
33	Oregon	19.9
35	North Carolina	19.2
35	Virginia	19.2
37	Kansas	18.4
38	Arizona	18.3
39	Minnesota	17.9
40	Texas	16.5
40	Washington	16.5
42	New Mexico	16.2
43	Hawaii	16.1
44	North Dakota	15.8
45	Alaska	15.5
46	Georgia	15.2
47	Idaho	14.9
48	California	14.2
49	Colorado	13.3
50	Utah	13.0
	District of Columbia	17.5

Source: Morgan Quitno Press using data from American Cancer Society
"Cancer Facts & Figures 2003" (Copyright 2003, Reprinted with permission from the American Cancer Society)
*Rates calculated using 2002 Census resident population estimates. Not age-adjusted.

Estimated Deaths by Leukemia in 2003

National Estimated Total = 21,900 Deaths

ALPHA ORDER

RANK	STATE	DEATHS	% of USA
23	Alabama	300	1.4%
NA	Alaska*	NA	NA
19	Arizona	400	1.8%
31	Arkansas	200	0.9%
1	California	2,100	9.6%
23	Colorado	300	1.4%
23	Connecticut	300	1.4%
37	Delaware	100	0.5%
2	Florida	1,600	7.3%
11	Georgia	500	2.3%
37	Hawaii	100	0.5%
37	Idaho	100	0.5%
6	Illinois	1,000	4.6%
11	Indiana	500	2.3%
23	Iowa	300	1.4%
31	Kansas	200	0.9%
23	Kentucky	300	1.4%
19	Louisiana	400	1.8%
37	Maine	100	0.5%
19	Maryland	400	1.8%
11	Massachusetts	500	2.3%
8	Michigan	800	3.7%
19	Minnesota	400	1.8%
31	Mississippi	200	0.9%
11	Missouri	500	2.3%
37	Montana	100	0.5%
31	Nebraska	200	0.9%
31	Nevada	200	0.9%
37	New Hampshire	100	0.5%
9	New Jersey	700	3.2%
37	New Mexico	100	0.5%
3	New York	1,400	6.4%
10	North Carolina	600	2.7%
37	North Dakota	100	0.5%
6	Ohio	1,000	4.6%
23	Oklahoma	300	1.4%
23	Oregon	300	1.4%
5	Pennsylvania	1,100	5.0%
37	Rhode Island	100	0.5%
23	South Carolina	300	1.4%
37	South Dakota	100	0.5%
11	Tennessee	500	2.3%
4	Texas	1,300	5.9%
37	Utah	100	0.5%
NA	Vermont*	NA	NA
11	Virginia	500	2.3%
11	Washington	500	2.3%
31	West Virginia	200	0.9%
11	Wisconsin	500	2.3%
NA	Wyoming*	NA	NA

RANK ORDER

RANK	STATE	DEATHS	% of USA
1	California	2,100	9.6%
2	Florida	1,600	7.3%
3	New York	1,400	6.4%
4	Texas	1,300	5.9%
5	Pennsylvania	1,100	5.0%
6	Illinois	1,000	4.6%
6	Ohio	1,000	4.6%
8	Michigan	800	3.7%
9	New Jersey	700	3.2%
10	North Carolina	600	2.7%
11	Georgia	500	2.3%
11	Indiana	500	2.3%
11	Massachusetts	500	2.3%
11	Missouri	500	2.3%
11	Tennessee	500	2.3%
11	Virginia	500	2.3%
11	Washington	500	2.3%
11	Wisconsin	500	2.3%
19	Arizona	400	1.8%
19	Louisiana	400	1.8%
19	Maryland	400	1.8%
19	Minnesota	400	1.8%
23	Alabama	300	1.4%
23	Colorado	300	1.4%
23	Connecticut	300	1.4%
23	Iowa	300	1.4%
23	Kentucky	300	1.4%
23	Oklahoma	300	1.4%
23	Oregon	300	1.4%
23	South Carolina	300	1.4%
31	Arkansas	200	0.9%
31	Kansas	200	0.9%
31	Mississippi	200	0.9%
31	Nebraska	200	0.9%
31	Nevada	200	0.9%
31	West Virginia	200	0.9%
37	Delaware	100	0.5%
37	Hawaii	100	0.5%
37	Idaho	100	0.5%
37	Maine	100	0.5%
37	Montana	100	0.5%
37	New Hampshire	100	0.5%
37	New Mexico	100	0.5%
37	North Dakota	100	0.5%
37	Rhode Island	100	0.5%
37	South Dakota	100	0.5%
37	Utah	100	0.5%
NA	Alaska*	NA	NA
NA	Vermont*	NA	NA
NA	Wyoming*	NA	NA
	District of Columbia*	NA	NA

Source: American Cancer Society
   "Cancer Facts & Figures 2003" (Copyright 2003, Reprinted with permission from the American Cancer Society)
*Fewer than 50 deaths.

Estimated Death Rate by Leukemia in 2003

National Estimated Rate = 7.6 Deaths per 100,000 Population*

ALPHA ORDER

RANK	STATE	RATE
41	Alabama	6.7
NA	Alaska**	NA
33	Arizona	7.3
31	Arkansas	7.4
43	California	6.0
41	Colorado	6.7
16	Connecticut	8.7
3	Delaware	12.4
8	Florida	9.6
45	Georgia	5.8
23	Hawaii	8.0
30	Idaho	7.5
26	Illinois	7.9
21	Indiana	8.1
7	Iowa	10.2
31	Kansas	7.4
33	Kentucky	7.3
12	Louisiana	8.9
29	Maine	7.7
33	Maryland	7.3
27	Massachusetts	7.8
23	Michigan	8.0
23	Minnesota	8.0
39	Mississippi	7.0
14	Missouri	8.8
6	Montana	11.0
4	Nebraska	11.6
10	Nevada	9.2
27	New Hampshire	7.8
21	New Jersey	8.1
46	New Mexico	5.4
33	New York	7.3
38	North Carolina	7.2
1	North Dakota	15.8
14	Ohio	8.8
17	Oklahoma	8.6
19	Oregon	8.5
12	Pennsylvania	8.9
9	Rhode Island	9.3
33	South Carolina	7.3
2	South Dakota	13.1
17	Tennessee	8.6
43	Texas	6.0
47	Utah	4.3
NA	Vermont**	NA
40	Virginia	6.9
20	Washington	8.2
5	West Virginia	11.1
10	Wisconsin	9.2
NA	Wyoming**	NA

RANK ORDER

RANK	STATE	RATE
1	North Dakota	15.8
2	South Dakota	13.1
3	Delaware	12.4
4	Nebraska	11.6
5	West Virginia	11.1
6	Montana	11.0
7	Iowa	10.2
8	Florida	9.6
9	Rhode Island	9.3
10	Nevada	9.2
10	Wisconsin	9.2
12	Louisiana	8.9
12	Pennsylvania	8.9
14	Missouri	8.8
14	Ohio	8.8
16	Connecticut	8.7
17	Oklahoma	8.6
17	Tennessee	8.6
19	Oregon	8.5
20	Washington	8.2
21	Indiana	8.1
21	New Jersey	8.1
23	Hawaii	8.0
23	Michigan	8.0
23	Minnesota	8.0
26	Illinois	7.9
27	Massachusetts	7.8
27	New Hampshire	7.8
29	Maine	7.7
30	Idaho	7.5
31	Arkansas	7.4
31	Kansas	7.4
33	Arizona	7.3
33	Kentucky	7.3
33	Maryland	7.3
33	New York	7.3
33	South Carolina	7.3
38	North Carolina	7.2
39	Mississippi	7.0
40	Virginia	6.9
41	Alabama	6.7
41	Colorado	6.7
43	California	6.0
43	Texas	6.0
45	Georgia	5.8
46	New Mexico	5.4
47	Utah	4.3
NA	Alaska**	NA
NA	Vermont**	NA
NA	Wyoming**	NA
	District of Columbia**	NA

Source: Morgan Quitno Press using data from American Cancer Society
"Cancer Facts & Figures 2003" (Copyright 2003, Reprinted with permission from the American Cancer Society)
Rates calculated using 2002 Census resident population estimates. Not age-adjusted.
**Fewer than 50 deaths.*

Estimated Deaths by Liver Cancer in 2003

National Estimated Total = 14,400 Deaths

ALPHA ORDER

RANK	STATE	DEATHS	% of USA
11	Alabama	300	2.1%
NA	Alaska*	NA	NA
11	Arizona	300	2.1%
22	Arkansas	200	1.4%
1	California	1,900	13.2%
30	Colorado	100	0.7%
22	Connecticut	200	1.4%
NA	Delaware*	NA	NA
3	Florida	1,000	6.9%
11	Georgia	300	2.1%
30	Hawaii	100	0.7%
NA	Idaho*	NA	NA
5	Illinois	700	4.9%
11	Indiana	300	2.1%
30	Iowa	100	0.7%
30	Kansas	100	0.7%
22	Kentucky	200	1.4%
11	Louisiana	300	2.1%
30	Maine	100	0.7%
22	Maryland	200	1.4%
11	Massachusetts	300	2.1%
7	Michigan	500	3.5%
22	Minnesota	200	1.4%
22	Mississippi	200	1.4%
11	Missouri	300	2.1%
NA	Montana*	NA	NA
30	Nebraska	100	0.7%
30	Nevada	100	0.7%
30	New Hampshire	100	0.7%
7	New Jersey	500	3.5%
30	New Mexico	100	0.7%
3	New York	1,000	6.9%
10	North Carolina	400	2.8%
NA	North Dakota*	NA	NA
7	Ohio	500	3.5%
22	Oklahoma	200	1.4%
30	Oregon	100	0.7%
5	Pennsylvania	700	4.9%
30	Rhode Island	100	0.7%
22	South Carolina	200	1.4%
NA	South Dakota*	NA	NA
11	Tennessee	300	2.1%
2	Texas	1,200	8.3%
30	Utah	100	0.7%
NA	Vermont*	NA	NA
11	Virginia	300	2.1%
11	Washington	300	2.1%
30	West Virginia	100	0.7%
11	Wisconsin	300	2.1%
NA	Wyoming*	NA	NA

RANK ORDER

RANK	STATE	DEATHS	% of USA
1	California	1,900	13.2%
2	Texas	1,200	8.3%
3	Florida	1,000	6.9%
3	New York	1,000	6.9%
5	Illinois	700	4.9%
5	Pennsylvania	700	4.9%
7	Michigan	500	3.5%
7	New Jersey	500	3.5%
7	Ohio	500	3.5%
10	North Carolina	400	2.8%
11	Alabama	300	2.1%
11	Arizona	300	2.1%
11	Georgia	300	2.1%
11	Indiana	300	2.1%
11	Louisiana	300	2.1%
11	Massachusetts	300	2.1%
11	Missouri	300	2.1%
11	Tennessee	300	2.1%
11	Virginia	300	2.1%
11	Washington	300	2.1%
11	Wisconsin	300	2.1%
22	Arkansas	200	1.4%
22	Connecticut	200	1.4%
22	Kentucky	200	1.4%
22	Maryland	200	1.4%
22	Minnesota	200	1.4%
22	Mississippi	200	1.4%
22	Oklahoma	200	1.4%
22	South Carolina	200	1.4%
30	Colorado	100	0.7%
30	Hawaii	100	0.7%
30	Iowa	100	0.7%
30	Kansas	100	0.7%
30	Maine	100	0.7%
30	Nebraska	100	0.7%
30	Nevada	100	0.7%
30	New Hampshire	100	0.7%
30	New Mexico	100	0.7%
30	Oregon	100	0.7%
30	Rhode Island	100	0.7%
30	Utah	100	0.7%
30	West Virginia	100	0.7%
NA	Alaska*	NA	NA
NA	Delaware*	NA	NA
NA	Idaho*	NA	NA
NA	Montana*	NA	NA
NA	North Dakota*	NA	NA
NA	South Dakota*	NA	NA
NA	Vermont*	NA	NA
NA	Wyoming*	NA	NA
	District of Columbia*	NA	NA

Source: American Cancer Society
   "Cancer Facts & Figures 2003" (Copyright 2003, Reprinted with permission from the American Cancer Society)
*Fewer than 50 deaths.

Estimated Death Rate by Liver Cancer in 2003

National Estimated Rate = 5.0 Deaths per 100,000 Population*

RANK	STATE	RATE
7	Alabama	6.7
NA	Alaska**	NA
16	Arizona	5.5
5	Arkansas	7.4
20	California	5.4
42	Colorado	2.2
10	Connecticut	5.8
NA	Delaware**	NA
9	Florida	6.0
39	Georgia	3.5
2	Hawaii	8.0
NA	Idaho**	NA
15	Illinois	5.6
26	Indiana	4.9
40	Iowa	3.4
37	Kansas	3.7
26	Kentucky	4.9
7	Louisiana	6.7
4	Maine	7.7
37	Maryland	3.7
31	Massachusetts	4.7
25	Michigan	5.0
36	Minnesota	4.0
6	Mississippi	7.0
22	Missouri	5.3
NA	Montana**	NA
10	Nebraska	5.8
32	Nevada	4.6
3	New Hampshire	7.8
10	New Jersey	5.8
20	New Mexico	5.4
23	New York	5.2
30	North Carolina	4.8
NA	North Dakota**	NA
33	Ohio	4.4
13	Oklahoma	5.7
41	Oregon	2.8
13	Pennsylvania	5.7
1	Rhode Island	9.3
26	South Carolina	4.9
NA	South Dakota**	NA
23	Tennessee	5.2
16	Texas	5.5
34	Utah	4.3
NA	Vermont**	NA
35	Virginia	4.1
26	Washington	4.9
16	West Virginia	5.5
16	Wisconsin	5.5
NA	Wyoming**	NA

RANK	STATE	RATE
1	Rhode Island	9.3
2	Hawaii	8.0
3	New Hampshire	7.8
4	Maine	7.7
5	Arkansas	7.4
6	Mississippi	7.0
7	Alabama	6.7
7	Louisiana	6.7
9	Florida	6.0
10	Connecticut	5.8
10	Nebraska	5.8
10	New Jersey	5.8
13	Oklahoma	5.7
13	Pennsylvania	5.7
15	Illinois	5.6
16	Arizona	5.5
16	Texas	5.5
16	West Virginia	5.5
16	Wisconsin	5.5
20	California	5.4
20	New Mexico	5.4
22	Missouri	5.3
23	New York	5.2
23	Tennessee	5.2
25	Michigan	5.0
26	Indiana	4.9
26	Kentucky	4.9
26	South Carolina	4.9
26	Washington	4.9
30	North Carolina	4.8
31	Massachusetts	4.7
32	Nevada	4.6
33	Ohio	4.4
34	Utah	4.3
35	Virginia	4.1
36	Minnesota	4.0
37	Kansas	3.7
37	Maryland	3.7
39	Georgia	3.5
40	Iowa	3.4
41	Oregon	2.8
42	Colorado	2.2
NA	Alaska**	NA
NA	Delaware**	NA
NA	Idaho**	NA
NA	Montana**	NA
NA	North Dakota**	NA
NA	South Dakota**	NA
NA	Vermont**	NA
NA	Wyoming**	NA
	District of Columbia**	NA

Source: Morgan Quitno Press using data from American Cancer Society
    "Cancer Facts & Figures 2003" (Copyright 2003, Reprinted with permission from the American Cancer Society)
Rates calculated using 2002 Census resident population estimates. Not age-adjusted.
**Fewer than 50 deaths.*

Estimated Deaths by Lung Cancer in 2003

National Estimated Total = 157,200 Deaths

ALPHA ORDER

RANK	STATE	DEATHS	% of USA
19	Alabama	3,000	1.9%
50	Alaska	200	0.1%
22	Arizona	2,700	1.7%
28	Arkansas	2,000	1.3%
1	California	13,200	8.4%
33	Colorado	1,500	1.0%
30	Connecticut	1,800	1.1%
42	Delaware	500	0.3%
2	Florida	12,100	7.7%
11	Georgia	4,200	2.7%
42	Hawaii	500	0.3%
41	Idaho	600	0.4%
7	Illinois	6,800	4.3%
13	Indiana	4,000	2.5%
31	Iowa	1,700	1.1%
33	Kansas	1,500	1.0%
17	Kentucky	3,200	2.0%
22	Louisiana	2,700	1.7%
36	Maine	900	0.6%
20	Maryland	2,900	1.8%
16	Massachusetts	3,700	2.4%
8	Michigan	5,600	3.6%
26	Minnesota	2,300	1.5%
28	Mississippi	2,000	1.3%
14	Missouri	3,900	2.5%
42	Montana	500	0.3%
36	Nebraska	900	0.6%
35	Nevada	1,300	0.8%
38	New Hampshire	700	0.4%
10	New Jersey	4,500	2.9%
38	New Mexico	700	0.4%
4	New York	9,200	5.9%
9	North Carolina	5,100	3.2%
48	North Dakota	300	0.2%
6	Ohio	7,400	4.7%
25	Oklahoma	2,400	1.5%
27	Oregon	2,100	1.3%
5	Pennsylvania	8,000	5.1%
38	Rhode Island	700	0.4%
24	South Carolina	2,500	1.6%
45	South Dakota	400	0.3%
12	Tennessee	4,100	2.6%
3	Texas	9,900	6.3%
45	Utah	400	0.3%
45	Vermont	400	0.3%
14	Virginia	3,900	2.5%
17	Washington	3,200	2.0%
32	West Virginia	1,600	1.0%
21	Wisconsin	2,800	1.8%
48	Wyoming	300	0.2%

RANK ORDER

RANK	STATE	DEATHS	% of USA
1	California	13,200	8.4%
2	Florida	12,100	7.7%
3	Texas	9,900	6.3%
4	New York	9,200	5.9%
5	Pennsylvania	8,000	5.1%
6	Ohio	7,400	4.7%
7	Illinois	6,800	4.3%
8	Michigan	5,600	3.6%
9	North Carolina	5,100	3.2%
10	New Jersey	4,500	2.9%
11	Georgia	4,200	2.7%
12	Tennessee	4,100	2.6%
13	Indiana	4,000	2.5%
14	Missouri	3,900	2.5%
14	Virginia	3,900	2.5%
16	Massachusetts	3,700	2.4%
17	Kentucky	3,200	2.0%
17	Washington	3,200	2.0%
19	Alabama	3,000	1.9%
20	Maryland	2,900	1.8%
21	Wisconsin	2,800	1.8%
22	Arizona	2,700	1.7%
22	Louisiana	2,700	1.7%
24	South Carolina	2,500	1.6%
25	Oklahoma	2,400	1.5%
26	Minnesota	2,300	1.5%
27	Oregon	2,100	1.3%
28	Arkansas	2,000	1.3%
28	Mississippi	2,000	1.3%
30	Connecticut	1,800	1.1%
31	Iowa	1,700	1.1%
32	West Virginia	1,600	1.0%
33	Colorado	1,500	1.0%
33	Kansas	1,500	1.0%
35	Nevada	1,300	0.8%
36	Maine	900	0.6%
36	Nebraska	900	0.6%
38	New Hampshire	700	0.4%
38	New Mexico	700	0.4%
38	Rhode Island	700	0.4%
41	Idaho	600	0.4%
42	Delaware	500	0.3%
42	Hawaii	500	0.3%
42	Montana	500	0.3%
45	South Dakota	400	0.3%
45	Utah	400	0.3%
45	Vermont	400	0.3%
48	North Dakota	300	0.2%
48	Wyoming	300	0.2%
50	Alaska	200	0.1%
	District of Columbia	300	0.2%

Source: American Cancer Society
"Cancer Facts & Figures 2003" (Copyright 2003, Reprinted with permission from the American Cancer Society)

Estimated Death Rate by Lung Cancer in 2003

National Estimated Rate = 54.5 Deaths per 100,000 Population*

ALPHA ORDER

RANK	STATE	RATE
10	Alabama	66.9
49	Alaska	31.1
38	Arizona	49.5
3	Arkansas	73.8
47	California	37.6
48	Colorado	33.3
35	Connecticut	52.0
16	Delaware	61.9
4	Florida	72.4
39	Georgia	49.1
45	Hawaii	40.2
44	Idaho	44.7
29	Illinois	54.0
12	Indiana	64.9
23	Iowa	57.9
26	Kansas	55.2
2	Kentucky	78.2
19	Louisiana	60.2
7	Maine	69.5
31	Maryland	53.1
24	Massachusetts	57.6
25	Michigan	55.7
42	Minnesota	45.8
6	Mississippi	69.6
8	Missouri	68.8
27	Montana	55.0
35	Nebraska	52.0
21	Nevada	59.8
28	New Hampshire	54.9
34	New Jersey	52.4
46	New Mexico	37.7
40	New York	48.0
17	North Carolina	61.3
41	North Dakota	47.3
15	Ohio	64.8
9	Oklahoma	68.7
22	Oregon	59.6
12	Pennsylvania	64.9
11	Rhode Island	65.4
18	South Carolina	60.9
33	South Dakota	52.6
5	Tennessee	70.7
43	Texas	45.5
50	Utah	17.3
12	Vermont	64.9
30	Virginia	53.5
32	Washington	52.7
1	West Virginia	88.8
37	Wisconsin	51.5
19	Wyoming	60.2

RANK ORDER

RANK	STATE	RATE
1	West Virginia	88.8
2	Kentucky	78.2
3	Arkansas	73.8
4	Florida	72.4
5	Tennessee	70.7
6	Mississippi	69.6
7	Maine	69.5
8	Missouri	68.8
9	Oklahoma	68.7
10	Alabama	66.9
11	Rhode Island	65.4
12	Indiana	64.9
12	Pennsylvania	64.9
12	Vermont	64.9
15	Ohio	64.8
16	Delaware	61.9
17	North Carolina	61.3
18	South Carolina	60.9
19	Louisiana	60.2
19	Wyoming	60.2
21	Nevada	59.8
22	Oregon	59.6
23	Iowa	57.9
24	Massachusetts	57.6
25	Michigan	55.7
26	Kansas	55.2
27	Montana	55.0
28	New Hampshire	54.9
29	Illinois	54.0
30	Virginia	53.5
31	Maryland	53.1
32	Washington	52.7
33	South Dakota	52.6
34	New Jersey	52.4
35	Connecticut	52.0
35	Nebraska	52.0
37	Wisconsin	51.5
38	Arizona	49.5
39	Georgia	49.1
40	New York	48.0
41	North Dakota	47.3
42	Minnesota	45.8
43	Texas	45.5
44	Idaho	44.7
45	Hawaii	40.2
46	New Mexico	37.7
47	California	37.6
48	Colorado	33.3
49	Alaska	31.1
50	Utah	17.3
	District of Columbia	52.5

Source: Morgan Quitno Press using data from American Cancer Society
   "Cancer Facts & Figures 2003" (Copyright 2003, Reprinted with permission from the American Cancer Society)
*Rates calculated using 2002 Census resident population estimates. Not age-adjusted.

Estimated Deaths by Non-Hodgkin's Lymphoma in 2003

National Estimated Total = 23,400 Deaths

ALPHA ORDER

RANK	STATE	DEATHS	% of USA
20	Alabama	400	1.7%
NA	Alaska*	NA	NA
20	Arizona	400	1.7%
25	Arkansas	300	1.3%
1	California	2,300	9.8%
25	Colorado	300	1.3%
25	Connecticut	300	1.3%
37	Delaware	100	0.4%
2	Florida	1,700	7.3%
13	Georgia	500	2.1%
37	Hawaii	100	0.4%
37	Idaho	100	0.4%
7	Illinois	1,000	4.3%
10	Indiana	600	2.6%
25	Iowa	300	1.3%
32	Kansas	200	0.9%
20	Kentucky	400	1.7%
20	Louisiana	400	1.7%
37	Maine	100	0.4%
20	Maryland	400	1.7%
10	Massachusetts	600	2.6%
8	Michigan	900	3.8%
13	Minnesota	500	2.1%
32	Mississippi	200	0.9%
13	Missouri	500	2.1%
37	Montana	100	0.4%
32	Nebraska	200	0.9%
37	Nevada	100	0.4%
37	New Hampshire	100	0.4%
9	New Jersey	800	3.4%
37	New Mexico	100	0.4%
3	New York	1,400	6.0%
10	North Carolina	600	2.6%
37	North Dakota	100	0.4%
6	Ohio	1,100	4.7%
25	Oklahoma	300	1.3%
25	Oregon	300	1.3%
5	Pennsylvania	1,300	5.6%
37	Rhode Island	100	0.4%
25	South Carolina	300	1.3%
37	South Dakota	100	0.4%
13	Tennessee	500	2.1%
3	Texas	1,400	6.0%
32	Utah	200	0.9%
37	Vermont	100	0.4%
13	Virginia	500	2.1%
13	Washington	500	2.1%
32	West Virginia	200	0.9%
13	Wisconsin	500	2.1%
NA	Wyoming*	NA	NA

RANK ORDER

RANK	STATE	DEATHS	% of USA
1	California	2,300	9.8%
2	Florida	1,700	7.3%
3	New York	1,400	6.0%
3	Texas	1,400	6.0%
5	Pennsylvania	1,300	5.6%
6	Ohio	1,100	4.7%
7	Illinois	1,000	4.3%
8	Michigan	900	3.8%
9	New Jersey	800	3.4%
10	Indiana	600	2.6%
10	Massachusetts	600	2.6%
10	North Carolina	600	2.6%
13	Georgia	500	2.1%
13	Minnesota	500	2.1%
13	Missouri	500	2.1%
13	Tennessee	500	2.1%
13	Virginia	500	2.1%
13	Washington	500	2.1%
13	Wisconsin	500	2.1%
20	Alabama	400	1.7%
20	Arizona	400	1.7%
20	Kentucky	400	1.7%
20	Louisiana	400	1.7%
20	Maryland	400	1.7%
25	Arkansas	300	1.3%
25	Colorado	300	1.3%
25	Connecticut	300	1.3%
25	Iowa	300	1.3%
25	Oklahoma	300	1.3%
25	Oregon	300	1.3%
25	South Carolina	300	1.3%
32	Kansas	200	0.9%
32	Mississippi	200	0.9%
32	Nebraska	200	0.9%
32	Utah	200	0.9%
32	West Virginia	200	0.9%
37	Delaware	100	0.4%
37	Hawaii	100	0.4%
37	Idaho	100	0.4%
37	Maine	100	0.4%
37	Montana	100	0.4%
37	Nevada	100	0.4%
37	New Hampshire	100	0.4%
37	New Mexico	100	0.4%
37	North Dakota	100	0.4%
37	Rhode Island	100	0.4%
37	South Dakota	100	0.4%
37	Vermont	100	0.4%
NA	Alaska*	NA	NA
NA	Wyoming*	NA	NA
	District of Columbia*	NA	NA

Source: American Cancer Society
"Cancer Facts & Figures 2003" (Copyright 2003, Reprinted with permission from the American Cancer Society)
*Fewer than 50 deaths.

Estimated Death Rate by Non-Hodgkin's Lymphoma in 2003

National Estimated Rate = 8.1 Deaths per 100,000 Population*

ALPHA ORDER

RANK	STATE	RATE
21	Alabama	8.9
NA	Alaska**	NA
36	Arizona	7.3
6	Arkansas	11.1
44	California	6.5
43	Colorado	6.7
24	Connecticut	8.7
4	Delaware	12.4
10	Florida	10.2
46	Georgia	5.8
30	Hawaii	8.0
34	Idaho	7.5
31	Illinois	7.9
14	Indiana	9.7
10	Iowa	10.2
35	Kansas	7.4
13	Kentucky	9.8
21	Louisiana	8.9
33	Maine	7.7
36	Maryland	7.3
16	Massachusetts	9.3
20	Michigan	9.0
12	Minnesota	10.0
41	Mississippi	7.0
23	Missouri	8.8
8	Montana	11.0
5	Nebraska	11.6
48	Nevada	4.6
32	New Hampshire	7.8
16	New Jersey	9.3
47	New Mexico	5.4
36	New York	7.3
40	North Carolina	7.2
2	North Dakota	15.8
15	Ohio	9.6
25	Oklahoma	8.6
28	Oregon	8.5
9	Pennsylvania	10.5
16	Rhode Island	9.3
36	South Carolina	7.3
3	South Dakota	13.1
25	Tennessee	8.6
45	Texas	6.4
25	Utah	8.6
1	Vermont	16.2
42	Virginia	6.9
29	Washington	8.2
6	West Virginia	11.1
19	Wisconsin	9.2
NA	Wyoming**	NA

RANK ORDER

RANK	STATE	RATE
1	Vermont	16.2
2	North Dakota	15.8
3	South Dakota	13.1
4	Delaware	12.4
5	Nebraska	11.6
6	Arkansas	11.1
6	West Virginia	11.1
8	Montana	11.0
9	Pennsylvania	10.5
10	Florida	10.2
10	Iowa	10.2
12	Minnesota	10.0
13	Kentucky	9.8
14	Indiana	9.7
15	Ohio	9.6
16	Massachusetts	9.3
16	New Jersey	9.3
16	Rhode Island	9.3
19	Wisconsin	9.2
20	Michigan	9.0
21	Alabama	8.9
21	Louisiana	8.9
23	Missouri	8.8
24	Connecticut	8.7
25	Oklahoma	8.6
25	Tennessee	8.6
25	Utah	8.6
28	Oregon	8.5
29	Washington	8.2
30	Hawaii	8.0
31	Illinois	7.9
32	New Hampshire	7.8
33	Maine	7.7
34	Idaho	7.5
35	Kansas	7.4
36	Arizona	7.3
36	Maryland	7.3
36	New York	7.3
36	South Carolina	7.3
40	North Carolina	7.2
41	Mississippi	7.0
42	Virginia	6.9
43	Colorado	6.7
44	California	6.5
45	Texas	6.4
46	Georgia	5.8
47	New Mexico	5.4
48	Nevada	4.6
NA	Alaska**	NA
NA	Wyoming**	NA
	District of Columbia**	NA

Source: Morgan Quitno Press using data from American Cancer Society
   "Cancer Facts & Figures 2003" (Copyright 2003, Reprinted with permission from the American Cancer Society)
*Rates calculated using 2002 Census resident population estimates. Not age-adjusted.
**Fewer than 50 deaths.

Estimated Deaths by Pancreatic Cancer in 2003

National Estimated Total = 30,000 Deaths

ALPHA ORDER

RANK	STATE	DEATHS	% of USA
20	Alabama	500	1.7%
NA	Alaska*	NA	NA
20	Arizona	500	1.7%
28	Arkansas	300	1.0%
1	California	2,900	9.7%
28	Colorado	300	1.0%
25	Connecticut	400	1.3%
40	Delaware	100	0.3%
2	Florida	2,200	7.3%
12	Georgia	700	2.3%
40	Hawaii	100	0.3%
40	Idaho	100	0.3%
6	Illinois	1,400	4.7%
14	Indiana	600	2.0%
28	Iowa	300	1.0%
28	Kansas	300	1.0%
25	Kentucky	400	1.3%
20	Louisiana	500	1.7%
34	Maine	200	0.7%
14	Maryland	600	2.0%
11	Massachusetts	800	2.7%
8	Michigan	1,100	3.7%
20	Minnesota	500	1.7%
28	Mississippi	300	1.0%
14	Missouri	600	2.0%
40	Montana	100	0.3%
34	Nebraska	200	0.7%
34	Nevada	200	0.7%
34	New Hampshire	200	0.7%
9	New Jersey	1,000	3.3%
34	New Mexico	200	0.7%
2	New York	2,200	7.3%
10	North Carolina	900	3.0%
40	North Dakota	100	0.3%
7	Ohio	1,300	4.3%
28	Oklahoma	300	1.0%
25	Oregon	400	1.3%
5	Pennsylvania	1,600	5.3%
40	Rhode Island	100	0.3%
20	South Carolina	500	1.7%
40	South Dakota	100	0.3%
14	Tennessee	600	2.0%
4	Texas	1,800	6.0%
40	Utah	100	0.3%
40	Vermont	100	0.3%
12	Virginia	700	2.3%
14	Washington	600	2.0%
34	West Virginia	200	0.7%
14	Wisconsin	600	2.0%
NA	Wyoming*	NA	NA

RANK ORDER

RANK	STATE	DEATHS	% of USA
1	California	2,900	9.7%
2	Florida	2,200	7.3%
2	New York	2,200	7.3%
4	Texas	1,800	6.0%
5	Pennsylvania	1,600	5.3%
6	Illinois	1,400	4.7%
7	Ohio	1,300	4.3%
8	Michigan	1,100	3.7%
9	New Jersey	1,000	3.3%
10	North Carolina	900	3.0%
11	Massachusetts	800	2.7%
12	Georgia	700	2.3%
12	Virginia	700	2.3%
14	Indiana	600	2.0%
14	Maryland	600	2.0%
14	Missouri	600	2.0%
14	Tennessee	600	2.0%
14	Washington	600	2.0%
14	Wisconsin	600	2.0%
20	Alabama	500	1.7%
20	Arizona	500	1.7%
20	Louisiana	500	1.7%
20	Minnesota	500	1.7%
20	South Carolina	500	1.7%
25	Connecticut	400	1.3%
25	Kentucky	400	1.3%
25	Oregon	400	1.3%
28	Arkansas	300	1.0%
28	Colorado	300	1.0%
28	Iowa	300	1.0%
28	Kansas	300	1.0%
28	Mississippi	300	1.0%
28	Oklahoma	300	1.0%
34	Maine	200	0.7%
34	Nebraska	200	0.7%
34	Nevada	200	0.7%
34	New Hampshire	200	0.7%
34	New Mexico	200	0.7%
34	West Virginia	200	0.7%
40	Delaware	100	0.3%
40	Hawaii	100	0.3%
40	Idaho	100	0.3%
40	Montana	100	0.3%
40	North Dakota	100	0.3%
40	Rhode Island	100	0.3%
40	South Dakota	100	0.3%
40	Utah	100	0.3%
40	Vermont	100	0.3%
NA	Alaska*	NA	NA
NA	Wyoming*	NA	NA
	District of Columbia	100	0.3%

Source: American Cancer Society
   "Cancer Facts & Figures 2003" (Copyright 2003, Reprinted with permission from the American Cancer Society)
*Fewer than 50 deaths.

Estimated Death Rate by Pancreatic Cancer in 2003

National Estimated Rate = 10.4 Deaths per 100,000 Population*

ALPHA ORDER

RANK	STATE	RATE
18	Alabama	11.1
NA	Alaska**	NA
39	Arizona	9.2
18	Arkansas	11.1
42	California	8.3
47	Colorado	6.7
11	Connecticut	11.6
8	Delaware	12.4
5	Florida	13.2
44	Georgia	8.2
45	Hawaii	8.0
46	Idaho	7.5
18	Illinois	11.1
36	Indiana	9.7
32	Iowa	10.2
22	Kansas	11.0
35	Kentucky	9.8
17	Louisiana	11.2
4	Maine	15.5
22	Maryland	11.0
8	Massachusetts	12.4
26	Michigan	10.9
33	Minnesota	10.0
30	Mississippi	10.4
29	Missouri	10.6
22	Montana	11.0
11	Nebraska	11.6
39	Nevada	9.2
3	New Hampshire	15.7
11	New Jersey	11.6
27	New Mexico	10.8
14	New York	11.5
27	North Carolina	10.8
2	North Dakota	15.8
15	Ohio	11.4
41	Oklahoma	8.6
15	Oregon	11.4
7	Pennsylvania	13.0
38	Rhode Island	9.3
10	South Carolina	12.2
6	South Dakota	13.1
31	Tennessee	10.3
42	Texas	8.3
48	Utah	4.3
1	Vermont	16.2
37	Virginia	9.6
34	Washington	9.9
18	West Virginia	11.1
22	Wisconsin	11.0
NA	Wyoming**	NA

RANK ORDER

RANK	STATE	RATE
1	Vermont	16.2
2	North Dakota	15.8
3	New Hampshire	15.7
4	Maine	15.5
5	Florida	13.2
6	South Dakota	13.1
7	Pennsylvania	13.0
8	Delaware	12.4
8	Massachusetts	12.4
10	South Carolina	12.2
11	Connecticut	11.6
11	Nebraska	11.6
11	New Jersey	11.6
14	New York	11.5
15	Ohio	11.4
15	Oregon	11.4
17	Louisiana	11.2
18	Alabama	11.1
18	Arkansas	11.1
18	Illinois	11.1
18	West Virginia	11.1
22	Kansas	11.0
22	Maryland	11.0
22	Montana	11.0
22	Wisconsin	11.0
26	Michigan	10.9
27	New Mexico	10.8
27	North Carolina	10.8
29	Missouri	10.6
30	Mississippi	10.4
31	Tennessee	10.3
32	Iowa	10.2
33	Minnesota	10.0
34	Washington	9.9
35	Kentucky	9.8
36	Indiana	9.7
37	Virginia	9.6
38	Rhode Island	9.3
39	Arizona	9.2
39	Nevada	9.2
41	Oklahoma	8.6
42	California	8.3
42	Texas	8.3
44	Georgia	8.2
45	Hawaii	8.0
46	Idaho	7.5
47	Colorado	6.7
48	Utah	4.3
NA	Alaska**	NA
NA	Wyoming**	NA
	District of Columbia	17.5

Source: Morgan Quitno Press using data from American Cancer Society
   "Cancer Facts & Figures 2003" (Copyright 2003, Reprinted with permission from the American Cancer Society)
Rates calculated using 2002 Census resident population estimates. Not age-adjusted.
**Fewer than 50 deaths.*

Estimated Deaths by Prostate Cancer in 2003

National Estimated Total = 28,900 Deaths

ALPHA ORDER

RANK	STATE	DEATHS	% of USA
15	Alabama	600	2.1%
NA	Alaska*	NA	NA
15	Arizona	600	2.1%
30	Arkansas	300	1.0%
1	California	2,700	9.3%
30	Colorado	300	1.0%
25	Connecticut	400	1.4%
39	Delaware	100	0.3%
2	Florida	2,100	7.3%
11	Georgia	700	2.4%
39	Hawaii	100	0.3%
39	Idaho	100	0.3%
6	Illinois	1,300	4.5%
11	Indiana	700	2.4%
25	Iowa	400	1.4%
30	Kansas	300	1.0%
25	Kentucky	400	1.4%
20	Louisiana	500	1.7%
39	Maine	100	0.3%
20	Maryland	500	1.7%
11	Massachusetts	700	2.4%
8	Michigan	1,100	3.8%
20	Minnesota	500	1.7%
25	Mississippi	400	1.4%
15	Missouri	600	2.1%
39	Montana	100	0.3%
34	Nebraska	200	0.7%
34	Nevada	200	0.7%
39	New Hampshire	100	0.3%
9	New Jersey	900	3.1%
34	New Mexico	200	0.7%
3	New York	1,800	6.2%
9	North Carolina	900	3.1%
39	North Dakota	100	0.3%
7	Ohio	1,200	4.2%
30	Oklahoma	300	1.0%
25	Oregon	400	1.4%
5	Pennsylvania	1,600	5.5%
39	Rhode Island	100	0.3%
20	South Carolina	500	1.7%
39	South Dakota	100	0.3%
15	Tennessee	600	2.1%
4	Texas	1,700	5.9%
34	Utah	200	0.7%
NA	Vermont*	NA	NA
11	Virginia	700	2.4%
20	Washington	500	1.7%
34	West Virginia	200	0.7%
15	Wisconsin	600	2.1%
39	Wyoming	100	0.3%

RANK ORDER

RANK	STATE	DEATHS	% of USA
1	California	2,700	9.3%
2	Florida	2,100	7.3%
3	New York	1,800	6.2%
4	Texas	1,700	5.9%
5	Pennsylvania	1,600	5.5%
6	Illinois	1,300	4.5%
7	Ohio	1,200	4.2%
8	Michigan	1,100	3.8%
9	New Jersey	900	3.1%
9	North Carolina	900	3.1%
11	Georgia	700	2.4%
11	Indiana	700	2.4%
11	Massachusetts	700	2.4%
11	Virginia	700	2.4%
15	Alabama	600	2.1%
15	Arizona	600	2.1%
15	Missouri	600	2.1%
15	Tennessee	600	2.1%
15	Wisconsin	600	2.1%
20	Louisiana	500	1.7%
20	Maryland	500	1.7%
20	Minnesota	500	1.7%
20	South Carolina	500	1.7%
20	Washington	500	1.7%
25	Connecticut	400	1.4%
25	Iowa	400	1.4%
25	Kentucky	400	1.4%
25	Mississippi	400	1.4%
25	Oregon	400	1.4%
30	Arkansas	300	1.0%
30	Colorado	300	1.0%
30	Kansas	300	1.0%
30	Oklahoma	300	1.0%
34	Nebraska	200	0.7%
34	Nevada	200	0.7%
34	New Mexico	200	0.7%
34	Utah	200	0.7%
34	West Virginia	200	0.7%
39	Delaware	100	0.3%
39	Hawaii	100	0.3%
39	Idaho	100	0.3%
39	Maine	100	0.3%
39	Montana	100	0.3%
39	New Hampshire	100	0.3%
39	North Dakota	100	0.3%
39	Rhode Island	100	0.3%
39	South Dakota	100	0.3%
39	Wyoming	100	0.3%
NA	Alaska*	NA	NA
NA	Vermont*	NA	NA
	District of Columbia	100	0.3%

Source: American Cancer Society
"Cancer Facts & Figures 2003" (Copyright 2003, Reprinted with permission from the American Cancer Society)
*Fewer than 50 deaths.

Age-Adjusted Death Rate by Prostate Cancer in 1999

National Rate = 33.9 Deaths per 100,000 Male Population*

ALPHA ORDER

RANK	STATE	RATE
4	Alabama	41.9
50	Alaska	22.6
46	Arizona	29.9
10	Arkansas	37.4
47	California	29.3
43	Colorado	30.8
42	Connecticut	31.0
8	Delaware	38.8
45	Florida	30.1
5	Georgia	41.6
49	Hawaii	22.7
22	Idaho	35.0
23	Illinois	34.9
16	Indiana	35.9
33	Iowa	33.1
40	Kansas	31.6
20	Kentucky	35.2
3	Louisiana	42.1
31	Maine	33.4
9	Maryland	38.2
34	Massachusetts	33.0
25	Michigan	34.7
19	Minnesota	35.3
1	Mississippi	46.0
37	Missouri	32.2
14	Montana	36.0
48	Nebraska	29.2
36	Nevada	32.8
35	New Hampshire	32.9
29	New Jersey	34.2
31	New Mexico	33.4
37	New York	32.2
6	North Carolina	39.9
17	North Dakota	35.5
26	Ohio	34.6
41	Oklahoma	31.2
21	Oregon	35.1
26	Pennsylvania	34.6
30	Rhode Island	33.9
2	South Carolina	43.2
23	South Dakota	34.9
12	Tennessee	37.1
28	Texas	34.3
13	Utah	37.0
14	Vermont	36.0
7	Virginia	39.1
44	Washington	30.4
39	West Virginia	31.9
17	Wisconsin	35.5
11	Wyoming	37.3

RANK ORDER

RANK	STATE	RATE
1	Mississippi	46.0
2	South Carolina	43.2
3	Louisiana	42.1
4	Alabama	41.9
5	Georgia	41.6
6	North Carolina	39.9
7	Virginia	39.1
8	Delaware	38.8
9	Maryland	38.2
10	Arkansas	37.4
11	Wyoming	37.3
12	Tennessee	37.1
13	Utah	37.0
14	Montana	36.0
14	Vermont	36.0
16	Indiana	35.9
17	North Dakota	35.5
17	Wisconsin	35.5
19	Minnesota	35.3
20	Kentucky	35.2
21	Oregon	35.1
22	Idaho	35.0
23	Illinois	34.9
23	South Dakota	34.9
25	Michigan	34.7
26	Ohio	34.6
26	Pennsylvania	34.6
28	Texas	34.3
29	New Jersey	34.2
30	Rhode Island	33.9
31	Maine	33.4
31	New Mexico	33.4
33	Iowa	33.1
34	Massachusetts	33.0
35	New Hampshire	32.9
36	Nevada	32.8
37	Missouri	32.2
37	New York	32.2
39	West Virginia	31.9
40	Kansas	31.6
41	Oklahoma	31.2
42	Connecticut	31.0
43	Colorado	30.8
44	Washington	30.4
45	Florida	30.1
46	Arizona	29.9
47	California	29.3
48	Nebraska	29.2
49	Hawaii	22.7
50	Alaska	22.6
	District of Columbia	53.7

Source: American Cancer Society
"Cancer Facts & Figures 2003" (Copyright 2003, Reprinted with permission from the American Cancer Society)
*For 1995 to 1999. Age-adjusted to the 2000 U.S. standard population.

Estimated Deaths by Ovarian Cancer in 2003

National Estimated Total = 14,300 Deaths

ALPHA ORDER

RANK	STATE	DEATHS	% of USA
20	Alabama	200	1.4%
NA	Alaska**	NA	NA
20	Arizona	200	1.4%
20	Arkansas	200	1.4%
1	California	1,500	10.5%
20	Colorado	200	1.4%
20	Connecticut	200	1.4%
NA	Delaware**	NA	NA
2	Florida	1,000	7.0%
10	Georgia	400	2.8%
NA	Hawaii**	NA	NA
33	Idaho	100	0.7%
6	Illinois	600	4.2%
10	Indiana	400	2.8%
20	Iowa	200	1.4%
33	Kansas	100	0.7%
20	Kentucky	200	1.4%
20	Louisiana	200	1.4%
33	Maine	100	0.7%
13	Maryland	300	2.1%
13	Massachusetts	300	2.1%
8	Michigan	500	3.5%
20	Minnesota	200	1.4%
20	Mississippi	200	1.4%
13	Missouri	300	2.1%
33	Montana	100	0.7%
33	Nebraska	100	0.7%
33	Nevada	100	0.7%
33	New Hampshire	100	0.7%
8	New Jersey	500	3.5%
33	New Mexico	100	0.7%
2	New York	1,000	7.0%
10	North Carolina	400	2.8%
NA	North Dakota**	NA	NA
6	Ohio	600	4.2%
20	Oklahoma	200	1.4%
20	Oregon	200	1.4%
5	Pennsylvania	700	4.9%
33	Rhode Island	100	0.7%
20	South Carolina	200	1.4%
33	South Dakota	100	0.7%
13	Tennessee	300	2.1%
4	Texas	900	6.3%
33	Utah	100	0.7%
NA	Vermont**	NA	NA
13	Virginia	300	2.1%
13	Washington	300	2.1%
33	West Virginia	100	0.7%
13	Wisconsin	300	2.1%
NA	Wyoming**	NA	NA

RANK ORDER

RANK	STATE	DEATHS	% of USA
1	California	1,500	10.5%
2	Florida	1,000	7.0%
2	New York	1,000	7.0%
4	Texas	900	6.3%
5	Pennsylvania	700	4.9%
6	Illinois	600	4.2%
6	Ohio	600	4.2%
8	Michigan	500	3.5%
8	New Jersey	500	3.5%
10	Georgia	400	2.8%
10	Indiana	400	2.8%
10	North Carolina	400	2.8%
13	Maryland	300	2.1%
13	Massachusetts	300	2.1%
13	Missouri	300	2.1%
13	Tennessee	300	2.1%
13	Virginia	300	2.1%
13	Washington	300	2.1%
13	Wisconsin	300	2.1%
20	Alabama	200	1.4%
20	Arizona	200	1.4%
20	Arkansas	200	1.4%
20	Colorado	200	1.4%
20	Connecticut	200	1.4%
20	Iowa	200	1.4%
20	Kentucky	200	1.4%
20	Louisiana	200	1.4%
20	Minnesota	200	1.4%
20	Mississippi	200	1.4%
20	Oklahoma	200	1.4%
20	Oregon	200	1.4%
20	South Carolina	200	1.4%
33	Idaho	100	0.7%
33	Kansas	100	0.7%
33	Maine	100	0.7%
33	Montana	100	0.7%
33	Nebraska	100	0.7%
33	Nevada	100	0.7%
33	New Hampshire	100	0.7%
33	New Mexico	100	0.7%
33	Rhode Island	100	0.7%
33	South Dakota	100	0.7%
33	Utah	100	0.7%
33	West Virginia	100	0.7%
NA	Alaska**	NA	NA
NA	Delaware**	NA	NA
NA	Hawaii**	NA	NA
NA	North Dakota**	NA	NA
NA	Vermont**	NA	NA
NA	Wyoming**	NA	NA
	District of Columbia**	NA	NA

Source: American Cancer Society
    "Cancer Facts & Figures 2003" (Copyright 2003, Reprinted with permission from the American Cancer Society)
*Fewer than 50 deaths.

Estimated Death Rate by Ovarian Cancer in 2003

National Estimated Rate = 10.0 Deaths per 100,000 Female Population*

ALPHA ORDER

RANK	STATE	RATE
38	Alabama	8.7
NA	Alaska**	NA
43	Arizona	7.8
7	Arkansas	14.6
37	California	8.8
34	Colorado	9.4
15	Connecticut	11.4
NA	Delaware**	NA
11	Florida	12.2
32	Georgia	9.6
NA	Hawaii**	NA
5	Idaho	15.5
33	Illinois	9.5
10	Indiana	12.9
9	Iowa	13.4
44	Kansas	7.4
29	Kentucky	9.7
38	Louisiana	8.7
6	Maine	15.3
18	Maryland	11.0
35	Massachusetts	9.1
28	Michigan	9.9
42	Minnesota	8.1
8	Mississippi	13.6
22	Missouri	10.4
2	Montana	22.1
13	Nebraska	11.5
25	Nevada	10.2
4	New Hampshire	15.9
13	New Jersey	11.5
20	New Mexico	10.8
25	New York	10.2
29	North Carolina	9.7
NA	North Dakota**	NA
23	Ohio	10.3
15	Oklahoma	11.4
12	Oregon	11.6
18	Pennsylvania	11.0
3	Rhode Island	18.4
29	South Carolina	9.7
1	South Dakota	26.3
23	Tennessee	10.3
40	Texas	8.6
36	Utah	9.0
NA	Vermont**	NA
41	Virginia	8.3
27	Washington	10.1
20	West Virginia	10.8
17	Wisconsin	11.1
NA	Wyoming**	NA

RANK ORDER

RANK	STATE	RATE
1	South Dakota	26.3
2	Montana	22.1
3	Rhode Island	18.4
4	New Hampshire	15.9
5	Idaho	15.5
6	Maine	15.3
7	Arkansas	14.6
8	Mississippi	13.6
9	Iowa	13.4
10	Indiana	12.9
11	Florida	12.2
12	Oregon	11.6
13	Nebraska	11.5
13	New Jersey	11.5
15	Connecticut	11.4
15	Oklahoma	11.4
17	Wisconsin	11.1
18	Maryland	11.0
18	Pennsylvania	11.0
20	New Mexico	10.8
20	West Virginia	10.8
22	Missouri	10.4
23	Ohio	10.3
23	Tennessee	10.3
25	Nevada	10.2
25	New York	10.2
27	Washington	10.1
28	Michigan	9.9
29	Kentucky	9.7
29	North Carolina	9.7
29	South Carolina	9.7
32	Georgia	9.6
33	Illinois	9.5
34	Colorado	9.4
35	Massachusetts	9.1
36	Utah	9.0
37	California	8.8
38	Alabama	8.7
38	Louisiana	8.7
40	Texas	8.6
41	Virginia	8.3
42	Minnesota	8.1
43	Arizona	7.8
44	Kansas	7.4
NA	Alaska**	NA
NA	Delaware**	NA
NA	Hawaii**	NA
NA	North Dakota**	NA
NA	Vermont**	NA
NA	Wyoming**	NA
	District of Columbia**	NA

Source: Morgan Quitno Press using data from American Cancer Society
   "Cancer Facts & Figures 2003" (Copyright 2003, Reprinted with permission from the American Cancer Society)
*Rates calculated using 2000 Census female population counts. Not age-adjusted.
**Fewer than 50 deaths.

Estimated Deaths by Brain Cancer in 2003

National Estimated Total = 13,100 Deaths

ALPHA ORDER

RANK	STATE	DEATHS	% of USA
20	Alabama	200	1.5%
NA	Alaska*	NA	NA
20	Arizona	200	1.5%
20	Arkansas	200	1.5%
1	California	1,500	11.5%
20	Colorado	200	1.5%
20	Connecticut	200	1.5%
NA	Delaware*	NA	NA
2	Florida	900	6.9%
11	Georgia	300	2.3%
NA	Hawaii*	NA	NA
33	Idaho	100	0.8%
7	Illinois	500	3.8%
11	Indiana	300	2.3%
20	Iowa	200	1.5%
33	Kansas	100	0.8%
20	Kentucky	200	1.5%
20	Louisiana	200	1.5%
33	Maine	100	0.8%
20	Maryland	200	1.5%
11	Massachusetts	300	2.3%
7	Michigan	500	3.8%
11	Minnesota	300	2.3%
20	Mississippi	200	1.5%
11	Missouri	300	2.3%
33	Montana	100	0.8%
33	Nebraska	100	0.8%
33	Nevada	100	0.8%
33	New Hampshire	100	0.8%
9	New Jersey	400	3.1%
33	New Mexico	100	0.8%
4	New York	800	6.1%
9	North Carolina	400	3.1%
NA	North Dakota*	NA	NA
5	Ohio	600	4.6%
20	Oklahoma	200	1.5%
20	Oregon	200	1.5%
5	Pennsylvania	600	4.6%
33	Rhode Island	100	0.8%
20	South Carolina	200	1.5%
33	South Dakota	100	0.8%
11	Tennessee	300	2.3%
2	Texas	900	6.9%
33	Utah	100	0.8%
NA	Vermont*	NA	NA
11	Virginia	300	2.3%
11	Washington	300	2.3%
33	West Virginia	100	0.8%
11	Wisconsin	300	2.3%
NA	Wyoming*	NA	NA

RANK ORDER

RANK	STATE	DEATHS	% of USA
1	California	1,500	11.5%
2	Florida	900	6.9%
2	Texas	900	6.9%
4	New York	800	6.1%
5	Ohio	600	4.6%
5	Pennsylvania	600	4.6%
7	Illinois	500	3.8%
7	Michigan	500	3.8%
9	New Jersey	400	3.1%
9	North Carolina	400	3.1%
11	Georgia	300	2.3%
11	Indiana	300	2.3%
11	Massachusetts	300	2.3%
11	Minnesota	300	2.3%
11	Missouri	300	2.3%
11	Tennessee	300	2.3%
11	Virginia	300	2.3%
11	Washington	300	2.3%
11	Wisconsin	300	2.3%
20	Alabama	200	1.5%
20	Arizona	200	1.5%
20	Arkansas	200	1.5%
20	Colorado	200	1.5%
20	Connecticut	200	1.5%
20	Iowa	200	1.5%
20	Kentucky	200	1.5%
20	Louisiana	200	1.5%
20	Maryland	200	1.5%
20	Mississippi	200	1.5%
20	Oklahoma	200	1.5%
20	Oregon	200	1.5%
20	South Carolina	200	1.5%
33	Idaho	100	0.8%
33	Kansas	100	0.8%
33	Maine	100	0.8%
33	Montana	100	0.8%
33	Nebraska	100	0.8%
33	Nevada	100	0.8%
33	New Hampshire	100	0.8%
33	New Mexico	100	0.8%
33	Rhode Island	100	0.8%
33	South Dakota	100	0.8%
33	Utah	100	0.8%
33	West Virginia	100	0.8%
NA	Alaska*	NA	NA
NA	Delaware*	NA	NA
NA	Hawaii*	NA	NA
NA	North Dakota*	NA	NA
NA	Vermont*	NA	NA
NA	Wyoming*	NA	NA
	District of Columbia*	NA	NA

Source: American Cancer Society
"Cancer Facts & Figures 2003" (Copyright 2003, Reprinted with permission from the American Cancer Society)
*Fewer than 50 deaths.

Estimated Death Rate by Brain Cancer in 2003

National Estimated Rate = 4.5 Deaths per 100,000 Population*

ALPHA ORDER

RANK	STATE	RATE
32	Alabama	4.5
NA	Alaska**	NA
41	Arizona	3.7
7	Arkansas	7.4
35	California	4.3
34	Colorado	4.4
11	Connecticut	5.8
NA	Delaware**	NA
17	Florida	5.4
44	Georgia	3.5
NA	Hawaii**	NA
6	Idaho	7.5
40	Illinois	4.0
23	Indiana	4.9
9	Iowa	6.8
41	Kansas	3.7
23	Kentucky	4.9
32	Louisiana	4.5
5	Maine	7.7
41	Maryland	3.7
29	Massachusetts	4.7
22	Michigan	5.0
10	Minnesota	6.0
8	Mississippi	7.0
19	Missouri	5.3
2	Montana	11.0
11	Nebraska	5.8
31	Nevada	4.6
4	New Hampshire	7.8
29	New Jersey	4.7
17	New Mexico	5.4
37	New York	4.2
28	North Carolina	4.8
NA	North Dakota**	NA
19	Ohio	5.3
13	Oklahoma	5.7
13	Oregon	5.7
23	Pennsylvania	4.9
3	Rhode Island	9.3
23	South Carolina	4.9
1	South Dakota	13.1
21	Tennessee	5.2
38	Texas	4.1
35	Utah	4.3
NA	Vermont**	NA
38	Virginia	4.1
23	Washington	4.9
15	West Virginia	5.5
15	Wisconsin	5.5
NA	Wyoming**	NA

RANK ORDER

RANK	STATE	RATE
1	South Dakota	13.1
2	Montana	11.0
3	Rhode Island	9.3
4	New Hampshire	7.8
5	Maine	7.7
6	Idaho	7.5
7	Arkansas	7.4
8	Mississippi	7.0
9	Iowa	6.8
10	Minnesota	6.0
11	Connecticut	5.8
11	Nebraska	5.8
13	Oklahoma	5.7
13	Oregon	5.7
15	West Virginia	5.5
15	Wisconsin	5.5
17	Florida	5.4
17	New Mexico	5.4
19	Missouri	5.3
19	Ohio	5.3
21	Tennessee	5.2
22	Michigan	5.0
23	Indiana	4.9
23	Kentucky	4.9
23	Pennsylvania	4.9
23	South Carolina	4.9
23	Washington	4.9
28	North Carolina	4.8
29	Massachusetts	4.7
29	New Jersey	4.7
31	Nevada	4.6
32	Alabama	4.5
32	Louisiana	4.5
34	Colorado	4.4
35	California	4.3
35	Utah	4.3
37	New York	4.2
38	Texas	4.1
38	Virginia	4.1
40	Illinois	4.0
41	Arizona	3.7
41	Kansas	3.7
41	Maryland	3.7
44	Georgia	3.5
NA	Alaska**	NA
NA	Delaware**	NA
NA	Hawaii**	NA
NA	North Dakota**	NA
NA	Vermont**	NA
NA	Wyoming**	NA
	District of Columbia**	NA

Source: Morgan Quitno Press using data from American Cancer Society
   "Cancer Facts & Figures 2003" (Copyright 2003, Reprinted with permission from the American Cancer Society)
*Rates calculated using 2000 Census female population counts. Not age-adjusted.
**Fewer than 50 deaths.

Deaths by Alzheimer's Disease in 2000

National Total = 49,558 Deaths*

ALPHA ORDER

RANK	STATE	DEATHS	% of USA
22	Alabama	895	1.8%
50	Alaska	47	0.1%
19	Arizona	1,045	2.1%
34	Arkansas	430	0.9%
1	California	4,419	8.9%
28	Colorado	712	1.4%
31	Connecticut	526	1.1%
48	Delaware	110	0.2%
2	Florida	3,265	6.6%
13	Georgia	1,235	2.5%
47	Hawaii	118	0.2%
40	Idaho	262	0.5%
6	Illinois	2,154	4.3%
14	Indiana	1,209	2.4%
27	Iowa	769	1.6%
30	Kansas	630	1.3%
24	Kentucky	845	1.7%
25	Louisiana	811	1.6%
32	Maine	466	0.9%
25	Maryland	811	1.6%
11	Massachusetts	1,433	2.9%
9	Michigan	1,646	3.3%
16	Minnesota	1,154	2.3%
33	Mississippi	443	0.9%
17	Missouri	1,096	2.2%
42	Montana	219	0.4%
36	Nebraska	353	0.7%
44	Nevada	195	0.4%
39	New Hampshire	273	0.6%
12	New Jersey	1,267	2.6%
38	New Mexico	275	0.6%
10	New York	1,539	3.1%
8	North Carolina	1,725	3.5%
43	North Dakota	209	0.4%
5	Ohio	2,295	4.6%
29	Oklahoma	638	1.3%
21	Oregon	910	1.8%
4	Pennsylvania	2,542	5.1%
41	Rhode Island	242	0.5%
23	South Carolina	874	1.8%
45	South Dakota	179	0.4%
20	Tennessee	1,024	2.1%
3	Texas	3,184	6.4%
37	Utah	342	0.7%
46	Vermont	134	0.3%
18	Virginia	1,094	2.2%
7	Washington	1,799	3.6%
35	West Virginia	361	0.7%
15	Wisconsin	1,177	2.4%
49	Wyoming	102	0.2%

RANK ORDER

RANK	STATE	DEATHS	% of USA
1	California	4,419	8.9%
2	Florida	3,265	6.6%
3	Texas	3,184	6.4%
4	Pennsylvania	2,542	5.1%
5	Ohio	2,295	4.6%
6	Illinois	2,154	4.3%
7	Washington	1,799	3.6%
8	North Carolina	1,725	3.5%
9	Michigan	1,646	3.3%
10	New York	1,539	3.1%
11	Massachusetts	1,433	2.9%
12	New Jersey	1,267	2.6%
13	Georgia	1,235	2.5%
14	Indiana	1,209	2.4%
15	Wisconsin	1,177	2.4%
16	Minnesota	1,154	2.3%
17	Missouri	1,096	2.2%
18	Virginia	1,094	2.2%
19	Arizona	1,045	2.1%
20	Tennessee	1,024	2.1%
21	Oregon	910	1.8%
22	Alabama	895	1.8%
23	South Carolina	874	1.8%
24	Kentucky	845	1.7%
25	Louisiana	811	1.6%
25	Maryland	811	1.6%
27	Iowa	769	1.6%
28	Colorado	712	1.4%
29	Oklahoma	638	1.3%
30	Kansas	630	1.3%
31	Connecticut	526	1.1%
32	Maine	466	0.9%
33	Mississippi	443	0.9%
34	Arkansas	430	0.9%
35	West Virginia	361	0.7%
36	Nebraska	353	0.7%
37	Utah	342	0.7%
38	New Mexico	275	0.6%
39	New Hampshire	273	0.6%
40	Idaho	262	0.5%
41	Rhode Island	242	0.5%
42	Montana	219	0.4%
43	North Dakota	209	0.4%
44	Nevada	195	0.4%
45	South Dakota	179	0.4%
46	Vermont	134	0.3%
47	Hawaii	118	0.2%
48	Delaware	110	0.2%
49	Wyoming	102	0.2%
50	Alaska	47	0.1%
	District of Columbia	75	0.2%

Source: U.S. Department of Health and Human Services, National Center for Health Statistics "National Vital Statistics Reports" (Vol. 50, No. 15, September 16, 2002)

*Final data by state of residence. A degenerative disease of the brain cells producing loss of memory and general intellectual impairment. It usually affects people over age 65. As the disease progresses, a variety of symptoms may become apparent, including confusion, irritability, and restlessness, as well as disorientation and impaired judgment and concentration.

Death Rate by Alzheimer's Disease in 2000

National Rate = 18.0 Deaths per 100,000 Population*

ALPHA ORDER

RANK	STATE	RATE
24	Alabama	20.4
50	Alaska	7.6
17	Arizona	21.4
34	Arkansas	16.7
46	California	13.1
33	Colorado	17.2
36	Connecticut	16.0
45	Delaware	14.4
18	Florida	21.3
42	Georgia	15.5
48	Hawaii	10.0
23	Idaho	20.6
32	Illinois	17.7
26	Indiana	20.2
5	Iowa	26.7
10	Kansas	23.6
19	Kentucky	21.2
30	Louisiana	18.5
1	Maine	37.0
42	Maryland	15.5
11	Massachusetts	23.1
35	Michigan	16.6
9	Minnesota	23.9
37	Mississippi	15.9
28	Missouri	19.9
6	Montana	24.7
22	Nebraska	21.1
47	Nevada	10.4
12	New Hampshire	22.5
44	New Jersey	15.4
39	New Mexico	15.7
49	New York	8.4
14	North Carolina	22.3
2	North Dakota	33.2
24	Ohio	20.4
29	Oklahoma	18.9
4	Oregon	27.2
19	Pennsylvania	21.2
7	Rhode Island	24.3
14	South Carolina	22.3
7	South Dakota	24.3
30	Tennessee	18.5
41	Texas	15.6
38	Utah	15.8
13	Vermont	22.4
39	Virginia	15.7
3	Washington	31.0
27	West Virginia	20.0
16	Wisconsin	22.2
19	Wyoming	21.2

RANK ORDER

RANK	STATE	RATE
1	Maine	37.0
2	North Dakota	33.2
3	Washington	31.0
4	Oregon	27.2
5	Iowa	26.7
6	Montana	24.7
7	Rhode Island	24.3
7	South Dakota	24.3
9	Minnesota	23.9
10	Kansas	23.6
11	Massachusetts	23.1
12	New Hampshire	22.5
13	Vermont	22.4
14	North Carolina	22.3
14	South Carolina	22.3
16	Wisconsin	22.2
17	Arizona	21.4
18	Florida	21.3
19	Kentucky	21.2
19	Pennsylvania	21.2
19	Wyoming	21.2
22	Nebraska	21.1
23	Idaho	20.6
24	Alabama	20.4
24	Ohio	20.4
26	Indiana	20.2
27	West Virginia	20.0
28	Missouri	19.9
29	Oklahoma	18.9
30	Louisiana	18.5
30	Tennessee	18.5
32	Illinois	17.7
33	Colorado	17.2
34	Arkansas	16.7
35	Michigan	16.6
36	Connecticut	16.0
37	Mississippi	15.9
38	Utah	15.8
39	New Mexico	15.7
39	Virginia	15.7
41	Texas	15.6
42	Georgia	15.5
42	Maryland	15.5
44	New Jersey	15.4
45	Delaware	14.4
46	California	13.1
47	Nevada	10.4
48	Hawaii	10.0
49	New York	8.4
50	Alaska	7.6

| | District of Columbia | 14.5 |

Source: U.S. Department of Health and Human Services, National Center for Health Statistics
"National Vital Statistics Reports" (Vol. 50, No. 15, September 16, 2002)
*Final data by state of residence. A degenerative disease of the brain cells producing loss of memory and general intellectual impairment. It usually affects people over age 65. As the disease progresses, a variety of symptoms may become apparent, including confusion, irritability, and restlessness, as well as disorientation and impaired judgment and concentration. Not age-adjusted.

Age-Adjusted Death Rate by Alzheimer's Disease in 2000

National Rate = 18.0 Deaths per 100,000 Population*

ALPHA ORDER

RANK	STATE	RATE
21	Alabama	20.5
18	Alaska	21.6
12	Arizona	22.4
45	Arkansas	14.9
43	California	15.1
10	Colorado	22.5
48	Connecticut	13.0
42	Delaware	15.3
43	Florida	15.1
17	Georgia	21.8
49	Hawaii	9.8
10	Idaho	22.5
36	Illinois	17.3
21	Indiana	20.5
24	Iowa	19.9
23	Kansas	20.3
14	Kentucky	22.2
19	Louisiana	21.2
2	Maine	32.5
32	Maryland	17.8
27	Massachusetts	19.6
39	Michigan	17.1
13	Minnesota	22.3
40	Mississippi	16.9
34	Missouri	17.7
14	Montana	22.2
36	Nebraska	17.3
46	Nevada	14.7
7	New Hampshire	23.6
47	New Jersey	14.2
31	New Mexico	18.2
50	New York	7.6
5	North Carolina	24.2
6	North Dakota	24.0
28	Ohio	19.5
34	Oklahoma	17.7
4	Oregon	25.1
41	Pennsylvania	16.6
32	Rhode Island	17.8
3	South Carolina	25.5
30	South Dakota	18.5
26	Tennessee	19.7
20	Texas	20.7
8	Utah	23.2
16	Vermont	22.1
29	Virginia	18.8
1	Washington	33.4
38	West Virginia	17.2
24	Wisconsin	19.9
8	Wyoming	23.2

RANK ORDER

RANK	STATE	RATE
1	Washington	33.4
2	Maine	32.5
3	South Carolina	25.5
4	Oregon	25.1
5	North Carolina	24.2
6	North Dakota	24.0
7	New Hampshire	23.6
8	Utah	23.2
8	Wyoming	23.2
10	Colorado	22.5
10	Idaho	22.5
12	Arizona	22.4
13	Minnesota	22.3
14	Kentucky	22.2
14	Montana	22.2
16	Vermont	22.1
17	Georgia	21.8
18	Alaska	21.6
19	Louisiana	21.2
20	Texas	20.7
21	Alabama	20.5
21	Indiana	20.5
23	Kansas	20.3
24	Iowa	19.9
24	Wisconsin	19.9
26	Tennessee	19.7
27	Massachusetts	19.6
28	Ohio	19.5
29	Virginia	18.8
30	South Dakota	18.5
31	New Mexico	18.2
32	Maryland	17.8
32	Rhode Island	17.8
34	Missouri	17.7
34	Oklahoma	17.7
36	Illinois	17.3
36	Nebraska	17.3
38	West Virginia	17.2
39	Michigan	17.1
40	Mississippi	16.9
41	Pennsylvania	16.6
42	Delaware	15.3
43	California	15.1
43	Florida	15.1
45	Arkansas	14.9
46	Nevada	14.7
47	New Jersey	14.2
48	Connecticut	13.0
49	Hawaii	9.8
50	New York	7.6
	District of Columbia	12.2

Source: U.S. Department of Health and Human Services, National Center for Health Statistics
"National Vital Statistics Reports" (Vol. 50, No. 15, September 16, 2002)
*Final data by state of residence. A degenerative disease of the brain cells producing loss of memory and general intellectual impairment. It usually affects people over age 65. As the disease progresses, a variety of symptoms may become apparent, including confusion, irritability, and restlessness, as well as disorientation and impaired judgment and concentration. Age-adjusted rates based on the year 2000 standard population.

Deaths by Atherosclerosis in 1999

National Total = 14,979 Deaths*

ALPHA ORDER

ALPHA ORDER

RANK	STATE	DEATHS	% of USA
25	Alabama	215	1.4%
49	Alaska	15	0.1%
21	Arizona	278	1.9%
33	Arkansas	156	1.0%
1	California	1,825	12.2%
9	Colorado	484	3.2%
30	Connecticut	170	1.1%
49	Delaware	15	0.1%
2	Florida	1,035	6.9%
11	Georgia	463	3.1%
45	Hawaii	32	0.2%
42	Idaho	46	0.3%
7	Illinois	611	4.1%
14	Indiana	404	2.7%
17	Iowa	326	2.2%
15	Kansas	345	2.3%
31	Kentucky	159	1.1%
24	Louisiana	219	1.5%
44	Maine	39	0.3%
28	Maryland	187	1.2%
19	Massachusetts	322	2.1%
8	Michigan	579	3.9%
26	Minnesota	209	1.4%
35	Mississippi	101	0.7%
20	Missouri	315	2.1%
41	Montana	51	0.3%
32	Nebraska	158	1.1%
40	Nevada	60	0.4%
38	New Hampshire	74	0.5%
12	New Jersey	439	2.9%
36	New Mexico	81	0.5%
5	New York	638	4.3%
13	North Carolina	423	2.8%
43	North Dakota	45	0.3%
6	Ohio	626	4.2%
10	Oklahoma	476	3.2%
27	Oregon	199	1.3%
4	Pennsylvania	641	4.3%
37	Rhode Island	77	0.5%
34	South Carolina	104	0.7%
45	South Dakota	32	0.2%
18	Tennessee	323	2.2%
3	Texas	838	5.6%
39	Utah	70	0.5%
47	Vermont	20	0.1%
22	Virginia	249	1.7%
15	Washington	345	2.3%
29	West Virginia	173	1.2%
23	Wisconsin	243	1.6%
48	Wyoming	18	0.1%

RANK ORDER

RANK	STATE	DEATHS	% of USA
1	California	1,825	12.2%
2	Florida	1,035	6.9%
3	Texas	838	5.6%
4	Pennsylvania	641	4.3%
5	New York	638	4.3%
6	Ohio	626	4.2%
7	Illinois	611	4.1%
8	Michigan	579	3.9%
9	Colorado	484	3.2%
10	Oklahoma	476	3.2%
11	Georgia	463	3.1%
12	New Jersey	439	2.9%
13	North Carolina	423	2.8%
14	Indiana	404	2.7%
15	Kansas	345	2.3%
15	Washington	345	2.3%
17	Iowa	326	2.2%
18	Tennessee	323	2.2%
19	Massachusetts	322	2.1%
20	Missouri	315	2.1%
21	Arizona	278	1.9%
22	Virginia	249	1.7%
23	Wisconsin	243	1.6%
24	Louisiana	219	1.5%
25	Alabama	215	1.4%
26	Minnesota	209	1.4%
27	Oregon	199	1.3%
28	Maryland	187	1.2%
29	West Virginia	173	1.2%
30	Connecticut	170	1.1%
31	Kentucky	159	1.1%
32	Nebraska	158	1.1%
33	Arkansas	156	1.0%
34	South Carolina	104	0.7%
35	Mississippi	101	0.7%
36	New Mexico	81	0.5%
37	Rhode Island	77	0.5%
38	New Hampshire	74	0.5%
39	Utah	70	0.5%
40	Nevada	60	0.4%
41	Montana	51	0.3%
42	Idaho	46	0.3%
43	North Dakota	45	0.3%
44	Maine	39	0.3%
45	Hawaii	32	0.2%
45	South Dakota	32	0.2%
47	Vermont	20	0.1%
48	Wyoming	18	0.1%
49	Alaska	15	0.1%
49	Delaware	15	0.1%
	District of Columbia	26	0.2%

*Source: U.S. Department of Health and Human Services, National Center for Health Statistics
(http://wonder.cdc.gov/WONDER/)*
Final data by state of residence. Atherosclerosis is a form of hardening of the arteries.

Death Rate by Atherosclerosis in 1999

National Rate = 5.5 Deaths per 100,000 Population*

ALPHA ORDER

RANK	STATE	RATE
30	Alabama	4.9
49	Alaska**	2.4
18	Arizona	5.8
12	Arkansas	6.1
22	California	5.5
3	Colorado	11.9
26	Connecticut	5.2
50	Delaware**	2.0
9	Florida	6.8
15	Georgia	5.9
47	Hawaii	2.7
38	Idaho	3.7
28	Illinois	5.0
9	Indiana	6.8
4	Iowa	11.4
2	Kansas	13.0
36	Kentucky	4.0
28	Louisiana	5.0
46	Maine	3.1
39	Maryland	3.6
26	Massachusetts	5.2
15	Michigan	5.9
33	Minnesota	4.4
39	Mississippi	3.6
18	Missouri	5.8
18	Montana	5.8
6	Nebraska	9.5
44	Nevada	3.3
11	New Hampshire	6.2
24	New Jersey	5.4
31	New Mexico	4.7
42	New York	3.5
22	North Carolina	5.5
8	North Dakota	7.1
21	Ohio	5.6
1	Oklahoma	14.2
13	Oregon	6.0
25	Pennsylvania	5.3
7	Rhode Island	7.8
47	South Carolina	2.7
33	South Dakota	4.4
15	Tennessee	5.9
35	Texas	4.2
44	Utah	3.3
43	Vermont	3.4
39	Virginia	3.6
13	Washington	6.0
5	West Virginia	9.6
32	Wisconsin	4.6
37	Wyoming**	3.8

RANK ORDER

RANK	STATE	RATE
1	Oklahoma	14.2
2	Kansas	13.0
3	Colorado	11.9
4	Iowa	11.4
5	West Virginia	9.6
6	Nebraska	9.5
7	Rhode Island	7.8
8	North Dakota	7.1
9	Florida	6.8
9	Indiana	6.8
11	New Hampshire	6.2
12	Arkansas	6.1
13	Oregon	6.0
13	Washington	6.0
15	Georgia	5.9
15	Michigan	5.9
15	Tennessee	5.9
18	Arizona	5.8
18	Missouri	5.8
18	Montana	5.8
21	Ohio	5.6
22	California	5.5
22	North Carolina	5.5
24	New Jersey	5.4
25	Pennsylvania	5.3
26	Connecticut	5.2
26	Massachusetts	5.2
28	Illinois	5.0
28	Louisiana	5.0
30	Alabama	4.9
31	New Mexico	4.7
32	Wisconsin	4.6
33	Minnesota	4.4
33	South Dakota	4.4
35	Texas	4.2
36	Kentucky	4.0
37	Wyoming**	3.8
38	Idaho	3.7
39	Maryland	3.6
39	Mississippi	3.6
39	Virginia	3.6
42	New York	3.5
43	Vermont	3.4
44	Nevada	3.3
44	Utah	3.3
46	Maine	3.1
47	Hawaii	2.7
47	South Carolina	2.7
49	Alaska**	2.4
50	Delaware**	2.0

| | District of Columbia | 5.0 |

Source: U.S. Department of Health and Human Services, National Center for Health Statistics
    (http://wonder.cdc.gov/WONDER/)
*Final data by state of residence. Atherosclerosis is a form of hardening of the arteries. Not age-adjusted.
**Due to low numbers of deaths, rates for these states should be interpreted with caution.

Age-Adjusted Death Rate by Atherosclerosis in 1999

National Rate = 5.5 Deaths per 100,000 Population*

ALPHA ORDER

RANK	STATE	RATE
27	Alabama	5.0
31	Alaska**	4.7
13	Arizona	6.1
19	Arkansas	5.5
9	California	6.5
1	Colorado	15.5
34	Connecticut	4.3
50	Delaware**	2.0
29	Florida	4.9
6	Georgia	8.0
49	Hawaii	2.7
42	Idaho	4.0
27	Illinois	5.0
8	Indiana	6.9
4	Iowa	8.5
3	Kansas	11.1
37	Kentucky	4.2
16	Louisiana	5.9
48	Maine	2.8
37	Maryland	4.2
32	Massachusetts	4.5
13	Michigan	6.1
41	Minnesota	4.1
43	Mississippi	3.9
24	Missouri	5.2
23	Montana	5.3
7	Nebraska	7.7
32	Nevada	4.5
9	New Hampshire	6.5
25	New Jersey	5.1
19	New Mexico	5.5
46	New York	3.3
15	North Carolina	6.0
25	North Dakota	5.1
21	Ohio	5.4
2	Oklahoma	13.3
18	Oregon	5.6
34	Pennsylvania	4.3
16	Rhode Island	5.9
47	South Carolina	3.1
44	South Dakota	3.5
12	Tennessee	6.2
21	Texas	5.4
29	Utah	4.9
45	Vermont	3.4
34	Virginia	4.3
9	Washington	6.5
5	West Virginia	8.3
37	Wisconsin	4.2
37	Wyoming**	4.2

RANK ORDER

RANK	STATE	RATE
1	Colorado	15.5
2	Oklahoma	13.3
3	Kansas	11.1
4	Iowa	8.5
5	West Virginia	8.3
6	Georgia	8.0
7	Nebraska	7.7
8	Indiana	6.9
9	California	6.5
9	New Hampshire	6.5
9	Washington	6.5
12	Tennessee	6.2
13	Arizona	6.1
13	Michigan	6.1
15	North Carolina	6.0
16	Louisiana	5.9
16	Rhode Island	5.9
18	Oregon	5.6
19	Arkansas	5.5
19	New Mexico	5.5
21	Ohio	5.4
21	Texas	5.4
23	Montana	5.3
24	Missouri	5.2
25	New Jersey	5.1
25	North Dakota	5.1
27	Alabama	5.0
27	Illinois	5.0
29	Florida	4.9
29	Utah	4.9
31	Alaska**	4.7
32	Massachusetts	4.5
32	Nevada	4.5
34	Connecticut	4.3
34	Pennsylvania	4.3
34	Virginia	4.3
37	Kentucky	4.2
37	Maryland	4.2
37	Wisconsin	4.2
37	Wyoming**	4.2
41	Minnesota	4.1
42	Idaho	4.0
43	Mississippi	3.9
44	South Dakota	3.5
45	Vermont	3.4
46	New York	3.3
47	South Carolina	3.1
48	Maine	2.8
49	Hawaii	2.7
50	Delaware**	2.0
	District of Columbia	4.5

Source: U.S. Department of Health and Human Services, National Center for Health Statistics
    (http://wonder.cdc.gov/WONDER/)
*Final data by state of residence. Atherosclerosis is a form of hardening of the arteries. Age-adjusted rates based on the year 2000 standard population.
**Due to low numbers of deaths, rates for these states should be interpreted with caution.

Deaths by Cerebrovascular Diseases in 2000

National Total = 167,661 Deaths*

ALPHA ORDER

RANK	STATE	DEATHS	% of USA
19	Alabama	3,183	1.9%
50	Alaska	170	0.1%
23	Arizona	2,648	1.6%
28	Arkansas	2,255	1.3%
1	California	18,185	10.8%
32	Colorado	1,907	1.1%
30	Connecticut	2,011	1.2%
47	Delaware	430	0.3%
3	Florida	10,532	6.3%
10	Georgia	4,625	2.8%
40	Hawaii	747	0.4%
41	Idaho	720	0.4%
6	Illinois	7,429	4.4%
13	Indiana	4,247	2.5%
29	Iowa	2,187	1.3%
33	Kansas	1,830	1.1%
24	Kentucky	2,637	1.6%
26	Louisiana	2,533	1.5%
38	Maine	833	0.5%
21	Maryland	2,955	1.8%
17	Massachusetts	3,669	2.2%
8	Michigan	5,864	3.5%
22	Minnesota	2,820	1.7%
31	Mississippi	1,999	1.2%
15	Missouri	3,940	2.3%
43	Montana	583	0.3%
35	Nebraska	1,091	0.7%
37	Nevada	872	0.5%
42	New Hampshire	662	0.4%
11	New Jersey	4,316	2.6%
39	New Mexico	813	0.5%
5	New York	8,006	4.8%
9	North Carolina	5,749	3.4%
46	North Dakota	456	0.3%
7	Ohio	7,175	4.3%
27	Oklahoma	2,493	1.5%
25	Oregon	2,585	1.5%
4	Pennsylvania	8,919	5.3%
44	Rhode Island	577	0.3%
20	South Carolina	2,956	1.8%
45	South Dakota	560	0.3%
12	Tennessee	4,266	2.5%
2	Texas	10,684	6.4%
36	Utah	975	0.6%
48	Vermont	343	0.2%
14	Virginia	4,104	2.4%
16	Washington	3,714	2.2%
34	West Virginia	1,296	0.8%
18	Wisconsin	3,598	2.1%
49	Wyoming	260	0.2%

RANK ORDER

RANK	STATE	DEATHS	% of USA
1	California	18,185	10.8%
2	Texas	10,684	6.4%
3	Florida	10,532	6.3%
4	Pennsylvania	8,919	5.3%
5	New York	8,006	4.8%
6	Illinois	7,429	4.4%
7	Ohio	7,175	4.3%
8	Michigan	5,864	3.5%
9	North Carolina	5,749	3.4%
10	Georgia	4,625	2.8%
11	New Jersey	4,316	2.6%
12	Tennessee	4,266	2.5%
13	Indiana	4,247	2.5%
14	Virginia	4,104	2.4%
15	Missouri	3,940	2.3%
16	Washington	3,714	2.2%
17	Massachusetts	3,669	2.2%
18	Wisconsin	3,598	2.1%
19	Alabama	3,183	1.9%
20	South Carolina	2,956	1.8%
21	Maryland	2,955	1.8%
22	Minnesota	2,820	1.7%
23	Arizona	2,648	1.6%
24	Kentucky	2,637	1.6%
25	Oregon	2,585	1.5%
26	Louisiana	2,533	1.5%
27	Oklahoma	2,493	1.5%
28	Arkansas	2,255	1.3%
29	Iowa	2,187	1.3%
30	Connecticut	2,011	1.2%
31	Mississippi	1,999	1.2%
32	Colorado	1,907	1.1%
33	Kansas	1,830	1.1%
34	West Virginia	1,296	0.8%
35	Nebraska	1,091	0.7%
36	Utah	975	0.6%
37	Nevada	872	0.5%
38	Maine	833	0.5%
39	New Mexico	813	0.5%
40	Hawaii	747	0.4%
41	Idaho	720	0.4%
42	New Hampshire	662	0.4%
43	Montana	583	0.3%
44	Rhode Island	577	0.3%
45	South Dakota	560	0.3%
46	North Dakota	456	0.3%
47	Delaware	430	0.3%
48	Vermont	343	0.2%
49	Wyoming	260	0.2%
50	Alaska	170	0.1%
	District of Columbia	252	0.2%

Source: U.S. Department of Health and Human Services, National Center for Health Statistics
   "National Vital Statistics Reports" (Vol. 50, No. 15, September 16, 2002)
*Final data by state of residence. Cerebrovascular diseases include stroke and other disorders of the blood vessels of the brain.

Death Rate by Cerebrovascular Diseases in 2000

National Rate = 60.9 Deaths per 100,000 Population*

ALPHA ORDER

RANK	STATE	RATE
10	Alabama	72.5
50	Alaska	27.3
40	Arizona	54.2
1	Arkansas	87.5
41	California	54.1
47	Colorado	46.1
26	Connecticut	61.0
38	Delaware	56.4
16	Florida	68.7
32	Georgia	58.2
25	Hawaii	63.3
37	Idaho	56.5
26	Illinois	61.0
15	Indiana	71.1
4	Iowa	76.0
17	Kansas	68.6
19	Kentucky	66.2
33	Louisiana	57.9
19	Maine	66.2
36	Maryland	56.6
28	Massachusetts	59.1
28	Michigan	59.1
31	Minnesota	58.4
13	Mississippi	71.7
14	Missouri	71.6
21	Montana	65.7
22	Nebraska	65.3
46	Nevada	46.4
39	New Hampshire	54.4
43	New Jersey	52.6
45	New Mexico	46.5
49	New York	43.8
8	North Carolina	74.2
10	North Dakota	72.5
24	Ohio	63.7
9	Oklahoma	73.8
2	Oregon	77.4
7	Pennsylvania	74.4
33	Rhode Island	57.9
6	South Carolina	75.3
4	South Dakota	76.0
3	Tennessee	77.1
44	Texas	52.4
48	Utah	45.0
35	Vermont	57.4
30	Virginia	58.9
23	Washington	63.9
12	West Virginia	71.9
18	Wisconsin	67.9
41	Wyoming	54.1

RANK ORDER

RANK	STATE	RATE
1	Arkansas	87.5
2	Oregon	77.4
3	Tennessee	77.1
4	Iowa	76.0
4	South Dakota	76.0
6	South Carolina	75.3
7	Pennsylvania	74.4
8	North Carolina	74.2
9	Oklahoma	73.8
10	Alabama	72.5
10	North Dakota	72.5
12	West Virginia	71.9
13	Mississippi	71.7
14	Missouri	71.6
15	Indiana	71.1
16	Florida	68.7
17	Kansas	68.6
18	Wisconsin	67.9
19	Kentucky	66.2
19	Maine	66.2
21	Montana	65.7
22	Nebraska	65.3
23	Washington	63.9
24	Ohio	63.7
25	Hawaii	63.3
26	Connecticut	61.0
26	Illinois	61.0
28	Massachusetts	59.1
28	Michigan	59.1
30	Virginia	58.9
31	Minnesota	58.4
32	Georgia	58.2
33	Louisiana	57.9
33	Rhode Island	57.9
35	Vermont	57.4
36	Maryland	56.6
37	Idaho	56.5
38	Delaware	56.4
39	New Hampshire	54.4
40	Arizona	54.2
41	California	54.1
41	Wyoming	54.1
43	New Jersey	52.6
44	Texas	52.4
45	New Mexico	46.5
46	Nevada	46.4
47	Colorado	46.1
48	Utah	45.0
49	New York	43.8
50	Alaska	27.3

District of Columbia	48.6

Source: U.S. Department of Health and Human Services, National Center for Health Statistics
    "National Vital Statistics Reports" (Vol. 50, No. 15, September 16, 2002)
*Final data by state of residence. Cerebrovascular diseases include stroke and other disorders of the blood vessels of the brain. Not age-adjusted.

Age-Adjusted Death Rate by Cerebrovascular Diseases in 2000

National Rate = 60.8 Deaths per 100,000 Population*

ALPHA ORDER

RANK	STATE	RATE
7	Alabama	72.1
15	Alaska	66.0
43	Arizona	55.6
3	Arkansas	78.9
23	California	61.6
36	Colorado	58.3
45	Connecticut	51.2
32	Delaware	58.8
47	Florida	50.5
5	Georgia	76.5
29	Hawaii	60.3
22	Idaho	61.7
27	Illinois	60.6
8	Indiana	71.9
32	Iowa	58.8
26	Kansas	60.7
12	Kentucky	68.1
18	Louisiana	64.4
35	Maine	58.7
19	Maryland	63.2
45	Massachusetts	51.2
28	Michigan	60.5
40	Minnesota	56.2
6	Mississippi	75.7
16	Missouri	65.3
30	Montana	59.9
41	Nebraska	55.8
37	Nevada	58.0
38	New Hampshire	57.2
48	New Jersey	48.8
44	New Mexico	52.2
50	New York	40.4
4	North Carolina	78.8
42	North Dakota	55.7
25	Ohio	60.9
10	Oklahoma	69.8
8	Oregon	71.9
31	Pennsylvania	59.5
49	Rhode Island	45.0
1	South Carolina	82.6
21	South Dakota	61.9
2	Tennessee	80.4
14	Texas	66.9
17	Utah	65.2
39	Vermont	57.0
13	Virginia	67.9
11	Washington	68.8
24	West Virginia	61.4
20	Wisconsin	62.6
32	Wyoming	58.8

RANK ORDER

RANK	STATE	RATE
1	South Carolina	82.6
2	Tennessee	80.4
3	Arkansas	78.9
4	North Carolina	78.8
5	Georgia	76.5
6	Mississippi	75.7
7	Alabama	72.1
8	Indiana	71.9
8	Oregon	71.9
10	Oklahoma	69.8
11	Washington	68.8
12	Kentucky	68.1
13	Virginia	67.9
14	Texas	66.9
15	Alaska	66.0
16	Missouri	65.3
17	Utah	65.2
18	Louisiana	64.4
19	Maryland	63.2
20	Wisconsin	62.6
21	South Dakota	61.9
22	Idaho	61.7
23	California	61.6
24	West Virginia	61.4
25	Ohio	60.9
26	Kansas	60.7
27	Illinois	60.6
28	Michigan	60.5
29	Hawaii	60.3
30	Montana	59.9
31	Pennsylvania	59.5
32	Delaware	58.8
32	Iowa	58.8
32	Wyoming	58.8
35	Maine	58.7
36	Colorado	58.3
37	Nevada	58.0
38	New Hampshire	57.2
39	Vermont	57.0
40	Minnesota	56.2
41	Nebraska	55.8
42	North Dakota	55.7
43	Arizona	55.6
44	New Mexico	52.2
45	Connecticut	51.2
45	Massachusetts	51.2
47	Florida	50.5
48	New Jersey	48.8
49	Rhode Island	45.0
50	New York	40.4
	District of Columbia	42.7

Source: U.S. Department of Health and Human Services, National Center for Health Statistics
   "National Vital Statistics Reports" (Vol. 50, No. 15, September 16, 2002)
*Final data by state of residence. Cerebrovascular diseases include stroke and other disorders of the blood vessels of the brain. Age-adjusted rates based on the year 2000 standard population.

Deaths by Chronic Liver Disease and Cirrhosis in 2000

National Total = 26,552 Deaths*

<table>
<tr><td colspan="4">ALPHA ORDER</td><td colspan="4">RANK ORDER</td></tr>
<tr><td>RANK</td><td>STATE</td><td>DEATHS</td><td>% of USA</td><td>RANK</td><td>STATE</td><td>DEATHS</td><td>% of USA</td></tr>
<tr><td>22</td><td>Alabama</td><td>407</td><td>1.5%</td><td>1</td><td>California</td><td>3,666</td><td>13.8%</td></tr>
<tr><td>49</td><td>Alaska</td><td>45</td><td>0.2%</td><td>2</td><td>Texas</td><td>2,092</td><td>7.9%</td></tr>
<tr><td>11</td><td>Arizona</td><td>656</td><td>2.5%</td><td>3</td><td>Florida</td><td>2,072</td><td>7.8%</td></tr>
<tr><td>34</td><td>Arkansas</td><td>228</td><td>0.9%</td><td>4</td><td>New York</td><td>1,409</td><td>5.3%</td></tr>
<tr><td>1</td><td>California</td><td>3,666</td><td>13.8%</td><td>5</td><td>Pennsylvania</td><td>1,089</td><td>4.1%</td></tr>
<tr><td>21</td><td>Colorado</td><td>421</td><td>1.6%</td><td>6</td><td>Illinois</td><td>1,065</td><td>4.0%</td></tr>
<tr><td>29</td><td>Connecticut</td><td>333</td><td>1.3%</td><td>7</td><td>Michigan</td><td>1,035</td><td>3.9%</td></tr>
<tr><td>46</td><td>Delaware</td><td>71</td><td>0.3%</td><td>8</td><td>Ohio</td><td>994</td><td>3.7%</td></tr>
<tr><td>3</td><td>Florida</td><td>2,072</td><td>7.8%</td><td>9</td><td>North Carolina</td><td>787</td><td>3.0%</td></tr>
<tr><td>12</td><td>Georgia</td><td>631</td><td>2.4%</td><td>10</td><td>New Jersey</td><td>765</td><td>2.9%</td></tr>
<tr><td>43</td><td>Hawaii</td><td>86</td><td>0.3%</td><td>11</td><td>Arizona</td><td>656</td><td>2.5%</td></tr>
<tr><td>40</td><td>Idaho</td><td>109</td><td>0.4%</td><td>12</td><td>Georgia</td><td>631</td><td>2.4%</td></tr>
<tr><td>6</td><td>Illinois</td><td>1,065</td><td>4.0%</td><td>13</td><td>Tennessee</td><td>595</td><td>2.2%</td></tr>
<tr><td>17</td><td>Indiana</td><td>490</td><td>1.8%</td><td>14</td><td>Virginia</td><td>571</td><td>2.2%</td></tr>
<tr><td>35</td><td>Iowa</td><td>191</td><td>0.7%</td><td>15</td><td>Massachusetts</td><td>540</td><td>2.0%</td></tr>
<tr><td>36</td><td>Kansas</td><td>175</td><td>0.7%</td><td>16</td><td>Washington</td><td>495</td><td>1.9%</td></tr>
<tr><td>24</td><td>Kentucky</td><td>370</td><td>1.4%</td><td>17</td><td>Indiana</td><td>490</td><td>1.8%</td></tr>
<tr><td>25</td><td>Louisiana</td><td>366</td><td>1.4%</td><td>18</td><td>South Carolina</td><td>460</td><td>1.7%</td></tr>
<tr><td>39</td><td>Maine</td><td>124</td><td>0.5%</td><td>19</td><td>Maryland</td><td>444</td><td>1.7%</td></tr>
<tr><td>19</td><td>Maryland</td><td>444</td><td>1.7%</td><td>19</td><td>Wisconsin</td><td>444</td><td>1.7%</td></tr>
<tr><td>15</td><td>Massachusetts</td><td>540</td><td>2.0%</td><td>21</td><td>Colorado</td><td>421</td><td>1.6%</td></tr>
<tr><td>7</td><td>Michigan</td><td>1,035</td><td>3.9%</td><td>22</td><td>Alabama</td><td>407</td><td>1.5%</td></tr>
<tr><td>26</td><td>Minnesota</td><td>350</td><td>1.3%</td><td>23</td><td>Missouri</td><td>405</td><td>1.5%</td></tr>
<tr><td>33</td><td>Mississippi</td><td>246</td><td>0.9%</td><td>24</td><td>Kentucky</td><td>370</td><td>1.4%</td></tr>
<tr><td>23</td><td>Missouri</td><td>405</td><td>1.5%</td><td>25</td><td>Louisiana</td><td>366</td><td>1.4%</td></tr>
<tr><td>44</td><td>Montana</td><td>85</td><td>0.3%</td><td>26</td><td>Minnesota</td><td>350</td><td>1.3%</td></tr>
<tr><td>41</td><td>Nebraska</td><td>95</td><td>0.4%</td><td>27</td><td>Oklahoma</td><td>348</td><td>1.3%</td></tr>
<tr><td>31</td><td>Nevada</td><td>290</td><td>1.1%</td><td>28</td><td>New Mexico</td><td>341</td><td>1.3%</td></tr>
<tr><td>42</td><td>New Hampshire</td><td>90</td><td>0.3%</td><td>29</td><td>Connecticut</td><td>333</td><td>1.3%</td></tr>
<tr><td>10</td><td>New Jersey</td><td>765</td><td>2.9%</td><td>30</td><td>Oregon</td><td>297</td><td>1.1%</td></tr>
<tr><td>28</td><td>New Mexico</td><td>341</td><td>1.3%</td><td>31</td><td>Nevada</td><td>290</td><td>1.1%</td></tr>
<tr><td>4</td><td>New York</td><td>1,409</td><td>5.3%</td><td>32</td><td>West Virginia</td><td>247</td><td>0.9%</td></tr>
<tr><td>9</td><td>North Carolina</td><td>787</td><td>3.0%</td><td>33</td><td>Mississippi</td><td>246</td><td>0.9%</td></tr>
<tr><td>48</td><td>North Dakota</td><td>48</td><td>0.2%</td><td>34</td><td>Arkansas</td><td>228</td><td>0.9%</td></tr>
<tr><td>8</td><td>Ohio</td><td>994</td><td>3.7%</td><td>35</td><td>Iowa</td><td>191</td><td>0.7%</td></tr>
<tr><td>27</td><td>Oklahoma</td><td>348</td><td>1.3%</td><td>36</td><td>Kansas</td><td>175</td><td>0.7%</td></tr>
<tr><td>30</td><td>Oregon</td><td>297</td><td>1.1%</td><td>37</td><td>Rhode Island</td><td>128</td><td>0.5%</td></tr>
<tr><td>5</td><td>Pennsylvania</td><td>1,089</td><td>4.1%</td><td>38</td><td>Utah</td><td>126</td><td>0.5%</td></tr>
<tr><td>37</td><td>Rhode Island</td><td>128</td><td>0.5%</td><td>39</td><td>Maine</td><td>124</td><td>0.5%</td></tr>
<tr><td>18</td><td>South Carolina</td><td>460</td><td>1.7%</td><td>40</td><td>Idaho</td><td>109</td><td>0.4%</td></tr>
<tr><td>45</td><td>South Dakota</td><td>82</td><td>0.3%</td><td>41</td><td>Nebraska</td><td>95</td><td>0.4%</td></tr>
<tr><td>13</td><td>Tennessee</td><td>595</td><td>2.2%</td><td>42</td><td>New Hampshire</td><td>90</td><td>0.3%</td></tr>
<tr><td>2</td><td>Texas</td><td>2,092</td><td>7.9%</td><td>43</td><td>Hawaii</td><td>86</td><td>0.3%</td></tr>
<tr><td>38</td><td>Utah</td><td>126</td><td>0.5%</td><td>44</td><td>Montana</td><td>85</td><td>0.3%</td></tr>
<tr><td>50</td><td>Vermont</td><td>41</td><td>0.2%</td><td>45</td><td>South Dakota</td><td>82</td><td>0.3%</td></tr>
<tr><td>14</td><td>Virginia</td><td>571</td><td>2.2%</td><td>46</td><td>Delaware</td><td>71</td><td>0.3%</td></tr>
<tr><td>16</td><td>Washington</td><td>495</td><td>1.9%</td><td>47</td><td>Wyoming</td><td>50</td><td>0.2%</td></tr>
<tr><td>32</td><td>West Virginia</td><td>247</td><td>0.9%</td><td>48</td><td>North Dakota</td><td>48</td><td>0.2%</td></tr>
<tr><td>19</td><td>Wisconsin</td><td>444</td><td>1.7%</td><td>49</td><td>Alaska</td><td>45</td><td>0.2%</td></tr>
<tr><td>47</td><td>Wyoming</td><td>50</td><td>0.2%</td><td>50</td><td>Vermont</td><td>41</td><td>0.2%</td></tr>
<tr><td></td><td></td><td></td><td></td><td></td><td>District of Columbia</td><td>57</td><td>0.2%</td></tr>
</table>

Source: U.S. Department of Health and Human Services, National Center for Health Statistics
    "National Vital Statistics Reports" (Vol. 50, No. 15, September 16, 2002)
*Final data by state of residence. Cirrhosis of the liver is characterized by the replacement of normal tissue with fibrous tissue and the loss of functional liver cells. It can result from alcohol abuse, nutritional deprivation, or infection especially by the hepatitis virus.

Death Rate by Chronic Liver Disease and Cirrhosis in 2000

National Rate = 9.6 Deaths per 100,000 Population*

ALPHA ORDER

RANK	STATE	RATE
20	Alabama	9.3
44	Alaska	7.2
5	Arizona	13.4
26	Arkansas	8.8
9	California	10.9
15	Colorado	10.2
17	Connecticut	10.1
20	Delaware	9.3
4	Florida	13.5
38	Georgia	7.9
43	Hawaii	7.3
31	Idaho	8.6
29	Illinois	8.7
36	Indiana	8.2
47	Iowa	6.6
47	Kansas	6.6
20	Kentucky	9.3
34	Louisiana	8.4
18	Maine	9.9
32	Maryland	8.5
29	Massachusetts	8.7
11	Michigan	10.4
44	Minnesota	7.2
26	Mississippi	8.8
41	Missouri	7.4
19	Montana	9.6
50	Nebraska	5.7
2	Nevada	15.4
41	New Hampshire	7.4
20	New Jersey	9.3
1	New Mexico	19.5
39	New York	7.7
15	North Carolina	10.2
40	North Dakota	7.6
26	Ohio	8.8
13	Oklahoma	10.3
25	Oregon	8.9
24	Pennsylvania	9.1
6	Rhode Island	12.9
7	South Carolina	11.7
8	South Dakota	11.1
10	Tennessee	10.8
13	Texas	10.3
49	Utah	5.8
46	Vermont	6.9
36	Virginia	8.2
32	Washington	8.5
3	West Virginia	13.7
34	Wisconsin	8.4
11	Wyoming	10.4

RANK ORDER

RANK	STATE	RATE
1	New Mexico	19.5
2	Nevada	15.4
3	West Virginia	13.7
4	Florida	13.5
5	Arizona	13.4
6	Rhode Island	12.9
7	South Carolina	11.7
8	South Dakota	11.1
9	California	10.9
10	Tennessee	10.8
11	Michigan	10.4
11	Wyoming	10.4
13	Oklahoma	10.3
13	Texas	10.3
15	Colorado	10.2
15	North Carolina	10.2
17	Connecticut	10.1
18	Maine	9.9
19	Montana	9.6
20	Alabama	9.3
20	Delaware	9.3
20	Kentucky	9.3
20	New Jersey	9.3
24	Pennsylvania	9.1
25	Oregon	8.9
26	Arkansas	8.8
26	Mississippi	8.8
26	Ohio	8.8
29	Illinois	8.7
29	Massachusetts	8.7
31	Idaho	8.6
32	Maryland	8.5
32	Washington	8.5
34	Louisiana	8.4
34	Wisconsin	8.4
36	Indiana	8.2
36	Virginia	8.2
38	Georgia	7.9
39	New York	7.7
40	North Dakota	7.6
41	Missouri	7.4
41	New Hampshire	7.4
43	Hawaii	7.3
44	Alaska	7.2
44	Minnesota	7.2
46	Vermont	6.9
47	Iowa	6.6
47	Kansas	6.6
49	Utah	5.8
50	Nebraska	5.7
	District of Columbia	11.0

Source: U.S. Department of Health and Human Services, National Center for Health Statistics
    "National Vital Statistics Reports" (Vol. 50, No. 15, September 16, 2002)
*Final data by state of residence. Cirrhosis of the liver is characterized by the replacement of normal tissue with fibrous tissue and the loss of functional liver cells. It can result from alcohol abuse, nutritional deprivation, or infection especially by the hepatitis virus. Not age-adjusted.

Age-Adjusted Death Rate by Chronic Liver Disease and Cirrhosis in 2000

National Rate = 9.6 Deaths per 100,000 Population*

ALPHA ORDER

RANK	STATE	RATE
24	Alabama	9.0
18	Alaska	9.4
3	Arizona	13.8
34	Arkansas	8.4
5	California	11.9
11	Colorado	10.6
17	Connecticut	9.5
19	Delaware	9.2
7	Florida	11.8
25	Georgia	8.9
46	Hawaii	6.8
21	Idaho	9.1
25	Illinois	8.9
38	Indiana	8.2
49	Iowa	6.1
48	Kansas	6.5
21	Kentucky	9.1
29	Louisiana	8.7
21	Maine	9.1
29	Maryland	8.7
36	Massachusetts	8.3
13	Michigan	10.4
42	Minnesota	7.4
19	Mississippi	9.2
45	Missouri	7.1
29	Montana	8.7
50	Nebraska	5.6
2	Nevada	15.5
41	New Hampshire	7.7
25	New Jersey	8.9
1	New Mexico	20.0
42	New York	7.4
15	North Carolina	10.1
44	North Dakota	7.3
32	Ohio	8.6
16	Oklahoma	10.0
34	Oregon	8.4
39	Pennsylvania	8.0
4	Rhode Island	12.0
8	South Carolina	11.6
10	South Dakota	11.1
12	Tennessee	10.5
9	Texas	11.4
40	Utah	7.8
47	Vermont	6.6
33	Virginia	8.5
28	Washington	8.8
5	West Virginia	11.9
36	Wisconsin	8.3
14	Wyoming	10.2

RANK ORDER

RANK	STATE	RATE
1	New Mexico	20.0
2	Nevada	15.5
3	Arizona	13.8
4	Rhode Island	12.0
5	California	11.9
5	West Virginia	11.9
7	Florida	11.8
8	South Carolina	11.6
9	Texas	11.4
10	South Dakota	11.1
11	Colorado	10.6
12	Tennessee	10.5
13	Michigan	10.4
14	Wyoming	10.2
15	North Carolina	10.1
16	Oklahoma	10.0
17	Connecticut	9.5
18	Alaska	9.4
19	Delaware	9.2
19	Mississippi	9.2
21	Idaho	9.1
21	Kentucky	9.1
21	Maine	9.1
24	Alabama	9.0
25	Georgia	8.9
25	Illinois	8.9
25	New Jersey	8.9
28	Washington	8.8
29	Louisiana	8.7
29	Maryland	8.7
29	Montana	8.7
32	Ohio	8.6
33	Virginia	8.5
34	Arkansas	8.4
34	Oregon	8.4
36	Massachusetts	8.3
36	Wisconsin	8.3
38	Indiana	8.2
39	Pennsylvania	8.0
40	Utah	7.8
41	New Hampshire	7.7
42	Minnesota	7.4
42	New York	7.4
44	North Dakota	7.3
45	Missouri	7.1
46	Hawaii	6.8
47	Vermont	6.6
48	Kansas	6.5
49	Iowa	6.1
50	Nebraska	5.6

District of Columbia   10.2

Source: U.S. Department of Health and Human Services, National Center for Health Statistics
"National Vital Statistics Reports" (Vol. 50, No. 15, September 16, 2002)
*Final data by state of residence. Cirrhosis of the liver is characterized by the replacement of normal tissue with fibrous tissue and the loss of functional liver cells. It can result from alcohol abuse, nutritional deprivation, or infection especially by the hepatitis virus. Age-adjusted rates based on the year 2000 standard population.

Deaths by Chronic Lower Respiratory Diseases in 2000

National Total = 122,009 Deaths*

RANK	STATE	DEATHS	% of USA		RANK	STATE	DEATHS	% of USA
21	Alabama	2,057	1.7%		1	California	12,756	10.5%
50	Alaska	132	0.1%		2	Florida	8,645	7.1%
18	Arizona	2,508	2.1%		3	Texas	7,286	6.0%
32	Arkansas	1,405	1.2%		4	New York	6,784	5.6%
1	California	12,756	10.5%		5	Pennsylvania	6,079	5.0%
25	Colorado	1,787	1.5%		6	Ohio	5,983	4.9%
29	Connecticut	1,533	1.3%		7	Illinois	4,768	3.9%
45	Delaware	341	0.3%		8	Michigan	4,352	3.6%
2	Florida	8,645	7.1%		9	North Carolina	3,699	3.0%
10	Georgia	3,067	2.5%		10	Georgia	3,067	2.5%
49	Hawaii	278	0.2%		11	Indiana	3,052	2.5%
40	Idaho	569	0.5%		12	New Jersey	3,007	2.5%
7	Illinois	4,768	3.9%		13	Massachusetts	2,925	2.4%
11	Indiana	3,052	2.5%		14	Tennessee	2,887	2.4%
30	Iowa	1,512	1.2%		15	Virginia	2,820	2.3%
31	Kansas	1,411	1.2%		16	Missouri	2,802	2.3%
20	Kentucky	2,170	1.8%		17	Washington	2,644	2.2%
27	Louisiana	1,684	1.4%		18	Arizona	2,508	2.1%
37	Maine	768	0.6%		19	Wisconsin	2,316	1.9%
23	Maryland	1,927	1.6%		20	Kentucky	2,170	1.8%
13	Massachusetts	2,925	2.4%		21	Alabama	2,057	1.7%
8	Michigan	4,352	3.6%		22	Oklahoma	1,980	1.6%
24	Minnesota	1,902	1.6%		23	Maryland	1,927	1.6%
34	Mississippi	1,257	1.0%		24	Minnesota	1,902	1.6%
16	Missouri	2,802	2.3%		25	Colorado	1,787	1.5%
42	Montana	517	0.4%		26	South Carolina	1,730	1.4%
36	Nebraska	838	0.7%		27	Louisiana	1,684	1.4%
35	Nevada	989	0.8%		28	Oregon	1,677	1.4%
39	New Hampshire	581	0.5%		29	Connecticut	1,533	1.3%
12	New Jersey	3,007	2.5%		30	Iowa	1,512	1.2%
38	New Mexico	767	0.6%		31	Kansas	1,411	1.2%
4	New York	6,784	5.6%		32	Arkansas	1,405	1.2%
9	North Carolina	3,699	3.0%		33	West Virginia	1,345	1.1%
47	North Dakota	295	0.2%		34	Mississippi	1,257	1.0%
6	Ohio	5,983	4.9%		35	Nevada	989	0.8%
22	Oklahoma	1,980	1.6%		36	Nebraska	838	0.7%
28	Oregon	1,677	1.4%		37	Maine	768	0.6%
5	Pennsylvania	6,079	5.0%		38	New Mexico	767	0.6%
43	Rhode Island	500	0.4%		39	New Hampshire	581	0.5%
26	South Carolina	1,730	1.4%		40	Idaho	569	0.5%
44	South Dakota	383	0.3%		41	Utah	524	0.4%
14	Tennessee	2,887	2.4%		42	Montana	517	0.4%
3	Texas	7,286	6.0%		43	Rhode Island	500	0.4%
41	Utah	524	0.4%		44	South Dakota	383	0.3%
46	Vermont	312	0.3%		45	Delaware	341	0.3%
15	Virginia	2,820	2.3%		46	Vermont	312	0.3%
17	Washington	2,644	2.2%		47	North Dakota	295	0.2%
33	West Virginia	1,345	1.1%		48	Wyoming	283	0.2%
19	Wisconsin	2,316	1.9%		49	Hawaii	278	0.2%
48	Wyoming	283	0.2%		50	Alaska	132	0.1%
						District of Columbia	175	0.1%

Source: U.S. Department of Health and Human Services, National Center for Health Statistics
    "National Vital Statistics Reports" (Vol. 50, No. 15, September 16, 2002)
*Final data by state of residence. Chronic lower respiratory diseases are diseases of the lungs including
bronchitis, emphysema and asthma. Includes allied conditions.

Death Rate by Chronic Lower Respiratory Diseases in 2000

National Rate = 44.3 Deaths per 100,000 Population*

ALPHA ORDER

RANK	STATE	RATE
26	Alabama	46.9
50	Alaska	21.2
16	Arizona	51.4
7	Arkansas	54.5
43	California	37.9
37	Colorado	43.2
28	Connecticut	46.5
31	Delaware	44.7
6	Florida	56.4
41	Georgia	38.6
49	Hawaii	23.6
31	Idaho	44.7
40	Illinois	39.1
17	Indiana	51.1
12	Iowa	52.5
10	Kansas	52.9
8	Kentucky	54.4
42	Louisiana	38.5
2	Maine	61.0
45	Maryland	36.9
25	Massachusetts	47.1
34	Michigan	43.9
39	Minnesota	39.4
30	Mississippi	45.1
18	Missouri	50.9
5	Montana	58.2
20	Nebraska	50.2
11	Nevada	52.6
23	New Hampshire	47.8
46	New Jersey	36.6
34	New Mexico	43.9
44	New York	37.1
24	North Carolina	47.7
26	North Dakota	46.9
9	Ohio	53.1
4	Oklahoma	58.6
20	Oregon	50.2
19	Pennsylvania	50.7
20	Rhode Island	50.2
33	South Carolina	44.1
15	South Dakota	51.9
13	Tennessee	52.2
47	Texas	35.7
48	Utah	24.2
13	Vermont	52.2
38	Virginia	40.5
29	Washington	45.5
1	West Virginia	74.6
36	Wisconsin	43.7
3	Wyoming	58.8

RANK ORDER

RANK	STATE	RATE
1	West Virginia	74.6
2	Maine	61.0
3	Wyoming	58.8
4	Oklahoma	58.6
5	Montana	58.2
6	Florida	56.4
7	Arkansas	54.5
8	Kentucky	54.4
9	Ohio	53.1
10	Kansas	52.9
11	Nevada	52.6
12	Iowa	52.5
13	Tennessee	52.2
13	Vermont	52.2
15	South Dakota	51.9
16	Arizona	51.4
17	Indiana	51.1
18	Missouri	50.9
19	Pennsylvania	50.7
20	Nebraska	50.2
20	Oregon	50.2
20	Rhode Island	50.2
23	New Hampshire	47.8
24	North Carolina	47.7
25	Massachusetts	47.1
26	Alabama	46.9
26	North Dakota	46.9
28	Connecticut	46.5
29	Washington	45.5
30	Mississippi	45.1
31	Delaware	44.7
31	Idaho	44.7
33	South Carolina	44.1
34	Michigan	43.9
34	New Mexico	43.9
36	Wisconsin	43.7
37	Colorado	43.2
38	Virginia	40.5
39	Minnesota	39.4
40	Illinois	39.1
41	Georgia	38.6
42	Louisiana	38.5
43	California	37.9
44	New York	37.1
45	Maryland	36.9
46	New Jersey	36.6
47	Texas	35.7
48	Utah	24.2
49	Hawaii	23.6
50	Alaska	21.2
	District of Columbia	33.8

Source: U.S. Department of Health and Human Services, National Center for Health Statistics
    "National Vital Statistics Reports" (Vol. 50, No. 15, September 16, 2002)
*Final data by state of residence. Chronic lower respiratory diseases are diseases of the lungs including
bronchitis, emphysema and asthma. Includes allied conditions. Not age-adjusted.

Age-Adjusted Death Rate by Chronic Lower Respiratory Diseases in 2000

National Rate = 44.3 Deaths per 100,000 Population*

ALPHA ORDER

RANK ORDER

RANK	STATE	RATE		RANK	STATE	RATE
27	Alabama	46.0		1	Nevada	63.1
25	Alaska	46.9		1	West Virginia	63.1
12	Arizona	51.6		1	Wyoming	63.1
18	Arkansas	49.2		4	Oklahoma	55.4
35	California	43.2		5	Kentucky	55.3
8	Colorado	53.6		6	Maine	55.0
42	Connecticut	40.2		7	Montana	53.9
30	Delaware	45.3		8	Colorado	53.6
39	Florida	41.3		9	Tennessee	53.3
15	Georgia	49.9		10	Vermont	52.9
50	Hawaii	22.1		11	Indiana	51.7
20	Idaho	49.1		12	Arizona	51.6
44	Illinois	39.5		13	New Hampshire	50.8
11	Indiana	51.7		14	Ohio	50.6
34	Iowa	43.3		15	Georgia	49.9
18	Kansas	49.2		16	North Carolina	49.3
5	Kentucky	55.3		16	Washington	49.3
36	Louisiana	42.4		18	Arkansas	49.2
6	Maine	55.0		18	Kansas	49.2
41	Maryland	40.8		20	Idaho	49.1
37	Massachusetts	42.1		21	New Mexico	48.5
32	Michigan	44.7		22	Mississippi	47.5
45	Minnesota	39.2		22	Oregon	47.5
22	Mississippi	47.5		24	Missouri	47.4
24	Missouri	47.4		25	Alaska	46.9
7	Montana	53.9		26	South Carolina	46.5
29	Nebraska	45.4		27	Alabama	46.0
1	Nevada	63.1		28	Virginia	45.6
13	New Hampshire	50.8		29	Nebraska	45.4
49	New Jersey	34.0		30	Delaware	45.3
21	New Mexico	48.5		31	Texas	45.1
47	New York	34.6		32	Michigan	44.7
16	North Carolina	49.3		33	South Dakota	44.2
46	North Dakota	38.9		34	Iowa	43.3
14	Ohio	50.6		35	California	43.2
4	Oklahoma	55.4		36	Louisiana	42.4
22	Oregon	47.5		37	Massachusetts	42.1
40	Pennsylvania	40.9		38	Wisconsin	41.6
43	Rhode Island	40.1		39	Florida	41.3
26	South Carolina	46.5		40	Pennsylvania	40.9
33	South Dakota	44.2		41	Maryland	40.8
9	Tennessee	53.3		42	Connecticut	40.2
31	Texas	45.1		43	Rhode Island	40.1
48	Utah	34.5		44	Illinois	39.5
10	Vermont	52.9		45	Minnesota	39.2
28	Virginia	45.6		46	North Dakota	38.9
16	Washington	49.3		47	New York	34.6
1	West Virginia	63.1		48	Utah	34.5
38	Wisconsin	41.6		49	New Jersey	34.0
1	Wyoming	63.1		50	Hawaii	22.1
					District of Columbia	30.0

Source: U.S. Department of Health and Human Services, National Center for Health Statistics
    "National Vital Statistics Reports" (Vol. 50, No. 15, September 16, 2002)
*Final data by state of residence. Chronic lower respiratory diseases are diseases of the lungs including bronchitis, emphysema and asthma. Includes allied conditions. Age-adjusted rates based on the year 2000 standard population.

Deaths by Diabetes Mellitus in 2000

National Total = 69,301 Deaths*

ALPHA ORDER

RANK	STATE	DEATHS	% of USA
20	Alabama	1,321	1.9%
50	Alaska	87	0.1%
25	Arizona	1,012	1.5%
29	Arkansas	714	1.0%
1	California	6,190	8.9%
33	Colorado	635	0.9%
30	Connecticut	683	1.0%
46	Delaware	193	0.3%
3	Florida	4,449	6.4%
16	Georgia	1,461	2.1%
44	Hawaii	203	0.3%
39	Idaho	304	0.4%
7	Illinois	2,995	4.3%
12	Indiana	1,673	2.4%
34	Iowa	630	0.9%
32	Kansas	668	1.0%
24	Kentucky	1,107	1.6%
11	Louisiana	1,694	2.4%
38	Maine	357	0.5%
15	Maryland	1,515	2.2%
18	Massachusetts	1,361	2.0%
8	Michigan	2,603	3.8%
22	Minnesota	1,209	1.7%
31	Mississippi	676	1.0%
17	Missouri	1,458	2.1%
43	Montana	227	0.3%
37	Nebraska	411	0.6%
42	Nevada	276	0.4%
40	New Hampshire	297	0.4%
9	New Jersey	2,483	3.6%
36	New Mexico	485	0.7%
4	New York	3,877	5.6%
10	North Carolina	2,084	3.0%
44	North Dakota	203	0.3%
6	Ohio	3,691	5.3%
26	Oklahoma	978	1.4%
27	Oregon	844	1.2%
5	Pennsylvania	3,794	5.5%
41	Rhode Island	292	0.4%
23	South Carolina	1,206	1.7%
47	South Dakota	180	0.3%
13	Tennessee	1,591	2.3%
2	Texas	5,196	7.5%
35	Utah	530	0.8%
48	Vermont	163	0.2%
14	Virginia	1,564	2.3%
19	Washington	1,331	1.9%
28	West Virginia	759	1.1%
21	Wisconsin	1,309	1.9%
49	Wyoming	111	0.2%

RANK ORDER

RANK	STATE	DEATHS	% of USA
1	California	6,190	8.9%
2	Texas	5,196	7.5%
3	Florida	4,449	6.4%
4	New York	3,877	5.6%
5	Pennsylvania	3,794	5.5%
6	Ohio	3,691	5.3%
7	Illinois	2,995	4.3%
8	Michigan	2,603	3.8%
9	New Jersey	2,483	3.6%
10	North Carolina	2,084	3.0%
11	Louisiana	1,694	2.4%
12	Indiana	1,673	2.4%
13	Tennessee	1,591	2.3%
14	Virginia	1,564	2.3%
15	Maryland	1,515	2.2%
16	Georgia	1,461	2.1%
17	Missouri	1,458	2.1%
18	Massachusetts	1,361	2.0%
19	Washington	1,331	1.9%
20	Alabama	1,321	1.9%
21	Wisconsin	1,309	1.9%
22	Minnesota	1,209	1.7%
23	South Carolina	1,206	1.7%
24	Kentucky	1,107	1.6%
25	Arizona	1,012	1.5%
26	Oklahoma	978	1.4%
27	Oregon	844	1.2%
28	West Virginia	759	1.1%
29	Arkansas	714	1.0%
30	Connecticut	683	1.0%
31	Mississippi	676	1.0%
32	Kansas	668	1.0%
33	Colorado	635	0.9%
34	Iowa	630	0.9%
35	Utah	530	0.8%
36	New Mexico	485	0.7%
37	Nebraska	411	0.6%
38	Maine	357	0.5%
39	Idaho	304	0.4%
40	New Hampshire	297	0.4%
41	Rhode Island	292	0.4%
42	Nevada	276	0.4%
43	Montana	227	0.3%
44	Hawaii	203	0.3%
44	North Dakota	203	0.3%
46	Delaware	193	0.3%
47	South Dakota	180	0.3%
48	Vermont	163	0.2%
49	Wyoming	111	0.2%
50	Alaska	87	0.1%
	District of Columbia	221	0.3%

Source: U.S. Department of Health and Human Services, National Center for Health Statistics
   "National Vital Statistics Reports" (Vol. 50, No. 15, September 16, 2002)
*Final data by state of residence. A severe, chronic form of diabetes caused by insufficient production of insulin and resulting in abnormal metabolism of carbohydrates, fats, and proteins. The disease, which typically appears in childhood or adolescence, is characterized by increased sugar levels in the blood and urine, excessive thirst and frequent urination.

Death Rate by Diabetes Mellitus in 2000

National Rate = 25.2 Deaths per 100,000 Population*

ALPHA ORDER

RANK ORDER

RANK	STATE	RATE		RANK	STATE	RATE
8	Alabama	30.1		1	West Virginia	42.1
50	Alaska	14.0		2	Louisiana	38.7
43	Arizona	20.7		3	Ohio	32.7
17	Arkansas	27.7		4	North Dakota	32.3
45	California	18.4		5	Pennsylvania	31.7
48	Colorado	15.4		6	South Carolina	30.7
43	Connecticut	20.7		7	New Jersey	30.3
25	Delaware	25.3		8	Alabama	30.1
10	Florida	29.0		9	Rhode Island	29.3
45	Georgia	18.4		10	Florida	29.0
47	Hawaii	17.2		10	Maryland	29.0
36	Idaho	23.9		12	Oklahoma	28.9
30	Illinois	24.6		13	Tennessee	28.8
15	Indiana	28.0		14	Maine	28.4
40	Iowa	21.9		15	Indiana	28.0
27	Kansas	25.1		16	Kentucky	27.8
16	Kentucky	27.8		17	Arkansas	27.7
2	Louisiana	38.7		17	New Mexico	27.7
14	Maine	28.4		19	Vermont	27.3
10	Maryland	29.0		20	North Carolina	26.9
40	Massachusetts	21.9		21	Missouri	26.5
22	Michigan	26.2		22	Michigan	26.2
28	Minnesota	25.0		23	Montana	25.6
35	Mississippi	24.3		24	Texas	25.5
21	Missouri	26.5		25	Delaware	25.3
23	Montana	25.6		25	Oregon	25.3
30	Nebraska	24.6		27	Kansas	25.1
49	Nevada	14.7		28	Minnesota	25.0
33	New Hampshire	24.4		29	Wisconsin	24.7
7	New Jersey	30.3		30	Illinois	24.6
17	New Mexico	27.7		30	Nebraska	24.6
42	New York	21.2		32	Utah	24.5
20	North Carolina	26.9		33	New Hampshire	24.4
4	North Dakota	32.3		33	South Dakota	24.4
3	Ohio	32.7		35	Mississippi	24.3
12	Oklahoma	28.9		36	Idaho	23.9
25	Oregon	25.3		37	Wyoming	23.1
5	Pennsylvania	31.7		38	Washington	22.9
9	Rhode Island	29.3		39	Virginia	22.4
6	South Carolina	30.7		40	Iowa	21.9
33	South Dakota	24.4		40	Massachusetts	21.9
13	Tennessee	28.8		42	New York	21.2
24	Texas	25.5		43	Arizona	20.7
32	Utah	24.5		43	Connecticut	20.7
19	Vermont	27.3		45	California	18.4
39	Virginia	22.4		45	Georgia	18.4
38	Washington	22.9		47	Hawaii	17.2
1	West Virginia	42.1		48	Colorado	15.4
29	Wisconsin	24.7		49	Nevada	14.7
37	Wyoming	23.1		50	Alaska	14.0
					District of Columbia	42.6

Source: U.S. Department of Health and Human Services, National Center for Health Statistics
    "National Vital Statistics Reports" (Vol. 50, No. 15, September 16, 2002)

*Final data by state of residence. A severe, chronic form of diabetes caused by insufficient production of insulin and resulting in abnormal metabolism of carbohydrates, fats, and proteins. The disease, which typically appears in childhood or adolescence, is characterized by increased sugar levels in the blood and urine, excessive thirst and frequent urination. Not age-adjusted.

Age-Adjusted Death Rate by Diabetes Mellitus in 2000

National Rate = 25.2 Deaths per 100,000 Population*

ALPHA ORDER				RANK ORDER		
RANK	STATE	RATE		RANK	STATE	RATE
9	Alabama	29.5		1	Louisiana	41.9
17	Alaska	26.9		2	West Virginia	35.9
41	Arizona	20.9		3	Utah	34.7
26	Arkansas	25.2		4	South Carolina	32.0
43	California	20.8		5	Maryland	31.5
46	Colorado	18.4		6	Ohio	31.4
47	Connecticut	18.3		7	Texas	31.2
24	Delaware	25.5		8	New Mexico	30.1
40	Florida	22.2		9	Alabama	29.5
38	Georgia	22.9		10	Tennessee	29.1
49	Hawaii	16.1		11	New Jersey	28.3
21	Idaho	25.9		12	Indiana	28.2
27	Illinois	24.9		13	Kentucky	28.1
12	Indiana	28.2		14	North Carolina	27.6
48	Iowa	18.2		15	Oklahoma	27.5
35	Kansas	23.6		16	Vermont	27.3
13	Kentucky	28.1		17	Alaska	26.9
1	Louisiana	41.9		18	North Dakota	26.8
23	Maine	25.6		19	Michigan	26.7
5	Maryland	31.5		20	Pennsylvania	26.2
44	Massachusetts	19.9		21	Idaho	25.9
19	Michigan	26.7		22	New Hampshire	25.8
29	Minnesota	24.8		23	Maine	25.6
25	Mississippi	25.4		24	Delaware	25.5
27	Missouri	24.9		25	Mississippi	25.4
35	Montana	23.6		26	Arkansas	25.2
39	Nebraska	22.3		27	Illinois	24.9
49	Nevada	16.1		27	Missouri	24.9
22	New Hampshire	25.8		29	Minnesota	24.8
11	New Jersey	28.3		29	Virginia	24.8
8	New Mexico	30.1		31	Washington	24.5
44	New York	19.9		32	Wyoming	24.3
14	North Carolina	27.6		33	Rhode Island	24.2
18	North Dakota	26.8		34	Oregon	23.9
6	Ohio	31.4		35	Kansas	23.6
15	Oklahoma	27.5		35	Montana	23.6
34	Oregon	23.9		37	Wisconsin	23.5
20	Pennsylvania	26.2		38	Georgia	22.9
33	Rhode Island	24.2		39	Nebraska	22.3
4	South Carolina	32.0		40	Florida	22.2
41	South Dakota	20.9		41	Arizona	20.9
10	Tennessee	29.1		41	South Dakota	20.9
7	Texas	31.2		43	California	20.8
3	Utah	34.7		44	Massachusetts	19.9
16	Vermont	27.3		44	New York	19.9
29	Virginia	24.8		46	Colorado	18.4
31	Washington	24.5		47	Connecticut	18.3
2	West Virginia	35.9		48	Iowa	18.2
37	Wisconsin	23.5		49	Hawaii	16.1
32	Wyoming	24.3		49	Nevada	16.1
					District of Columbia	38.3

Source: U.S. Department of Health and Human Services, National Center for Health Statistics
"National Vital Statistics Reports" (Vol. 50, No. 15, September 16, 2002)
*Final data by state of residence. A severe, chronic form of diabetes caused by insufficient production of insulin and resulting in abnormal metabolism of carbohydrates, fats, and proteins. The disease, which typically appears in childhood or adolescence, is characterized by increased sugar levels in the blood and urine, excessive thirst and frequent urination. Age-adjusted rates based on the year 2000 standard population.

Deaths by Diseases of the Heart in 2000

National Total = 710,760 Deaths*

ALPHA ORDER

RANK	STATE	DEATHS	% of USA
18	Alabama	13,406	1.9%
50	Alaska	607	0.1%
24	Arizona	10,584	1.5%
30	Arkansas	8,278	1.2%
1	California	68,426	9.6%
34	Colorado	6,184	0.9%
27	Connecticut	8,993	1.3%
46	Delaware	1,983	0.3%
3	Florida	50,336	7.1%
11	Georgia	17,406	2.4%
43	Hawaii	2,390	0.3%
42	Idaho	2,519	0.4%
7	Illinois	31,844	4.5%
13	Indiana	16,210	2.3%
29	Iowa	8,559	1.2%
32	Kansas	6,931	1.0%
20	Kentucky	11,936	1.7%
21	Louisiana	11,629	1.6%
37	Maine	3,400	0.5%
19	Maryland	12,348	1.7%
15	Massachusetts	15,314	2.2%
8	Michigan	27,325	3.8%
28	Minnesota	8,885	1.3%
26	Mississippi	9,256	1.3%
12	Missouri	17,235	2.4%
45	Montana	1,995	0.3%
35	Nebraska	4,197	0.6%
36	Nevada	4,089	0.6%
41	New Hampshire	2,811	0.4%
9	New Jersey	23,724	3.3%
38	New Mexico	3,191	0.4%
2	New York	57,474	8.1%
10	North Carolina	19,723	2.8%
47	North Dakota	1,679	0.2%
6	Ohio	32,722	4.6%
23	Oklahoma	11,297	1.6%
31	Oregon	7,094	1.0%
5	Pennsylvania	40,708	5.7%
39	Rhode Island	3,115	0.4%
25	South Carolina	9,893	1.4%
44	South Dakota	2,105	0.3%
14	Tennessee	16,174	2.3%
4	Texas	43,020	6.1%
40	Utah	2,909	0.4%
48	Vermont	1,438	0.2%
16	Virginia	15,264	2.1%
22	Washington	11,370	1.6%
33	West Virginia	6,435	0.9%
17	Wisconsin	13,601	1.9%
49	Wyoming	992	0.1%

RANK ORDER

RANK	STATE	DEATHS	% of USA
1	California	68,426	9.6%
2	New York	57,474	8.1%
3	Florida	50,336	7.1%
4	Texas	43,020	6.1%
5	Pennsylvania	40,708	5.7%
6	Ohio	32,722	4.6%
7	Illinois	31,844	4.5%
8	Michigan	27,325	3.8%
9	New Jersey	23,724	3.3%
10	North Carolina	19,723	2.8%
11	Georgia	17,406	2.4%
12	Missouri	17,235	2.4%
13	Indiana	16,210	2.3%
14	Tennessee	16,174	2.3%
15	Massachusetts	15,314	2.2%
16	Virginia	15,264	2.1%
17	Wisconsin	13,601	1.9%
18	Alabama	13,406	1.9%
19	Maryland	12,348	1.7%
20	Kentucky	11,936	1.7%
21	Louisiana	11,629	1.6%
22	Washington	11,370	1.6%
23	Oklahoma	11,297	1.6%
24	Arizona	10,584	1.5%
25	South Carolina	9,893	1.4%
26	Mississippi	9,256	1.3%
27	Connecticut	8,993	1.3%
28	Minnesota	8,885	1.3%
29	Iowa	8,559	1.2%
30	Arkansas	8,278	1.2%
31	Oregon	7,094	1.0%
32	Kansas	6,931	1.0%
33	West Virginia	6,435	0.9%
34	Colorado	6,184	0.9%
35	Nebraska	4,197	0.6%
36	Nevada	4,089	0.6%
37	Maine	3,400	0.5%
38	New Mexico	3,191	0.4%
39	Rhode Island	3,115	0.4%
40	Utah	2,909	0.4%
41	New Hampshire	2,811	0.4%
42	Idaho	2,519	0.4%
43	Hawaii	2,390	0.3%
44	South Dakota	2,105	0.3%
45	Montana	1,995	0.3%
46	Delaware	1,983	0.3%
47	North Dakota	1,679	0.2%
48	Vermont	1,438	0.2%
49	Wyoming	992	0.1%
50	Alaska	607	0.1%
	District of Columbia	1,756	0.2%

Source: U.S. Department of Health and Human Services, National Center for Health Statistics
   "National Vital Statistics Reports" (Vol. 50, No. 15, September 16, 2002)
*Final data by state of residence.

Death Rate by Diseases of the Heart in 2000

National Rate = 258.2 Deaths per 100,000 Population*

ALPHA ORDER

RANK	STATE	RATE
10	Alabama	305.5
50	Alaska	97.6
38	Arizona	216.8
6	Arkansas	321.3
42	California	203.5
48	Colorado	149.5
18	Connecticut	272.7
24	Delaware	260.2
5	Florida	328.3
35	Georgia	219.1
43	Hawaii	202.7
44	Idaho	197.8
23	Illinois	261.3
19	Indiana	271.2
12	Iowa	297.5
25	Kansas	260.0
11	Kentucky	299.5
22	Louisiana	265.8
20	Maine	270.1
32	Maryland	236.6
30	Massachusetts	246.8
17	Michigan	275.5
46	Minnesota	184.0
4	Mississippi	332.1
8	Missouri	313.2
34	Montana	224.7
29	Nebraska	251.3
37	Nevada	217.5
33	New Hampshire	231.2
15	New Jersey	289.2
47	New Mexico	182.6
7	New York	314.4
27	North Carolina	254.6
21	North Dakota	266.8
14	Ohio	290.3
3	Oklahoma	334.2
39	Oregon	212.3
2	Pennsylvania	339.7
9	Rhode Island	312.7
28	South Carolina	252.1
16	South Dakota	285.5
13	Tennessee	292.3
40	Texas	211.0
49	Utah	134.4
31	Vermont	240.5
36	Virginia	219.0
45	Washington	195.7
1	West Virginia	357.0
26	Wisconsin	256.8
41	Wyoming	206.3

RANK ORDER

RANK	STATE	RATE
1	West Virginia	357.0
2	Pennsylvania	339.7
3	Oklahoma	334.2
4	Mississippi	332.1
5	Florida	328.3
6	Arkansas	321.3
7	New York	314.4
8	Missouri	313.2
9	Rhode Island	312.7
10	Alabama	305.5
11	Kentucky	299.5
12	Iowa	297.5
13	Tennessee	292.3
14	Ohio	290.3
15	New Jersey	289.2
16	South Dakota	285.5
17	Michigan	275.5
18	Connecticut	272.7
19	Indiana	271.2
20	Maine	270.1
21	North Dakota	266.8
22	Louisiana	265.8
23	Illinois	261.3
24	Delaware	260.2
25	Kansas	260.0
26	Wisconsin	256.8
27	North Carolina	254.6
28	South Carolina	252.1
29	Nebraska	251.3
30	Massachusetts	246.8
31	Vermont	240.5
32	Maryland	236.6
33	New Hampshire	231.2
34	Montana	224.7
35	Georgia	219.1
36	Virginia	219.0
37	Nevada	217.5
38	Arizona	216.8
39	Oregon	212.3
40	Texas	211.0
41	Wyoming	206.3
42	California	203.5
43	Hawaii	202.7
44	Idaho	197.8
45	Washington	195.7
46	Minnesota	184.0
47	New Mexico	182.6
48	Colorado	149.5
49	Utah	134.4
50	Alaska	97.6
	District of Columbia	338.8

Source: U.S. Department of Health and Human Services, National Center for Health Statistics
        "National Vital Statistics Reports" (Vol. 50, No. 15, September 16, 2002)
*Final data by state of residence. Not age-adjusted.

Age-Adjusted Death Rate by Diseases of the Heart in 2000

National Rate = 257.9 Deaths per 100,000 Population*

ALPHA ORDER

RANK	STATE	RATE
5	Alabama	302.1
43	Alaska	209.8
36	Arizona	221.9
8	Arkansas	290.6
35	California	231.7
49	Colorado	183.6
34	Connecticut	232.9
17	Delaware	268.8
26	Florida	243.5
11	Georgia	282.1
48	Hawaii	191.9
40	Idaho	215.2
23	Illinois	260.9
15	Indiana	274.0
31	Iowa	238.2
33	Kansas	234.5
3	Kentucky	305.1
7	Louisiana	292.6
28	Maine	241.6
22	Maryland	261.4
38	Massachusetts	217.4
12	Michigan	281.4
50	Minnesota	178.7
1	Mississippi	348.9
10	Missouri	287.5
44	Montana	204.8
39	Nebraska	217.3
21	Nevada	263.3
27	New Hampshire	242.7
18	New Jersey	268.5
45	New Mexico	203.0
9	New York	290.0
19	North Carolina	266.6
41	North Dakota	213.6
13	Ohio	278.3
2	Oklahoma	315.7
46	Oregon	198.7
14	Pennsylvania	275.0
24	Rhode Island	248.1
16	South Carolina	269.8
32	South Dakota	235.9
6	Tennessee	300.5
20	Texas	264.6
47	Utah	192.2
30	Vermont	238.7
25	Virginia	248.0
42	Washington	210.1
3	West Virginia	305.1
29	Wisconsin	239.2
37	Wyoming	218.8

RANK ORDER

RANK	STATE	RATE
1	Mississippi	348.9
2	Oklahoma	315.7
3	Kentucky	305.1
3	West Virginia	305.1
5	Alabama	302.1
6	Tennessee	300.5
7	Louisiana	292.6
8	Arkansas	290.6
9	New York	290.0
10	Missouri	287.5
11	Georgia	282.1
12	Michigan	281.4
13	Ohio	278.3
14	Pennsylvania	275.0
15	Indiana	274.0
16	South Carolina	269.8
17	Delaware	268.8
18	New Jersey	268.5
19	North Carolina	266.6
20	Texas	264.6
21	Nevada	263.3
22	Maryland	261.4
23	Illinois	260.9
24	Rhode Island	248.1
25	Virginia	248.0
26	Florida	243.5
27	New Hampshire	242.7
28	Maine	241.6
29	Wisconsin	239.2
30	Vermont	238.7
31	Iowa	238.2
32	South Dakota	235.9
33	Kansas	234.5
34	Connecticut	232.9
35	California	231.7
36	Arizona	221.9
37	Wyoming	218.8
38	Massachusetts	217.4
39	Nebraska	217.3
40	Idaho	215.2
41	North Dakota	213.6
42	Washington	210.1
43	Alaska	209.8
44	Montana	204.8
45	New Mexico	203.0
46	Oregon	198.7
47	Utah	192.2
48	Hawaii	191.9
49	Colorado	183.6
50	Minnesota	178.7
	District of Columbia	298.6

Source: U.S. Department of Health and Human Services, National Center for Health Statistics
   "National Vital Statistics Reports" (Vol. 50, No. 15, September 16, 2002)
*Final data by state of residence. Age-adjusted rates based on the year 2000 standard population.

Deaths by Malignant Neoplasms in 2000

National Total = 553,091 Deaths*

RANK	STATE	DEATHS	% of USA
20	Alabama	9,807	1.8%
50	Alaska	704	0.1%
24	Arizona	9,073	1.6%
30	Arkansas	6,090	1.1%
1	California	53,158	9.6%
32	Colorado	5,922	1.1%
27	Connecticut	7,065	1.3%
45	Delaware	1,609	0.3%
2	Florida	39,183	7.1%
12	Georgia	13,690	2.5%
43	Hawaii	1,943	0.4%
42	Idaho	2,128	0.4%
6	Illinois	25,365	4.6%
14	Indiana	12,842	2.3%
29	Iowa	6,448	1.2%
33	Kansas	5,223	0.9%
23	Kentucky	9,207	1.7%
21	Louisiana	9,400	1.7%
37	Maine	3,070	0.6%
19	Maryland	10,290	1.9%
11	Massachusetts	14,027	2.5%
8	Michigan	19,798	3.6%
22	Minnesota	9,215	1.7%
31	Mississippi	6,075	1.1%
16	Missouri	12,144	2.2%
44	Montana	1,867	0.3%
36	Nebraska	3,382	0.6%
35	Nevada	3,763	0.7%
39	New Hampshire	2,484	0.4%
9	New Jersey	18,073	3.3%
38	New Mexico	2,906	0.5%
3	New York	37,198	6.7%
10	North Carolina	15,786	2.9%
47	North Dakota	1,346	0.2%
7	Ohio	24,988	4.5%
26	Oklahoma	7,402	1.3%
28	Oregon	6,951	1.3%
5	Pennsylvania	30,161	5.5%
40	Rhode Island	2,433	0.4%
25	South Carolina	8,250	1.5%
46	South Dakota	1,597	0.3%
15	Tennessee	12,339	2.2%
4	Texas	33,300	6.0%
41	Utah	2,359	0.4%
48	Vermont	1,240	0.2%
13	Virginia	13,528	2.4%
17	Washington	10,668	1.9%
34	West Virginia	4,753	0.9%
18	Wisconsin	10,638	1.9%
49	Wyoming	868	0.2%

RANK	STATE	DEATHS	% of USA
1	California	53,158	9.6%
2	Florida	39,183	7.1%
3	New York	37,198	6.7%
4	Texas	33,300	6.0%
5	Pennsylvania	30,161	5.5%
6	Illinois	25,365	4.6%
7	Ohio	24,988	4.5%
8	Michigan	19,798	3.6%
9	New Jersey	18,073	3.3%
10	North Carolina	15,786	2.9%
11	Massachusetts	14,027	2.5%
12	Georgia	13,690	2.5%
13	Virginia	13,528	2.4%
14	Indiana	12,842	2.3%
15	Tennessee	12,339	2.2%
16	Missouri	12,144	2.2%
17	Washington	10,668	1.9%
18	Wisconsin	10,638	1.9%
19	Maryland	10,290	1.9%
20	Alabama	9,807	1.8%
21	Louisiana	9,400	1.7%
22	Minnesota	9,215	1.7%
23	Kentucky	9,207	1.7%
24	Arizona	9,073	1.6%
25	South Carolina	8,250	1.5%
26	Oklahoma	7,402	1.3%
27	Connecticut	7,065	1.3%
28	Oregon	6,951	1.3%
29	Iowa	6,448	1.2%
30	Arkansas	6,090	1.1%
31	Mississippi	6,075	1.1%
32	Colorado	5,922	1.1%
33	Kansas	5,223	0.9%
34	West Virginia	4,753	0.9%
35	Nevada	3,763	0.7%
36	Nebraska	3,382	0.6%
37	Maine	3,070	0.6%
38	New Mexico	2,906	0.5%
39	New Hampshire	2,484	0.4%
40	Rhode Island	2,433	0.4%
41	Utah	2,359	0.4%
42	Idaho	2,128	0.4%
43	Hawaii	1,943	0.4%
44	Montana	1,867	0.3%
45	Delaware	1,609	0.3%
46	South Dakota	1,597	0.3%
47	North Dakota	1,346	0.2%
48	Vermont	1,240	0.2%
49	Wyoming	868	0.2%
50	Alaska	704	0.1%
	District of Columbia	1,335	0.2%

Source: U.S. Department of Health and Human Services, National Center for Health Statistics
"National Vital Statistics Reports" (Vol. 50, No. 15, September 16, 2002)
Final data by state of residence. Neoplasms are abnormal tissue, tumors. Includes many cancers.

Death Rate by Malignant Neoplasms in 2000

National Rate = 200.9 Deaths per 100,000 Population*

ALPHA ORDER

RANK	STATE	RATE
10	Alabama	223.5
49	Alaska	113.2
39	Arizona	185.8
6	Arkansas	236.4
47	California	158.1
48	Colorado	143.2
20	Connecticut	214.3
22	Delaware	211.1
2	Florida	255.6
42	Georgia	172.4
45	Hawaii	164.8
43	Idaho	167.1
25	Illinois	208.2
18	Indiana	214.9
9	Iowa	224.1
36	Kansas	195.9
7	Kentucky	231.0
18	Louisiana	214.9
5	Maine	243.9
35	Maryland	197.2
8	Massachusetts	226.1
34	Michigan	199.6
38	Minnesota	190.9
16	Mississippi	218.0
13	Missouri	220.7
23	Montana	210.3
31	Nebraska	202.5
33	Nevada	200.1
28	New Hampshire	204.3
14	New Jersey	220.3
44	New Mexico	166.3
30	New York	203.5
29	North Carolina	203.8
21	North Dakota	213.9
12	Ohio	221.7
15	Oklahoma	219.0
26	Oregon	208.0
3	Pennsylvania	251.7
4	Rhode Island	244.3
24	South Carolina	210.2
17	South Dakota	216.6
11	Tennessee	223.0
46	Texas	163.3
50	Utah	109.0
27	Vermont	207.4
37	Virginia	194.1
40	Washington	183.6
1	West Virginia	263.7
32	Wisconsin	200.9
41	Wyoming	180.5

RANK ORDER

RANK	STATE	RATE
1	West Virginia	263.7
2	Florida	255.6
3	Pennsylvania	251.7
4	Rhode Island	244.3
5	Maine	243.9
6	Arkansas	236.4
7	Kentucky	231.0
8	Massachusetts	226.1
9	Iowa	224.1
10	Alabama	223.5
11	Tennessee	223.0
12	Ohio	221.7
13	Missouri	220.7
14	New Jersey	220.3
15	Oklahoma	219.0
16	Mississippi	218.0
17	South Dakota	216.6
18	Indiana	214.9
18	Louisiana	214.9
20	Connecticut	214.3
21	North Dakota	213.9
22	Delaware	211.1
23	Montana	210.3
24	South Carolina	210.2
25	Illinois	208.2
26	Oregon	208.0
27	Vermont	207.4
28	New Hampshire	204.3
29	North Carolina	203.8
30	New York	203.5
31	Nebraska	202.5
32	Wisconsin	200.9
33	Nevada	200.1
34	Michigan	199.6
35	Maryland	197.2
36	Kansas	195.9
37	Virginia	194.1
38	Minnesota	190.9
39	Arizona	185.8
40	Washington	183.6
41	Wyoming	180.5
42	Georgia	172.4
43	Idaho	167.1
44	New Mexico	166.3
45	Hawaii	164.8
46	Texas	163.3
47	California	158.1
48	Colorado	143.2
49	Alaska	113.2
50	Utah	109.0
	District of Columbia	257.5

Source: U.S. Department of Health and Human Services, National Center for Health Statistics
"National Vital Statistics Reports" (Vol. 50, No. 15, September 16, 2002)
*Final data by state of residence. Neoplasms are abnormal tissue, tumors. Includes many cancers. Not age-adjusted.

Age-Adjusted Death Rate by Malignant Neoplasms in 2000

National Rate = 201.0 Deaths per 100,000 Population*

RANK	STATE	RATE
8	Alabama	217.7
27	Alaska	203.3
42	Arizona	187.0
11	Arkansas	215.7
47	California	178.3
48	Colorado	167.7
38	Connecticut	192.0
18	Delaware	210.7
29	Florida	197.5
17	Georgia	211.1
49	Hawaii	154.0
45	Idaho	181.3
16	Illinois	211.5
9	Indiana	216.5
35	Iowa	193.5
41	Kansas	187.2
2	Kentucky	230.3
1	Louisiana	230.6
6	Maine	222.2
14	Maryland	211.7
22	Massachusetts	208.3
28	Michigan	202.4
37	Minnesota	193.1
3	Mississippi	228.1
21	Missouri	208.7
33	Montana	194.3
40	Nebraska	187.9
7	Nevada	222.1
12	New Hampshire	215.4
26	New Jersey	206.7
46	New Mexico	178.4
38	New York	192.0
24	North Carolina	207.2
44	North Dakota	185.0
13	Ohio	212.7
23	Oklahoma	207.7
30	Oregon	197.4
19	Pennsylvania	210.4
20	Rhode Island	210.0
10	South Carolina	215.9
36	South Dakota	193.2
5	Tennessee	223.7
31	Texas	196.6
50	Utah	151.4
25	Vermont	207.1
14	Virginia	211.7
32	Washington	196.2
4	West Virginia	224.4
34	Wisconsin	194.1
43	Wyoming	186.7

RANK	STATE	RATE
1	Louisiana	230.6
2	Kentucky	230.3
3	Mississippi	228.1
4	West Virginia	224.4
5	Tennessee	223.7
6	Maine	222.2
7	Nevada	222.1
8	Alabama	217.7
9	Indiana	216.5
10	South Carolina	215.9
11	Arkansas	215.7
12	New Hampshire	215.4
13	Ohio	212.7
14	Maryland	211.7
14	Virginia	211.7
16	Illinois	211.5
17	Georgia	211.1
18	Delaware	210.7
19	Pennsylvania	210.4
20	Rhode Island	210.0
21	Missouri	208.7
22	Massachusetts	208.3
23	Oklahoma	207.7
24	North Carolina	207.2
25	Vermont	207.1
26	New Jersey	206.7
27	Alaska	203.3
28	Michigan	202.4
29	Florida	197.5
30	Oregon	197.4
31	Texas	196.6
32	Washington	196.2
33	Montana	194.3
34	Wisconsin	194.1
35	Iowa	193.5
36	South Dakota	193.2
37	Minnesota	193.1
38	Connecticut	192.0
38	New York	192.0
40	Nebraska	187.9
41	Kansas	187.2
42	Arizona	187.0
43	Wyoming	186.7
44	North Dakota	185.0
45	Idaho	181.3
46	New Mexico	178.4
47	California	178.3
48	Colorado	167.7
49	Hawaii	154.0
50	Utah	151.4
	District of Columbia	231.9

Source: U.S. Department of Health and Human Services, National Center for Health Statistics
"National Vital Statistics Reports" (Vol. 50, No. 15, September 16, 2002)
Final data by state of residence. Neoplasms are abnormal tissue, tumors. Includes many cancers. Age-adjusted rates based on the year 2000 standard population.

Deaths by Pneumonia and Influenza in 2000

National Total = 65,313 Deaths*

ALPHA ORDER

ALPHA ORDER

RANK	STATE	DEATHS	% of USA
20	Alabama	1,138	1.7%
50	Alaska	45	0.1%
18	Arizona	1,222	1.9%
29	Arkansas	798	1.2%
1	California	8,324	12.7%
33	Colorado	607	0.9%
25	Connecticut	890	1.4%
42	Delaware	229	0.4%
4	Florida	3,365	5.2%
12	Georgia	1,792	2.7%
43	Hawaii	221	0.3%
41	Idaho	288	0.4%
6	Illinois	2,917	4.5%
16	Indiana	1,270	1.9%
24	Iowa	937	1.4%
30	Kansas	743	1.1%
19	Kentucky	1,157	1.8%
23	Louisiana	972	1.5%
38	Maine	336	0.5%
21	Maryland	1,116	1.7%
8	Massachusetts	2,078	3.2%
9	Michigan	2,052	3.1%
27	Minnesota	845	1.3%
28	Mississippi	809	1.2%
14	Missouri	1,629	2.5%
45	Montana	202	0.3%
35	Nebraska	433	0.7%
39	Nevada	320	0.5%
46	New Hampshire	194	0.3%
10	New Jersey	2,044	3.1%
40	New Mexico	290	0.4%
2	New York	5,201	8.0%
11	North Carolina	1,945	3.0%
47	North Dakota	166	0.3%
7	Ohio	2,533	3.9%
26	Oklahoma	885	1.4%
32	Oregon	642	1.0%
5	Pennsylvania	3,069	4.7%
37	Rhode Island	342	0.5%
31	South Carolina	699	1.1%
44	South Dakota	212	0.3%
13	Tennessee	1,672	2.6%
3	Texas	3,706	5.7%
36	Utah	388	0.6%
49	Vermont	119	0.2%
15	Virginia	1,510	2.3%
22	Washington	1,010	1.5%
34	West Virginia	456	0.7%
17	Wisconsin	1,258	1.9%
48	Wyoming	126	0.2%

RANK ORDER

RANK	STATE	DEATHS	% of USA
1	California	8,324	12.7%
2	New York	5,201	8.0%
3	Texas	3,706	5.7%
4	Florida	3,365	5.2%
5	Pennsylvania	3,069	4.7%
6	Illinois	2,917	4.5%
7	Ohio	2,533	3.9%
8	Massachusetts	2,078	3.2%
9	Michigan	2,052	3.1%
10	New Jersey	2,044	3.1%
11	North Carolina	1,945	3.0%
12	Georgia	1,792	2.7%
13	Tennessee	1,672	2.6%
14	Missouri	1,629	2.5%
15	Virginia	1,510	2.3%
16	Indiana	1,270	1.9%
17	Wisconsin	1,258	1.9%
18	Arizona	1,222	1.9%
19	Kentucky	1,157	1.8%
20	Alabama	1,138	1.7%
21	Maryland	1,116	1.7%
22	Washington	1,010	1.5%
23	Louisiana	972	1.5%
24	Iowa	937	1.4%
25	Connecticut	890	1.4%
26	Oklahoma	885	1.4%
27	Minnesota	845	1.3%
28	Mississippi	809	1.2%
29	Arkansas	798	1.2%
30	Kansas	743	1.1%
31	South Carolina	699	1.1%
32	Oregon	642	1.0%
33	Colorado	607	0.9%
34	West Virginia	456	0.7%
35	Nebraska	433	0.7%
36	Utah	388	0.6%
37	Rhode Island	342	0.5%
38	Maine	336	0.5%
39	Nevada	320	0.5%
40	New Mexico	290	0.4%
41	Idaho	288	0.4%
42	Delaware	229	0.4%
43	Hawaii	221	0.3%
44	South Dakota	212	0.3%
45	Montana	202	0.3%
46	New Hampshire	194	0.3%
47	North Dakota	166	0.3%
48	Wyoming	126	0.2%
49	Vermont	119	0.2%
50	Alaska	45	0.1%
	District of Columbia	111	0.2%

Source: U.S. Department of Health and Human Services, National Center for Health Statistics
     "National Vital Statistics Reports" (Vol. 50, No. 15, September 16, 2002)
*Final data by state of residence.

Death Rate by Pneumonia and Influenza in 2000

National Rate = 23.7 Deaths per 100,000 Population*

ALPHA ORDER

RANK ORDER

RANK	STATE	RATE		RANK	STATE	RATE
18	Alabama	25.9		1	Rhode Island	34.3
50	Alaska	7.2		2	Massachusetts	33.5
23	Arizona	25.0		3	Iowa	32.6
4	Arkansas	31.0		4	Arkansas	31.0
25	California	24.8		5	Tennessee	30.2
49	Colorado	14.7		6	Delaware	30.0
13	Connecticut	27.0		7	Missouri	29.6
6	Delaware	30.0		8	Kentucky	29.0
33	Florida	21.9		8	Mississippi	29.0
29	Georgia	22.6		10	South Dakota	28.8
40	Hawaii	18.7		11	New York	28.5
29	Idaho	22.6		12	Kansas	27.9
26	Illinois	23.9		13	Connecticut	27.0
36	Indiana	21.3		14	Maine	26.7
3	Iowa	32.6		15	North Dakota	26.4
12	Kansas	27.9		16	Oklahoma	26.2
8	Kentucky	29.0		16	Wyoming	26.2
32	Louisiana	22.2		18	Alabama	25.9
14	Maine	26.7		18	Nebraska	25.9
35	Maryland	21.4		20	Pennsylvania	25.6
2	Massachusetts	33.5		21	West Virginia	25.3
37	Michigan	20.7		22	North Carolina	25.1
44	Minnesota	17.5		23	Arizona	25.0
8	Mississippi	29.0		24	New Jersey	24.9
7	Missouri	29.6		25	California	24.8
28	Montana	22.8		26	Illinois	23.9
18	Nebraska	25.9		27	Wisconsin	23.8
46	Nevada	17.0		28	Montana	22.8
48	New Hampshire	16.0		29	Georgia	22.6
24	New Jersey	24.9		29	Idaho	22.6
47	New Mexico	16.6		31	Ohio	22.5
11	New York	28.5		32	Louisiana	22.2
22	North Carolina	25.1		33	Florida	21.9
15	North Dakota	26.4		34	Virginia	21.7
31	Ohio	22.5		35	Maryland	21.4
16	Oklahoma	26.2		36	Indiana	21.3
39	Oregon	19.2		37	Michigan	20.7
20	Pennsylvania	25.6		38	Vermont	19.9
1	Rhode Island	34.3		39	Oregon	19.2
43	South Carolina	17.8		40	Hawaii	18.7
10	South Dakota	28.8		41	Texas	18.2
5	Tennessee	30.2		42	Utah	17.9
41	Texas	18.2		43	South Carolina	17.8
42	Utah	17.9		44	Minnesota	17.5
38	Vermont	19.9		45	Washington	17.4
34	Virginia	21.7		46	Nevada	17.0
45	Washington	17.4		47	New Mexico	16.6
21	West Virginia	25.3		48	New Hampshire	16.0
27	Wisconsin	23.8		49	Colorado	14.7
16	Wyoming	26.2		50	Alaska	7.2
					District of Columbia	21.4

Source: U.S. Department of Health and Human Services, National Center for Health Statistics
    "National Vital Statistics Reports" (Vol. 50, No. 15, September 16, 2002)
*Final data by state of residence. Not age-adjusted.

Age-Adjusted Death Rate by Pneumonia and Influenza in 2000

National Rate = 23.7 Deaths per 100,000 Population*

<table>
<tr><td colspan="3">ALPHA ORDER</td><td colspan="3">RANK ORDER</td></tr>
<tr><td>RANK</td><td>STATE</td><td>RATE</td><td>RANK</td><td>STATE</td><td>RATE</td></tr>
<tr><td>14</td><td>Alabama</td><td>25.9</td><td>1</td><td>Tennessee</td><td>31.7</td></tr>
<tr><td>50</td><td>Alaska</td><td>16.0</td><td>2</td><td>Delaware</td><td>31.5</td></tr>
<tr><td>14</td><td>Arizona</td><td>25.9</td><td>3</td><td>Mississippi</td><td>30.6</td></tr>
<tr><td>9</td><td>Arkansas</td><td>27.9</td><td>4</td><td>Georgia</td><td>30.1</td></tr>
<tr><td>8</td><td>California</td><td>28.3</td><td>5</td><td>Kentucky</td><td>30.0</td></tr>
<tr><td>44</td><td>Colorado</td><td>18.5</td><td>6</td><td>Massachusetts</td><td>28.7</td></tr>
<tr><td>29</td><td>Connecticut</td><td>22.4</td><td>7</td><td>Wyoming</td><td>28.5</td></tr>
<tr><td>2</td><td>Delaware</td><td>31.5</td><td>8</td><td>California</td><td>28.3</td></tr>
<tr><td>49</td><td>Florida</td><td>16.2</td><td>9</td><td>Arkansas</td><td>27.9</td></tr>
<tr><td>4</td><td>Georgia</td><td>30.1</td><td>10</td><td>North Carolina</td><td>26.9</td></tr>
<tr><td>45</td><td>Hawaii</td><td>17.9</td><td>11</td><td>Missouri</td><td>26.7</td></tr>
<tr><td>21</td><td>Idaho</td><td>24.5</td><td>12</td><td>New York</td><td>26.1</td></tr>
<tr><td>24</td><td>Illinois</td><td>23.6</td><td>12</td><td>Rhode Island</td><td>26.1</td></tr>
<tr><td>35</td><td>Indiana</td><td>21.5</td><td>14</td><td>Alabama</td><td>25.9</td></tr>
<tr><td>19</td><td>Iowa</td><td>24.9</td><td>14</td><td>Arizona</td><td>25.9</td></tr>
<tr><td>22</td><td>Kansas</td><td>24.3</td><td>16</td><td>Utah</td><td>25.7</td></tr>
<tr><td>5</td><td>Kentucky</td><td>30.0</td><td>17</td><td>Virginia</td><td>25.3</td></tr>
<tr><td>18</td><td>Louisiana</td><td>25.0</td><td>18</td><td>Louisiana</td><td>25.0</td></tr>
<tr><td>25</td><td>Maine</td><td>23.5</td><td>19</td><td>Iowa</td><td>24.9</td></tr>
<tr><td>23</td><td>Maryland</td><td>23.9</td><td>20</td><td>Oklahoma</td><td>24.7</td></tr>
<tr><td>6</td><td>Massachusetts</td><td>28.7</td><td>21</td><td>Idaho</td><td>24.5</td></tr>
<tr><td>36</td><td>Michigan</td><td>21.2</td><td>22</td><td>Kansas</td><td>24.3</td></tr>
<tr><td>48</td><td>Minnesota</td><td>16.4</td><td>23</td><td>Maryland</td><td>23.9</td></tr>
<tr><td>3</td><td>Mississippi</td><td>30.6</td><td>24</td><td>Illinois</td><td>23.6</td></tr>
<tr><td>11</td><td>Missouri</td><td>26.7</td><td>25</td><td>Maine</td><td>23.5</td></tr>
<tr><td>37</td><td>Montana</td><td>20.8</td><td>26</td><td>Texas</td><td>23.2</td></tr>
<tr><td>31</td><td>Nebraska</td><td>21.7</td><td>27</td><td>New Jersey</td><td>23.1</td></tr>
<tr><td>30</td><td>Nevada</td><td>22.0</td><td>28</td><td>South Dakota</td><td>22.7</td></tr>
<tr><td>47</td><td>New Hampshire</td><td>16.7</td><td>29</td><td>Connecticut</td><td>22.4</td></tr>
<tr><td>27</td><td>New Jersey</td><td>23.1</td><td>30</td><td>Nevada</td><td>22.0</td></tr>
<tr><td>42</td><td>New Mexico</td><td>18.8</td><td>31</td><td>Nebraska</td><td>21.7</td></tr>
<tr><td>12</td><td>New York</td><td>26.1</td><td>31</td><td>West Virginia</td><td>21.7</td></tr>
<tr><td>10</td><td>North Carolina</td><td>26.9</td><td>33</td><td>Ohio</td><td>21.6</td></tr>
<tr><td>39</td><td>North Dakota</td><td>19.8</td><td>33</td><td>Wisconsin</td><td>21.6</td></tr>
<tr><td>33</td><td>Ohio</td><td>21.6</td><td>35</td><td>Indiana</td><td>21.5</td></tr>
<tr><td>20</td><td>Oklahoma</td><td>24.7</td><td>36</td><td>Michigan</td><td>21.2</td></tr>
<tr><td>46</td><td>Oregon</td><td>17.8</td><td>37</td><td>Montana</td><td>20.8</td></tr>
<tr><td>38</td><td>Pennsylvania</td><td>20.5</td><td>38</td><td>Pennsylvania</td><td>20.5</td></tr>
<tr><td>12</td><td>Rhode Island</td><td>26.1</td><td>39</td><td>North Dakota</td><td>19.8</td></tr>
<tr><td>39</td><td>South Carolina</td><td>19.8</td><td>39</td><td>South Carolina</td><td>19.8</td></tr>
<tr><td>28</td><td>South Dakota</td><td>22.7</td><td>41</td><td>Vermont</td><td>19.7</td></tr>
<tr><td>1</td><td>Tennessee</td><td>31.7</td><td>42</td><td>New Mexico</td><td>18.8</td></tr>
<tr><td>26</td><td>Texas</td><td>23.2</td><td>43</td><td>Washington</td><td>18.7</td></tr>
<tr><td>16</td><td>Utah</td><td>25.7</td><td>44</td><td>Colorado</td><td>18.5</td></tr>
<tr><td>41</td><td>Vermont</td><td>19.7</td><td>45</td><td>Hawaii</td><td>17.9</td></tr>
<tr><td>17</td><td>Virginia</td><td>25.3</td><td>46</td><td>Oregon</td><td>17.8</td></tr>
<tr><td>43</td><td>Washington</td><td>18.7</td><td>47</td><td>New Hampshire</td><td>16.7</td></tr>
<tr><td>31</td><td>West Virginia</td><td>21.7</td><td>48</td><td>Minnesota</td><td>16.4</td></tr>
<tr><td>33</td><td>Wisconsin</td><td>21.6</td><td>49</td><td>Florida</td><td>16.2</td></tr>
<tr><td>7</td><td>Wyoming</td><td>28.5</td><td>50</td><td>Alaska</td><td>16.0</td></tr>
<tr><td></td><td></td><td></td><td></td><td>District of Columbia</td><td>18.6</td></tr>
</table>

Source: U.S. Department of Health and Human Services, National Center for Health Statistics
"National Vital Statistics Reports" (Vol. 50, No. 15, September 16, 2002)
*Final data by state of residence. Age-adjusted rates based on the year 2000 standard population.

Deaths by Tuberculosis in 1999

National Total = 930 Deaths*

ALPHA ORDER

RANK	STATE	DEATHS	% of USA
19	Alabama	16	1.7%
40	Alaska	2	0.2%
14	Arizona	21	2.3%
24	Arkansas	12	1.3%
1	California	157	16.9%
28	Colorado	8	0.9%
32	Connecticut	5	0.5%
40	Delaware	2	0.2%
3	Florida	69	7.4%
6	Georgia	37	4.0%
33	Hawaii	4	0.4%
33	Idaho	4	0.4%
5	Illinois	38	4.1%
23	Indiana	13	1.4%
37	Iowa	3	0.3%
33	Kansas	4	0.4%
20	Kentucky	15	1.6%
11	Louisiana	23	2.5%
37	Maine	3	0.3%
15	Maryland	20	2.2%
26	Massachusetts	9	1.0%
9	Michigan	27	2.9%
30	Minnesota	6	0.6%
20	Mississippi	15	1.6%
17	Missouri	19	2.0%
40	Montana	2	0.2%
40	Nebraska	2	0.2%
29	Nevada	7	0.8%
46	New Hampshire	1	0.1%
10	New Jersey	25	2.7%
25	New Mexico	11	1.2%
4	New York	61	6.6%
11	North Carolina	23	2.5%
49	North Dakota	0	0.0%
8	Ohio	30	3.2%
20	Oklahoma	15	1.6%
40	Oregon	2	0.2%
6	Pennsylvania	37	4.0%
33	Rhode Island	4	0.4%
18	South Carolina	17	1.8%
37	South Dakota	3	0.3%
11	Tennessee	23	2.5%
2	Texas	91	9.8%
40	Utah	2	0.2%
46	Vermont	1	0.1%
15	Virginia	20	2.2%
26	Washington	9	1.0%
46	West Virginia	1	0.1%
30	Wisconsin	6	0.6%
49	Wyoming	0	0.0%

RANK ORDER

RANK	STATE	DEATHS	% of USA
1	California	157	16.9%
2	Texas	91	9.8%
3	Florida	69	7.4%
4	New York	61	6.6%
5	Illinois	38	4.1%
6	Georgia	37	4.0%
6	Pennsylvania	37	4.0%
8	Ohio	30	3.2%
9	Michigan	27	2.9%
10	New Jersey	25	2.7%
11	Louisiana	23	2.5%
11	North Carolina	23	2.5%
11	Tennessee	23	2.5%
14	Arizona	21	2.3%
15	Maryland	20	2.2%
15	Virginia	20	2.2%
17	Missouri	19	2.0%
18	South Carolina	17	1.8%
19	Alabama	16	1.7%
20	Kentucky	15	1.6%
20	Mississippi	15	1.6%
20	Oklahoma	15	1.6%
23	Indiana	13	1.4%
24	Arkansas	12	1.3%
25	New Mexico	11	1.2%
26	Massachusetts	9	1.0%
26	Washington	9	1.0%
28	Colorado	8	0.9%
29	Nevada	7	0.8%
30	Minnesota	6	0.6%
30	Wisconsin	6	0.6%
32	Connecticut	5	0.5%
33	Hawaii	4	0.4%
33	Idaho	4	0.4%
33	Kansas	4	0.4%
33	Rhode Island	4	0.4%
37	Iowa	3	0.3%
37	Maine	3	0.3%
37	South Dakota	3	0.3%
40	Alaska	2	0.2%
40	Delaware	2	0.2%
40	Montana	2	0.2%
40	Nebraska	2	0.2%
40	Oregon	2	0.2%
40	Utah	2	0.2%
46	New Hampshire	1	0.1%
46	Vermont	1	0.1%
46	West Virginia	1	0.1%
49	North Dakota	0	0.0%
49	Wyoming	0	0.0%
	District of Columbia	5	0.5%

Source: U.S. Department of Health and Human Services, National Center for Health Statistics
(http://wonder.cdc.gov/WONDER/)
By state of residence.

Death Rate by Tuberculosis in 1999

National Rate = 0.3 Deaths per 100,000 Population*

ALPHA ORDER

RANK	STATE	RATE
9	Alabama	0.4
19	Alaska	0.3
9	Arizona	0.4
2	Arkansas	0.5
2	California	0.5
32	Colorado	0.2
32	Connecticut	0.2
19	Delaware	0.3
2	Florida	0.5
2	Georgia	0.5
19	Hawaii	0.3
19	Idaho	0.3
19	Illinois	0.3
32	Indiana	0.2
40	Iowa	0.1
32	Kansas	0.2
9	Kentucky	0.4
2	Louisiana	0.5
32	Maine	0.2
9	Maryland	0.4
40	Massachusetts	0.1
19	Michigan	0.3
40	Minnesota	0.1
2	Mississippi	0.5
19	Missouri	0.3
32	Montana	0.2
40	Nebraska	0.1
9	Nevada	0.4
40	New Hampshire	0.1
19	New Jersey	0.3
1	New Mexico	0.6
19	New York	0.3
19	North Carolina	0.3
49	North Dakota	0.0
19	Ohio	0.3
9	Oklahoma	0.4
40	Oregon	0.1
19	Pennsylvania	0.3
9	Rhode Island	0.4
9	South Carolina	0.4
9	South Dakota	0.4
9	Tennessee	0.4
2	Texas	0.5
40	Utah	0.1
32	Vermont	0.2
19	Virginia	0.3
32	Washington	0.2
40	West Virginia	0.1
40	Wisconsin	0.1
49	Wyoming	0.0

RANK ORDER

RANK	STATE	RATE
1	New Mexico	0.6
2	Arkansas	0.5
2	California	0.5
2	Florida	0.5
2	Georgia	0.5
2	Louisiana	0.5
2	Mississippi	0.5
2	Texas	0.5
9	Alabama	0.4
9	Arizona	0.4
9	Kentucky	0.4
9	Maryland	0.4
9	Nevada	0.4
9	Oklahoma	0.4
9	Rhode Island	0.4
9	South Carolina	0.4
9	South Dakota	0.4
9	Tennessee	0.4
19	Alaska	0.3
19	Delaware	0.3
19	Hawaii	0.3
19	Idaho	0.3
19	Illinois	0.3
19	Michigan	0.3
19	Missouri	0.3
19	New Jersey	0.3
19	New York	0.3
19	North Carolina	0.3
19	Ohio	0.3
19	Pennsylvania	0.3
19	Virginia	0.3
32	Colorado	0.2
32	Connecticut	0.2
32	Indiana	0.2
32	Kansas	0.2
32	Maine	0.2
32	Montana	0.2
32	Vermont	0.2
32	Washington	0.2
40	Iowa	0.1
40	Massachusetts	0.1
40	Minnesota	0.1
40	Nebraska	0.1
40	New Hampshire	0.1
40	Oregon	0.1
40	Utah	0.1
40	West Virginia	0.1
40	Wisconsin	0.1
49	North Dakota	0.0
49	Wyoming	0.0
	District of Columbia	1.0

Source: U.S. Department of Health and Human Services, National Center for Health Statistics
(http://wonder.cdc.gov/WONDER/)
*By state of residence. Not age-adjusted. Due to low numbers of deaths, rates for all states should be interpreted with caution.

Age-Adjusted Death Rate by Tuberculosis in 1999

National Rate = 0.3 Deaths per 100,000 Population*

ALPHA ORDER

RANK	STATE	RATE
9	Alabama	0.4
9	Alaska	0.4
4	Arizona	0.5
9	Arkansas	0.4
4	California	0.5
32	Colorado	0.2
38	Connecticut	0.1
20	Delaware	0.3
9	Florida	0.4
4	Georgia	0.5
20	Hawaii	0.3
20	Idaho	0.3
20	Illinois	0.3
32	Indiana	0.2
38	Iowa	0.1
38	Kansas	0.1
9	Kentucky	0.4
2	Louisiana	0.6
32	Maine	0.2
9	Maryland	0.4
38	Massachusetts	0.1
20	Michigan	0.3
38	Minnesota	0.1
2	Mississippi	0.6
20	Missouri	0.3
32	Montana	0.2
38	Nebraska	0.1
9	Nevada	0.4
38	New Hampshire	0.1
20	New Jersey	0.3
1	New Mexico	0.7
20	New York	0.3
20	North Carolina	0.3
48	North Dakota	0.0
20	Ohio	0.3
9	Oklahoma	0.4
38	Oregon	0.1
20	Pennsylvania	0.3
9	Rhode Island	0.4
4	South Carolina	0.5
9	South Dakota	0.4
9	Tennessee	0.4
4	Texas	0.5
38	Utah	0.1
32	Vermont	0.2
20	Virginia	0.3
32	Washington	0.2
48	West Virginia	0.0
38	Wisconsin	0.1
48	Wyoming	0.0

RANK ORDER

RANK	STATE	RATE
1	New Mexico	0.7
2	Louisiana	0.6
2	Mississippi	0.6
4	Arizona	0.5
4	California	0.5
4	Georgia	0.5
4	South Carolina	0.5
4	Texas	0.5
9	Alabama	0.4
9	Alaska	0.4
9	Arkansas	0.4
9	Florida	0.4
9	Kentucky	0.4
9	Maryland	0.4
9	Nevada	0.4
9	Oklahoma	0.4
9	Rhode Island	0.4
9	South Dakota	0.4
9	Tennessee	0.4
20	Delaware	0.3
20	Hawaii	0.3
20	Idaho	0.3
20	Illinois	0.3
20	Michigan	0.3
20	Missouri	0.3
20	New Jersey	0.3
20	New York	0.3
20	North Carolina	0.3
20	Ohio	0.3
20	Pennsylvania	0.3
20	Virginia	0.3
32	Colorado	0.2
32	Indiana	0.2
32	Maine	0.2
32	Montana	0.2
32	Vermont	0.2
32	Washington	0.2
38	Connecticut	0.1
38	Iowa	0.1
38	Kansas	0.1
38	Massachusetts	0.1
38	Minnesota	0.1
38	Nebraska	0.1
38	New Hampshire	0.1
38	Oregon	0.1
38	Utah	0.1
38	Wisconsin	0.1
48	North Dakota	0.0
48	West Virginia	0.0
48	Wyoming	0.0
	District of Columbia	0.9

Source: U.S. Department of Health and Human Services, National Center for Health Statistics
    (http://wonder.cdc.gov/WONDER/)
*By state of residence. Due to low numbers of deaths, rates for all states should be interpreted with caution.
Age-adjusted rates based on the year 2000 standard population.

Deaths by Injury in 1999

National Total = 143,948 Deaths*

ALPHA ORDER

RANK	STATE	DEATHS	% of USA
16	Alabama	3,306	2.3%
45	Alaska	441	0.3%
13	Arizona	3,450	2.4%
29	Arkansas	1,802	1.3%
1	California	14,341	10.0%
25	Colorado	2,292	1.6%
34	Connecticut	1,428	1.0%
46	Delaware	377	0.3%
3	Florida	8,954	6.2%
10	Georgia	4,585	3.2%
44	Hawaii	467	0.3%
39	Idaho	809	0.6%
6	Illinois	6,168	4.3%
15	Indiana	3,323	2.3%
32	Iowa	1,481	1.0%
31	Kansas	1,562	1.1%
22	Kentucky	2,410	1.7%
18	Louisiana	2,942	2.0%
40	Maine	658	0.5%
26	Maryland	2,262	1.6%
28	Massachusetts	1,867	1.3%
8	Michigan	4,921	3.4%
23	Minnesota	2,348	1.6%
27	Mississippi	2,258	1.6%
12	Missouri	3,550	2.5%
41	Montana	656	0.5%
38	Nebraska	906	0.6%
35	Nevada	1,281	0.9%
42	New Hampshire	487	0.3%
17	New Jersey	3,088	2.1%
33	New Mexico	1,454	1.0%
4	New York	6,962	4.8%
9	North Carolina	4,825	3.4%
49	North Dakota	353	0.2%
7	Ohio	5,182	3.6%
24	Oklahoma	2,332	1.6%
30	Oregon	1,784	1.2%
5	Pennsylvania	6,537	4.5%
47	Rhode Island	375	0.3%
21	South Carolina	2,632	1.8%
43	South Dakota	477	0.3%
11	Tennessee	3,826	2.7%
2	Texas	10,551	7.3%
37	Utah	983	0.7%
50	Vermont	289	0.2%
14	Virginia	3,424	2.4%
19	Washington	2,920	2.0%
36	West Virginia	1,126	0.8%
20	Wisconsin	2,750	1.9%
48	Wyoming	369	0.3%

RANK ORDER

RANK	STATE	DEATHS	% of USA
1	California	14,341	10.0%
2	Texas	10,551	7.3%
3	Florida	8,954	6.2%
4	New York	6,962	4.8%
5	Pennsylvania	6,537	4.5%
6	Illinois	6,168	4.3%
7	Ohio	5,182	3.6%
8	Michigan	4,921	3.4%
9	North Carolina	4,825	3.4%
10	Georgia	4,585	3.2%
11	Tennessee	3,826	2.7%
12	Missouri	3,550	2.5%
13	Arizona	3,450	2.4%
14	Virginia	3,424	2.4%
15	Indiana	3,323	2.3%
16	Alabama	3,306	2.3%
17	New Jersey	3,088	2.1%
18	Louisiana	2,942	2.0%
19	Washington	2,920	2.0%
20	Wisconsin	2,750	1.9%
21	South Carolina	2,632	1.8%
22	Kentucky	2,410	1.7%
23	Minnesota	2,348	1.6%
24	Oklahoma	2,332	1.6%
25	Colorado	2,292	1.6%
26	Maryland	2,262	1.6%
27	Mississippi	2,258	1.6%
28	Massachusetts	1,867	1.3%
29	Arkansas	1,802	1.3%
30	Oregon	1,784	1.2%
31	Kansas	1,562	1.1%
32	Iowa	1,481	1.0%
33	New Mexico	1,454	1.0%
34	Connecticut	1,428	1.0%
35	Nevada	1,281	0.9%
36	West Virginia	1,126	0.8%
37	Utah	983	0.7%
38	Nebraska	906	0.6%
39	Idaho	809	0.6%
40	Maine	658	0.5%
41	Montana	656	0.5%
42	New Hampshire	487	0.3%
43	South Dakota	477	0.3%
44	Hawaii	467	0.3%
45	Alaska	441	0.3%
46	Delaware	377	0.3%
47	Rhode Island	375	0.3%
48	Wyoming	369	0.3%
49	North Dakota	353	0.2%
50	Vermont	289	0.2%
	District of Columbia	377	0.3%

Source: U.S. Department of Health and Human Services, National Center for Health Statistics
    (http://wonder.cdc.gov/WONDER/)
*By state of residence. Injury as used here includes Accidents (including motor vehicle), Suicides, Homicides and
"Other" undetermined.

Death Rate by Injury in 1999

National Rate = 52.8 Deaths per 100,000 Population*

ALPHA ORDER

RANK	STATE	RATE
4	Alabama	75.7
7	Alaska	71.2
6	Arizona	72.2
9	Arkansas	70.6
44	California	43.3
23	Colorado	56.5
43	Connecticut	43.5
35	Delaware	50.0
20	Florida	59.3
21	Georgia	58.9
46	Hawaii	39.4
16	Idaho	64.6
33	Illinois	50.9
24	Indiana	55.9
32	Iowa	51.6
21	Kansas	58.9
19	Kentucky	60.8
13	Louisiana	67.3
30	Maine	52.5
42	Maryland	43.7
50	Massachusetts	30.2
36	Michigan	49.9
38	Minnesota	49.2
2	Mississippi	81.6
15	Missouri	64.9
5	Montana	74.3
27	Nebraska	54.4
8	Nevada	70.8
45	New Hampshire	40.5
48	New Jersey	37.9
1	New Mexico	83.6
47	New York	38.3
17	North Carolina	63.1
25	North Dakota	55.7
41	Ohio	46.0
11	Oklahoma	69.4
28	Oregon	53.8
26	Pennsylvania	54.5
49	Rhode Island	37.8
12	South Carolina	67.7
14	South Dakota	65.1
10	Tennessee	69.8
29	Texas	52.6
40	Utah	46.2
39	Vermont	48.7
37	Virginia	49.8
34	Washington	50.7
18	West Virginia	62.3
31	Wisconsin	52.4
3	Wyoming	76.9

RANK ORDER

RANK	STATE	RATE
1	New Mexico	83.6
2	Mississippi	81.6
3	Wyoming	76.9
4	Alabama	75.7
5	Montana	74.3
6	Arizona	72.2
7	Alaska	71.2
8	Nevada	70.8
9	Arkansas	70.6
10	Tennessee	69.8
11	Oklahoma	69.4
12	South Carolina	67.7
13	Louisiana	67.3
14	South Dakota	65.1
15	Missouri	64.9
16	Idaho	64.6
17	North Carolina	63.1
18	West Virginia	62.3
19	Kentucky	60.8
20	Florida	59.3
21	Georgia	58.9
21	Kansas	58.9
23	Colorado	56.5
24	Indiana	55.9
25	North Dakota	55.7
26	Pennsylvania	54.5
27	Nebraska	54.4
28	Oregon	53.8
29	Texas	52.6
30	Maine	52.5
31	Wisconsin	52.4
32	Iowa	51.6
33	Illinois	50.9
34	Washington	50.7
35	Delaware	50.0
36	Michigan	49.9
37	Virginia	49.8
38	Minnesota	49.2
39	Vermont	48.7
40	Utah	46.2
41	Ohio	46.0
42	Maryland	43.7
43	Connecticut	43.5
44	California	43.3
45	New Hampshire	40.5
46	Hawaii	39.4
47	New York	38.3
48	New Jersey	37.9
49	Rhode Island	37.8
50	Massachusetts	30.2

| | District of Columbia | 72.6 |

Source: U.S. Department of Health and Human Services, National Center for Health Statistics (http://wonder.cdc.gov/WONDER/)

*By state of residence. Injury as used here includes Accidents (including motor vehicle), Suicides, Homicides and "Other" undetermined. Not age-adjusted.

Age-Adjusted Death Rate by Injury in 1999

National Rate = 52.7 Deaths per 100,000 Population*

ALPHA ORDER

RANK	STATE	RATE
5	Alabama	75.0
2	Alaska	83.5
6	Arizona	73.5
9	Arkansas	69.7
43	California	44.4
21	Colorado	59.3
44	Connecticut	42.1
36	Delaware	50.3
23	Florida	56.9
18	Georgia	61.9
46	Hawaii	39.2
14	Idaho	66.2
32	Illinois	51.0
24	Indiana	55.9
39	Iowa	48.1
22	Kansas	57.3
19	Kentucky	60.7
13	Louisiana	68.6
35	Maine	50.5
42	Maryland	44.7
50	Massachusetts	28.9
37	Michigan	50.1
38	Minnesota	48.3
3	Mississippi	82.3
15	Missouri	63.6
8	Montana	72.5
27	Nebraska	52.4
7	Nevada	73.4
45	New Hampshire	40.9
48	New Jersey	37.2
1	New Mexico	86.7
47	New York	37.6
15	North Carolina	63.6
28	North Dakota	52.3
41	Ohio	45.5
11	Oklahoma	69.0
26	Oregon	52.7
29	Pennsylvania	51.9
49	Rhode Island	35.5
12	South Carolina	68.7
17	South Dakota	63.0
10	Tennessee	69.6
25	Texas	55.2
30	Utah	51.4
39	Vermont	48.1
32	Virginia	51.0
31	Washington	51.1
20	West Virginia	59.7
32	Wisconsin	51.0
4	Wyoming	77.5

RANK ORDER

RANK	STATE	RATE
1	New Mexico	86.7
2	Alaska	83.5
3	Mississippi	82.3
4	Wyoming	77.5
5	Alabama	75.0
6	Arizona	73.5
7	Nevada	73.4
8	Montana	72.5
9	Arkansas	69.7
10	Tennessee	69.6
11	Oklahoma	69.0
12	South Carolina	68.7
13	Louisiana	68.6
14	Idaho	66.2
15	Missouri	63.6
15	North Carolina	63.6
17	South Dakota	63.0
18	Georgia	61.9
19	Kentucky	60.7
20	West Virginia	59.7
21	Colorado	59.3
22	Kansas	57.3
23	Florida	56.9
24	Indiana	55.9
25	Texas	55.2
26	Oregon	52.7
27	Nebraska	52.4
28	North Dakota	52.3
29	Pennsylvania	51.9
30	Utah	51.4
31	Washington	51.1
32	Illinois	51.0
32	Virginia	51.0
32	Wisconsin	51.0
35	Maine	50.5
36	Delaware	50.3
37	Michigan	50.1
38	Minnesota	48.3
39	Iowa	48.1
39	Vermont	48.1
41	Ohio	45.5
42	Maryland	44.7
43	California	44.4
44	Connecticut	42.1
45	New Hampshire	40.9
46	Hawaii	39.2
47	New York	37.6
48	New Jersey	37.2
49	Rhode Island	35.5
50	Massachusetts	28.9
	District of Columbia	71.3

Source: U.S. Department of Health and Human Services, National Center for Health Statistics
(http://wonder.cdc.gov/WONDER/)
*By state of residence. Injury as used here includes Accidents (including motor vehicle), Suicides, Homicides and
"Other" undetermined. Age-adjusted rates based on the year 2000 standard population.

Deaths by Accidents in 2000

National Total = 97,900 Deaths*

ALPHA ORDER

ALPHA ORDER

RANK	STATE	DEATHS	% of USA
18	Alabama	2,093	2.1%
42	Alaska	343	0.4%
14	Arizona	2,326	2.4%
28	Arkansas	1,267	1.3%
1	California	8,577	8.8%
24	Colorado	1,702	1.7%
31	Connecticut	1,175	1.2%
46	Delaware	290	0.3%
3	Florida	6,267	6.4%
10	Georgia	3,103	3.2%
42	Hawaii	343	0.4%
39	Idaho	518	0.5%
6	Illinois	4,041	4.1%
17	Indiana	2,139	2.2%
32	Iowa	1,070	1.1%
33	Kansas	1,054	1.1%
22	Kentucky	1,838	1.9%
20	Louisiana	2,006	2.0%
41	Maine	407	0.4%
30	Maryland	1,182	1.2%
27	Massachusetts	1,357	1.4%
9	Michigan	3,220	3.3%
23	Minnesota	1,711	1.7%
25	Mississippi	1,653	1.7%
12	Missouri	2,398	2.4%
40	Montana	495	0.5%
38	Nebraska	640	0.7%
36	Nevada	730	0.7%
44	New Hampshire	321	0.3%
15	New Jersey	2,284	2.3%
34	New Mexico	995	1.0%
5	New York	4,244	4.3%
7	North Carolina	3,525	3.6%
47	North Dakota	248	0.3%
8	Ohio	3,492	3.6%
26	Oklahoma	1,566	1.6%
29	Oregon	1,248	1.3%
4	Pennsylvania	4,583	4.7%
49	Rhode Island	235	0.2%
21	South Carolina	1,974	2.0%
44	South Dakota	321	0.3%
11	Tennessee	2,743	2.8%
2	Texas	7,407	7.6%
37	Utah	665	0.7%
50	Vermont	234	0.2%
13	Virginia	2,396	2.4%
19	Washington	2,049	2.1%
35	West Virginia	817	0.8%
16	Wisconsin	2,159	2.2%
48	Wyoming	245	0.3%

RANK ORDER

RANK	STATE	DEATHS	% of USA
1	California	8,577	8.8%
2	Texas	7,407	7.6%
3	Florida	6,267	6.4%
4	Pennsylvania	4,583	4.7%
5	New York	4,244	4.3%
6	Illinois	4,041	4.1%
7	North Carolina	3,525	3.6%
8	Ohio	3,492	3.6%
9	Michigan	3,220	3.3%
10	Georgia	3,103	3.2%
11	Tennessee	2,743	2.8%
12	Missouri	2,398	2.4%
13	Virginia	2,396	2.4%
14	Arizona	2,326	2.4%
15	New Jersey	2,284	2.3%
16	Wisconsin	2,159	2.2%
17	Indiana	2,139	2.2%
18	Alabama	2,093	2.1%
19	Washington	2,049	2.1%
20	Louisiana	2,006	2.0%
21	South Carolina	1,974	2.0%
22	Kentucky	1,838	1.9%
23	Minnesota	1,711	1.7%
24	Colorado	1,702	1.7%
25	Mississippi	1,653	1.7%
26	Oklahoma	1,566	1.6%
27	Massachusetts	1,357	1.4%
28	Arkansas	1,267	1.3%
29	Oregon	1,248	1.3%
30	Maryland	1,182	1.2%
31	Connecticut	1,175	1.2%
32	Iowa	1,070	1.1%
33	Kansas	1,054	1.1%
34	New Mexico	995	1.0%
35	West Virginia	817	0.8%
36	Nevada	730	0.7%
37	Utah	665	0.7%
38	Nebraska	640	0.7%
39	Idaho	518	0.5%
40	Montana	495	0.5%
41	Maine	407	0.4%
42	Alaska	343	0.4%
42	Hawaii	343	0.4%
44	New Hampshire	321	0.3%
44	South Dakota	321	0.3%
46	Delaware	290	0.3%
47	North Dakota	248	0.3%
48	Wyoming	245	0.3%
49	Rhode Island	235	0.2%
50	Vermont	234	0.2%
	District of Columbia	204	0.2%

*Source: U.S. Department of Health and Human Services, National Center for Health Statistics
"National Vital Statistics Reports" (Vol. 50, No. 15, September 16, 2002)*
Final data by state of residence. Includes motor vehicle deaths, poisoning, falls, drowning and other accidents.

Death Rate by Accidents in 2000

National Rate = 35.6 Deaths per 100,000 Population*

<table>
<tr><td colspan="3">ALPHA ORDER</td><td colspan="3">RANK ORDER</td></tr>
<tr><td>RANK</td><td>STATE</td><td>RATE</td><td>RANK</td><td>STATE</td><td>RATE</td></tr>
<tr><td>9</td><td>Alabama</td><td>47.7</td><td>1</td><td>Mississippi</td><td>59.3</td></tr>
<tr><td>4</td><td>Alaska</td><td>55.1</td><td>2</td><td>New Mexico</td><td>56.9</td></tr>
<tr><td>10</td><td>Arizona</td><td>47.6</td><td>3</td><td>Montana</td><td>55.8</td></tr>
<tr><td>8</td><td>Arkansas</td><td>49.2</td><td>4</td><td>Alaska</td><td>55.1</td></tr>
<tr><td>46</td><td>California</td><td>25.5</td><td>5</td><td>Wyoming</td><td>50.9</td></tr>
<tr><td>18</td><td>Colorado</td><td>41.1</td><td>6</td><td>South Carolina</td><td>50.3</td></tr>
<tr><td>34</td><td>Connecticut</td><td>35.6</td><td>7</td><td>Tennessee</td><td>49.6</td></tr>
<tr><td>29</td><td>Delaware</td><td>38.0</td><td>8</td><td>Arkansas</td><td>49.2</td></tr>
<tr><td>19</td><td>Florida</td><td>40.9</td><td>9</td><td>Alabama</td><td>47.7</td></tr>
<tr><td>24</td><td>Georgia</td><td>39.1</td><td>10</td><td>Arizona</td><td>47.6</td></tr>
<tr><td>43</td><td>Hawaii</td><td>29.1</td><td>11</td><td>Oklahoma</td><td>46.3</td></tr>
<tr><td>21</td><td>Idaho</td><td>40.7</td><td>12</td><td>Kentucky</td><td>46.1</td></tr>
<tr><td>38</td><td>Illinois</td><td>33.2</td><td>13</td><td>Louisiana</td><td>45.9</td></tr>
<tr><td>33</td><td>Indiana</td><td>35.8</td><td>14</td><td>North Carolina</td><td>45.5</td></tr>
<tr><td>31</td><td>Iowa</td><td>37.2</td><td>15</td><td>West Virginia</td><td>45.3</td></tr>
<tr><td>22</td><td>Kansas</td><td>39.5</td><td>16</td><td>Missouri</td><td>43.6</td></tr>
<tr><td>12</td><td>Kentucky</td><td>46.1</td><td>17</td><td>South Dakota</td><td>43.5</td></tr>
<tr><td>13</td><td>Louisiana</td><td>45.9</td><td>18</td><td>Colorado</td><td>41.1</td></tr>
<tr><td>40</td><td>Maine</td><td>32.3</td><td>19</td><td>Florida</td><td>40.9</td></tr>
<tr><td>49</td><td>Maryland</td><td>22.6</td><td>20</td><td>Wisconsin</td><td>40.8</td></tr>
<tr><td>50</td><td>Massachusetts</td><td>21.9</td><td>21</td><td>Idaho</td><td>40.7</td></tr>
<tr><td>39</td><td>Michigan</td><td>32.5</td><td>22</td><td>Kansas</td><td>39.5</td></tr>
<tr><td>35</td><td>Minnesota</td><td>35.4</td><td>23</td><td>North Dakota</td><td>39.4</td></tr>
<tr><td>1</td><td>Mississippi</td><td>59.3</td><td>24</td><td>Georgia</td><td>39.1</td></tr>
<tr><td>16</td><td>Missouri</td><td>43.6</td><td>24</td><td>Vermont</td><td>39.1</td></tr>
<tr><td>3</td><td>Montana</td><td>55.8</td><td>26</td><td>Nevada</td><td>38.8</td></tr>
<tr><td>27</td><td>Nebraska</td><td>38.3</td><td>27</td><td>Nebraska</td><td>38.3</td></tr>
<tr><td>26</td><td>Nevada</td><td>38.8</td><td>28</td><td>Pennsylvania</td><td>38.2</td></tr>
<tr><td>45</td><td>New Hampshire</td><td>26.4</td><td>29</td><td>Delaware</td><td>38.0</td></tr>
<tr><td>44</td><td>New Jersey</td><td>27.8</td><td>30</td><td>Oregon</td><td>37.4</td></tr>
<tr><td>2</td><td>New Mexico</td><td>56.9</td><td>31</td><td>Iowa</td><td>37.2</td></tr>
<tr><td>48</td><td>New York</td><td>23.2</td><td>32</td><td>Texas</td><td>36.3</td></tr>
<tr><td>14</td><td>North Carolina</td><td>45.5</td><td>33</td><td>Indiana</td><td>35.8</td></tr>
<tr><td>23</td><td>North Dakota</td><td>39.4</td><td>34</td><td>Connecticut</td><td>35.6</td></tr>
<tr><td>41</td><td>Ohio</td><td>31.0</td><td>35</td><td>Minnesota</td><td>35.4</td></tr>
<tr><td>11</td><td>Oklahoma</td><td>46.3</td><td>36</td><td>Washington</td><td>35.3</td></tr>
<tr><td>30</td><td>Oregon</td><td>37.4</td><td>37</td><td>Virginia</td><td>34.4</td></tr>
<tr><td>28</td><td>Pennsylvania</td><td>38.2</td><td>38</td><td>Illinois</td><td>33.2</td></tr>
<tr><td>47</td><td>Rhode Island</td><td>23.6</td><td>39</td><td>Michigan</td><td>32.5</td></tr>
<tr><td>6</td><td>South Carolina</td><td>50.3</td><td>40</td><td>Maine</td><td>32.3</td></tr>
<tr><td>17</td><td>South Dakota</td><td>43.5</td><td>41</td><td>Ohio</td><td>31.0</td></tr>
<tr><td>7</td><td>Tennessee</td><td>49.6</td><td>42</td><td>Utah</td><td>30.7</td></tr>
<tr><td>32</td><td>Texas</td><td>36.3</td><td>43</td><td>Hawaii</td><td>29.1</td></tr>
<tr><td>42</td><td>Utah</td><td>30.7</td><td>44</td><td>New Jersey</td><td>27.8</td></tr>
<tr><td>24</td><td>Vermont</td><td>39.1</td><td>45</td><td>New Hampshire</td><td>26.4</td></tr>
<tr><td>37</td><td>Virginia</td><td>34.4</td><td>46</td><td>California</td><td>25.5</td></tr>
<tr><td>36</td><td>Washington</td><td>35.3</td><td>47</td><td>Rhode Island</td><td>23.6</td></tr>
<tr><td>15</td><td>West Virginia</td><td>45.3</td><td>48</td><td>New York</td><td>23.2</td></tr>
<tr><td>20</td><td>Wisconsin</td><td>40.8</td><td>49</td><td>Maryland</td><td>22.6</td></tr>
<tr><td>5</td><td>Wyoming</td><td>50.9</td><td>50</td><td>Massachusetts</td><td>21.9</td></tr>
<tr><td></td><td></td><td></td><td></td><td>District of Columbia</td><td>39.4</td></tr>
</table>

Source: U.S. Department of Health and Human Services, National Center for Health Statistics
"National Vital Statistics Reports" (Vol. 50, No. 15, September 16, 2002)
*Final data by state of residence. Includes motor vehicle deaths, poisoning, falls, drowning and other accidents.
Not age-adjusted.

Age-Adjusted Death Rate by Accidents in 2000

National Rate = 35.5 Deaths per 100,000 Population*

ALPHA ORDER			RANK ORDER		
RANK	STATE	RATE	RANK	STATE	RATE
10	Alabama	47.4	1	Alaska	64.9
1	Alaska	64.9	2	Mississippi	60.0
8	Arizona	48.8	3	New Mexico	59.1
9	Arkansas	48.0	4	Montana	54.7
46	California	26.3	5	Wyoming	52.3
15	Colorado	43.8	6	South Carolina	50.7
38	Connecticut	33.5	7	Tennessee	49.9
26	Delaware	38.3	8	Arizona	48.8
23	Florida	39.0	9	Arkansas	48.0
18	Georgia	42.0	10	Alabama	47.4
43	Hawaii	28.3	11	Louisiana	46.7
20	Idaho	41.9	12	North Carolina	46.3
39	Illinois	33.2	13	Kentucky	46.1
30	Indiana	35.8	14	Oklahoma	45.7
37	Iowa	33.9	15	Colorado	43.8
27	Kansas	38.2	16	West Virginia	43.3
13	Kentucky	46.1	17	Missouri	42.4
11	Louisiana	46.7	18	Georgia	42.0
41	Maine	31.1	18	South Dakota	42.0
47	Maryland	23.4	20	Idaho	41.9
50	Massachusetts	20.5	21	Nevada	40.9
40	Michigan	32.6	22	Wisconsin	39.2
36	Minnesota	34.7	23	Florida	39.0
2	Mississippi	60.0	24	Vermont	38.6
17	Missouri	42.4	25	Texas	38.4
4	Montana	54.7	26	Delaware	38.3
30	Nebraska	35.8	27	Kansas	38.2
21	Nevada	40.9	28	Oregon	36.4
45	New Hampshire	26.7	29	Pennsylvania	35.9
44	New Jersey	27.2	30	Indiana	35.8
3	New Mexico	59.1	30	Nebraska	35.8
48	New York	22.6	30	North Dakota	35.8
12	North Carolina	46.3	30	Washington	35.8
30	North Dakota	35.8	34	Virginia	35.6
42	Ohio	30.5	35	Utah	34.9
14	Oklahoma	45.7	36	Minnesota	34.7
28	Oregon	36.4	37	Iowa	33.9
29	Pennsylvania	35.9	38	Connecticut	33.5
49	Rhode Island	21.2	39	Illinois	33.2
6	South Carolina	50.7	40	Michigan	32.6
18	South Dakota	42.0	41	Maine	31.1
7	Tennessee	49.9	42	Ohio	30.5
25	Texas	38.4	43	Hawaii	28.3
35	Utah	34.9	44	New Jersey	27.2
24	Vermont	38.6	45	New Hampshire	26.7
34	Virginia	35.6	46	California	26.3
30	Washington	35.8	47	Maryland	23.4
16	West Virginia	43.3	48	New York	22.6
22	Wisconsin	39.2	49	Rhode Island	21.2
5	Wyoming	52.3	50	Massachusetts	20.5
				District of Columbia	36.8

Source: U.S. Department of Health and Human Services, National Center for Health Statistics
    "National Vital Statistics Reports" (Vol. 50, No. 15, September 16, 2002)
*Final data by state of residence. Includes motor vehicle deaths, poisoning, falls, drowning and other accidents.
Age-adjusted rates based on the year 2000 standard population.

Deaths by Motor Vehicle Accidents in 2000

National Total = 43,354 Deaths*

ALPHA ORDER

RANK	STATE	DEATHS	% of USA
13	Alabama	1,064	2.5%
44	Alaska	132	0.3%
16	Arizona	999	2.3%
26	Arkansas	680	1.6%
2	California	3,743	8.6%
23	Colorado	751	1.7%
36	Connecticut	340	0.8%
46	Delaware	126	0.3%
3	Florida	3,057	7.1%
7	Georgia	1,536	3.5%
45	Hawaii	129	0.3%
39	Idaho	271	0.6%
5	Illinois	1,568	3.6%
19	Indiana	918	2.1%
32	Iowa	474	1.1%
29	Kansas	495	1.1%
21	Kentucky	832	1.9%
15	Louisiana	1,014	2.3%
42	Maine	175	0.4%
28	Maryland	612	1.4%
30	Massachusetts	493	1.1%
9	Michigan	1,507	3.5%
25	Minnesota	689	1.6%
18	Mississippi	935	2.2%
12	Missouri	1,097	2.5%
40	Montana	234	0.5%
38	Nebraska	285	0.7%
37	Nevada	303	0.7%
43	New Hampshire	134	0.3%
22	New Jersey	772	1.8%
33	New Mexico	418	1.0%
6	New York	1,541	3.6%
4	North Carolina	1,693	3.9%
48	North Dakota	105	0.2%
10	Ohio	1,456	3.4%
27	Oklahoma	679	1.6%
31	Oregon	478	1.1%
8	Pennsylvania	1,522	3.5%
49	Rhode Island	81	0.2%
14	South Carolina	1,025	2.4%
41	South Dakota	178	0.4%
11	Tennessee	1,395	3.2%
1	Texas	3,824	8.8%
35	Utah	364	0.8%
50	Vermont	76	0.2%
17	Virginia	981	2.3%
24	Washington	711	1.6%
34	West Virginia	394	0.9%
20	Wisconsin	890	2.1%
47	Wyoming	122	0.3%

RANK ORDER

RANK	STATE	DEATHS	% of USA
1	Texas	3,824	8.8%
2	California	3,743	8.6%
3	Florida	3,057	7.1%
4	North Carolina	1,693	3.9%
5	Illinois	1,568	3.6%
6	New York	1,541	3.6%
7	Georgia	1,536	3.5%
8	Pennsylvania	1,522	3.5%
9	Michigan	1,507	3.5%
10	Ohio	1,456	3.4%
11	Tennessee	1,395	3.2%
12	Missouri	1,097	2.5%
13	Alabama	1,064	2.5%
14	South Carolina	1,025	2.4%
15	Louisiana	1,014	2.3%
16	Arizona	999	2.3%
17	Virginia	981	2.3%
18	Mississippi	935	2.2%
19	Indiana	918	2.1%
20	Wisconsin	890	2.1%
21	Kentucky	832	1.9%
22	New Jersey	772	1.8%
23	Colorado	751	1.7%
24	Washington	711	1.6%
25	Minnesota	689	1.6%
26	Arkansas	680	1.6%
27	Oklahoma	679	1.6%
28	Maryland	612	1.4%
29	Kansas	495	1.1%
30	Massachusetts	493	1.1%
31	Oregon	478	1.1%
32	Iowa	474	1.1%
33	New Mexico	418	1.0%
34	West Virginia	394	0.9%
35	Utah	364	0.8%
36	Connecticut	340	0.8%
37	Nevada	303	0.7%
38	Nebraska	285	0.7%
39	Idaho	271	0.6%
40	Montana	234	0.5%
41	South Dakota	178	0.4%
42	Maine	175	0.4%
43	New Hampshire	134	0.3%
44	Alaska	132	0.3%
45	Hawaii	129	0.3%
46	Delaware	126	0.3%
47	Wyoming	122	0.3%
48	North Dakota	105	0.2%
49	Rhode Island	81	0.2%
50	Vermont	76	0.2%
	District of Columbia	56	0.1%

Source: U.S. Department of Health and Human Services, National Center for Health Statistics
   "National Vital Statistics Reports" (Vol. 50, No. 15, September 16, 2002)

*Final data by state of residence. These numbers are compiled from death certificates by the Centers for Disease Control and Prevention. They may differ from motor vehicle deaths collected by the U.S. Department of Transportation from other sources.

Death Rate by Motor Vehicle Accidents in 2000

National Rate = 15.7 Deaths per 100,000 Population*

ALPHA ORDER

RANK	STATE	RATE
7	Alabama	24.2
14	Alaska	21.2
16	Arizona	20.5
2	Arkansas	26.4
43	California	11.1
23	Colorado	18.2
46	Connecticut	10.3
28	Delaware	16.5
18	Florida	19.9
20	Georgia	19.3
45	Hawaii	10.9
13	Idaho	21.3
37	Illinois	12.9
31	Indiana	15.4
28	Iowa	16.5
22	Kansas	18.6
15	Kentucky	20.9
10	Louisiana	23.2
36	Maine	13.9
42	Maryland	11.7
50	Massachusetts	7.9
32	Michigan	15.2
33	Minnesota	14.3
1	Mississippi	33.5
18	Missouri	19.9
2	Montana	26.4
24	Nebraska	17.1
30	Nevada	16.1
44	New Hampshire	11.0
47	New Jersey	9.4
9	New Mexico	23.9
48	New York	8.4
11	North Carolina	21.9
27	North Dakota	16.7
37	Ohio	12.9
17	Oklahoma	20.1
33	Oregon	14.3
39	Pennsylvania	12.7
49	Rhode Island	8.1
4	South Carolina	26.1
8	South Dakota	24.1
6	Tennessee	25.2
21	Texas	18.8
25	Utah	16.8
39	Vermont	12.7
35	Virginia	14.1
41	Washington	12.2
11	West Virginia	21.9
25	Wisconsin	16.8
5	Wyoming	25.4

RANK ORDER

RANK	STATE	RATE
1	Mississippi	33.5
2	Arkansas	26.4
2	Montana	26.4
4	South Carolina	26.1
5	Wyoming	25.4
6	Tennessee	25.2
7	Alabama	24.2
8	South Dakota	24.1
9	New Mexico	23.9
10	Louisiana	23.2
11	North Carolina	21.9
11	West Virginia	21.9
13	Idaho	21.3
14	Alaska	21.2
15	Kentucky	20.9
16	Arizona	20.5
17	Oklahoma	20.1
18	Florida	19.9
18	Missouri	19.9
20	Georgia	19.3
21	Texas	18.8
22	Kansas	18.6
23	Colorado	18.2
24	Nebraska	17.1
25	Utah	16.8
25	Wisconsin	16.8
27	North Dakota	16.7
28	Delaware	16.5
28	Iowa	16.5
30	Nevada	16.1
31	Indiana	15.4
32	Michigan	15.2
33	Minnesota	14.3
33	Oregon	14.3
35	Virginia	14.1
36	Maine	13.9
37	Illinois	12.9
37	Ohio	12.9
39	Pennsylvania	12.7
39	Vermont	12.7
41	Washington	12.2
42	Maryland	11.7
43	California	11.1
44	New Hampshire	11.0
45	Hawaii	10.9
46	Connecticut	10.3
47	New Jersey	9.4
48	New York	8.4
49	Rhode Island	8.1
50	Massachusetts	7.9
	District of Columbia	10.8

Source: U.S. Department of Health and Human Services, National Center for Health Statistics
    "National Vital Statistics Reports" (Vol. 50, No. 15, September 16, 2002)
*Final data by state of residence. These numbers are compiled from death certificates by the Centers for Disease Control and Prevention. They may differ from motor vehicle deaths collected by the U.S. Department of Transportation from other sources. Not age-adjusted.

Age-Adjusted Death Rate by Motor Vehicle Accidents in 2000

National Rate = 15.7 Deaths per 100,000 Population*

ALPHA ORDER

RANK	STATE	RATE
8	Alabama	24.0
10	Alaska	23.4
15	Arizona	20.8
3	Arkansas	26.2
43	California	11.3
22	Colorado	18.4
46	Connecticut	10.3
27	Delaware	16.5
17	Florida	19.9
19	Georgia	19.8
45	Hawaii	10.7
14	Idaho	21.4
37	Illinois	12.9
31	Indiana	15.3
30	Iowa	16.0
23	Kansas	18.3
16	Kentucky	20.6
11	Louisiana	23.1
36	Maine	13.7
42	Maryland	11.9
50	Massachusetts	7.9
32	Michigan	15.2
33	Minnesota	14.2
1	Mississippi	33.5
19	Missouri	19.8
2	Montana	26.6
25	Nebraska	16.7
27	Nevada	16.5
44	New Hampshire	11.1
47	New Jersey	9.4
7	New Mexico	24.3
48	New York	8.4
12	North Carolina	22.0
29	North Dakota	16.3
38	Ohio	12.8
17	Oklahoma	19.9
33	Oregon	14.2
40	Pennsylvania	12.5
49	Rhode Island	8.1
4	South Carolina	25.8
9	South Dakota	23.9
6	Tennessee	25.2
21	Texas	19.0
24	Utah	17.8
39	Vermont	12.6
35	Virginia	14.0
41	Washington	12.2
13	West Virginia	21.6
26	Wisconsin	16.6
5	Wyoming	25.7

RANK ORDER

RANK	STATE	RATE
1	Mississippi	33.5
2	Montana	26.6
3	Arkansas	26.2
4	South Carolina	25.8
5	Wyoming	25.7
6	Tennessee	25.2
7	New Mexico	24.3
8	Alabama	24.0
9	South Dakota	23.9
10	Alaska	23.4
11	Louisiana	23.1
12	North Carolina	22.0
13	West Virginia	21.6
14	Idaho	21.4
15	Arizona	20.8
16	Kentucky	20.6
17	Florida	19.9
17	Oklahoma	19.9
19	Georgia	19.8
19	Missouri	19.8
21	Texas	19.0
22	Colorado	18.4
23	Kansas	18.3
24	Utah	17.8
25	Nebraska	16.7
26	Wisconsin	16.6
27	Delaware	16.5
27	Nevada	16.5
29	North Dakota	16.3
30	Iowa	16.0
31	Indiana	15.3
32	Michigan	15.2
33	Minnesota	14.2
33	Oregon	14.2
35	Virginia	14.0
36	Maine	13.7
37	Illinois	12.9
38	Ohio	12.8
39	Vermont	12.6
40	Pennsylvania	12.5
41	Washington	12.2
42	Maryland	11.9
43	California	11.3
44	New Hampshire	11.1
45	Hawaii	10.7
46	Connecticut	10.3
47	New Jersey	9.4
48	New York	8.4
49	Rhode Island	8.1
50	Massachusetts	7.9
	District of Columbia	10.6

Source: U.S. Department of Health and Human Services, National Center for Health Statistics
        "National Vital Statistics Reports" (Vol. 50, No. 15, September 16, 2002)
*Final data by state of residence. These numbers are compiled from death certificates by the Centers for Disease Control and Prevention. They may differ from motor vehicle deaths collected by the U.S. Department of Transportation from other sources. Age-adjusted rates based on the year 2000 standard population.

Deaths by Homicide in 2000

National Total = 16,765 Homicides*

ALPHA ORDER

ALPHA ORDER

RANK	STATE	HOMICIDES	% of USA
14	Alabama	444	2.6%
40	Alaska	37	0.2%
16	Arizona	410	2.4%
22	Arkansas	204	1.2%
1	California	2,064	12.3%
28	Colorado	151	0.9%
33	Connecticut	95	0.6%
44	Delaware	23	0.1%
5	Florida	937	5.6%
7	Georgia	659	3.9%
41	Hawaii	35	0.2%
43	Idaho	24	0.1%
3	Illinois	991	5.9%
18	Indiana	367	2.2%
37	Iowa	58	0.3%
29	Kansas	141	0.8%
22	Kentucky	204	1.2%
10	Louisiana	600	3.6%
45	Maine	18	0.1%
11	Maryland	503	3.0%
32	Massachusetts	122	0.7%
6	Michigan	722	4.3%
30	Minnesota	139	0.8%
21	Mississippi	312	1.9%
17	Missouri	398	2.4%
41	Montana	35	0.2%
36	Nebraska	64	0.4%
31	Nevada	134	0.8%
46	New Hampshire	15	0.1%
20	New Jersey	320	1.9%
27	New Mexico	160	1.0%
3	New York	991	5.9%
8	North Carolina	657	3.9%
48	North Dakota	12	0.1%
13	Ohio	465	2.8%
24	Oklahoma	200	1.2%
34	Oregon	91	0.5%
9	Pennsylvania	650	3.9%
39	Rhode Island	39	0.2%
19	South Carolina	326	1.9%
47	South Dakota	14	0.1%
12	Tennessee	471	2.8%
2	Texas	1,317	7.9%
38	Utah	52	0.3%
49	Vermont	11	0.1%
15	Virginia	435	2.6%
24	Washington	200	1.2%
35	West Virginia	80	0.5%
26	Wisconsin	174	1.0%
50	Wyoming	10	0.1%

RANK ORDER

RANK	STATE	HOMICIDES	% of USA
1	California	2,064	12.3%
2	Texas	1,317	7.9%
3	Illinois	991	5.9%
3	New York	991	5.9%
5	Florida	937	5.6%
6	Michigan	722	4.3%
7	Georgia	659	3.9%
8	North Carolina	657	3.9%
9	Pennsylvania	650	3.9%
10	Louisiana	600	3.6%
11	Maryland	503	3.0%
12	Tennessee	471	2.8%
13	Ohio	465	2.8%
14	Alabama	444	2.6%
15	Virginia	435	2.6%
16	Arizona	410	2.4%
17	Missouri	398	2.4%
18	Indiana	367	2.2%
19	South Carolina	326	1.9%
20	New Jersey	320	1.9%
21	Mississippi	312	1.9%
22	Arkansas	204	1.2%
22	Kentucky	204	1.2%
24	Oklahoma	200	1.2%
24	Washington	200	1.2%
26	Wisconsin	174	1.0%
27	New Mexico	160	1.0%
28	Colorado	151	0.9%
29	Kansas	141	0.8%
30	Minnesota	139	0.8%
31	Nevada	134	0.8%
32	Massachusetts	122	0.7%
33	Connecticut	95	0.6%
34	Oregon	91	0.5%
35	West Virginia	80	0.5%
36	Nebraska	64	0.4%
37	Iowa	58	0.3%
38	Utah	52	0.3%
39	Rhode Island	39	0.2%
40	Alaska	37	0.2%
41	Hawaii	35	0.2%
41	Montana	35	0.2%
43	Idaho	24	0.1%
44	Delaware	23	0.1%
45	Maine	18	0.1%
46	New Hampshire	15	0.1%
47	South Dakota	14	0.1%
48	North Dakota	12	0.1%
49	Vermont	11	0.1%
50	Wyoming	10	0.1%
	District of Columbia	184	1.1%

Source: U.S. Department of Health and Human Services, National Center for Health Statistics
   "National Vital Statistics Reports" (Vol. 50, No. 15, September 16, 2002)
*By state of residence. Includes legal intervention. Homicide data shown here are collected by the Centers for Disease Control and Prevention based on death certificates and differ from murder data collected by the F.B.I. from other sources.

Death Rate by Homicide in 2000

National Rate = 6.1 Deaths per 100,000 Population*

ALPHA ORDER				RANK ORDER		
RANK	STATE	RATE		RANK	STATE	RATE
3	Alabama	10.1		1	Louisiana	13.7
21	Alaska	5.9		2	Mississippi	11.2
8	Arizona	8.4		3	Alabama	10.1
12	Arkansas	7.9		4	Maryland	9.6
18	California	6.1		5	New Mexico	9.2
33	Colorado	3.7		6	North Carolina	8.5
38	Connecticut	2.9		6	Tennessee	8.5
36	Delaware	3.0		8	Arizona	8.4
18	Florida	6.1		9	Georgia	8.3
9	Georgia	8.3		9	South Carolina	8.3
36	Hawaii	3.0		11	Illinois	8.1
44	Idaho	1.9		12	Arkansas	7.9
11	Illinois	8.1		13	Michigan	7.3
18	Indiana	6.1		14	Missouri	7.2
42	Iowa	2.0		15	Nevada	7.1
25	Kansas	5.3		16	Texas	6.5
26	Kentucky	5.1		17	Virginia	6.2
1	Louisiana	13.7		18	California	6.1
NA	Maine**	NA		18	Florida	6.1
4	Maryland	9.6		18	Indiana	6.1
42	Massachusetts	2.0		21	Alaska	5.9
13	Michigan	7.3		21	Oklahoma	5.9
38	Minnesota	2.9		23	New York	5.4
2	Mississippi	11.2		23	Pennsylvania	5.4
14	Missouri	7.2		25	Kansas	5.3
29	Montana	3.9		26	Kentucky	5.1
32	Nebraska	3.8		27	West Virginia	4.4
15	Nevada	7.1		28	Ohio	4.1
NA	New Hampshire**	NA		29	Montana	3.9
29	New Jersey	3.9		29	New Jersey	3.9
5	New Mexico	9.2		29	Rhode Island	3.9
23	New York	5.4		32	Nebraska	3.8
6	North Carolina	8.5		33	Colorado	3.7
NA	North Dakota**	NA		34	Washington	3.4
28	Ohio	4.1		35	Wisconsin	3.3
21	Oklahoma	5.9		36	Delaware	3.0
40	Oregon	2.7		36	Hawaii	3.0
23	Pennsylvania	5.4		38	Connecticut	2.9
29	Rhode Island	3.9		38	Minnesota	2.9
9	South Carolina	8.3		40	Oregon	2.7
NA	South Dakota**	NA		41	Utah	2.4
6	Tennessee	8.5		42	Iowa	2.0
16	Texas	6.5		42	Massachusetts	2.0
41	Utah	2.4		44	Idaho	1.9
NA	Vermont**	NA		NA	Maine**	NA
17	Virginia	6.2		NA	New Hampshire**	NA
34	Washington	3.4		NA	North Dakota**	NA
27	West Virginia	4.4		NA	South Dakota**	NA
35	Wisconsin	3.3		NA	Vermont**	NA
NA	Wyoming**	NA		NA	Wyoming**	NA
					District of Columbia	35.5

Source: U.S. Department of Health and Human Services, National Center for Health Statistics
   "National Vital Statistics Reports" (Vol. 50, No. 15, September 16, 2002)
*By state of residence. Includes legal intervention. Homicide data shown here are collected by the Centers for Disease Control and Prevention based on death certificates and differ from murder data collected by the F.B.I. from other sources. Not age-adjusted.
**Insufficient data to determine a reliable rate.

Age-Adjusted Death Rate by Homicide in 2000

National Rate = 6.1 Deaths per 100,000 Population*

RANK	STATE	RATE		RANK	STATE	RATE
	ALPHA ORDER				RANK ORDER	
3	Alabama	10.0		1	Louisiana	13.5
22	Alaska	5.9		2	Mississippi	11.1
6	Arizona	8.6		3	Alabama	10.0
12	Arkansas	7.9		4	Maryland	9.6
20	California	6.0		5	New Mexico	9.1
33	Colorado	3.6		6	Arizona	8.6
36	Connecticut	3.0		7	North Carolina	8.5
36	Delaware	3.0		7	Tennessee	8.5
16	Florida	6.4		9	Illinois	8.1
11	Georgia	8.0		9	South Carolina	8.1
38	Hawaii	2.9		11	Georgia	8.0
43	Idaho	2.0		12	Arkansas	7.9
9	Illinois	8.1		13	Missouri	7.3
18	Indiana	6.1		13	Nevada	7.3
42	Iowa	2.1		15	Michigan	7.2
25	Kansas	5.3		16	Florida	6.4
26	Kentucky	5.1		16	Texas	6.4
1	Louisiana	13.5		18	Indiana	6.1
NA	Maine**	NA		18	Virginia	6.1
4	Maryland	9.6		20	California	6.0
43	Massachusetts	2.0		20	Oklahoma	6.0
15	Michigan	7.2		22	Alaska	5.9
38	Minnesota	2.9		23	Pennsylvania	5.6
2	Mississippi	11.1		24	New York	5.5
13	Missouri	7.3		25	Kansas	5.3
29	Montana	4.0		26	Kentucky	5.1
32	Nebraska	3.8		27	West Virginia	4.5
13	Nevada	7.3		28	Ohio	4.1
NA	New Hampshire**	NA		29	Montana	4.0
29	New Jersey	4.0		29	New Jersey	4.0
5	New Mexico	9.1		29	Rhode Island	4.0
24	New York	5.5		32	Nebraska	3.8
7	North Carolina	8.5		33	Colorado	3.6
NA	North Dakota**	NA		34	Washington	3.4
28	Ohio	4.1		35	Wisconsin	3.2
20	Oklahoma	6.0		36	Connecticut	3.0
40	Oregon	2.7		36	Delaware	3.0
23	Pennsylvania	5.6		38	Hawaii	2.9
29	Rhode Island	4.0		38	Minnesota	2.9
9	South Carolina	8.1		40	Oregon	2.7
NA	South Dakota**	NA		41	Utah	2.4
7	Tennessee	8.5		42	Iowa	2.1
16	Texas	6.4		43	Idaho	2.0
41	Utah	2.4		43	Massachusetts	2.0
NA	Vermont**	NA		NA	Maine**	NA
18	Virginia	6.1		NA	New Hampshire**	NA
34	Washington	3.4		NA	North Dakota**	NA
27	West Virginia	4.5		NA	South Dakota**	NA
35	Wisconsin	3.2		NA	Vermont**	NA
NA	Wyoming**	NA		NA	Wyoming**	NA
					District of Columbia	36.2

Source: U.S. Department of Health and Human Services, National Center for Health Statistics
    "National Vital Statistics Reports" (Vol. 50, No. 15, September 16, 2002)
*By state of residence. Includes legal intervention. Homicide data shown here are collected by the Centers for Disease Control and Prevention based on death certificates and differ from murder data collected by the F.B.I. from other sources. Age-adjusted rates based on the year 2000 standard population.
**Insufficient data to determine a reliable rate.

Deaths by Suicide in 2000

National Total = 29,350 Suicides*

ALPHA ORDER

RANK	STATE	SUICIDES	% of USA
19	Alabama	583	2.0%
42	Alaska	137	0.5%
11	Arizona	784	2.7%
30	Arkansas	349	1.2%
1	California	2,969	10.1%
17	Colorado	613	2.1%
33	Connecticut	304	1.0%
47	Delaware	82	0.3%
2	Florida	2,086	7.1%
10	Georgia	847	2.9%
42	Hawaii	137	0.5%
39	Idaho	167	0.6%
7	Illinois	1,003	3.4%
16	Indiana	683	2.3%
36	Iowa	289	1.0%
32	Kansas	325	1.1%
21	Kentucky	521	1.8%
25	Louisiana	468	1.6%
41	Maine	154	0.5%
24	Maryland	474	1.6%
29	Massachusetts	387	1.3%
8	Michigan	974	3.3%
27	Minnesota	440	1.5%
35	Mississippi	294	1.0%
15	Missouri	699	2.4%
40	Montana	158	0.5%
38	Nebraska	193	0.7%
28	Nevada	400	1.4%
44	New Hampshire	131	0.4%
20	New Jersey	560	1.9%
31	New Mexico	327	1.1%
5	New York	1,132	3.9%
9	North Carolina	971	3.3%
50	North Dakota	68	0.2%
6	Ohio	1,088	3.7%
22	Oklahoma	497	1.7%
23	Oregon	493	1.7%
4	Pennsylvania	1,356	4.6%
49	Rhode Island	75	0.3%
26	South Carolina	443	1.5%
45	South Dakota	95	0.3%
13	Tennessee	730	2.5%
3	Texas	2,053	7.0%
34	Utah	298	1.0%
48	Vermont	77	0.3%
12	Virginia	768	2.6%
14	Washington	727	2.5%
37	West Virginia	245	0.8%
18	Wisconsin	590	2.0%
46	Wyoming	83	0.3%

RANK ORDER

RANK	STATE	SUICIDES	% of USA
1	California	2,969	10.1%
2	Florida	2,086	7.1%
3	Texas	2,053	7.0%
4	Pennsylvania	1,356	4.6%
5	New York	1,132	3.9%
6	Ohio	1,088	3.7%
7	Illinois	1,003	3.4%
8	Michigan	974	3.3%
9	North Carolina	971	3.3%
10	Georgia	847	2.9%
11	Arizona	784	2.7%
12	Virginia	768	2.6%
13	Tennessee	730	2.5%
14	Washington	727	2.5%
15	Missouri	699	2.4%
16	Indiana	683	2.3%
17	Colorado	613	2.1%
18	Wisconsin	590	2.0%
19	Alabama	583	2.0%
20	New Jersey	560	1.9%
21	Kentucky	521	1.8%
22	Oklahoma	497	1.7%
23	Oregon	493	1.7%
24	Maryland	474	1.6%
25	Louisiana	468	1.6%
26	South Carolina	443	1.5%
27	Minnesota	440	1.5%
28	Nevada	400	1.4%
29	Massachusetts	387	1.3%
30	Arkansas	349	1.2%
31	New Mexico	327	1.1%
32	Kansas	325	1.1%
33	Connecticut	304	1.0%
34	Utah	298	1.0%
35	Mississippi	294	1.0%
36	Iowa	289	1.0%
37	West Virginia	245	0.8%
38	Nebraska	193	0.7%
39	Idaho	167	0.6%
40	Montana	158	0.5%
41	Maine	154	0.5%
42	Alaska	137	0.5%
42	Hawaii	137	0.5%
44	New Hampshire	131	0.4%
45	South Dakota	95	0.3%
46	Wyoming	83	0.3%
47	Delaware	82	0.3%
48	Vermont	77	0.3%
49	Rhode Island	75	0.3%
50	North Dakota	68	0.2%
	District of Columbia	23	0.1%

*Source: U.S. Department of Health and Human Services, National Center for Health Statistics
"National Vital Statistics Reports" (Vol. 50, No. 15, September 16, 2002)
Final data by state of residence.

Death Rate by Suicide in 2000

National Rate = 10.7 Suicides per 100,000 Population*

ALPHA ORDER

RANK	STATE	RATE
14	Alabama	13.3
1	Alaska	22.0
6	Arizona	16.1
13	Arkansas	13.5
45	California	8.8
7	Colorado	14.8
42	Connecticut	9.2
32	Delaware	10.8
11	Florida	13.6
35	Georgia	10.7
25	Hawaii	11.6
16	Idaho	13.1
46	Illinois	8.2
27	Indiana	11.4
39	Iowa	10.0
23	Kansas	12.2
16	Kentucky	13.1
35	Louisiana	10.7
23	Maine	12.2
43	Maryland	9.1
49	Massachusetts	6.2
40	Michigan	9.8
43	Minnesota	9.1
37	Mississippi	10.5
20	Missouri	12.7
4	Montana	17.8
25	Nebraska	11.6
2	Nevada	21.3
32	New Hampshire	10.8
48	New Jersey	6.8
3	New Mexico	18.7
49	New York	6.2
21	North Carolina	12.5
32	North Dakota	10.8
41	Ohio	9.7
9	Oklahoma	14.7
7	Oregon	14.8
28	Pennsylvania	11.3
47	Rhode Island	7.5
28	South Carolina	11.3
18	South Dakota	12.9
15	Tennessee	13.2
38	Texas	10.1
10	Utah	13.8
18	Vermont	12.9
31	Virginia	11.0
21	Washington	12.5
11	West Virginia	13.6
30	Wisconsin	11.1
5	Wyoming	17.3

RANK ORDER

RANK	STATE	RATE
1	Alaska	22.0
2	Nevada	21.3
3	New Mexico	18.7
4	Montana	17.8
5	Wyoming	17.3
6	Arizona	16.1
7	Colorado	14.8
7	Oregon	14.8
9	Oklahoma	14.7
10	Utah	13.8
11	Florida	13.6
11	West Virginia	13.6
13	Arkansas	13.5
14	Alabama	13.3
15	Tennessee	13.2
16	Idaho	13.1
16	Kentucky	13.1
18	South Dakota	12.9
18	Vermont	12.9
20	Missouri	12.7
21	North Carolina	12.5
21	Washington	12.5
23	Kansas	12.2
23	Maine	12.2
25	Hawaii	11.6
25	Nebraska	11.6
27	Indiana	11.4
28	Pennsylvania	11.3
28	South Carolina	11.3
30	Wisconsin	11.1
31	Virginia	11.0
32	Delaware	10.8
32	New Hampshire	10.8
32	North Dakota	10.8
35	Georgia	10.7
35	Louisiana	10.7
37	Mississippi	10.5
38	Texas	10.1
39	Iowa	10.0
40	Michigan	9.8
41	Ohio	9.7
42	Connecticut	9.2
43	Maryland	9.1
43	Minnesota	9.1
45	California	8.8
46	Illinois	8.2
47	Rhode Island	7.5
48	New Jersey	6.8
49	Massachusetts	6.2
49	New York	6.2
	District of Columbia	4.4

Source: U.S. Department of Health and Human Services, National Center for Health Statistics
    "National Vital Statistics Reports" (Vol. 50, No. 15, September 16, 2002)
*Final data by state of residence. Not age-adjusted.

Age-Adjusted Death Rate by Suicide in 2000

National Rate = 10.6 Deaths per 100,000 Population*

ALPHA ORDER

RANK	STATE	RATE
14	Alabama	13.1
2	Alaska	21.4
6	Arizona	16.6
11	Arkansas	13.5
42	California	9.1
8	Colorado	15.0
45	Connecticut	9.0
35	Delaware	10.6
16	Florida	13.0
30	Georgia	11.0
25	Hawaii	11.6
11	Idaho	13.5
46	Illinois	8.3
27	Indiana	11.4
39	Iowa	10.0
23	Kansas	12.3
18	Kentucky	12.9
32	Louisiana	10.9
24	Maine	11.8
42	Maryland	9.1
49	Massachusetts	6.1
40	Michigan	9.8
42	Minnesota	9.1
34	Mississippi	10.7
19	Missouri	12.6
4	Montana	17.9
26	Nebraska	11.5
1	Nevada	21.7
37	New Hampshire	10.5
48	New Jersey	6.7
3	New Mexico	19.1
49	New York	6.1
19	North Carolina	12.6
35	North Dakota	10.6
41	Ohio	9.5
9	Oklahoma	14.9
10	Oregon	14.4
30	Pennsylvania	11.0
47	Rhode Island	7.5
28	South Carolina	11.2
16	South Dakota	13.0
14	Tennessee	13.1
38	Texas	10.4
7	Utah	15.4
22	Vermont	12.4
32	Virginia	10.9
21	Washington	12.5
13	West Virginia	13.2
29	Wisconsin	11.1
5	Wyoming	17.4

RANK ORDER

RANK	STATE	RATE
1	Nevada	21.7
2	Alaska	21.4
3	New Mexico	19.1
4	Montana	17.9
5	Wyoming	17.4
6	Arizona	16.6
7	Utah	15.4
8	Colorado	15.0
9	Oklahoma	14.9
10	Oregon	14.4
11	Arkansas	13.5
11	Idaho	13.5
13	West Virginia	13.2
14	Alabama	13.1
14	Tennessee	13.1
16	Florida	13.0
16	South Dakota	13.0
18	Kentucky	12.9
19	Missouri	12.6
19	North Carolina	12.6
21	Washington	12.5
22	Vermont	12.4
23	Kansas	12.3
24	Maine	11.8
25	Hawaii	11.6
26	Nebraska	11.5
27	Indiana	11.4
28	South Carolina	11.2
29	Wisconsin	11.1
30	Georgia	11.0
30	Pennsylvania	11.0
32	Louisiana	10.9
32	Virginia	10.9
34	Mississippi	10.7
35	Delaware	10.6
35	North Dakota	10.6
37	New Hampshire	10.5
38	Texas	10.4
39	Iowa	10.0
40	Michigan	9.8
41	Ohio	9.5
42	California	9.1
42	Maryland	9.1
42	Minnesota	9.1
45	Connecticut	9.0
46	Illinois	8.3
47	Rhode Island	7.5
48	New Jersey	6.7
49	Massachusetts	6.1
49	New York	6.1
	District of Columbia	4.4

Source: U.S. Department of Health and Human Services, National Center for Health Statistics
    "National Vital Statistics Reports" (Vol. 50, No. 15, September 16, 2002)
*Final data by state of residence. Age-adjusted rates based on the year 2000 standard population.

Years Lost by Premature Death in 1999

National Average = 7,734 Years Lost per 100,000 Population*

ALPHA ORDER

RANK	STATE	YEARS
3	Alabama	10,128
26	Alaska	7,690
17	Arizona	8,216
5	Arkansas	9,524
39	California	6,618
37	Colorado	6,686
42	Connecticut	6,525
21	Delaware	7,867
16	Florida	8,391
8	Georgia	9,028
47	Hawaii	6,215
34	Idaho	6,825
19	Illinois	8,011
18	Indiana	8,036
46	Iowa	6,343
30	Kansas	7,306
12	Kentucky	8,582
2	Louisiana	10,228
40	Maine	6,588
15	Maryland	8,397
49	Massachusetts	6,148
20	Michigan	8,010
50	Minnesota	5,985
1	Mississippi	11,083
14	Missouri	8,420
29	Montana	7,393
33	Nebraska	6,854
9	Nevada	8,970
48	New Hampshire	6,204
32	New Jersey	7,166
13	New Mexico	8,505
31	New York	7,223
10	North Carolina	8,844
41	North Dakota	6,562
24	Ohio	7,781
7	Oklahoma	9,181
35	Oregon	6,798
23	Pennsylvania	7,784
36	Rhode Island	6,750
4	South Carolina	9,915
25	South Dakota	7,777
6	Tennessee	9,346
27	Texas	7,669
43	Utah	6,503
44	Vermont	6,443
28	Virginia	7,417
45	Washington	6,401
11	West Virginia	8,750
38	Wisconsin	6,623
22	Wyoming	7,844

RANK ORDER

RANK	STATE	YEARS
1	Mississippi	11,083
2	Louisiana	10,228
3	Alabama	10,128
4	South Carolina	9,915
5	Arkansas	9,524
6	Tennessee	9,346
7	Oklahoma	9,181
8	Georgia	9,028
9	Nevada	8,970
10	North Carolina	8,844
11	West Virginia	8,750
12	Kentucky	8,582
13	New Mexico	8,505
14	Missouri	8,420
15	Maryland	8,397
16	Florida	8,391
17	Arizona	8,216
18	Indiana	8,036
19	Illinois	8,011
20	Michigan	8,010
21	Delaware	7,867
22	Wyoming	7,844
23	Pennsylvania	7,784
24	Ohio	7,781
25	South Dakota	7,777
26	Alaska	7,690
27	Texas	7,669
28	Virginia	7,417
29	Montana	7,393
30	Kansas	7,306
31	New York	7,223
32	New Jersey	7,166
33	Nebraska	6,854
34	Idaho	6,825
35	Oregon	6,798
36	Rhode Island	6,750
37	Colorado	6,686
38	Wisconsin	6,623
39	California	6,618
40	Maine	6,588
41	North Dakota	6,562
42	Connecticut	6,525
43	Utah	6,503
44	Vermont	6,443
45	Washington	6,401
46	Iowa	6,343
47	Hawaii	6,215
48	New Hampshire	6,204
49	Massachusetts	6,148
50	Minnesota	5,985
	District of Columbia	14,645

Source: U.S. Department of Health and Human Services, National Center for Health Statistics
   unpublished data
*Age-adjusted years of potential life lost due to death before age 75.

Years Lost by Premature Death from Cancer in 1999

National Average = 1,724 Years Lost per 100,000 Population*

<table>
<tr><td colspan="3">ALPHA ORDER</td><td colspan="3">RANK ORDER</td></tr>
<tr><td>RANK</td><td>STATE</td><td>YEARS</td><td>RANK</td><td>STATE</td><td>YEARS</td></tr>
<tr><td>8</td><td>Alabama</td><td>1,892</td><td>1</td><td>Mississippi</td><td>2,144</td></tr>
<tr><td>47</td><td>Alaska</td><td>1,411</td><td>2</td><td>Louisiana</td><td>2,041</td></tr>
<tr><td>35</td><td>Arizona</td><td>1,606</td><td>3</td><td>West Virginia</td><td>2,002</td></tr>
<tr><td>7</td><td>Arkansas</td><td>1,965</td><td>4</td><td>South Carolina</td><td>1,994</td></tr>
<tr><td>42</td><td>California</td><td>1,546</td><td>5</td><td>Kentucky</td><td>1,969</td></tr>
<tr><td>50</td><td>Colorado</td><td>1,308</td><td>6</td><td>Tennessee</td><td>1,966</td></tr>
<tr><td>36</td><td>Connecticut</td><td>1,605</td><td>7</td><td>Arkansas</td><td>1,965</td></tr>
<tr><td>9</td><td>Delaware</td><td>1,886</td><td>8</td><td>Alabama</td><td>1,892</td></tr>
<tr><td>18</td><td>Florida</td><td>1,797</td><td>9</td><td>Delaware</td><td>1,886</td></tr>
<tr><td>17</td><td>Georgia</td><td>1,801</td><td>10</td><td>North Carolina</td><td>1,868</td></tr>
<tr><td>48</td><td>Hawaii</td><td>1,399</td><td>11</td><td>Rhode Island</td><td>1,853</td></tr>
<tr><td>43</td><td>Idaho</td><td>1,530</td><td>12</td><td>Ohio</td><td>1,847</td></tr>
<tr><td>25</td><td>Illinois</td><td>1,743</td><td>13</td><td>Maine</td><td>1,840</td></tr>
<tr><td>15</td><td>Indiana</td><td>1,821</td><td>14</td><td>Missouri</td><td>1,826</td></tr>
<tr><td>41</td><td>Iowa</td><td>1,550</td><td>15</td><td>Indiana</td><td>1,821</td></tr>
<tr><td>31</td><td>Kansas</td><td>1,657</td><td>16</td><td>Pennsylvania</td><td>1,817</td></tr>
<tr><td>5</td><td>Kentucky</td><td>1,969</td><td>17</td><td>Georgia</td><td>1,801</td></tr>
<tr><td>2</td><td>Louisiana</td><td>2,041</td><td>18</td><td>Florida</td><td>1,797</td></tr>
<tr><td>13</td><td>Maine</td><td>1,840</td><td>19</td><td>Oklahoma</td><td>1,793</td></tr>
<tr><td>21</td><td>Maryland</td><td>1,774</td><td>20</td><td>Virginia</td><td>1,789</td></tr>
<tr><td>30</td><td>Massachusetts</td><td>1,673</td><td>21</td><td>Maryland</td><td>1,774</td></tr>
<tr><td>26</td><td>Michigan</td><td>1,738</td><td>22</td><td>Vermont</td><td>1,757</td></tr>
<tr><td>40</td><td>Minnesota</td><td>1,553</td><td>23</td><td>New Hampshire</td><td>1,748</td></tr>
<tr><td>1</td><td>Mississippi</td><td>2,144</td><td>23</td><td>New Jersey</td><td>1,748</td></tr>
<tr><td>14</td><td>Missouri</td><td>1,826</td><td>25</td><td>Illinois</td><td>1,743</td></tr>
<tr><td>44</td><td>Montana</td><td>1,500</td><td>26</td><td>Michigan</td><td>1,738</td></tr>
<tr><td>38</td><td>Nebraska</td><td>1,577</td><td>27</td><td>Nevada</td><td>1,737</td></tr>
<tr><td>27</td><td>Nevada</td><td>1,737</td><td>28</td><td>New York</td><td>1,714</td></tr>
<tr><td>23</td><td>New Hampshire</td><td>1,748</td><td>29</td><td>South Dakota</td><td>1,702</td></tr>
<tr><td>23</td><td>New Jersey</td><td>1,748</td><td>30</td><td>Massachusetts</td><td>1,673</td></tr>
<tr><td>45</td><td>New Mexico</td><td>1,432</td><td>31</td><td>Kansas</td><td>1,657</td></tr>
<tr><td>28</td><td>New York</td><td>1,714</td><td>32</td><td>Texas</td><td>1,649</td></tr>
<tr><td>10</td><td>North Carolina</td><td>1,868</td><td>33</td><td>Wyoming</td><td>1,644</td></tr>
<tr><td>46</td><td>North Dakota</td><td>1,412</td><td>34</td><td>Wisconsin</td><td>1,621</td></tr>
<tr><td>12</td><td>Ohio</td><td>1,847</td><td>35</td><td>Arizona</td><td>1,606</td></tr>
<tr><td>19</td><td>Oklahoma</td><td>1,793</td><td>36</td><td>Connecticut</td><td>1,605</td></tr>
<tr><td>37</td><td>Oregon</td><td>1,580</td><td>37</td><td>Oregon</td><td>1,580</td></tr>
<tr><td>16</td><td>Pennsylvania</td><td>1,817</td><td>38</td><td>Nebraska</td><td>1,577</td></tr>
<tr><td>11</td><td>Rhode Island</td><td>1,853</td><td>39</td><td>Washington</td><td>1,570</td></tr>
<tr><td>4</td><td>South Carolina</td><td>1,994</td><td>40</td><td>Minnesota</td><td>1,553</td></tr>
<tr><td>29</td><td>South Dakota</td><td>1,702</td><td>41</td><td>Iowa</td><td>1,550</td></tr>
<tr><td>6</td><td>Tennessee</td><td>1,966</td><td>42</td><td>California</td><td>1,546</td></tr>
<tr><td>32</td><td>Texas</td><td>1,649</td><td>43</td><td>Idaho</td><td>1,530</td></tr>
<tr><td>49</td><td>Utah</td><td>1,325</td><td>44</td><td>Montana</td><td>1,500</td></tr>
<tr><td>22</td><td>Vermont</td><td>1,757</td><td>45</td><td>New Mexico</td><td>1,432</td></tr>
<tr><td>20</td><td>Virginia</td><td>1,789</td><td>46</td><td>North Dakota</td><td>1,412</td></tr>
<tr><td>39</td><td>Washington</td><td>1,570</td><td>47</td><td>Alaska</td><td>1,411</td></tr>
<tr><td>3</td><td>West Virginia</td><td>2,002</td><td>48</td><td>Hawaii</td><td>1,399</td></tr>
<tr><td>34</td><td>Wisconsin</td><td>1,621</td><td>49</td><td>Utah</td><td>1,325</td></tr>
<tr><td>33</td><td>Wyoming</td><td>1,644</td><td>50</td><td>Colorado</td><td>1,308</td></tr>
<tr><td></td><td></td><td></td><td></td><td>District of Columbia</td><td>2,123</td></tr>
</table>

Source: U.S. Department of Health and Human Services, National Center for Health Statistics
   unpublished data
*Age-adjusted years of potential life lost due to death before age 75.

Years Lost by Premature Death from Heart Disease in 1999

National Average = 1,317 Years Lost per 100,000 Population*

ALPHA ORDER

RANK	STATE	YEARS
2	Alabama	1,848
45	Alaska	961
27	Arizona	1,171
8	Arkansas	1,686
35	California	1,092
49	Colorado	859
33	Connecticut	1,105
19	Delaware	1,369
23	Florida	1,293
10	Georgia	1,614
25	Hawaii	1,185
40	Idaho	1,002
16	Illinois	1,450
14	Indiana	1,461
32	Iowa	1,114
36	Kansas	1,077
9	Kentucky	1,629
3	Louisiana	1,776
37	Maine	1,065
20	Maryland	1,347
39	Massachusetts	1,055
13	Michigan	1,486
48	Minnesota	886
1	Mississippi	2,173
12	Missouri	1,536
41	Montana	999
31	Nebraska	1,121
11	Nevada	1,581
38	New Hampshire	1,059
28	New Jersey	1,152
46	New Mexico	960
24	New York	1,279
15	North Carolina	1,457
26	North Dakota	1,184
17	Ohio	1,425
6	Oklahoma	1,703
42	Oregon	998
18	Pennsylvania	1,380
29	Rhode Island	1,128
4	South Carolina	1,721
29	South Dakota	1,128
5	Tennessee	1,720
21	Texas	1,330
50	Utah	759
43	Vermont	997
22	Virginia	1,301
44	Washington	965
7	West Virginia	1,692
34	Wisconsin	1,102
47	Wyoming	929

RANK ORDER

RANK	STATE	YEARS
1	Mississippi	2,173
2	Alabama	1,848
3	Louisiana	1,776
4	South Carolina	1,721
5	Tennessee	1,720
6	Oklahoma	1,703
7	West Virginia	1,692
8	Arkansas	1,686
9	Kentucky	1,629
10	Georgia	1,614
11	Nevada	1,581
12	Missouri	1,536
13	Michigan	1,486
14	Indiana	1,461
15	North Carolina	1,457
16	Illinois	1,450
17	Ohio	1,425
18	Pennsylvania	1,380
19	Delaware	1,369
20	Maryland	1,347
21	Texas	1,330
22	Virginia	1,301
23	Florida	1,293
24	New York	1,279
25	Hawaii	1,185
26	North Dakota	1,184
27	Arizona	1,171
28	New Jersey	1,152
29	Rhode Island	1,128
29	South Dakota	1,128
31	Nebraska	1,121
32	Iowa	1,114
33	Connecticut	1,105
34	Wisconsin	1,102
35	California	1,092
36	Kansas	1,077
37	Maine	1,065
38	New Hampshire	1,059
39	Massachusetts	1,055
40	Idaho	1,002
41	Montana	999
42	Oregon	998
43	Vermont	997
44	Washington	965
45	Alaska	961
46	New Mexico	960
47	Wyoming	929
48	Minnesota	886
49	Colorado	859
50	Utah	759
	District of Columbia	1,823

Source: U.S. Department of Health and Human Services, National Center for Health Statistics
unpublished data
*Age-adjusted years of potential life lost due to death before age 75.

Years Lost by Premature Death from Homicide in 1999

National Average = 279 Years Lost per 100,000 Population*

ALPHA ORDER				RANK ORDER		
RANK	STATE	YEARS		RANK	STATE	YEARS
6	Alabama	421		1	Maryland	508
10	Alaska	356		2	Louisiana	486
4	Arizona	438		3	Mississippi	485
16	Arkansas	308		4	Arizona	438
21	California	276		5	New Mexico	431
25	Colorado	230		6	Alabama	421
32	Connecticut	169		7	Illinois	405
39	Delaware	134		8	Nevada	397
18	Florida	300		9	North Carolina	373
12	Georgia	351		10	Alaska	356
42	Hawaii	109		11	South Carolina	353
41	Idaho	115		12	Georgia	351
7	Illinois	405		13	Michigan	346
17	Indiana	304		14	Tennessee	337
46	Iowa	76		15	Missouri	331
26	Kansas	226		16	Arkansas	308
28	Kentucky	218		17	Indiana	304
2	Louisiana	486		18	Florida	300
45	Maine	91		19	Oklahoma	291
1	Maryland	508		20	Texas	283
43	Massachusetts	105		21	California	276
13	Michigan	346		22	Pennsylvania	265
40	Minnesota	128		23	Virginia	258
3	Mississippi	485		24	New York	246
15	Missouri	331		25	Colorado	230
35	Montana	162		26	Kansas	226
34	Nebraska	164		27	West Virginia	223
8	Nevada	397		28	Kentucky	218
NA	New Hampshire**	NA		29	Wisconsin	193
33	New Jersey	168		30	Rhode Island	180
5	New Mexico	431		31	Ohio	173
24	New York	246		32	Connecticut	169
9	North Carolina	373		33	New Jersey	168
NA	North Dakota**	NA		34	Nebraska	164
31	Ohio	173		35	Montana	162
19	Oklahoma	291		36	South Dakota	155
37	Oregon	153		37	Oregon	153
22	Pennsylvania	265		38	Washington	148
30	Rhode Island	180		39	Delaware	134
11	South Carolina	353		40	Minnesota	128
36	South Dakota	155		41	Idaho	115
14	Tennessee	337		42	Hawaii	109
20	Texas	283		43	Massachusetts	105
44	Utah	98		44	Utah	98
NA	Vermont**	NA		45	Maine	91
23	Virginia	258		46	Iowa	76
38	Washington	148		NA	New Hampshire**	NA
27	West Virginia	223		NA	North Dakota**	NA
29	Wisconsin	193		NA	Vermont**	NA
NA	Wyoming**	NA		NA	Wyoming**	NA
					District of Columbia	1,875

Source: U.S. Department of Health and Human Services, National Center for Health Statistics
unpublished data

*Age-adjusted years of potential life lost due to death before age 75.

**Data for states with fewer than 20 deaths from homicide for persons under 75 years of age are considered unreliable and are not shown.

179

Years Lost by Premature Death from Suicide in 1999

National Average = 343 Years Lost per 100,000 Population*

ALPHA ORDER

RANK	STATE	YEARS
19	Alabama	401
4	Alaska	584
8	Arizona	501
12	Arkansas	448
44	California	277
10	Colorado	467
47	Connecticut	255
20	Delaware	400
23	Florida	394
33	Georgia	353
18	Hawaii	404
11	Idaho	455
45	Illinois	275
31	Indiana	357
34	Iowa	351
21	Kansas	399
30	Kentucky	376
24	Louisiana	393
16	Maine	426
46	Maryland	271
48	Massachusetts	231
38	Michigan	334
41	Minnesota	315
37	Mississippi	338
16	Missouri	426
5	Montana	551
27	Nebraska	391
2	Nevada	660
26	New Hampshire	392
49	New Jersey	215
3	New Mexico	642
50	New York	209
28	North Carolina	388
24	North Dakota	393
42	Ohio	310
6	Oklahoma	527
14	Oregon	433
32	Pennsylvania	354
39	Rhode Island	330
36	South Carolina	350
7	South Dakota	513
15	Tennessee	427
39	Texas	330
9	Utah	494
43	Vermont	301
34	Virginia	351
13	Washington	445
22	West Virginia	395
29	Wisconsin	378
1	Wyoming	662

RANK ORDER

RANK	STATE	YEARS
1	Wyoming	662
2	Nevada	660
3	New Mexico	642
4	Alaska	584
5	Montana	551
6	Oklahoma	527
7	South Dakota	513
8	Arizona	501
9	Utah	494
10	Colorado	467
11	Idaho	455
12	Arkansas	448
13	Washington	445
14	Oregon	433
15	Tennessee	427
16	Maine	426
16	Missouri	426
18	Hawaii	404
19	Alabama	401
20	Delaware	400
21	Kansas	399
22	West Virginia	395
23	Florida	394
24	Louisiana	393
24	North Dakota	393
26	New Hampshire	392
27	Nebraska	391
28	North Carolina	388
29	Wisconsin	378
30	Kentucky	376
31	Indiana	357
32	Pennsylvania	354
33	Georgia	353
34	Iowa	351
34	Virginia	351
36	South Carolina	350
37	Mississippi	338
38	Michigan	334
39	Rhode Island	330
39	Texas	330
41	Minnesota	315
42	Ohio	310
43	Vermont	301
44	California	277
45	Illinois	275
46	Maryland	271
47	Connecticut	255
48	Massachusetts	231
49	New Jersey	215
50	New York	209
	District of Columbia	186

Source: U.S. Department of Health and Human Services, National Center for Health Statistics
    unpublished data
*Age-adjusted years of potential life lost due to death before age 75.

Years Lost by Premature Death from Unintentional Injuries in 1999

National Average = 1,048 Years Lost per 100,000 Population*

ALPHA ORDER

RANK	STATE	YEARS
4	Alabama	1,651
3	Alaska	1,683
12	Arizona	1,435
6	Arkansas	1,577
41	California	864
26	Colorado	1,071
42	Connecticut	849
34	Delaware	969
19	Florida	1,236
21	Georgia	1,189
48	Hawaii	666
14	Idaho	1,385
30	Illinois	1,000
25	Indiana	1,124
31	Iowa	990
23	Kansas	1,162
15	Kentucky	1,295
10	Louisiana	1,459
29	Maine	1,003
45	Maryland	719
50	Massachusetts	471
37	Michigan	953
43	Minnesota	828
1	Mississippi	1,912
20	Missouri	1,228
7	Montana	1,554
27	Nebraska	1,053
16	Nevada	1,284
44	New Hampshire	729
46	New Jersey	718
2	New Mexico	1,812
47	New York	713
18	North Carolina	1,255
22	North Dakota	1,184
39	Ohio	887
13	Oklahoma	1,412
33	Oregon	980
28	Pennsylvania	1,041
49	Rhode Island	530
8	South Carolina	1,500
11	South Dakota	1,446
9	Tennessee	1,490
24	Texas	1,150
35	Utah	968
36	Vermont	960
40	Virginia	865
32	Washington	989
17	West Virginia	1,280
38	Wisconsin	949
5	Wyoming	1,644

RANK ORDER

RANK	STATE	YEARS
1	Mississippi	1,912
2	New Mexico	1,812
3	Alaska	1,683
4	Alabama	1,651
5	Wyoming	1,644
6	Arkansas	1,577
7	Montana	1,554
8	South Carolina	1,500
9	Tennessee	1,490
10	Louisiana	1,459
11	South Dakota	1,446
12	Arizona	1,435
13	Oklahoma	1,412
14	Idaho	1,385
15	Kentucky	1,295
16	Nevada	1,284
17	West Virginia	1,280
18	North Carolina	1,255
19	Florida	1,236
20	Missouri	1,228
21	Georgia	1,189
22	North Dakota	1,184
23	Kansas	1,162
24	Texas	1,150
25	Indiana	1,124
26	Colorado	1,071
27	Nebraska	1,053
28	Pennsylvania	1,041
29	Maine	1,003
30	Illinois	1,000
31	Iowa	990
32	Washington	989
33	Oregon	980
34	Delaware	969
35	Utah	968
36	Vermont	960
37	Michigan	953
38	Wisconsin	949
39	Ohio	887
40	Virginia	865
41	California	864
42	Connecticut	849
43	Minnesota	828
44	New Hampshire	729
45	Maryland	719
46	New Jersey	718
47	New York	713
48	Hawaii	666
49	Rhode Island	530
50	Massachusetts	471
	District of Columbia	729

Source: U.S. Department of Health and Human Services, National Center for Health Statistics
   unpublished data

*Age-adjusted years of potential life lost due to death before age 75. Includes such subcategories as falls, drowning, fires/burns, poisonings and motor vehicle injuries.

Alcohol-Induced Deaths in 1999

National Total = 19,171 Deaths*

ALPHA ORDER

RANK	STATE	DEATHS	% of USA
28	Alabama	242	1.3%
39	Alaska	93	0.5%
10	Arizona	466	2.4%
36	Arkansas	118	0.6%
1	California	3,245	16.9%
12	Colorado	462	2.4%
31	Connecticut	174	0.9%
46	Delaware	59	0.3%
2	Florida	1,266	6.6%
11	Georgia	463	2.4%
49	Hawaii	37	0.2%
44	Idaho	74	0.4%
6	Illinois	636	3.3%
24	Indiana	301	1.6%
32	Iowa	150	0.8%
34	Kansas	130	0.7%
30	Kentucky	230	1.2%
26	Louisiana	291	1.5%
38	Maine	105	0.5%
21	Maryland	314	1.6%
18	Massachusetts	351	1.8%
7	Michigan	614	3.2%
23	Minnesota	302	1.6%
32	Mississippi	150	0.8%
16	Missouri	392	2.0%
43	Montana	75	0.4%
40	Nebraska	90	0.5%
27	Nevada	250	1.3%
41	New Hampshire	89	0.5%
13	New Jersey	456	2.4%
25	New Mexico	292	1.5%
3	New York	1,220	6.4%
5	North Carolina	670	3.5%
48	North Dakota	51	0.3%
9	Ohio	548	2.9%
29	Oklahoma	240	1.3%
22	Oregon	305	1.6%
14	Pennsylvania	450	2.3%
45	Rhode Island	69	0.4%
15	South Carolina	419	2.2%
42	South Dakota	80	0.4%
17	Tennessee	391	2.0%
4	Texas	1,163	6.1%
35	Utah	127	0.7%
50	Vermont	36	0.2%
20	Virginia	329	1.7%
8	Washington	557	2.9%
37	West Virginia	116	0.6%
19	Wisconsin	349	1.8%
47	Wyoming	57	0.3%

RANK ORDER

RANK	STATE	DEATHS	% of USA
1	California	3,245	16.9%
2	Florida	1,266	6.6%
3	New York	1,220	6.4%
4	Texas	1,163	6.1%
5	North Carolina	670	3.5%
6	Illinois	636	3.3%
7	Michigan	614	3.2%
8	Washington	557	2.9%
9	Ohio	548	2.9%
10	Arizona	466	2.4%
11	Georgia	463	2.4%
12	Colorado	462	2.4%
13	New Jersey	456	2.4%
14	Pennsylvania	450	2.3%
15	South Carolina	419	2.2%
16	Missouri	392	2.0%
17	Tennessee	391	2.0%
18	Massachusetts	351	1.8%
19	Wisconsin	349	1.8%
20	Virginia	329	1.7%
21	Maryland	314	1.6%
22	Oregon	305	1.6%
23	Minnesota	302	1.6%
24	Indiana	301	1.6%
25	New Mexico	292	1.5%
26	Louisiana	291	1.5%
27	Nevada	250	1.3%
28	Alabama	242	1.3%
29	Oklahoma	240	1.3%
30	Kentucky	230	1.2%
31	Connecticut	174	0.9%
32	Iowa	150	0.8%
32	Mississippi	150	0.8%
34	Kansas	130	0.7%
35	Utah	127	0.7%
36	Arkansas	118	0.6%
37	West Virginia	116	0.6%
38	Maine	105	0.5%
39	Alaska	93	0.5%
40	Nebraska	90	0.5%
41	New Hampshire	89	0.5%
42	South Dakota	80	0.4%
43	Montana	75	0.4%
44	Idaho	74	0.4%
45	Rhode Island	69	0.4%
46	Delaware	59	0.3%
47	Wyoming	57	0.3%
48	North Dakota	51	0.3%
49	Hawaii	37	0.2%
50	Vermont	36	0.2%
	District of Columbia	77	0.4%

Source: U.S. Department of Health and Human Services, National Center for Health Statistics
    (http://wonder.cdc.gov/WONDER/)
*By state of residence. Includes excessive blood level of alcohol, accidental poisoning by alcohol and the following alcohol-related causes: psychoses, dependence syndrome, polyneuropathy, cardiomyopathy, gastritis, chronic liver disease and cirrhosis. Excludes accidents, homicides and other causes indirectly related to alcohol use.

Death Rate by Alcohol-Induced Deaths in 1999

National Rate = 7.0 Deaths per 100,000 Population*

ALPHA ORDER

RANK	STATE	RATE
38	Alabama	5.5
2	Alaska	15.0
8	Arizona	9.8
48	Arkansas	4.6
8	California	9.8
5	Colorado	11.4
41	Connecticut	5.3
17	Delaware	7.8
14	Florida	8.4
32	Georgia	5.9
50	Hawaii	3.1
32	Idaho	5.9
42	Illinois	5.2
44	Indiana	5.1
42	Iowa	5.2
45	Kansas	4.9
34	Kentucky	5.8
23	Louisiana	6.7
14	Maine	8.4
29	Maryland	6.1
36	Massachusetts	5.7
28	Michigan	6.2
27	Minnesota	6.3
39	Mississippi	5.4
19	Missouri	7.2
13	Montana	8.5
39	Nebraska	5.4
3	Nevada	13.8
18	New Hampshire	7.4
37	New Jersey	5.6
1	New Mexico	16.8
23	New York	6.7
12	North Carolina	8.8
16	North Dakota	8.0
45	Ohio	4.9
20	Oklahoma	7.1
11	Oregon	9.2
49	Pennsylvania	3.8
22	Rhode Island	7.0
7	South Carolina	10.8
6	South Dakota	10.9
20	Tennessee	7.1
34	Texas	5.8
31	Utah	6.0
29	Vermont	6.1
47	Virginia	4.8
10	Washington	9.7
26	West Virginia	6.4
25	Wisconsin	6.6
4	Wyoming	11.9

RANK ORDER

RANK	STATE	RATE
1	New Mexico	16.8
2	Alaska	15.0
3	Nevada	13.8
4	Wyoming	11.9
5	Colorado	11.4
6	South Dakota	10.9
7	South Carolina	10.8
8	Arizona	9.8
8	California	9.8
10	Washington	9.7
11	Oregon	9.2
12	North Carolina	8.8
13	Montana	8.5
14	Florida	8.4
14	Maine	8.4
16	North Dakota	8.0
17	Delaware	7.8
18	New Hampshire	7.4
19	Missouri	7.2
20	Oklahoma	7.1
20	Tennessee	7.1
22	Rhode Island	7.0
23	Louisiana	6.7
23	New York	6.7
25	Wisconsin	6.6
26	West Virginia	6.4
27	Minnesota	6.3
28	Michigan	6.2
29	Maryland	6.1
29	Vermont	6.1
31	Utah	6.0
32	Georgia	5.9
32	Idaho	5.9
34	Kentucky	5.8
34	Texas	5.8
36	Massachusetts	5.7
37	New Jersey	5.6
38	Alabama	5.5
39	Mississippi	5.4
39	Nebraska	5.4
41	Connecticut	5.3
42	Illinois	5.2
42	Iowa	5.2
44	Indiana	5.1
45	Kansas	4.9
45	Ohio	4.9
47	Virginia	4.8
48	Arkansas	4.6
49	Pennsylvania	3.8
50	Hawaii	3.1

District of Columbia   14.8

Source: U.S. Department of Health and Human Services, National Center for Health Statistics
(http://wonder.cdc.gov/WONDER/)
By state of residence. Includes excessive blood level of alcohol, accidental poisoning by alcohol and the
following alcohol-related causes: psychoses, dependence syndrome, polyneuropathy, cardiomyopathy, gastritis,
chronic liver disease and cirrhosis. Excludes accidents, homicides and other causes indirectly related to alcohol
use. Not age-adjusted.

Age-Adjusted Death Rate by Alcohol-Induced Deaths in 1999

National Rate = 7.1 Deaths per 100,000 Population*

ALPHA ORDER

RANK	STATE	RATE
39	Alabama	5.4
2	Alaska	16.3
9	Arizona	10.1
48	Arkansas	4.6
7	California	10.7
5	Colorado	11.4
42	Connecticut	5.2
17	Delaware	7.7
13	Florida	7.9
28	Georgia	6.3
50	Hawaii	3.0
31	Idaho	6.2
41	Illinois	5.3
43	Indiana	5.1
44	Iowa	5.0
44	Kansas	5.0
35	Kentucky	5.7
23	Louisiana	6.9
13	Maine	7.9
32	Maryland	6.1
37	Massachusetts	5.6
28	Michigan	6.3
27	Minnesota	6.5
35	Mississippi	5.7
20	Missouri	7.1
13	Montana	7.9
38	Nebraska	5.5
3	Nevada	13.8
19	New Hampshire	7.6
39	New Jersey	5.4
1	New Mexico	17.4
25	New York	6.6
12	North Carolina	8.7
13	North Dakota	7.9
46	Ohio	4.8
20	Oklahoma	7.1
11	Oregon	8.8
49	Pennsylvania	3.5
23	Rhode Island	6.9
7	South Carolina	10.7
5	South Dakota	11.4
22	Tennessee	7.0
28	Texas	6.3
17	Utah	7.7
34	Vermont	5.8
46	Virginia	4.8
10	Washington	10.0
33	West Virginia	5.9
25	Wisconsin	6.6
4	Wyoming	11.7

RANK ORDER

RANK	STATE	RATE
1	New Mexico	17.4
2	Alaska	16.3
3	Nevada	13.8
4	Wyoming	11.7
5	Colorado	11.4
5	South Dakota	11.4
7	California	10.7
7	South Carolina	10.7
9	Arizona	10.1
10	Washington	10.0
11	Oregon	8.8
12	North Carolina	8.7
13	Florida	7.9
13	Maine	7.9
13	Montana	7.9
13	North Dakota	7.9
17	Delaware	7.7
17	Utah	7.7
19	New Hampshire	7.6
20	Missouri	7.1
20	Oklahoma	7.1
22	Tennessee	7.0
23	Louisiana	6.9
23	Rhode Island	6.9
25	New York	6.6
25	Wisconsin	6.6
27	Minnesota	6.5
28	Georgia	6.3
28	Michigan	6.3
28	Texas	6.3
31	Idaho	6.2
32	Maryland	6.1
33	West Virginia	5.9
34	Vermont	5.8
35	Kentucky	5.7
35	Mississippi	5.7
37	Massachusetts	5.6
38	Nebraska	5.5
39	Alabama	5.4
39	New Jersey	5.4
41	Illinois	5.3
42	Connecticut	5.2
43	Indiana	5.1
44	Iowa	5.0
44	Kansas	5.0
46	Ohio	4.8
46	Virginia	4.8
48	Arkansas	4.6
49	Pennsylvania	3.5
50	Hawaii	3.0

District of Columbia	13.9

Source: U.S. Department of Health and Human Services, National Center for Health Statistics
    (http://wonder.cdc.gov/WONDER/)
*By state of residence. Includes excessive blood level of alcohol, accidental poisoning by alcohol and the following alcohol-related causes: psychoses, dependence syndrome, polyneuropathy, cardiomyopathy, gastritis, chronic liver disease and cirrhosis. Excludes accidents, homicides and other causes indirectly related to alcohol use. Age-adjusted rates based on the year 2000 standard population.

Drug-Induced Deaths in 1999

National Total = 19,102 Deaths*

ALPHA ORDER

RANK	STATE	DEATHS	% of USA
29	Alabama	195	1.0%
43	Alaska	56	0.3%
11	Arizona	557	2.9%
33	Arkansas	121	0.6%
1	California	3,089	16.2%
16	Colorado	375	2.0%
19	Connecticut	330	1.7%
44	Delaware	54	0.3%
4	Florida	1,058	5.5%
18	Georgia	345	1.8%
36	Hawaii	83	0.4%
39	Idaho	66	0.3%
6	Illinois	872	4.6%
23	Indiana	249	1.3%
42	Iowa	59	0.3%
35	Kansas	99	0.5%
27	Kentucky	214	1.1%
24	Louisiana	245	1.3%
38	Maine	70	0.4%
9	Maryland	660	3.5%
13	Massachusetts	512	2.7%
8	Michigan	708	3.7%
32	Minnesota	167	0.9%
34	Mississippi	101	0.5%
21	Missouri	293	1.5%
45	Montana	48	0.3%
46	Nebraska	41	0.2%
26	Nevada	236	1.2%
40	New Hampshire	62	0.3%
7	New Jersey	757	4.0%
22	New Mexico	275	1.4%
3	New York	1,099	5.8%
14	North Carolina	401	2.1%
50	North Dakota	15	0.1%
12	Ohio	534	2.8%
30	Oklahoma	189	1.0%
20	Oregon	328	1.7%
5	Pennsylvania	1,048	5.5%
41	Rhode Island	61	0.3%
31	South Carolina	168	0.9%
49	South Dakota	20	0.1%
17	Tennessee	372	1.9%
2	Texas	1,250	6.5%
28	Utah	210	1.1%
47	Vermont	31	0.2%
15	Virginia	390	2.0%
10	Washington	596	3.1%
37	West Virginia	80	0.4%
25	Wisconsin	237	1.2%
48	Wyoming	21	0.1%

RANK ORDER

RANK	STATE	DEATHS	% of USA
1	California	3,089	16.2%
2	Texas	1,250	6.5%
3	New York	1,099	5.8%
4	Florida	1,058	5.5%
5	Pennsylvania	1,048	5.5%
6	Illinois	872	4.6%
7	New Jersey	757	4.0%
8	Michigan	708	3.7%
9	Maryland	660	3.5%
10	Washington	596	3.1%
11	Arizona	557	2.9%
12	Ohio	534	2.8%
13	Massachusetts	512	2.7%
14	North Carolina	401	2.1%
15	Virginia	390	2.0%
16	Colorado	375	2.0%
17	Tennessee	372	1.9%
18	Georgia	345	1.8%
19	Connecticut	330	1.7%
20	Oregon	328	1.7%
21	Missouri	293	1.5%
22	New Mexico	275	1.4%
23	Indiana	249	1.3%
24	Louisiana	245	1.3%
25	Wisconsin	237	1.2%
26	Nevada	236	1.2%
27	Kentucky	214	1.1%
28	Utah	210	1.1%
29	Alabama	195	1.0%
30	Oklahoma	189	1.0%
31	South Carolina	168	0.9%
32	Minnesota	167	0.9%
33	Arkansas	121	0.6%
34	Mississippi	101	0.5%
35	Kansas	99	0.5%
36	Hawaii	83	0.4%
37	West Virginia	80	0.4%
38	Maine	70	0.4%
39	Idaho	66	0.3%
40	New Hampshire	62	0.3%
41	Rhode Island	61	0.3%
42	Iowa	59	0.3%
43	Alaska	56	0.3%
44	Delaware	54	0.3%
45	Montana	48	0.3%
46	Nebraska	41	0.2%
47	Vermont	31	0.2%
48	Wyoming	21	0.1%
49	South Dakota	20	0.1%
50	North Dakota	15	0.1%
	District of Columbia	55	0.3%

Source: U.S. Department of Health and Human Services, National Center for Health Statistics (http://wonder.cdc.gov/WONDER/)

By state of residence. Includes drug psychoses, drug dependence, nondependent use excluding alcohol and tobacco, accidental poisoning or suicide by drugs, medicaments and biologicals. Excludes accidents, homicides and other causes indirectly related to drug use.

Death Rate from Drug-Induced Deaths in 1999

National Rate = 7.0 Deaths per 100,000 Population*

ALPHA ORDER

RANK	STATE	RATE
37	Alabama	4.5
12	Alaska	9.0
4	Arizona	11.7
35	Arkansas	4.7
9	California	9.3
11	Colorado	9.2
6	Connecticut	10.1
15	Delaware	7.2
18	Florida	7.0
39	Georgia	4.4
18	Hawaii	7.0
31	Idaho	5.3
15	Illinois	7.2
43	Indiana	4.2
50	Iowa	2.1
44	Kansas	3.7
28	Kentucky	5.4
25	Louisiana	5.6
25	Maine	5.6
3	Maryland	12.8
14	Massachusetts	8.3
15	Michigan	7.2
46	Minnesota	3.5
45	Mississippi	3.6
28	Missouri	5.4
28	Montana	5.4
48	Nebraska	2.5
2	Nevada	13.0
32	New Hampshire	5.2
9	New Jersey	9.3
1	New Mexico	15.8
23	New York	6.0
32	North Carolina	5.2
49	North Dakota**	2.4
35	Ohio	4.7
25	Oklahoma	5.6
7	Oregon	9.9
13	Pennsylvania	8.7
21	Rhode Island	6.2
42	South Carolina	4.3
47	South Dakota	2.7
20	Tennessee	6.8
21	Texas	6.2
7	Utah	9.9
32	Vermont	5.2
24	Virginia	5.7
5	Washington	10.4
39	West Virginia	4.4
37	Wisconsin	4.5
39	Wyoming	4.4

RANK ORDER

RANK	STATE	RATE
1	New Mexico	15.8
2	Nevada	13.0
3	Maryland	12.8
4	Arizona	11.7
5	Washington	10.4
6	Connecticut	10.1
7	Oregon	9.9
7	Utah	9.9
9	California	9.3
9	New Jersey	9.3
11	Colorado	9.2
12	Alaska	9.0
13	Pennsylvania	8.7
14	Massachusetts	8.3
15	Delaware	7.2
15	Illinois	7.2
15	Michigan	7.2
18	Florida	7.0
18	Hawaii	7.0
20	Tennessee	6.8
21	Rhode Island	6.2
21	Texas	6.2
23	New York	6.0
24	Virginia	5.7
25	Louisiana	5.6
25	Maine	5.6
25	Oklahoma	5.6
28	Kentucky	5.4
28	Missouri	5.4
28	Montana	5.4
31	Idaho	5.3
32	New Hampshire	5.2
32	North Carolina	5.2
32	Vermont	5.2
35	Arkansas	4.7
35	Ohio	4.7
37	Alabama	4.5
37	Wisconsin	4.5
39	Georgia	4.4
39	West Virginia	4.4
39	Wyoming	4.4
42	South Carolina	4.3
43	Indiana	4.2
44	Kansas	3.7
45	Mississippi	3.6
46	Minnesota	3.5
47	South Dakota	2.7
48	Nebraska	2.5
49	North Dakota**	2.4
50	Iowa	2.1

	District of Columbia	10.6

Source: U.S. Department of Health and Human Services, National Center for Health Statistics (http://wonder.cdc.gov/WONDER/)

By state of residence. Includes drug psychoses, drug dependence, nondependent use excluding alcohol and tobacco, accidental poisoning or suicide by drugs, medicaments and biologicals. Excludes accidents, homicides and other causes indirectly related to drug use. Not age-adjusted.

**Due to low numbers of deaths, rates for this state should be interpreted with caution.*

Age-Adjusted Death Rate from Drug-Induced Deaths in 1999

National Rate = 7.0 Deaths per 100,000 Population*

ALPHA ORDER

RANK ORDER

RANK	STATE	RATE
39	Alabama	4.4
9	Alaska	9.6
3	Arizona	12.2
35	Arkansas	4.9
10	California	9.4
12	Colorado	9.0
7	Connecticut	9.9
18	Delaware	7.0
15	Florida	7.2
39	Georgia	4.4
19	Hawaii	6.9
27	Idaho	5.5
15	Illinois	7.2
43	Indiana	4.2
50	Iowa	2.1
44	Kansas	3.8
31	Kentucky	5.3
25	Louisiana	5.8
29	Maine	5.4
4	Maryland	12.0
14	Massachusetts	8.0
17	Michigan	7.1
46	Minnesota	3.5
44	Mississippi	3.8
29	Missouri	5.4
26	Montana	5.6
48	Nebraska	2.5
2	Nevada	13.0
33	New Hampshire	5.0
11	New Jersey	9.1
1	New Mexico	16.2
23	New York	5.9
31	North Carolina	5.3
49	North Dakota**	2.3
36	Ohio	4.7
23	Oklahoma	5.9
7	Oregon	9.9
13	Pennsylvania	8.7
22	Rhode Island	6.1
42	South Carolina	4.3
47	South Dakota	2.8
20	Tennessee	6.7
21	Texas	6.4
5	Utah	11.5
33	Vermont	5.0
27	Virginia	5.5
6	Washington	10.2
39	West Virginia	4.4
37	Wisconsin	4.5
37	Wyoming	4.5

RANK	STATE	RATE
1	New Mexico	16.2
2	Nevada	13.0
3	Arizona	12.2
4	Maryland	12.0
5	Utah	11.5
6	Washington	10.2
7	Connecticut	9.9
7	Oregon	9.9
9	Alaska	9.6
10	California	9.4
11	New Jersey	9.1
12	Colorado	9.0
13	Pennsylvania	8.7
14	Massachusetts	8.0
15	Florida	7.2
15	Illinois	7.2
17	Michigan	7.1
18	Delaware	7.0
19	Hawaii	6.9
20	Tennessee	6.7
21	Texas	6.4
22	Rhode Island	6.1
23	New York	5.9
23	Oklahoma	5.9
25	Louisiana	5.8
26	Montana	5.6
27	Idaho	5.5
27	Virginia	5.5
29	Maine	5.4
29	Missouri	5.4
31	Kentucky	5.3
31	North Carolina	5.3
33	New Hampshire	5.0
33	Vermont	5.0
35	Arkansas	4.9
36	Ohio	4.7
37	Wisconsin	4.5
37	Wyoming	4.5
39	Alabama	4.4
39	Georgia	4.4
39	West Virginia	4.4
42	South Carolina	4.3
43	Indiana	4.2
44	Kansas	3.8
44	Mississippi	3.8
46	Minnesota	3.5
47	South Dakota	2.8
48	Nebraska	2.5
49	North Dakota**	2.3
50	Iowa	2.1

| | District of Columbia | 9.7 |

Source: U.S. Department of Health and Human Services, National Center for Health Statistics
     (http://wonder.cdc.gov/WONDER/)

*By state of residence. Includes drug psychoses, drug dependence, nondependent use excluding alcohol and tobacco, accidental poisoning or suicide by drugs, medicaments and biologicals. Excludes accidents, homicides and other causes indirectly related to drug use. Age-adjusted rates based on the year 2000 standard population.
**Due to low numbers of deaths, rates for this state should be interpreted with caution.

Occupational Fatalities in 2001

National Total = 5,900 Deaths*

RANK	STATE	DEATHS	% of USA
15	Alabama	138	2.3%
30	Alaska	64	1.1%
26	Arizona	87	1.5%
28	Arkansas	68	1.2%
2	California	510	8.6%
14	Colorado	139	2.4%
41	Connecticut	40	0.7%
48	Delaware	10	0.2%
3	Florida	368	6.2%
4	Georgia	235	4.0%
40	Hawaii	41	0.7%
38	Idaho	45	0.8%
5	Illinois	231	3.9%
11	Indiana	152	2.6%
33	Iowa	62	1.1%
24	Kansas	93	1.6%
22	Kentucky	105	1.8%
18	Louisiana	117	2.0%
46	Maine	23	0.4%
30	Maryland	64	1.1%
37	Massachusetts	53	0.9%
10	Michigan	175	3.0%
27	Minnesota	76	1.3%
20	Mississippi	111	1.9%
13	Missouri	143	2.4%
35	Montana	58	1.0%
36	Nebraska	57	1.0%
41	Nevada	40	0.7%
49	New Hampshire	9	0.2%
17	New Jersey	129	2.2%
34	New Mexico	59	1.0%
7	New York	220	3.7%
9	North Carolina	203	3.4%
45	North Dakota	25	0.4%
8	Ohio	209	3.5%
19	Oklahoma	115	1.9%
39	Oregon	44	0.7%
6	Pennsylvania	225	3.8%
47	Rhode Island	17	0.3%
25	South Carolina	89	1.5%
44	South Dakota	35	0.6%
16	Tennessee	136	2.3%
1	Texas	534	9.1%
29	Utah	65	1.1%
50	Vermont	6	0.1%
12	Virginia	146	2.5%
23	Washington	102	1.7%
32	West Virginia	63	1.1%
21	Wisconsin	110	1.9%
41	Wyoming	40	0.7%

RANK	STATE	DEATHS	% of USA
1	Texas	534	9.1%
2	California	510	8.6%
3	Florida	368	6.2%
4	Georgia	235	4.0%
5	Illinois	231	3.9%
6	Pennsylvania	225	3.8%
7	New York	220	3.7%
8	Ohio	209	3.5%
9	North Carolina	203	3.4%
10	Michigan	175	3.0%
11	Indiana	152	2.6%
12	Virginia	146	2.5%
13	Missouri	143	2.4%
14	Colorado	139	2.4%
15	Alabama	138	2.3%
16	Tennessee	136	2.3%
17	New Jersey	129	2.2%
18	Louisiana	117	2.0%
19	Oklahoma	115	1.9%
20	Mississippi	111	1.9%
21	Wisconsin	110	1.9%
22	Kentucky	105	1.8%
23	Washington	102	1.7%
24	Kansas	93	1.6%
25	South Carolina	89	1.5%
26	Arizona	87	1.5%
27	Minnesota	76	1.3%
28	Arkansas	68	1.2%
29	Utah	65	1.1%
30	Alaska	64	1.1%
30	Maryland	64	1.1%
32	West Virginia	63	1.1%
33	Iowa	62	1.1%
34	New Mexico	59	1.0%
35	Montana	58	1.0%
36	Nebraska	57	1.0%
37	Massachusetts	53	0.9%
38	Idaho	45	0.8%
39	Oregon	44	0.7%
40	Hawaii	41	0.7%
41	Connecticut	40	0.7%
41	Nevada	40	0.7%
41	Wyoming	40	0.7%
44	South Dakota	35	0.6%
45	North Dakota	25	0.4%
46	Maine	23	0.4%
47	Rhode Island	17	0.3%
48	Delaware	10	0.2%
49	New Hampshire	9	0.2%
50	Vermont	6	0.1%
	District of Columbia	11	0.2%

Source: U.S. Department of Labor, Bureau of Labor Statistics
"National Census of Fatal Occupational Injuries, 2001" (press release, September 25, 2002)
*Includes three fatalities that occurred within the territorial boundaries of the United States but for which a state of incident could not be determined. Does not include 2,886 fatal work injuries resulting from the attacks of September 11th.

Occupational Fatality Rate in 2001

National Rate = 4.4 Deaths per 100,000 Workers*

ALPHA ORDER

RANK	STATE	RATE
13	Alabama	6.8
1	Alaska	21.2
33	Arizona	3.8
19	Arkansas	5.8
41	California	3.1
14	Colorado	6.3
46	Connecticut	2.4
45	Delaware	2.5
26	Florida	5.0
18	Georgia	5.9
10	Hawaii	7.1
12	Idaho	6.9
33	Illinois	3.8
23	Indiana	5.1
30	Iowa	4.0
11	Kansas	7.0
20	Kentucky	5.6
16	Louisiana	6.1
38	Maine	3.5
46	Maryland	2.4
49	Massachusetts	1.7
36	Michigan	3.6
42	Minnesota	2.8
4	Mississippi	9.1
23	Missouri	5.1
3	Montana	13.1
14	Nebraska	6.3
28	Nevada	4.1
50	New Hampshire	1.4
40	New Jersey	3.2
8	New Mexico	7.4
43	New York	2.6
21	North Carolina	5.4
7	North Dakota	7.6
35	Ohio	3.7
9	Oklahoma	7.2
43	Oregon	2.6
31	Pennsylvania	3.9
38	Rhode Island	3.5
27	South Carolina	4.8
5	South Dakota	8.9
23	Tennessee	5.1
21	Texas	5.4
16	Utah	6.1
48	Vermont	1.9
28	Virginia	4.1
36	Washington	3.6
6	West Virginia	8.0
31	Wisconsin	3.9
2	Wyoming	15.3

RANK ORDER

RANK	STATE	RATE
1	Alaska	21.2
2	Wyoming	15.3
3	Montana	13.1
4	Mississippi	9.1
5	South Dakota	8.9
6	West Virginia	8.0
7	North Dakota	7.6
8	New Mexico	7.4
9	Oklahoma	7.2
10	Hawaii	7.1
11	Kansas	7.0
12	Idaho	6.9
13	Alabama	6.8
14	Colorado	6.3
14	Nebraska	6.3
16	Louisiana	6.1
16	Utah	6.1
18	Georgia	5.9
19	Arkansas	5.8
20	Kentucky	5.6
21	North Carolina	5.4
21	Texas	5.4
23	Indiana	5.1
23	Missouri	5.1
23	Tennessee	5.1
26	Florida	5.0
27	South Carolina	4.8
28	Nevada	4.1
28	Virginia	4.1
30	Iowa	4.0
31	Pennsylvania	3.9
31	Wisconsin	3.9
33	Arizona	3.8
33	Illinois	3.8
35	Ohio	3.7
36	Michigan	3.6
36	Washington	3.6
38	Maine	3.5
38	Rhode Island	3.5
40	New Jersey	3.2
41	California	3.1
42	Minnesota	2.8
43	New York	2.6
43	Oregon	2.6
45	Delaware	2.5
46	Connecticut	2.4
46	Maryland	2.4
48	Vermont	1.9
49	Massachusetts	1.7
50	New Hampshire	1.4

District of Columbia 4.2

Source: Morgan Quitno Press using data from U.S. Department of Labor, Bureau of Labor Statistics
  "National Census of Fatal Occupational Injuries, 2001" (press release, September 25, 2002)
*Based on employed civilian labor force. Does not include 2,886 fatal work injuries resulting from the attacks of
September 11th.

189

III. FACILITIES

Community Hospitals in 2001

National Total = 4,908 Hospitals*

RANK	STATE	HOSPITALS	% of USA
20	Alabama	107	2.2%
47	Alaska	19	0.4%
31	Arizona	61	1.2%
26	Arkansas	83	1.7%
2	California	384	7.8%
29	Colorado	66	1.3%
41	Connecticut	35	0.7%
50	Delaware	5	0.1%
5	Florida	202	4.1%
8	Georgia	147	3.0%
46	Hawaii	23	0.5%
38	Idaho	40	0.8%
6	Illinois	192	3.9%
18	Indiana	110	2.2%
16	Iowa	116	2.4%
10	Kansas	133	2.7%
21	Kentucky	103	2.1%
12	Louisiana	125	2.5%
40	Maine	37	0.8%
36	Maryland	49	1.0%
27	Massachusetts	80	1.6%
9	Michigan	145	3.0%
10	Minnesota	133	2.7%
22	Mississippi	96	2.0%
15	Missouri	117	2.4%
34	Montana	53	1.1%
24	Nebraska	84	1.7%
44	Nevada	24	0.5%
43	New Hampshire	28	0.6%
28	New Jersey	78	1.6%
41	New Mexico	35	0.7%
3	New York	212	4.3%
17	North Carolina	111	2.3%
38	North Dakota	40	0.8%
7	Ohio	166	3.4%
19	Oklahoma	108	2.2%
32	Oregon	60	1.2%
4	Pennsylvania	205	4.2%
49	Rhode Island	11	0.2%
30	South Carolina	62	1.3%
35	South Dakota	50	1.0%
13	Tennessee	123	2.5%
1	Texas	411	8.4%
37	Utah	42	0.9%
48	Vermont	14	0.3%
23	Virginia	87	1.8%
24	Washington	84	1.7%
33	West Virginia	57	1.2%
14	Wisconsin	121	2.5%
44	Wyoming	24	0.5%

RANK	STATE	HOSPITALS	% of USA
1	Texas	411	8.4%
2	California	384	7.8%
3	New York	212	4.3%
4	Pennsylvania	205	4.2%
5	Florida	202	4.1%
6	Illinois	192	3.9%
7	Ohio	166	3.4%
8	Georgia	147	3.0%
9	Michigan	145	3.0%
10	Kansas	133	2.7%
10	Minnesota	133	2.7%
12	Louisiana	125	2.5%
13	Tennessee	123	2.5%
14	Wisconsin	121	2.5%
15	Missouri	117	2.4%
16	Iowa	116	2.4%
17	North Carolina	111	2.3%
18	Indiana	110	2.2%
19	Oklahoma	108	2.2%
20	Alabama	107	2.2%
21	Kentucky	103	2.1%
22	Mississippi	96	2.0%
23	Virginia	87	1.8%
24	Nebraska	84	1.7%
24	Washington	84	1.7%
26	Arkansas	83	1.7%
27	Massachusetts	80	1.6%
28	New Jersey	78	1.6%
29	Colorado	66	1.3%
30	South Carolina	62	1.3%
31	Arizona	61	1.2%
32	Oregon	60	1.2%
33	West Virginia	57	1.2%
34	Montana	53	1.1%
35	South Dakota	50	1.0%
36	Maryland	49	1.0%
37	Utah	42	0.9%
38	Idaho	40	0.8%
38	North Dakota	40	0.8%
40	Maine	37	0.8%
41	Connecticut	35	0.7%
41	New Mexico	35	0.7%
43	New Hampshire	28	0.6%
44	Nevada	24	0.5%
44	Wyoming	24	0.5%
46	Hawaii	23	0.5%
47	Alaska	19	0.4%
48	Vermont	14	0.3%
49	Rhode Island	11	0.2%
50	Delaware	5	0.1%
	District of Columbia	10	0.2%

Source: American Hospital Association (Chicago, IL)
    "Hospital Statistics" (2003 edition)
*Community hospitals are all nonfederal, short-term, general and special hospitals whose facilities and services are available to the public.

Rate of Community Hospitals in 2001

National Rate = 1.7 Community Hospitals per 100,000 Population*

ALPHA ORDER

RANK	STATE	RATE
18	Alabama	2.4
12	Alaska	3.0
42	Arizona	1.1
10	Arkansas	3.1
42	California	1.1
32	Colorado	1.5
46	Connecticut	1.0
50	Delaware	0.6
39	Florida	1.2
29	Georgia	1.7
24	Hawaii	1.9
12	Idaho	3.0
32	Illinois	1.5
27	Indiana	1.8
7	Iowa	4.0
4	Kansas	4.9
17	Kentucky	2.5
15	Louisiana	2.8
14	Maine	2.9
48	Maryland	0.9
39	Massachusetts	1.2
36	Michigan	1.4
16	Minnesota	2.7
8	Mississippi	3.4
22	Missouri	2.1
3	Montana	5.9
4	Nebraska	4.9
42	Nevada	1.1
20	New Hampshire	2.2
48	New Jersey	0.9
24	New Mexico	1.9
42	New York	1.1
36	North Carolina	1.4
2	North Dakota	6.3
32	Ohio	1.5
10	Oklahoma	3.1
29	Oregon	1.7
29	Pennsylvania	1.7
46	Rhode Island	1.0
32	South Carolina	1.5
1	South Dakota	6.6
22	Tennessee	2.1
24	Texas	1.9
27	Utah	1.8
19	Vermont	2.3
39	Virginia	1.2
36	Washington	1.4
9	West Virginia	3.2
20	Wisconsin	2.2
4	Wyoming	4.9

RANK ORDER

RANK	STATE	RATE
1	South Dakota	6.6
2	North Dakota	6.3
3	Montana	5.9
4	Kansas	4.9
4	Nebraska	4.9
4	Wyoming	4.9
7	Iowa	4.0
8	Mississippi	3.4
9	West Virginia	3.2
10	Arkansas	3.1
10	Oklahoma	3.1
12	Alaska	3.0
12	Idaho	3.0
14	Maine	2.9
15	Louisiana	2.8
16	Minnesota	2.7
17	Kentucky	2.5
18	Alabama	2.4
19	Vermont	2.3
20	New Hampshire	2.2
20	Wisconsin	2.2
22	Missouri	2.1
22	Tennessee	2.1
24	Hawaii	1.9
24	New Mexico	1.9
24	Texas	1.9
27	Indiana	1.8
27	Utah	1.8
29	Georgia	1.7
29	Oregon	1.7
29	Pennsylvania	1.7
32	Colorado	1.5
32	Illinois	1.5
32	Ohio	1.5
32	South Carolina	1.5
36	Michigan	1.4
36	North Carolina	1.4
36	Washington	1.4
39	Florida	1.2
39	Massachusetts	1.2
39	Virginia	1.2
42	Arizona	1.1
42	California	1.1
42	Nevada	1.1
42	New York	1.1
46	Connecticut	1.0
46	Rhode Island	1.0
48	Maryland	0.9
48	New Jersey	0.9
50	Delaware	0.6
	District of Columbia	1.7

Source: Morgan Quitno Press using data from American Hospital Association (Chicago, IL)
   "Hospital Statistics" (2003 edition)
*Community hospitals are all nonfederal, short-term, general and special hospitals whose facilities and services are available to the public.

Community Hospitals per 1,000 Square Miles in 2001

National Rate = 1.3 Community Hospitals*

ALPHA ORDER

RANK ORDER

RANK	STATE	RATE		RANK	STATE	RATE
24	Alabama	2.0		1	New Jersey	9.5
50	Alaska**	0.0		2	Rhode Island	8.9
43	Arizona	0.5		3	Massachusetts	8.7
29	Arkansas	1.6		4	Connecticut	6.3
18	California	2.4		5	Pennsylvania	4.5
39	Colorado	0.6		6	Maryland	4.0
4	Connecticut	6.3		7	New York	3.9
20	Delaware	2.1		8	Ohio	3.7
10	Florida	3.4		9	Hawaii	3.6
15	Georgia	2.5		10	Florida	3.4
9	Hawaii	3.6		11	Illinois	3.3
43	Idaho	0.5		12	Indiana	3.0
11	Illinois	3.3		12	New Hampshire	3.0
12	Indiana	3.0		14	Tennessee	2.9
20	Iowa	2.1		15	Georgia	2.5
29	Kansas	1.6		15	Kentucky	2.5
15	Kentucky	2.5		15	Louisiana	2.5
15	Louisiana	2.5		18	California	2.4
37	Maine	1.1		18	West Virginia	2.4
6	Maryland	4.0		20	Delaware	2.1
3	Massachusetts	8.7		20	Iowa	2.1
31	Michigan	1.5		20	North Carolina	2.1
31	Minnesota	1.5		20	Virginia	2.1
24	Mississippi	2.0		24	Alabama	2.0
28	Missouri	1.7		24	Mississippi	2.0
46	Montana	0.4		24	South Carolina	2.0
37	Nebraska	1.1		27	Wisconsin	1.8
48	Nevada	0.2		28	Missouri	1.7
12	New Hampshire	3.0		29	Arkansas	1.6
1	New Jersey	9.5		29	Kansas	1.6
47	New Mexico	0.3		31	Michigan	1.5
7	New York	3.9		31	Minnesota	1.5
20	North Carolina	2.1		31	Oklahoma	1.5
39	North Dakota	0.6		31	Texas	1.5
8	Ohio	3.7		31	Vermont	1.5
31	Oklahoma	1.5		36	Washington	1.2
39	Oregon	0.6		37	Maine	1.1
5	Pennsylvania	4.5		37	Nebraska	1.1
2	Rhode Island	8.9		39	Colorado	0.6
24	South Carolina	2.0		39	North Dakota	0.6
39	South Dakota	0.6		39	Oregon	0.6
14	Tennessee	2.9		39	South Dakota	0.6
31	Texas	1.5		43	Arizona	0.5
43	Utah	0.5		43	Idaho	0.5
31	Vermont	1.5		43	Utah	0.5
20	Virginia	2.1		46	Montana	0.4
36	Washington	1.2		47	New Mexico	0.3
18	West Virginia	2.4		48	Nevada	0.2
27	Wisconsin	1.8		48	Wyoming	0.2
48	Wyoming	0.2		50	Alaska**	0.0
					District of Columbia***	NA

Source: Morgan Quitno Press using data from American Hospital Association (Chicago, IL)
"Hospital Statistics" (2003 edition)

*Based on 1990 Census land and water area figures. Community hospitals are nonfederal short-term general and other special hospitals, whose facilities and services are available to the public.

**Alaska has 19 community hospitals for its 615,230 square miles.

***The District of Columbia has 10 community hospitals for its 68 square miles.

Community Hospitals in Urban Areas in 2001

National Total = 2,741 Hospitals*

ALPHA ORDER

RANK ORDER

RANK	STATE	HOSPITALS	% of USA	RANK	STATE	HOSPITALS	% of USA
16	Alabama	57	2.1%	1	California	344	12.6%
47	Alaska	3	0.1%	2	Texas	250	9.1%
20	Arizona	46	1.7%	3	New York	176	6.4%
29	Arkansas	28	1.0%	4	Florida	170	6.2%
1	California	344	12.6%	5	Pennsylvania	161	5.9%
27	Colorado	31	1.1%	6	Illinois	120	4.4%
28	Connecticut	29	1.1%	7	Ohio	114	4.2%
47	Delaware	3	0.1%	8	Michigan	86	3.1%
4	Florida	170	6.2%	9	New Jersey	78	2.8%
12	Georgia	64	2.3%	10	Louisiana	76	2.8%
38	Hawaii	13	0.5%	11	Massachusetts	69	2.5%
43	Idaho	7	0.3%	12	Georgia	64	2.3%
6	Illinois	120	4.4%	12	Indiana	64	2.3%
12	Indiana	64	2.3%	14	Missouri	60	2.2%
32	Iowa	21	0.8%	14	Tennessee	60	2.2%
29	Kansas	28	1.0%	16	Alabama	57	2.1%
26	Kentucky	32	1.2%	17	Wisconsin	56	2.0%
10	Louisiana	76	2.8%	18	Virginia	52	1.9%
42	Maine	8	0.3%	19	North Carolina	50	1.8%
23	Maryland	40	1.5%	20	Arizona	46	1.7%
11	Massachusetts	69	2.5%	21	Minnesota	45	1.6%
8	Michigan	86	3.1%	22	Washington	44	1.6%
21	Minnesota	45	1.6%	23	Maryland	40	1.5%
34	Mississippi	20	0.7%	23	Oklahoma	40	1.5%
14	Missouri	60	2.2%	25	South Carolina	35	1.3%
46	Montana	5	0.2%	26	Kentucky	32	1.2%
37	Nebraska	14	0.5%	27	Colorado	31	1.1%
36	Nevada	15	0.5%	28	Connecticut	29	1.1%
40	New Hampshire	10	0.4%	29	Arkansas	28	1.0%
9	New Jersey	78	2.8%	29	Kansas	28	1.0%
38	New Mexico	13	0.5%	29	Oregon	28	1.0%
3	New York	176	6.4%	32	Iowa	21	0.8%
19	North Carolina	50	1.8%	32	Utah	21	0.8%
43	North Dakota	7	0.3%	34	Mississippi	20	0.7%
7	Ohio	114	4.2%	35	West Virginia	18	0.7%
23	Oklahoma	40	1.5%	36	Nevada	15	0.5%
29	Oregon	28	1.0%	37	Nebraska	14	0.5%
5	Pennsylvania	161	5.9%	38	Hawaii	13	0.5%
40	Rhode Island	10	0.4%	38	New Mexico	13	0.5%
25	South Carolina	35	1.3%	40	New Hampshire	10	0.4%
45	South Dakota	6	0.2%	40	Rhode Island	10	0.4%
14	Tennessee	60	2.2%	42	Maine	8	0.3%
2	Texas	250	9.1%	43	Idaho	7	0.3%
32	Utah	21	0.8%	43	North Dakota	7	0.3%
49	Vermont	2	0.1%	45	South Dakota	6	0.2%
18	Virginia	52	1.9%	46	Montana	5	0.2%
22	Washington	44	1.6%	47	Alaska	3	0.1%
35	West Virginia	18	0.7%	47	Delaware	3	0.1%
17	Wisconsin	56	2.0%	49	Vermont	2	0.1%
49	Wyoming	2	0.1%	49	Wyoming	2	0.1%
					District of Columbia	10	0.4%

Source: American Hospital Association (Chicago, IL)
   "Hospital Statistics" (2003 edition)

*Community hospitals are all nonfederal, short-term, general and special hospitals whose facilities and services are available to the public. Urban is defined as any area inside a metropolitan statistical area as defined by the U.S. Office of Management and Budget.

Percent of Community Hospitals in Urban Areas in 2001

National Percent = 55.8% of Community Hospitals*

ALPHA ORDER

RANK	STATE	PERCENT
22	Alabama	53.3
46	Alaska	15.8
10	Arizona	75.4
36	Arkansas	33.7
3	California	89.6
27	Colorado	47.0
7	Connecticut	82.9
16	Delaware	60.0
5	Florida	84.2
31	Georgia	43.5
20	Hawaii	56.5
43	Idaho	17.5
12	Illinois	62.5
19	Indiana	58.2
42	Iowa	18.1
40	Kansas	21.1
38	Kentucky	31.1
14	Louisiana	60.8
39	Maine	21.6
8	Maryland	81.6
4	Massachusetts	86.3
18	Michigan	59.3
35	Minnesota	33.8
41	Mississippi	20.8
24	Missouri	51.3
49	Montana	9.4
45	Nebraska	16.7
12	Nevada	62.5
34	New Hampshire	35.7
1	New Jersey	100.0
32	New Mexico	37.1
6	New York	83.0
30	North Carolina	45.0
43	North Dakota	17.5
11	Ohio	68.7
33	Oklahoma	37.0
28	Oregon	46.7
9	Pennsylvania	78.5
2	Rhode Island	90.9
20	South Carolina	56.5
48	South Dakota	12.0
26	Tennessee	48.8
14	Texas	60.8
25	Utah *	50.0
47	Vermont	14.3
17	Virginia	59.8
23	Washington	52.4
37	West Virginia	31.6
29	Wisconsin	46.3
50	Wyoming	8.3

RANK ORDER

RANK	STATE	PERCENT
1	New Jersey	100.0
2	Rhode Island	90.9
3	California	89.6
4	Massachusetts	86.3
5	Florida	84.2
6	New York	83.0
7	Connecticut	82.9
8	Maryland	81.6
9	Pennsylvania	78.5
10	Arizona	75.4
11	Ohio	68.7
12	Illinois	62.5
12	Nevada	62.5
14	Louisiana	60.8
14	Texas	60.8
16	Delaware	60.0
17	Virginia	59.8
18	Michigan	59.3
19	Indiana	58.2
20	Hawaii	56.5
20	South Carolina	56.5
22	Alabama	53.3
23	Washington	52.4
24	Missouri	51.3
25	Utah	50.0
26	Tennessee	48.8
27	Colorado	47.0
28	Oregon	46.7
29	Wisconsin	46.3
30	North Carolina	45.0
31	Georgia	43.5
32	New Mexico	37.1
33	Oklahoma	37.0
34	New Hampshire	35.7
35	Minnesota	33.8
36	Arkansas	33.7
37	West Virginia	31.6
38	Kentucky	31.1
39	Maine	21.6
40	Kansas	21.1
41	Mississippi	20.8
42	Iowa	18.1
43	Idaho	17.5
43	North Dakota	17.5
45	Nebraska	16.7
46	Alaska	15.8
47	Vermont	14.3
48	South Dakota	12.0
49	Montana	9.4
50	Wyoming	8.3
	District of Columbia	100.0

Source: Morgan Quitno Press using data from American Hospital Association (Chicago, IL)
"Hospital Statistics" (2003 edition)
*Community hospitals are all nonfederal, short-term, general and special hospitals whose facilities and services are available to the public. Urban is defined as any area inside a metropolitan statistical area as defined by the U.S. Office of Management and Budget.

Community Hospitals in Rural Areas in 2001

National Total = 2,167 Hospitals*

ALPHA ORDER

RANK	STATE	HOSPITALS	% of USA
18	Alabama	50	2.3%
40	Alaska	16	0.7%
41	Arizona	15	0.7%
16	Arkansas	55	2.5%
24	California	40	1.8%
28	Colorado	35	1.6%
47	Connecticut	6	0.3%
48	Delaware	2	0.1%
32	Florida	32	1.5%
5	Georgia	83	3.8%
44	Hawaii	10	0.5%
30	Idaho	33	1.5%
7	Illinois	72	3.3%
21	Indiana	46	2.1%
3	Iowa	95	4.4%
2	Kansas	105	4.8%
8	Kentucky	71	3.3%
19	Louisiana	49	2.3%
34	Maine	29	1.3%
45	Maryland	9	0.4%
43	Massachusetts	11	0.5%
14	Michigan	59	2.7%
4	Minnesota	88	4.1%
6	Mississippi	76	3.5%
15	Missouri	57	2.6%
20	Montana	48	2.2%
9	Nebraska	70	3.2%
45	Nevada	9	0.4%
39	New Hampshire	18	0.8%
50	New Jersey	0	0.0%
36	New Mexico	22	1.0%
27	New York	36	1.7%
13	North Carolina	61	2.8%
30	North Dakota	33	1.5%
17	Ohio	52	2.4%
10	Oklahoma	68	3.1%
32	Oregon	32	1.5%
22	Pennsylvania	44	2.0%
49	Rhode Island	1	0.0%
35	South Carolina	27	1.2%
22	South Dakota	44	2.0%
12	Tennessee	63	2.9%
1	Texas	161	7.4%
38	Utah	21	1.0%
42	Vermont	12	0.6%
28	Virginia	35	1.6%
24	Washington	40	1.8%
26	West Virginia	39	1.8%
11	Wisconsin	65	3.0%
36	Wyoming	22	1.0%

RANK ORDER

RANK	STATE	HOSPITALS	% of USA
1	Texas	161	7.4%
2	Kansas	105	4.8%
3	Iowa	95	4.4%
4	Minnesota	88	4.1%
5	Georgia	83	3.8%
6	Mississippi	76	3.5%
7	Illinois	72	3.3%
8	Kentucky	71	3.3%
9	Nebraska	70	3.2%
10	Oklahoma	68	3.1%
11	Wisconsin	65	3.0%
12	Tennessee	63	2.9%
13	North Carolina	61	2.8%
14	Michigan	59	2.7%
15	Missouri	57	2.6%
16	Arkansas	55	2.5%
17	Ohio	52	2.4%
18	Alabama	50	2.3%
19	Louisiana	49	2.3%
20	Montana	48	2.2%
21	Indiana	46	2.1%
22	Pennsylvania	44	2.0%
22	South Dakota	44	2.0%
24	California	40	1.8%
24	Washington	40	1.8%
26	West Virginia	39	1.8%
27	New York	36	1.7%
28	Colorado	35	1.6%
28	Virginia	35	1.6%
30	Idaho	33	1.5%
30	North Dakota	33	1.5%
32	Florida	32	1.5%
32	Oregon	32	1.5%
34	Maine	29	1.3%
35	South Carolina	27	1.2%
36	New Mexico	22	1.0%
36	Wyoming	22	1.0%
38	Utah	21	1.0%
39	New Hampshire	18	0.8%
40	Alaska	16	0.7%
41	Arizona	15	0.7%
42	Vermont	12	0.6%
43	Massachusetts	11	0.5%
44	Hawaii	10	0.5%
45	Maryland	9	0.4%
45	Nevada	9	0.4%
47	Connecticut	6	0.3%
48	Delaware	2	0.1%
49	Rhode Island	1	0.0%
50	New Jersey	0	0.0%
	District of Columbia	0	0.0%

Source: American Hospital Association (Chicago, IL)
   "Hospital Statistics" (2003 edition)
*Community hospitals are all nonfederal, short-term, general and special hospitals whose facilities and services are available to the public. Rural is defined as any area outside a metropolitan statistical area as defined by the U.S. Office of Management and Budget.

Percent of Community Hospitals in Rural Areas in 2001

National Percent = 44.2% of Community Hospitals*

ALPHA ORDER

RANK	STATE	PERCENT
29	Alabama	46.7
5	Alaska	84.2
41	Arizona	24.6
15	Arkansas	66.3
48	California	10.4
24	Colorado	53.0
44	Connecticut	17.1
35	Delaware	40.0
46	Florida	15.8
20	Georgia	56.5
30	Hawaii	43.5
7	Idaho	82.5
38	Illinois	37.5
32	Indiana	41.8
9	Iowa	81.9
11	Kansas	78.9
13	Kentucky	68.9
36	Louisiana	39.2
12	Maine	78.4
43	Maryland	18.4
47	Massachusetts	13.8
33	Michigan	40.7
16	Minnesota	66.2
10	Mississippi	79.2
27	Missouri	48.7
2	Montana	90.6
6	Nebraska	83.3
38	Nevada	37.5
17	New Hampshire	64.3
50	New Jersey	0.0
19	New Mexico	62.9
45	New York	17.0
21	North Carolina	55.0
7	North Dakota	82.5
40	Ohio	31.3
18	Oklahoma	63.0
23	Oregon	53.3
42	Pennsylvania	21.5
49	Rhode Island	9.1
30	South Carolina	43.5
3	South Dakota	88.0
25	Tennessee	51.2
36	Texas	39.2
26	Utah	50.0
4	Vermont	85.7
34	Virginia	40.2
28	Washington	47.6
14	West Virginia	68.4
22	Wisconsin	53.7
1	Wyoming	91.7

RANK ORDER

RANK	STATE	PERCENT
1	Wyoming	91.7
2	Montana	90.6
3	South Dakota	88.0
4	Vermont	85.7
5	Alaska	84.2
6	Nebraska	83.3
7	Idaho	82.5
7	North Dakota	82.5
9	Iowa	81.9
10	Mississippi	79.2
11	Kansas	78.9
12	Maine	78.4
13	Kentucky	68.9
14	West Virginia	68.4
15	Arkansas	66.3
16	Minnesota	66.2
17	New Hampshire	64.3
18	Oklahoma	63.0
19	New Mexico	62.9
20	Georgia	56.5
21	North Carolina	55.0
22	Wisconsin	53.7
23	Oregon	53.3
24	Colorado	53.0
25	Tennessee	51.2
26	Utah	50.0
27	Missouri	48.7
28	Washington	47.6
29	Alabama	46.7
30	Hawaii	43.5
30	South Carolina	43.5
32	Indiana	41.8
33	Michigan	40.7
34	Virginia	40.2
35	Delaware	40.0
36	Louisiana	39.2
36	Texas	39.2
38	Illinois	37.5
38	Nevada	37.5
40	Ohio	31.3
41	Arizona	24.6
42	Pennsylvania	21.5
43	Maryland	18.4
44	Connecticut	17.1
45	New York	17.0
46	Florida	15.8
47	Massachusetts	13.8
48	California	10.4
49	Rhode Island	9.1
50	New Jersey	0.0
	District of Columbia	0.0

Source: Morgan Quitno Press using data from American Hospital Association (Chicago, IL)
      "Hospital Statistics" (2003 edition)
*Community hospitals are all nonfederal, short-term, general and special hospitals whose facilities and services are available to the public. Rural is defined as any area outside a metropolitan statistical area as defined by the U.S. Office of Management and Budget.

Nongovernment Not-For-Profit Hospitals in 2001

National Total = 2,998 Hospitals*

ALPHA ORDER

RANK	STATE	HOSPITALS	% of USA
31	Alabama	37	1.2%
47	Alaska	10	0.3%
31	Arizona	37	1.2%
22	Arkansas	49	1.6%
1	California	220	7.3%
37	Colorado	32	1.1%
33	Connecticut	34	1.1%
49	Delaware	5	0.2%
10	Florida	87	2.9%
17	Georgia	62	2.1%
43	Hawaii	14	0.5%
45	Idaho	11	0.4%
4	Illinois	156	5.2%
20	Indiana	57	1.9%
21	Iowa	56	1.9%
17	Kansas	62	2.1%
12	Kentucky	71	2.4%
34	Louisiana	33	1.1%
34	Maine	33	1.1%
24	Maryland	47	1.6%
13	Massachusetts	70	2.3%
7	Michigan	122	4.1%
9	Minnesota	90	3.0%
38	Mississippi	27	0.9%
15	Missouri	69	2.3%
28	Montana	42	1.4%
26	Nebraska	43	1.4%
48	Nevada	7	0.2%
39	New Hampshire	24	0.8%
11	New Jersey	74	2.5%
42	New Mexico	19	0.6%
3	New York	181	6.0%
13	North Carolina	70	2.3%
30	North Dakota	39	1.3%
6	Ohio	139	4.6%
23	Oklahoma	48	1.6%
25	Oregon	44	1.5%
2	Pennsylvania	189	6.3%
45	Rhode Island	11	0.4%
41	South Carolina	20	0.7%
26	South Dakota	43	1.4%
19	Tennessee	61	2.0%
5	Texas	146	4.9%
40	Utah	22	0.7%
43	Vermont	14	0.5%
16	Virginia	67	2.2%
29	Washington	41	1.4%
34	West Virginia	33	1.1%
8	Wisconsin	118	3.9%
49	Wyoming	5	0.2%

RANK ORDER

RANK	STATE	HOSPITALS	% of USA
1	California	220	7.3%
2	Pennsylvania	189	6.3%
3	New York	181	6.0%
4	Illinois	156	5.2%
5	Texas	146	4.9%
6	Ohio	139	4.6%
7	Michigan	122	4.1%
8	Wisconsin	118	3.9%
9	Minnesota	90	3.0%
10	Florida	87	2.9%
11	New Jersey	74	2.5%
12	Kentucky	71	2.4%
13	Massachusetts	70	2.3%
13	North Carolina	70	2.3%
15	Missouri	69	2.3%
16	Virginia	67	2.2%
17	Georgia	62	2.1%
17	Kansas	62	2.1%
19	Tennessee	61	2.0%
20	Indiana	57	1.9%
21	Iowa	56	1.9%
22	Arkansas	49	1.6%
23	Oklahoma	48	1.6%
24	Maryland	47	1.6%
25	Oregon	44	1.5%
26	Nebraska	43	1.4%
26	South Dakota	43	1.4%
28	Montana	42	1.4%
29	Washington	41	1.4%
30	North Dakota	39	1.3%
31	Alabama	37	1.2%
31	Arizona	37	1.2%
33	Connecticut	34	1.1%
34	Louisiana	33	1.1%
34	Maine	33	1.1%
34	West Virginia	33	1.1%
37	Colorado	32	1.1%
38	Mississippi	27	0.9%
39	New Hampshire	24	0.8%
40	Utah	22	0.7%
41	South Carolina	20	0.7%
42	New Mexico	19	0.6%
43	Hawaii	14	0.5%
43	Vermont	14	0.5%
45	Idaho	11	0.4%
45	Rhode Island	11	0.4%
47	Alaska	10	0.3%
48	Nevada	7	0.2%
49	Delaware	5	0.2%
49	Wyoming	5	0.2%
	District of Columbia	7	0.2%

Source: American Hospital Association (Chicago, IL)
   "Hospital Statistics" (2003 edition)
*Nongovernment not-for-profit hospitals are a subset of community hospitals.

Investor-Owned (For-Profit) Hospitals in 2001

National Total = 754 Hospitals*

ALPHA ORDER

RANK	STATE	HOSPITALS	% of USA
7	Alabama	30	4.0%
38	Alaska	1	0.1%
9	Arizona	20	2.7%
11	Arkansas	19	2.5%
3	California	89	11.8%
23	Colorado	8	1.1%
45	Connecticut	0	0.0%
45	Delaware	0	0.0%
2	Florida	95	12.6%
6	Georgia	32	4.2%
38	Hawaii	1	0.1%
34	Idaho	2	0.3%
23	Illinois	8	1.1%
18	Indiana	12	1.6%
38	Iowa	1	0.1%
21	Kansas	9	1.2%
12	Kentucky	18	2.4%
4	Louisiana	37	4.9%
38	Maine	1	0.1%
34	Maryland	2	0.3%
25	Massachusetts	6	0.8%
32	Michigan	3	0.4%
45	Minnesota	0	0.0%
8	Mississippi	24	3.2%
18	Missouri	12	1.6%
45	Montana	0	0.0%
34	Nebraska	2	0.3%
20	Nevada	10	1.3%
28	New Hampshire	4	0.5%
34	New Jersey	2	0.3%
25	New Mexico	6	0.8%
25	New York	6	0.8%
21	North Carolina	9	1.2%
38	North Dakota	1	0.1%
28	Ohio	4	0.5%
13	Oklahoma	15	2.0%
28	Oregon	4	0.5%
15	Pennsylvania	14	1.9%
45	Rhode Island	0	0.0%
9	South Carolina	20	2.7%
38	South Dakota	1	0.1%
5	Tennessee	36	4.8%
1	Texas	137	18.2%
17	Utah	13	1.7%
45	Vermont	0	0.0%
13	Virginia	15	2.0%
28	Washington	4	0.5%
15	West Virginia	14	1.9%
38	Wisconsin	1	0.1%
32	Wyoming	3	0.4%

RANK ORDER

RANK	STATE	HOSPITALS	% of USA
1	Texas	137	18.2%
2	Florida	95	12.6%
3	California	89	11.8%
4	Louisiana	37	4.9%
5	Tennessee	36	4.8%
6	Georgia	32	4.2%
7	Alabama	30	4.0%
8	Mississippi	24	3.2%
9	Arizona	20	2.7%
9	South Carolina	20	2.7%
11	Arkansas	19	2.5%
12	Kentucky	18	2.4%
13	Oklahoma	15	2.0%
13	Virginia	15	2.0%
15	Pennsylvania	14	1.9%
15	West Virginia	14	1.9%
17	Utah	13	1.7%
18	Indiana	12	1.6%
18	Missouri	12	1.6%
20	Nevada	10	1.3%
21	Kansas	9	1.2%
21	North Carolina	9	1.2%
23	Colorado	8	1.1%
23	Illinois	8	1.1%
25	Massachusetts	6	0.8%
25	New Mexico	6	0.8%
25	New York	6	0.8%
28	New Hampshire	4	0.5%
28	Ohio	4	0.5%
28	Oregon	4	0.5%
28	Washington	4	0.5%
32	Michigan	3	0.4%
32	Wyoming	3	0.4%
34	Idaho	2	0.3%
34	Maryland	2	0.3%
34	Nebraska	2	0.3%
34	New Jersey	2	0.3%
38	Alaska	1	0.1%
38	Hawaii	1	0.1%
38	Iowa	1	0.1%
38	Maine	1	0.1%
38	North Dakota	1	0.1%
38	South Dakota	1	0.1%
38	Wisconsin	1	0.1%
45	Connecticut	0	0.0%
45	Delaware	0	0.0%
45	Minnesota	0	0.0%
45	Montana	0	0.0%
45	Rhode Island	0	0.0%
45	Vermont	0	0.0%
	District of Columbia	3	0.4%

Source: American Hospital Association (Chicago, IL)
    "Hospital Statistics" (2003 edition)
*Investor-owned (for-profit) hospitals are a subset of community hospitals.

State and Local Government-Owned Hospitals in 2001

National Total = 1,156 Hospitals*

ALPHA ORDER

RANK	STATE	HOSPITALS	% of USA
11	Alabama	40	3.5%
32	Alaska	8	0.7%
38	Arizona	4	0.3%
26	Arkansas	15	1.3%
2	California	75	6.5%
18	Colorado	26	2.2%
44	Connecticut	1	0.1%
45	Delaware	0	0.0%
23	Florida	20	1.7%
6	Georgia	53	4.6%
32	Hawaii	8	0.7%
17	Idaho	27	2.3%
16	Illinois	28	2.4%
10	Indiana	41	3.5%
4	Iowa	59	5.1%
3	Kansas	62	5.4%
27	Kentucky	14	1.2%
5	Louisiana	55	4.8%
40	Maine	3	0.3%
45	Maryland	0	0.0%
38	Massachusetts	4	0.3%
23	Michigan	20	1.7%
9	Minnesota	43	3.7%
7	Mississippi	45	3.9%
14	Missouri	36	3.1%
29	Montana	11	1.0%
12	Nebraska	39	3.4%
34	Nevada	7	0.6%
45	New Hampshire	0	0.0%
41	New Jersey	2	0.2%
30	New Mexico	10	0.9%
20	New York	25	2.2%
15	North Carolina	32	2.8%
45	North Dakota	0	0.0%
21	Ohio	23	2.0%
7	Oklahoma	45	3.9%
28	Oregon	12	1.0%
41	Pennsylvania	2	0.2%
45	Rhode Island	0	0.0%
22	South Carolina	22	1.9%
36	South Dakota	6	0.5%
18	Tennessee	26	2.2%
1	Texas	128	11.1%
34	Utah	7	0.6%
45	Vermont	0	0.0%
37	Virginia	5	0.4%
12	Washington	39	3.4%
30	West Virginia	10	0.9%
41	Wisconsin	2	0.2%
25	Wyoming	16	1.4%

RANK ORDER

RANK	STATE	HOSPITALS	% of USA
1	Texas	128	11.1%
2	California	75	6.5%
3	Kansas	62	5.4%
4	Iowa	59	5.1%
5	Louisiana	55	4.8%
6	Georgia	53	4.6%
7	Mississippi	45	3.9%
7	Oklahoma	45	3.9%
9	Minnesota	43	3.7%
10	Indiana	41	3.5%
11	Alabama	40	3.5%
12	Nebraska	39	3.4%
12	Washington	39	3.4%
14	Missouri	36	3.1%
15	North Carolina	32	2.8%
16	Illinois	28	2.4%
17	Idaho	27	2.3%
18	Colorado	26	2.2%
18	Tennessee	26	2.2%
20	New York	25	2.2%
21	Ohio	23	2.0%
22	South Carolina	22	1.9%
23	Florida	20	1.7%
23	Michigan	20	1.7%
25	Wyoming	16	1.4%
26	Arkansas	15	1.3%
27	Kentucky	14	1.2%
28	Oregon	12	1.0%
29	Montana	11	1.0%
30	New Mexico	10	0.9%
30	West Virginia	10	0.9%
32	Alaska	8	0.7%
32	Hawaii	8	0.7%
34	Nevada	7	0.6%
34	Utah	7	0.6%
36	South Dakota	6	0.5%
37	Virginia	5	0.4%
38	Arizona	4	0.3%
38	Massachusetts	4	0.3%
40	Maine	3	0.3%
41	New Jersey	2	0.2%
41	Pennsylvania	2	0.2%
41	Wisconsin	2	0.2%
44	Connecticut	1	0.1%
45	Delaware	0	0.0%
45	Maryland	0	0.0%
45	New Hampshire	0	0.0%
45	North Dakota	0	0.0%
45	Rhode Island	0	0.0%
45	Vermont	0	0.0%
	District of Columbia	0	0.0%

Source: American Hospital Association (Chicago, IL)
 "Hospital Statistics" (2003 edition)
*State and local government-owned hospitals are a subset of community hospitals.

Beds in Community Hospitals in 2001

National Total = 825,966 Beds*

ALPHA ORDER

RANK	STATE	BEDS	% of USA
17	Alabama	16,627	2.0%
50	Alaska	1,442	0.2%
29	Arizona	10,732	1.3%
30	Arkansas	9,535	1.2%
1	California	73,291	8.9%
31	Colorado	9,442	1.1%
33	Connecticut	8,041	1.0%
48	Delaware	1,853	0.2%
4	Florida	51,762	6.3%
10	Georgia	24,113	2.9%
44	Hawaii	3,235	0.4%
43	Idaho	3,439	0.4%
6	Illinois	36,834	4.5%
14	Indiana	19,036	2.3%
23	Iowa	11,538	1.4%
27	Kansas	11,211	1.4%
21	Kentucky	15,001	1.8%
15	Louisiana	17,975	2.2%
40	Maine	3,844	0.5%
26	Maryland	11,234	1.4%
19	Massachusetts	16,504	2.0%
8	Michigan	25,630	3.1%
18	Minnesota	16,508	2.0%
22	Mississippi	13,670	1.7%
13	Missouri	19,257	2.3%
37	Montana	4,463	0.5%
32	Nebraska	8,324	1.0%
39	Nevada	4,099	0.5%
45	New Hampshire	2,853	0.3%
9	New Jersey	24,580	3.0%
42	New Mexico	3,584	0.4%
2	New York	67,296	8.1%
11	North Carolina	23,755	2.9%
41	North Dakota	3,717	0.5%
7	Ohio	33,310	4.0%
28	Oklahoma	11,207	1.4%
35	Oregon	6,660	0.8%
5	Pennsylvania	42,131	5.1%
46	Rhode Island	2,449	0.3%
25	South Carolina	11,282	1.4%
36	South Dakota	4,465	0.5%
12	Tennessee	20,600	2.5%
3	Texas	56,354	6.8%
38	Utah	4,437	0.5%
49	Vermont	1,694	0.2%
16	Virginia	16,775	2.0%
24	Washington	11,382	1.4%
34	West Virginia	7,906	1.0%
20	Wisconsin	15,597	1.9%
47	Wyoming	1,920	0.2%

RANK ORDER

RANK	STATE	BEDS	% of USA
1	California	73,291	8.9%
2	New York	67,296	8.1%
3	Texas	56,354	6.8%
4	Florida	51,762	6.3%
5	Pennsylvania	42,131	5.1%
6	Illinois	36,834	4.5%
7	Ohio	33,310	4.0%
8	Michigan	25,630	3.1%
9	New Jersey	24,580	3.0%
10	Georgia	24,113	2.9%
11	North Carolina	23,755	2.9%
12	Tennessee	20,600	2.5%
13	Missouri	19,257	2.3%
14	Indiana	19,036	2.3%
15	Louisiana	17,975	2.2%
16	Virginia	16,775	2.0%
17	Alabama	16,627	2.0%
18	Minnesota	16,508	2.0%
19	Massachusetts	16,504	2.0%
20	Wisconsin	15,597	1.9%
21	Kentucky	15,001	1.8%
22	Mississippi	13,670	1.7%
23	Iowa	11,538	1.4%
24	Washington	11,382	1.4%
25	South Carolina	11,282	1.4%
26	Maryland	11,234	1.4%
27	Kansas	11,211	1.4%
28	Oklahoma	11,207	1.4%
29	Arizona	10,732	1.3%
30	Arkansas	9,535	1.2%
31	Colorado	9,442	1.1%
32	Nebraska	8,324	1.0%
33	Connecticut	8,041	1.0%
34	West Virginia	7,906	1.0%
35	Oregon	6,660	0.8%
36	South Dakota	4,465	0.5%
37	Montana	4,463	0.5%
38	Utah	4,437	0.5%
39	Nevada	4,099	0.5%
40	Maine	3,844	0.5%
41	North Dakota	3,717	0.5%
42	New Mexico	3,584	0.4%
43	Idaho	3,439	0.4%
44	Hawaii	3,235	0.4%
45	New Hampshire	2,853	0.3%
46	Rhode Island	2,449	0.3%
47	Wyoming	1,920	0.2%
48	Delaware	1,853	0.2%
49	Vermont	1,694	0.2%
50	Alaska	1,442	0.2%
	District of Columbia	3,372	0.4%

Source: American Hospital Association (Chicago, IL)
       "Hospital Statistics" (2003 edition)
*All nonfederal short-term general and other special hospitals, whose facilities and services are available to the public. Includes beds in hospital and nursing home units.

Rate of Beds in Community Hospitals in 2001

National Rate = 289 Beds per 100,000 Population*

ALPHA ORDER

RANK	STATE	RATE
11	Alabama	372
40	Alaska	228
45	Arizona	202
14	Arkansas	354
43	California	212
42	Colorado	213
36	Connecticut	234
37	Delaware	233
20	Florida	316
28	Georgia	287
31	Hawaii	264
33	Idaho	260
23	Illinois	294
21	Indiana	311
9	Iowa	394
7	Kansas	415
12	Kentucky	369
8	Louisiana	402
22	Maine	299
44	Maryland	209
34	Massachusetts	258
35	Michigan	256
18	Minnesota	331
5	Mississippi	478
16	Missouri	342
3	Montana	493
4	Nebraska	484
47	Nevada	195
41	New Hampshire	227
25	New Jersey	289
46	New Mexico	196
15	New York	353
25	North Carolina	289
2	North Dakota	584
24	Ohio	292
19	Oklahoma	323
49	Oregon	192
16	Pennsylvania	342
39	Rhode Island	231
29	South Carolina	278
1	South Dakota	589
13	Tennessee	358
31	Texas	264
47	Utah	195
30	Vermont	276
37	Virginia	233
50	Washington	190
6	West Virginia	439
25	Wisconsin	289
10	Wyoming	389

RANK ORDER

RANK	STATE	RATE
1	South Dakota	589
2	North Dakota	584
3	Montana	493
4	Nebraska	484
5	Mississippi	478
6	West Virginia	439
7	Kansas	415
8	Louisiana	402
9	Iowa	394
10	Wyoming	389
11	Alabama	372
12	Kentucky	369
13	Tennessee	358
14	Arkansas	354
15	New York	353
16	Missouri	342
16	Pennsylvania	342
18	Minnesota	331
19	Oklahoma	323
20	Florida	316
21	Indiana	311
22	Maine	299
23	Illinois	294
24	Ohio	292
25	New Jersey	289
25	North Carolina	289
25	Wisconsin	289
28	Georgia	287
29	South Carolina	278
30	Vermont	276
31	Hawaii	264
31	Texas	264
33	Idaho	260
34	Massachusetts	258
35	Michigan	256
36	Connecticut	234
37	Delaware	233
37	Virginia	233
39	Rhode Island	231
40	Alaska	228
41	New Hampshire	227
42	Colorado	213
43	California	212
44	Maryland	209
45	Arizona	202
46	New Mexico	196
47	Nevada	195
47	Utah	195
49	Oregon	192
50	Washington	190

District of Columbia 588

Source: Morgan Quitno Press using data from American Hospital Association (Chicago, IL)
    "Hospital Statistics" (2003 edition)
*All nonfederal short-term general and other special hospitals, whose facilities and services are available to the
public. Includes beds in hospital and nursing home units.

Average Number of Beds per Community Hospital in 2001

National Average = 168 Beds per Community Hospital*

ALPHA ORDER

RANK	STATE	BEDS
23	Alabama	155
50	Alaska	76
17	Arizona	176
35	Arkansas	115
14	California	191
26	Colorado	143
5	Connecticut	230
1	Delaware	371
4	Florida	256
22	Georgia	164
28	Hawaii	141
46	Idaho	86
13	Illinois	192
18	Indiana	173
42	Iowa	99
47	Kansas	84
24	Kentucky	146
25	Louisiana	144
38	Maine	104
6	Maryland	229
9	Massachusetts	206
16	Michigan	177
33	Minnesota	124
27	Mississippi	142
21	Missouri	165
47	Montana	84
42	Nebraska	99
19	Nevada	171
40	New Hampshire	102
3	New Jersey	315
40	New Mexico	102
2	New York	317
8	North Carolina	214
44	North Dakota	93
11	Ohio	201
38	Oklahoma	104
36	Oregon	111
9	Pennsylvania	206
7	Rhode Island	223
15	South Carolina	182
45	South Dakota	89
20	Tennessee	167
30	Texas	137
37	Utah	106
34	Vermont	121
12	Virginia	193
31	Washington	136
29	West Virginia	139
32	Wisconsin	129
49	Wyoming	80

RANK ORDER

RANK	STATE	BEDS
1	Delaware	371
2	New York	317
3	New Jersey	315
4	Florida	256
5	Connecticut	230
6	Maryland	229
7	Rhode Island	223
8	North Carolina	214
9	Massachusetts	206
9	Pennsylvania	206
11	Ohio	201
12	Virginia	193
13	Illinois	192
14	California	191
15	South Carolina	182
16	Michigan	177
17	Arizona	176
18	Indiana	173
19	Nevada	171
20	Tennessee	167
21	Missouri	165
22	Georgia	164
23	Alabama	155
24	Kentucky	146
25	Louisiana	144
26	Colorado	143
27	Mississippi	142
28	Hawaii	141
29	West Virginia	139
30	Texas	137
31	Washington	136
32	Wisconsin	129
33	Minnesota	124
34	Vermont	121
35	Arkansas	115
36	Oregon	111
37	Utah	106
38	Maine	104
38	Oklahoma	104
40	New Hampshire	102
40	New Mexico	102
42	Iowa	99
42	Nebraska	99
44	North Dakota	93
45	South Dakota	89
46	Idaho	86
47	Kansas	84
47	Montana	84
49	Wyoming	80
50	Alaska	76
	District of Columbia	337

*Source: Morgan Quitno Press using data from American Hospital Association (Chicago, IL)
 "Hospital Statistics" (2003 edition)*
*All nonfederal short-term general and other special hospitals, whose facilities and services are available to the public. Includes beds in hospital and nursing home units.

Admissions to Community Hospitals in 2001

National Total = 33,813,589 Admissions*

ALPHA ORDER

RANK	STATE	ADMISSIONS	% of USA
17	Alabama	684,923	2.0%
49	Alaska	49,065	0.1%
23	Arizona	562,824	1.7%
29	Arkansas	371,080	1.1%
1	California	3,332,839	9.9%
28	Colorado	413,605	1.2%
31	Connecticut	360,007	1.1%
47	Delaware	83,047	0.2%
4	Florida	2,207,147	6.5%
11	Georgia	903,663	2.7%
43	Hawaii	108,252	0.3%
40	Idaho	122,510	0.4%
6	Illinois	1,559,357	4.6%
16	Indiana	718,369	2.1%
30	Iowa	370,885	1.1%
33	Kansas	322,067	1.0%
20	Kentucky	594,899	1.8%
18	Louisiana	682,586	2.0%
39	Maine	148,612	0.4%
19	Maryland	608,165	1.8%
13	Massachusetts	766,708	2.3%
8	Michigan	1,122,004	3.3%
21	Minnesota	586,016	1.7%
26	Mississippi	436,100	1.3%
12	Missouri	800,648	2.4%
45	Montana	103,346	0.3%
36	Nebraska	206,700	0.6%
35	Nevada	207,844	0.6%
42	New Hampshire	116,071	0.3%
9	New Jersey	1,083,798	3.2%
38	New Mexico	164,461	0.5%
3	New York	2,410,906	7.1%
10	North Carolina	973,451	2.9%
46	North Dakota	91,530	0.3%
7	Ohio	1,439,252	4.3%
27	Oklahoma	434,831	1.3%
32	Oregon	334,862	1.0%
5	Pennsylvania	1,808,531	5.3%
41	Rhode Island	120,901	0.4%
25	South Carolina	505,294	1.5%
44	South Dakota	103,907	0.3%
14	Tennessee	751,495	2.2%
2	Texas	2,461,016	7.3%
37	Utah	203,037	0.6%
48	Vermont	54,701	0.2%
15	Virginia	743,992	2.2%
24	Washington	522,624	1.5%
34	West Virginia	297,079	0.9%
22	Wisconsin	579,089	1.7%
50	Wyoming	47,587	0.1%

RANK ORDER

RANK	STATE	ADMISSIONS	% of USA
1	California	3,332,839	9.9%
2	Texas	2,461,016	7.3%
3	New York	2,410,906	7.1%
4	Florida	2,207,147	6.5%
5	Pennsylvania	1,808,531	5.3%
6	Illinois	1,559,357	4.6%
7	Ohio	1,439,252	4.3%
8	Michigan	1,122,004	3.3%
9	New Jersey	1,083,798	3.2%
10	North Carolina	973,451	2.9%
11	Georgia	903,663	2.7%
12	Missouri	800,648	2.4%
13	Massachusetts	766,708	2.3%
14	Tennessee	751,495	2.2%
15	Virginia	743,992	2.2%
16	Indiana	718,369	2.1%
17	Alabama	684,923	2.0%
18	Louisiana	682,586	2.0%
19	Maryland	608,165	1.8%
20	Kentucky	594,899	1.8%
21	Minnesota	586,016	1.7%
22	Wisconsin	579,089	1.7%
23	Arizona	562,824	1.7%
24	Washington	522,624	1.5%
25	South Carolina	505,294	1.5%
26	Mississippi	436,100	1.3%
27	Oklahoma	434,831	1.3%
28	Colorado	413,605	1.2%
29	Arkansas	371,080	1.1%
30	Iowa	370,885	1.1%
31	Connecticut	360,007	1.1%
32	Oregon	334,862	1.0%
33	Kansas	322,067	1.0%
34	West Virginia	297,079	0.9%
35	Nevada	207,844	0.6%
36	Nebraska	206,700	0.6%
37	Utah	203,037	0.6%
38	New Mexico	164,461	0.5%
39	Maine	148,612	0.4%
40	Idaho	122,510	0.4%
41	Rhode Island	120,901	0.4%
42	New Hampshire	116,071	0.3%
43	Hawaii	108,252	0.3%
44	South Dakota	103,907	0.3%
45	Montana	103,346	0.3%
46	North Dakota	91,530	0.3%
47	Delaware	83,047	0.2%
48	Vermont	54,701	0.2%
49	Alaska	49,065	0.1%
50	Wyoming	47,587	0.1%
	District of Columbia	131,906	0.4%

Source: American Hospital Association (Chicago, IL)
    "Hospital Statistics" (2003 edition)
*Admissions to all nonfederal short-term general and other special hospitals, whose facilities and services are available to the public. Includes admissions to hospital and nursing home units.

Inpatient Days in Community Hospitals in 2001

National Total = 194,106,316 Inpatient Days*

ALPHA ORDER   RANK ORDER

RANK	STATE	DAYS	% of USA
19	Alabama	3,570,273	1.8%
50	Alaska	303,092	0.2%
25	Arizona	2,520,301	1.3%
32	Arkansas	2,034,589	1.0%
2	California	17,835,799	9.2%
31	Colorado	2,111,549	1.1%
29	Connecticut	2,184,918	1.1%
47	Delaware	502,238	0.3%
4	Florida	11,521,025	5.9%
11	Georgia	5,484,805	2.8%
41	Hawaii	879,258	0.5%
44	Idaho	682,010	0.4%
6	Illinois	8,215,380	4.2%
17	Indiana	3,944,457	2.0%
27	Iowa	2,491,172	1.3%
30	Kansas	2,175,989	1.1%
21	Kentucky	3,315,218	1.7%
18	Louisiana	3,736,536	1.9%
40	Maine	898,059	0.5%
23	Maryland	2,981,003	1.5%
12	Massachusetts	4,382,048	2.3%
9	Michigan	6,108,896	3.1%
16	Minnesota	4,102,576	2.1%
22	Mississippi	2,990,906	1.5%
14	Missouri	4,219,659	2.2%
36	Montana	1,058,079	0.5%
33	Nebraska	1,826,566	0.9%
38	Nevada	1,019,835	0.5%
46	New Hampshire	637,239	0.3%
8	New Jersey	6,165,019	3.2%
43	New Mexico	758,923	0.4%
1	New York	19,021,960	9.8%
10	North Carolina	5,959,143	3.1%
42	North Dakota	787,722	0.4%
7	Ohio	7,483,873	3.9%
28	Oklahoma	2,360,979	1.2%
35	Oregon	1,449,556	0.7%
5	Pennsylvania	10,395,360	5.4%
45	Rhode Island	638,571	0.3%
24	South Carolina	2,940,707	1.5%
37	South Dakota	1,046,760	0.5%
15	Tennessee	4,122,419	2.1%
3	Texas	12,650,063	6.5%
39	Utah	902,313	0.5%
48	Vermont	403,993	0.2%
13	Virginia	4,239,227	2.2%
26	Washington	2,501,066	1.3%
34	West Virginia	1,806,411	0.9%
20	Wisconsin	3,455,633	1.8%
49	Wyoming	379,674	0.2%

RANK	STATE	DAYS	% of USA
1	New York	19,021,960	9.8%
2	California	17,835,799	9.2%
3	Texas	12,650,063	6.5%
4	Florida	11,521,025	5.9%
5	Pennsylvania	10,395,360	5.4%
6	Illinois	8,215,380	4.2%
7	Ohio	7,483,873	3.9%
8	New Jersey	6,165,019	3.2%
9	Michigan	6,108,896	3.1%
10	North Carolina	5,959,143	3.1%
11	Georgia	5,484,805	2.8%
12	Massachusetts	4,382,048	2.3%
13	Virginia	4,239,227	2.2%
14	Missouri	4,219,659	2.2%
15	Tennessee	4,122,419	2.1%
16	Minnesota	4,102,576	2.1%
17	Indiana	3,944,457	2.0%
18	Louisiana	3,736,536	1.9%
19	Alabama	3,570,273	1.8%
20	Wisconsin	3,455,633	1.8%
21	Kentucky	3,315,218	1.7%
22	Mississippi	2,990,906	1.5%
23	Maryland	2,981,003	1.5%
24	South Carolina	2,940,707	1.5%
25	Arizona	2,520,301	1.3%
26	Washington	2,501,066	1.3%
27	Iowa	2,491,172	1.3%
28	Oklahoma	2,360,979	1.2%
29	Connecticut	2,184,918	1.1%
30	Kansas	2,175,989	1.1%
31	Colorado	2,111,549	1.1%
32	Arkansas	2,034,589	1.0%
33	Nebraska	1,826,566	0.9%
34	West Virginia	1,806,411	0.9%
35	Oregon	1,449,556	0.7%
36	Montana	1,058,079	0.5%
37	South Dakota	1,046,760	0.5%
38	Nevada	1,019,835	0.5%
39	Utah	902,313	0.5%
40	Maine	898,059	0.5%
41	Hawaii	879,258	0.5%
42	North Dakota	787,722	0.4%
43	New Mexico	758,923	0.4%
44	Idaho	682,010	0.4%
45	Rhode Island	638,571	0.3%
46	New Hampshire	637,239	0.3%
47	Delaware	502,238	0.3%
48	Vermont	403,993	0.2%
49	Wyoming	379,674	0.2%
50	Alaska	303,092	0.2%
	District of Columbia	903,469	0.5%

Source: American Hospital Association (Chicago, IL)
    "Hospital Statistics" (2003 edition)
*Inpatient days in all nonfederal short-term general and other special hospitals, whose facilities and services are available to the public. Includes days in hospital and nursing home units.

Average Daily Census in Community Hospitals in 2001

National Average = 531,798 Inpatients*

RANK	STATE (ALPHA ORDER)	INPATIENTS		RANK	STATE (RANK ORDER)	INPATIENTS
19	Alabama	9,782		1	New York	52,115
50	Alaska	830		2	California	48,865
25	Arizona	6,905		3	Texas	34,658
32	Arkansas	5,574		4	Florida	31,564
2	California	48,865		5	Pennsylvania	28,480
31	Colorado	5,785		6	Illinois	22,508
29	Connecticut	5,986		7	Ohio	20,504
47	Delaware	1,376		8	New Jersey	16,890
4	Florida	31,564		9	Michigan	16,737
11	Georgia	15,027		10	North Carolina	16,326
41	Hawaii	2,409		11	Georgia	15,027
44	Idaho	1,869		12	Massachusetts	12,006
6	Illinois	22,508		13	Virginia	11,614
17	Indiana	10,807		14	Missouri	11,561
27	Iowa	6,825		15	Tennessee	11,294
30	Kansas	5,962		16	Minnesota	11,240
21	Kentucky	9,083		17	Indiana	10,807
18	Louisiana	10,237		18	Louisiana	10,237
40	Maine	2,460		19	Alabama	9,782
23	Maryland	8,167		20	Wisconsin	9,467
12	Massachusetts	12,006		21	Kentucky	9,083
9	Michigan	16,737		22	Mississippi	8,194
16	Minnesota	11,240		23	Maryland	8,167
22	Mississippi	8,194		24	South Carolina	8,057
14	Missouri	11,561		25	Arizona	6,905
36	Montana	2,899		26	Washington	6,852
33	Nebraska	5,004		27	Iowa	6,825
38	Nevada	2,794		28	Oklahoma	6,468
46	New Hampshire	1,746		29	Connecticut	5,986
8	New Jersey	16,890		30	Kansas	5,962
43	New Mexico	2,079		31	Colorado	5,785
1	New York	52,115		32	Arkansas	5,574
10	North Carolina	16,326		33	Nebraska	5,004
42	North Dakota	2,158		34	West Virginia	4,949
7	Ohio	20,504		35	Oregon	3,971
28	Oklahoma	6,468		36	Montana	2,899
35	Oregon	3,971		37	South Dakota	2,868
5	Pennsylvania	28,480		38	Nevada	2,794
45	Rhode Island	1,750		39	Utah	2,472
24	South Carolina	8,057		40	Maine	2,460
37	South Dakota	2,868		41	Hawaii	2,409
15	Tennessee	11,294		42	North Dakota	2,158
3	Texas	34,658		43	New Mexico	2,079
39	Utah	2,472		44	Idaho	1,869
48	Vermont	1,107		45	Rhode Island	1,750
13	Virginia	11,614		46	New Hampshire	1,746
26	Washington	6,852		47	Delaware	1,376
34	West Virginia	4,949		48	Vermont	1,107
20	Wisconsin	9,467		49	Wyoming	1,040
49	Wyoming	1,040		50	Alaska	830
					District of Columbia	2,475

Source: Morgan Quitno Press using data from American Hospital Association (Chicago, IL)
"Hospital Statistics" (2003 edition)
Average total of inpatients receiving care in all nonfederal short-term general and other special hospitals, whose facilities and services are available to the public. Excludes newborns.

Average Stay in Community Hospitals in 2001

National Average = 5.7 Days*

ALPHA ORDER

RANK	STATE	DAYS
39	Alabama	5.2
13	Alaska	6.2
48	Arizona	4.5
28	Arkansas	5.5
33	California	5.4
42	Colorado	5.1
14	Connecticut	6.1
18	Delaware	6.0
39	Florida	5.2
14	Georgia	6.1
5	Hawaii	8.1
26	Idaho	5.6
36	Illinois	5.3
28	Indiana	5.5
12	Iowa	6.7
11	Kansas	6.8
26	Kentucky	5.6
28	Louisiana	5.5
18	Maine	6.0
44	Maryland	4.9
22	Massachusetts	5.7
33	Michigan	5.4
9	Minnesota	7.0
10	Mississippi	6.9
36	Missouri	5.3
1	Montana	10.2
3	Nebraska	8.8
44	Nevada	4.9
28	New Hampshire	5.5
22	New Jersey	5.7
47	New Mexico	4.6
7	New York	7.9
14	North Carolina	6.1
4	North Dakota	8.6
39	Ohio	5.2
33	Oklahoma	5.4
50	Oregon	4.3
22	Pennsylvania	5.7
36	Rhode Island	5.3
21	South Carolina	5.8
2	South Dakota	10.1
28	Tennessee	5.5
42	Texas	5.1
49	Utah	4.4
8	Vermont	7.4
22	Virginia	5.7
46	Washington	4.8
14	West Virginia	6.1
18	Wisconsin	6.0
6	Wyoming	8.0

RANK ORDER

RANK	STATE	DAYS
1	Montana	10.2
2	South Dakota	10.1
3	Nebraska	8.8
4	North Dakota	8.6
5	Hawaii	8.1
6	Wyoming	8.0
7	New York	7.9
8	Vermont	7.4
9	Minnesota	7.0
10	Mississippi	6.9
11	Kansas	6.8
12	Iowa	6.7
13	Alaska	6.2
14	Connecticut	6.1
14	Georgia	6.1
14	North Carolina	6.1
14	West Virginia	6.1
18	Delaware	6.0
18	Maine	6.0
18	Wisconsin	6.0
21	South Carolina	5.8
22	Massachusetts	5.7
22	New Jersey	5.7
22	Pennsylvania	5.7
22	Virginia	5.7
26	Idaho	5.6
26	Kentucky	5.6
28	Arkansas	5.5
28	Indiana	5.5
28	Louisiana	5.5
28	New Hampshire	5.5
28	Tennessee	5.5
33	California	5.4
33	Michigan	5.4
33	Oklahoma	5.4
36	Illinois	5.3
36	Missouri	5.3
36	Rhode Island	5.3
39	Alabama	5.2
39	Florida	5.2
39	Ohio	5.2
42	Colorado	5.1
42	Texas	5.1
44	Maryland	4.9
44	Nevada	4.9
46	Washington	4.8
47	New Mexico	4.6
48	Arizona	4.5
49	Utah	4.4
50	Oregon	4.3
	District of Columbia	6.8

Source: American Hospital Association (Chicago, IL)
   "Hospital Statistics" (2003 edition)
*All nonfederal short-term general and other special hospitals, whose facilities and services are available to the public.

Occupancy Rate in Community Hospitals in 2001

National Rate = 64.4% of Community Hospital Beds Occupied*

ALPHA ORDER

RANK ORDER

RANK	STATE	PERCENT		RANK	STATE	PERCENT
38	Alabama	58.8		1	New York	77.4
43	Alaska	57.6		2	Hawaii	74.5
19	Arizona	64.3		3	Connecticut	74.4
39	Arkansas	58.5		4	Delaware	74.3
15	California	66.7		5	Maryland	72.7
26	Colorado	61.3		5	Massachusetts	72.7
3	Connecticut	74.4		7	Rhode Island	71.5
4	Delaware	74.3		8	South Carolina	71.4
29	Florida	61.0		9	Virginia	69.2
23	Georgia	62.3		10	New Jersey	68.7
2	Hawaii	74.5		10	North Carolina	68.7
48	Idaho	54.3		12	Nevada	68.2
28	Illinois	61.1		13	Minnesota	68.1
45	Indiana	56.8		14	Pennsylvania	67.6
37	Iowa	59.2		15	California	66.7
50	Kansas	53.2		16	Michigan	65.3
31	Kentucky	60.5		16	Vermont	65.3
44	Louisiana	57.0		18	Montana	65.0
21	Maine	64.0		19	Arizona	64.3
5	Maryland	72.7		20	South Dakota	64.2
5	Massachusetts	72.7		21	Maine	64.0
16	Michigan	65.3		22	West Virginia	62.6
13	Minnesota	68.1		23	Georgia	62.3
35	Mississippi	59.9		24	Ohio	61.6
34	Missouri	60.0		25	Texas	61.5
18	Montana	65.0		26	Colorado	61.3
33	Nebraska	60.1		27	New Hampshire	61.2
12	Nevada	68.2		28	Illinois	61.1
27	New Hampshire	61.2		29	Florida	61.0
10	New Jersey	68.7		30	Wisconsin	60.7
41	New Mexico	58.0		31	Kentucky	60.5
1	New York	77.4		32	Washington	60.2
10	North Carolina	68.7		33	Nebraska	60.1
40	North Dakota	58.1		34	Missouri	60.0
24	Ohio	61.6		35	Mississippi	59.9
42	Oklahoma	57.7		36	Oregon	59.6
36	Oregon	59.6		37	Iowa	59.2
14	Pennsylvania	67.6		38	Alabama	58.8
7	Rhode Island	71.5		39	Arkansas	58.5
8	South Carolina	71.4		40	North Dakota	58.1
20	South Dakota	64.2		41	New Mexico	58.0
47	Tennessee	54.8		42	Oklahoma	57.7
25	Texas	61.5		43	Alaska	57.6
46	Utah	55.7		44	Louisiana	57.0
16	Vermont	65.3		45	Indiana	56.8
9	Virginia	69.2		46	Utah	55.7
32	Washington	60.2		47	Tennessee	54.8
22	West Virginia	62.6		48	Idaho	54.3
30	Wisconsin	60.7		49	Wyoming	54.2
49	Wyoming	54.2		50	Kansas	53.2

District of Columbia   73.4

Source: Morgan Quitno Press using data from American Hospital Association (Chicago, IL)
"Hospital Statistics" (2003 edition)
*Average daily census compared to number of community hospital beds.

Outpatient Visits to Community Hospitals in 2001

National Total = 538,480,378 Visits*

ALPHA ORDER

RANK	STATE	VISITS	% of USA
23	Alabama	7,786,063	1.4%
48	Alaska	1,387,626	0.3%
31	Arizona	5,071,628	0.9%
33	Arkansas	4,493,774	0.8%
1	California	48,547,534	9.0%
26	Colorado	6,912,525	1.3%
27	Connecticut	6,489,426	1.2%
47	Delaware	1,484,918	0.3%
8	Florida	20,770,794	3.9%
14	Georgia	12,015,054	2.2%
39	Hawaii	3,167,587	0.6%
42	Idaho	2,640,078	0.5%
7	Illinois	25,269,913	4.7%
11	Indiana	14,393,285	2.7%
20	Iowa	9,399,353	1.7%
30	Kansas	5,394,028	1.0%
21	Kentucky	8,677,388	1.6%
16	Louisiana	10,060,381	1.9%
36	Maine	3,512,598	0.7%
28	Maryland	6,266,389	1.2%
9	Massachusetts	18,778,137	3.5%
6	Michigan	25,984,089	4.8%
22	Minnesota	8,565,860	1.6%
35	Mississippi	4,102,499	0.8%
12	Missouri	14,198,807	2.6%
41	Montana	2,648,345	0.5%
37	Nebraska	3,429,842	0.6%
44	Nevada	2,126,113	0.4%
40	New Hampshire	2,929,626	0.5%
10	New Jersey	18,444,560	3.4%
38	New Mexico	3,409,228	0.6%
2	New York	45,645,773	8.5%
13	North Carolina	13,430,676	2.5%
45	North Dakota	1,858,738	0.3%
5	Ohio	28,377,274	5.3%
32	Oklahoma	4,569,904	0.8%
24	Oregon	7,658,130	1.4%
3	Pennsylvania	32,063,424	6.0%
43	Rhode Island	2,151,240	0.4%
25	South Carolina	7,629,295	1.4%
46	South Dakota	1,828,098	0.3%
18	Tennessee	9,536,927	1.8%
4	Texas	31,453,948	5.8%
34	Utah	4,418,349	0.8%
49	Vermont	1,291,504	0.2%
17	Virginia	9,748,533	1.8%
19	Washington	9,432,504	1.8%
29	West Virginia	5,762,260	1.1%
15	Wisconsin	11,029,283	2.0%
50	Wyoming	818,022	0.2%

RANK ORDER

RANK	STATE	VISITS	% of USA
1	California	48,547,534	9.0%
2	New York	45,645,773	8.5%
3	Pennsylvania	32,063,424	6.0%
4	Texas	31,453,948	5.8%
5	Ohio	28,377,274	5.3%
6	Michigan	25,984,089	4.8%
7	Illinois	25,269,913	4.7%
8	Florida	20,770,794	3.9%
9	Massachusetts	18,778,137	3.5%
10	New Jersey	18,444,560	3.4%
11	Indiana	14,393,285	2.7%
12	Missouri	14,198,807	2.6%
13	North Carolina	13,430,676	2.5%
14	Georgia	12,015,054	2.2%
15	Wisconsin	11,029,283	2.0%
16	Louisiana	10,060,381	1.9%
17	Virginia	9,748,533	1.8%
18	Tennessee	9,536,927	1.8%
19	Washington	9,432,504	1.8%
20	Iowa	9,399,353	1.7%
21	Kentucky	8,677,388	1.6%
22	Minnesota	8,565,860	1.6%
23	Alabama	7,786,063	1.4%
24	Oregon	7,658,130	1.4%
25	South Carolina	7,629,295	1.4%
26	Colorado	6,912,525	1.3%
27	Connecticut	6,489,426	1.2%
28	Maryland	6,266,389	1.2%
29	West Virginia	5,762,260	1.1%
30	Kansas	5,394,028	1.0%
31	Arizona	5,071,628	0.9%
32	Oklahoma	4,569,904	0.8%
33	Arkansas	4,493,774	0.8%
34	Utah	4,418,349	0.8%
35	Mississippi	4,102,499	0.8%
36	Maine	3,512,598	0.7%
37	Nebraska	3,429,842	0.6%
38	New Mexico	3,409,228	0.6%
39	Hawaii	3,167,587	0.6%
40	New Hampshire	2,929,626	0.5%
41	Montana	2,648,345	0.5%
42	Idaho	2,640,078	0.5%
43	Rhode Island	2,151,240	0.4%
44	Nevada	2,126,113	0.4%
45	North Dakota	1,858,738	0.3%
46	South Dakota	1,828,098	0.3%
47	Delaware	1,484,918	0.3%
48	Alaska	1,387,626	0.3%
49	Vermont	1,291,504	0.2%
50	Wyoming	818,022	0.2%
	District of Columbia	1,419,048	0.3%

Source: American Hospital Association (Chicago, IL)
   "Hospital Statistics" (2003 edition)
*All nonfederal short-term general and other special hospitals, whose facilities and services are available to the public. Includes emergency and other visits.

Emergency Outpatient Visits to Community Hospitals in 2001

National Total = 105,957,778 Visits*

ALPHA ORDER

RANK ORDER

RANK	STATE	VISITS	% of USA	RANK	STATE	VISITS	% of USA
20	Alabama	1,959,967	1.8%	1	California	10,262,726	9.7%
49	Alaska	205,595	0.2%	2	Texas	7,806,334	7.4%
26	Arizona	1,401,509	1.3%	3	New York	7,452,574	7.0%
30	Arkansas	1,152,995	1.1%	4	Florida	5,879,596	5.5%
1	California	10,262,726	9.7%	5	Ohio	5,124,561	4.8%
27	Colorado	1,380,740	1.3%	6	Pennsylvania	4,873,595	4.6%
28	Connecticut	1,328,651	1.3%	7	Illinois	4,582,408	4.3%
45	Delaware	268,517	0.3%	8	Michigan	3,753,945	3.5%
4	Florida	5,879,596	5.5%	9	North Carolina	3,230,198	3.0%
10	Georgia	3,149,115	3.0%	10	Georgia	3,149,115	3.0%
43	Hawaii	287,017	0.3%	11	New Jersey	2,936,620	2.8%
42	Idaho	411,533	0.4%	12	Massachusetts	2,717,815	2.6%
7	Illinois	4,582,408	4.3%	13	Tennessee	2,710,481	2.6%
16	Indiana	2,385,242	2.3%	14	Virginia	2,482,380	2.3%
32	Iowa	1,063,304	1.0%	15	Missouri	2,443,744	2.3%
34	Kansas	907,083	0.9%	16	Indiana	2,385,242	2.3%
19	Kentucky	1,985,284	1.9%	17	Louisiana	2,267,490	2.1%
17	Louisiana	2,267,490	2.1%	18	Washington	2,063,313	1.9%
35	Maine	700,510	0.7%	19	Kentucky	1,985,284	1.9%
22	Maryland	1,854,562	1.8%	20	Alabama	1,959,967	1.8%
12	Massachusetts	2,717,815	2.6%	21	Wisconsin	1,866,201	1.8%
8	Michigan	3,753,945	3.5%	22	Maryland	1,854,562	1.8%
24	Minnesota	1,506,825	1.4%	23	South Carolina	1,840,819	1.7%
25	Mississippi	1,501,052	1.4%	24	Minnesota	1,506,825	1.4%
15	Missouri	2,443,744	2.3%	25	Mississippi	1,501,052	1.4%
44	Montana	276,175	0.3%	26	Arizona	1,401,509	1.3%
38	Nebraska	545,607	0.5%	27	Colorado	1,380,740	1.3%
37	Nevada	548,798	0.5%	28	Connecticut	1,328,651	1.3%
39	New Hampshire	537,367	0.5%	29	Oklahoma	1,226,716	1.2%
11	New Jersey	2,936,620	2.8%	30	Arkansas	1,152,995	1.1%
40	New Mexico	528,979	0.5%	31	Oregon	1,098,201	1.0%
3	New York	7,452,574	7.0%	32	Iowa	1,063,304	1.0%
9	North Carolina	3,230,198	3.0%	33	West Virginia	1,057,155	1.0%
46	North Dakota	259,673	0.2%	34	Kansas	907,083	0.9%
5	Ohio	5,124,561	4.8%	35	Maine	700,510	0.7%
29	Oklahoma	1,226,716	1.2%	36	Utah	699,934	0.7%
31	Oregon	1,098,201	1.0%	37	Nevada	548,798	0.5%
6	Pennsylvania	4,873,595	4.6%	38	Nebraska	545,607	0.5%
41	Rhode Island	451,325	0.4%	39	New Hampshire	537,367	0.5%
23	South Carolina	1,840,819	1.7%	40	New Mexico	528,979	0.5%
48	South Dakota	211,200	0.2%	41	Rhode Island	451,325	0.4%
13	Tennessee	2,710,481	2.6%	42	Idaho	411,533	0.4%
2	Texas	7,806,334	7.4%	43	Hawaii	287,017	0.3%
36	Utah	699,934	0.7%	44	Montana	276,175	0.3%
47	Vermont	237,773	0.2%	45	Delaware	268,517	0.3%
14	Virginia	2,482,380	2.3%	46	North Dakota	259,673	0.2%
18	Washington	2,063,313	1.9%	47	Vermont	237,773	0.2%
33	West Virginia	1,057,155	1.0%	48	South Dakota	211,200	0.2%
21	Wisconsin	1,866,201	1.8%	49	Alaska	205,595	0.2%
50	Wyoming	196,723	0.2%	50	Wyoming	196,723	0.2%
					District of Columbia	337,851	0.3%

Source: American Hospital Association (Chicago, IL)
    "Hospital Statistics" (2003 edition)
*All nonfederal short-term general and other special hospitals, whose facilities and services are available to the public.

Surgical Operations in Community Hospitals in 2001

National Total = 26,464,309 Surgical Operations*

ALPHA ORDER

RANK	STATE	OPERATIONS	% of USA
20	Alabama	484,083	1.8%
48	Alaska	53,737	0.2%
26	Arizona	356,918	1.3%
33	Arkansas	260,895	1.0%
1	California	2,152,812	8.1%
27	Colorado	325,599	1.2%
28	Connecticut	295,397	1.1%
44	Delaware	81,663	0.3%
5	Florida	1,517,602	5.7%
9	Georgia	781,897	3.0%
43	Hawaii	83,627	0.3%
42	Idaho	98,948	0.4%
7	Illinois	1,124,467	4.2%
16	Indiana	581,910	2.2%
25	Iowa	396,899	1.5%
34	Kansas	248,738	0.9%
18	Kentucky	526,436	2.0%
22	Louisiana	458,751	1.7%
38	Maine	159,828	0.6%
19	Maryland	513,858	1.9%
13	Massachusetts	680,456	2.6%
8	Michigan	1,023,833	3.9%
23	Minnesota	443,246	1.7%
32	Mississippi	270,609	1.0%
15	Missouri	599,128	2.3%
47	Montana	69,318	0.3%
35	Nebraska	197,546	0.7%
37	Nevada	168,175	0.6%
41	New Hampshire	109,169	0.4%
12	New Jersey	693,414	2.6%
40	New Mexico	123,442	0.5%
2	New York	1,947,693	7.4%
10	North Carolina	749,805	2.8%
46	North Dakota	69,532	0.3%
6	Ohio	1,211,012	4.6%
29	Oklahoma	294,169	1.1%
31	Oregon	280,424	1.1%
4	Pennsylvania	1,578,445	6.0%
39	Rhode Island	134,966	0.5%
24	South Carolina	435,354	1.6%
45	South Dakota	77,058	0.3%
14	Tennessee	645,162	2.4%
3	Texas	1,775,921	6.7%
36	Utah	182,117	0.7%
49	Vermont	52,490	0.2%
11	Virginia	703,536	2.7%
21	Washington	475,620	1.8%
30	West Virginia	286,558	1.1%
17	Wisconsin	543,578	2.1%
50	Wyoming	40,188	0.2%

RANK ORDER

RANK	STATE	OPERATIONS	% of USA
1	California	2,152,812	8.1%
2	New York	1,947,693	7.4%
3	Texas	1,775,921	6.7%
4	Pennsylvania	1,578,445	6.0%
5	Florida	1,517,602	5.7%
6	Ohio	1,211,012	4.6%
7	Illinois	1,124,467	4.2%
8	Michigan	1,023,833	3.9%
9	Georgia	781,897	3.0%
10	North Carolina	749,805	2.8%
11	Virginia	703,536	2.7%
12	New Jersey	693,414	2.6%
13	Massachusetts	680,456	2.6%
14	Tennessee	645,162	2.4%
15	Missouri	599,128	2.3%
16	Indiana	581,910	2.2%
17	Wisconsin	543,578	2.1%
18	Kentucky	526,436	2.0%
19	Maryland	513,858	1.9%
20	Alabama	484,083	1.8%
21	Washington	475,620	1.8%
22	Louisiana	458,751	1.7%
23	Minnesota	443,246	1.7%
24	South Carolina	435,354	1.6%
25	Iowa	396,899	1.5%
26	Arizona	356,918	1.3%
27	Colorado	325,599	1.2%
28	Connecticut	295,397	1.1%
29	Oklahoma	294,169	1.1%
30	West Virginia	286,558	1.1%
31	Oregon	280,424	1.1%
32	Mississippi	270,609	1.0%
33	Arkansas	260,895	1.0%
34	Kansas	248,738	0.9%
35	Nebraska	197,546	0.7%
36	Utah	182,117	0.7%
37	Nevada	168,175	0.6%
38	Maine	159,828	0.6%
39	Rhode Island	134,966	0.5%
40	New Mexico	123,442	0.5%
41	New Hampshire	109,169	0.4%
42	Idaho	98,948	0.4%
43	Hawaii	83,627	0.3%
44	Delaware	81,663	0.3%
45	South Dakota	77,058	0.3%
46	North Dakota	69,532	0.3%
47	Montana	69,318	0.3%
48	Alaska	53,737	0.2%
49	Vermont	52,490	0.2%
50	Wyoming	40,188	0.2%
	District of Columbia	98,280	0.4%

Source: American Hospital Association (Chicago, IL)
"Hospital Statistics" (2003 edition)
Includes inpatient and outpatient surgeries.

Medicare and Medicaid Certified Facilities in 2003

National Total = 235,360 Facilities*

ALPHA ORDER

RANK	STATE	FACILITIES	% of USA
19	Alabama	4,107	1.7%
49	Alaska	532	0.2%
27	Arizona	3,367	1.4%
32	Arkansas	2,692	1.1%
1	California	22,967	9.8%
30	Colorado	3,027	1.3%
28	Connecticut	3,210	1.4%
47	Delaware	761	0.3%
3	Florida	14,929	6.3%
9	Georgia	7,419	3.2%
45	Hawaii	934	0.4%
40	Idaho	1,110	0.5%
6	Illinois	10,089	4.3%
11	Indiana	6,306	2.7%
26	Iowa	3,563	1.5%
29	Kansas	3,204	1.4%
23	Kentucky	3,754	1.6%
14	Louisiana	5,232	2.2%
38	Maine	1,343	0.6%
18	Maryland	4,273	1.8%
17	Massachusetts	4,530	1.9%
8	Michigan	7,660	3.3%
25	Minnesota	3,633	1.5%
31	Mississippi	2,719	1.2%
13	Missouri	5,732	2.4%
43	Montana	966	0.4%
35	Nebraska	1,933	0.8%
39	Nevada	1,242	0.5%
41	New Hampshire	1,109	0.5%
12	New Jersey	6,038	2.6%
36	New Mexico	1,544	0.7%
4	New York	12,267	5.2%
10	North Carolina	6,956	3.0%
46	North Dakota	842	0.4%
5	Ohio	11,262	4.8%
22	Oklahoma	3,783	1.6%
33	Oregon	2,551	1.1%
7	Pennsylvania	9,701	4.1%
44	Rhode Island	946	0.4%
21	South Carolina	3,816	1.6%
42	South Dakota	986	0.4%
15	Tennessee	5,204	2.2%
2	Texas	19,085	8.1%
37	Utah	1,392	0.6%
48	Vermont	553	0.2%
16	Virginia	5,146	2.2%
24	Washington	3,728	1.6%
34	West Virginia	2,128	0.9%
20	Wisconsin	3,896	1.7%
50	Wyoming	523	0.2%

RANK ORDER

RANK	STATE	FACILITIES	% of USA
1	California	22,967	9.8%
2	Texas	19,085	8.1%
3	Florida	14,929	6.3%
4	New York	12,267	5.2%
5	Ohio	11,262	4.8%
6	Illinois	10,089	4.3%
7	Pennsylvania	9,701	4.1%
8	Michigan	7,660	3.3%
9	Georgia	7,419	3.2%
10	North Carolina	6,956	3.0%
11	Indiana	6,306	2.7%
12	New Jersey	6,038	2.6%
13	Missouri	5,732	2.4%
14	Louisiana	5,232	2.2%
15	Tennessee	5,204	2.2%
16	Virginia	5,146	2.2%
17	Massachusetts	4,530	1.9%
18	Maryland	4,273	1.8%
19	Alabama	4,107	1.7%
20	Wisconsin	3,896	1.7%
21	South Carolina	3,816	1.6%
22	Oklahoma	3,783	1.6%
23	Kentucky	3,754	1.6%
24	Washington	3,728	1.6%
25	Minnesota	3,633	1.5%
26	Iowa	3,563	1.5%
27	Arizona	3,367	1.4%
28	Connecticut	3,210	1.4%
29	Kansas	3,204	1.4%
30	Colorado	3,027	1.3%
31	Mississippi	2,719	1.2%
32	Arkansas	2,692	1.1%
33	Oregon	2,551	1.1%
34	West Virginia	2,128	0.9%
35	Nebraska	1,933	0.8%
36	New Mexico	1,544	0.7%
37	Utah	1,392	0.6%
38	Maine	1,343	0.6%
39	Nevada	1,242	0.5%
40	Idaho	1,110	0.5%
41	New Hampshire	1,109	0.5%
42	South Dakota	986	0.4%
43	Montana	966	0.4%
44	Rhode Island	946	0.4%
45	Hawaii	934	0.4%
46	North Dakota	842	0.4%
47	Delaware	761	0.3%
48	Vermont	553	0.2%
49	Alaska	532	0.2%
50	Wyoming	523	0.2%
	District of Columbia	670	0.3%

Source: U.S. Department of Health and Human Services, Centers for Medicare and Medicaid Services
    OSCAR Report 10 (February 5, 2003)
*Certified by CMS to participate in the Medicare/Medicaid programs. All provider groups including hospitals, home health agencies, rural health centers, community mental health centers, nursing facilities, outpatient physical therapy facilities, hospices and laboratories. National total does not include 1,342 certified facilities in U.S. territories.

Medicare and Medicaid Certified Hospitals in 2003

National Total = 5,959 Hospitals*

ALPHA ORDER

RANK	STATE	HOSPITALS	% of USA
19	Alabama	121	2.0%
47	Alaska	24	0.4%
29	Arizona	84	1.4%
26	Arkansas	104	1.7%
2	California	447	7.5%
30	Colorado	83	1.4%
40	Connecticut	46	0.8%
50	Delaware	11	0.2%
5	Florida	229	3.8%
9	Georgia	176	3.0%
46	Hawaii	27	0.5%
41	Idaho	45	0.8%
6	Illinois	216	3.6%
11	Indiana	153	2.6%
20	Iowa	120	2.0%
12	Kansas	152	2.6%
21	Kentucky	116	1.9%
8	Louisiana	193	3.2%
43	Maine	41	0.7%
32	Maryland	67	1.1%
21	Massachusetts	116	1.9%
9	Michigan	176	3.0%
14	Minnesota	148	2.5%
25	Mississippi	106	1.8%
17	Missouri	138	2.3%
35	Montana	65	1.1%
28	Nebraska	95	1.6%
42	Nevada	42	0.7%
44	New Hampshire	30	0.5%
24	New Jersey	107	1.8%
37	New Mexico	52	0.9%
3	New York	256	4.3%
18	North Carolina	134	2.2%
38	North Dakota	50	0.8%
7	Ohio	211	3.5%
15	Oklahoma	147	2.5%
36	Oregon	62	1.0%
4	Pennsylvania	249	4.2%
49	Rhode Island	15	0.3%
31	South Carolina	75	1.3%
33	South Dakota	66	1.1%
13	Tennessee	149	2.5%
1	Texas	488	8.2%
39	Utah	49	0.8%
48	Vermont	16	0.3%
23	Virginia	111	1.9%
27	Washington	100	1.7%
33	West Virginia	66	1.1%
16	Wisconsin	142	2.4%
45	Wyoming	29	0.5%

RANK ORDER

RANK	STATE	HOSPITALS	% of USA
1	Texas	488	8.2%
2	California	447	7.5%
3	New York	256	4.3%
4	Pennsylvania	249	4.2%
5	Florida	229	3.8%
6	Illinois	216	3.6%
7	Ohio	211	3.5%
8	Louisiana	193	3.2%
9	Georgia	176	3.0%
9	Michigan	176	3.0%
11	Indiana	153	2.6%
12	Kansas	152	2.6%
13	Tennessee	149	2.5%
14	Minnesota	148	2.5%
15	Oklahoma	147	2.5%
16	Wisconsin	142	2.4%
17	Missouri	138	2.3%
18	North Carolina	134	2.2%
19	Alabama	121	2.0%
20	Iowa	120	2.0%
21	Kentucky	116	1.9%
21	Massachusetts	116	1.9%
23	Virginia	111	1.9%
24	New Jersey	107	1.8%
25	Mississippi	106	1.8%
26	Arkansas	104	1.7%
27	Washington	100	1.7%
28	Nebraska	95	1.6%
29	Arizona	84	1.4%
30	Colorado	83	1.4%
31	South Carolina	75	1.3%
32	Maryland	67	1.1%
33	South Dakota	66	1.1%
33	West Virginia	66	1.1%
35	Montana	65	1.1%
36	Oregon	62	1.0%
37	New Mexico	52	0.9%
38	North Dakota	50	0.8%
39	Utah	49	0.8%
40	Connecticut	46	0.8%
41	Idaho	45	0.8%
42	Nevada	42	0.7%
43	Maine	41	0.7%
44	New Hampshire	30	0.5%
45	Wyoming	29	0.5%
46	Hawaii	27	0.5%
47	Alaska	24	0.4%
48	Vermont	16	0.3%
49	Rhode Island	15	0.3%
50	Delaware	11	0.2%
	District of Columbia	14	0.2%

Source: U.S. Department of Health and Human Services, Centers for Medicare and Medicaid Services
    OSCAR Database (February 5, 2003)
*Certified by CMS to participate in the Medicare/Medicaid programs. Excludes licensed facilities that do not
accept federal funding and facilities managed by the Department of Veterans Affairs. National total does not
include 64 certified hospitals in U.S. territories.

Beds in Medicare and Medicaid Certified Hospitals in 2003

National Total = 944,933 Beds*

ALPHA ORDER					RANK ORDER			
RANK	STATE	BEDS	% of USA		RANK	STATE	BEDS	% of USA
17	Alabama	19,924	2.1%		1	California	83,100	8.8%
49	Alaska	1,526	0.2%		2	New York	75,621	8.0%
28	Arizona	11,872	1.3%		3	Texas	57,260	6.1%
31	Arkansas	11,024	1.2%		4	Florida	53,095	5.6%
1	California	83,100	8.8%		5	Illinois	47,378	5.0%
29	Colorado	11,408	1.2%		6	Ohio	47,071	5.0%
32	Connecticut	10,372	1.1%		7	Pennsylvania	42,780	4.5%
47	Delaware	2,321	0.2%		8	New Jersey	31,665	3.4%
4	Florida	53,095	5.6%		9	Michigan	30,834	3.3%
11	Georgia	25,257	2.7%		10	North Carolina	26,079	2.8%
46	Hawaii	2,738	0.3%		11	Georgia	25,257	2.7%
45	Idaho	2,874	0.3%		12	Tennessee	24,765	2.6%
5	Illinois	47,378	5.0%		13	Missouri	24,642	2.6%
16	Indiana	21,228	2.2%		14	Louisiana	22,487	2.4%
27	Iowa	12,000	1.3%		15	Virginia	21,371	2.3%
30	Kansas	11,369	1.2%		16	Indiana	21,228	2.2%
20	Kentucky	17,340	1.8%		17	Alabama	19,924	2.1%
14	Louisiana	22,487	2.4%		18	Massachusetts	19,741	2.1%
39	Maine	4,078	0.4%		19	Wisconsin	19,560	2.1%
22	Maryland	16,563	1.8%		20	Kentucky	17,340	1.8%
18	Massachusetts	19,741	2.1%		21	Minnesota	16,703	1.8%
9	Michigan	30,834	3.3%		22	Maryland	16,563	1.8%
21	Minnesota	16,703	1.8%		23	Oklahoma	14,833	1.6%
25	Mississippi	12,944	1.4%		24	Washington	13,973	1.5%
13	Missouri	24,642	2.6%		25	Mississippi	12,944	1.4%
44	Montana	2,919	0.3%		26	South Carolina	12,577	1.3%
35	Nebraska	7,089	0.8%		27	Iowa	12,000	1.3%
36	Nevada	5,197	0.5%		28	Arizona	11,872	1.3%
41	New Hampshire	3,366	0.4%		29	Colorado	11,408	1.2%
8	New Jersey	31,665	3.4%		30	Kansas	11,369	1.2%
38	New Mexico	4,944	0.5%		31	Arkansas	11,024	1.2%
2	New York	75,621	8.0%		32	Connecticut	10,372	1.1%
10	North Carolina	26,079	2.8%		33	West Virginia	9,481	1.0%
43	North Dakota	3,244	0.3%		34	Oregon	7,962	0.8%
6	Ohio	47,071	5.0%		35	Nebraska	7,089	0.8%
23	Oklahoma	14,833	1.6%		36	Nevada	5,197	0.5%
34	Oregon	7,962	0.8%		37	Utah	5,146	0.5%
7	Pennsylvania	42,780	4.5%		38	New Mexico	4,944	0.5%
40	Rhode Island	3,785	0.4%		39	Maine	4,078	0.4%
26	South Carolina	12,577	1.3%		40	Rhode Island	3,785	0.4%
42	South Dakota	3,324	0.4%		41	New Hampshire	3,366	0.4%
12	Tennessee	24,765	2.6%		42	South Dakota	3,324	0.4%
3	Texas	57,260	6.1%		43	North Dakota	3,244	0.3%
37	Utah	5,146	0.5%		44	Montana	2,919	0.3%
48	Vermont	2,061	0.2%		45	Idaho	2,874	0.3%
15	Virginia	21,371	2.3%		46	Hawaii	2,738	0.3%
24	Washington	13,973	1.5%		47	Delaware	2,321	0.2%
33	West Virginia	9,481	1.0%		48	Vermont	2,061	0.2%
19	Wisconsin	19,560	2.1%		49	Alaska	1,526	0.2%
50	Wyoming	1,511	0.2%		50	Wyoming	1,511	0.2%
						District of Columbia	4,531	0.5%

Source: U.S. Department of Health and Human Services, Centers for Medicare and Medicaid Services
    OSCAR Database (February 5, 2003)
*Beds in hospitals certified by CMS to participate in the Medicare/Medicaid programs. Excludes licensed facilities
that do not accept federal funding and facilities managed by the Department of Veterans Affairs. National total
does not include 11,133 beds in U.S. territories.

Medicare and Medicaid Certified Children's Hospitals in 2003

National Total = 80 Hospitals*

ALPHA ORDER

RANK	STATE	HOSPITALS	% of USA
9	Alabama	2	2.5%
33	Alaska	0	0.0%
9	Arizona	2	2.5%
21	Arkansas	1	1.3%
1	California	9	11.3%
21	Colorado	1	1.3%
21	Connecticut	1	1.3%
21	Delaware	1	1.3%
9	Florida	2	2.5%
9	Georgia	2	2.5%
21	Hawaii	1	1.3%
33	Idaho	0	0.0%
9	Illinois	2	2.5%
21	Indiana	1	1.3%
33	Iowa	0	0.0%
21	Kansas	1	1.3%
33	Kentucky	0	0.0%
21	Louisiana	1	1.3%
33	Maine	0	0.0%
9	Maryland	2	2.5%
9	Massachusetts	2	2.5%
21	Michigan	1	1.3%
5	Minnesota	3	3.8%
33	Mississippi	0	0.0%
5	Missouri	3	3.8%
33	Montana	0	0.0%
9	Nebraska	2	2.5%
33	Nevada	0	0.0%
33	New Hampshire	0	0.0%
21	New Jersey	1	1.3%
21	New Mexico	1	1.3%
9	New York	2	2.5%
33	North Carolina	0	0.0%
33	North Dakota	0	0.0%
2	Ohio	8	10.0%
9	Oklahoma	2	2.5%
33	Oregon	0	0.0%
4	Pennsylvania	6	7.5%
33	Rhode Island	0	0.0%
33	South Carolina	0	0.0%
33	South Dakota	0	0.0%
9	Tennessee	2	2.5%
2	Texas	8	10.0%
21	Utah	1	1.3%
33	Vermont	0	0.0%
5	Virginia	3	3.8%
9	Washington	2	2.5%
33	West Virginia	0	0.0%
5	Wisconsin	3	3.8%
33	Wyoming	0	0.0%

RANK ORDER

RANK	STATE	HOSPITALS	% of USA
1	California	9	11.3%
2	Ohio	8	10.0%
2	Texas	8	10.0%
4	Pennsylvania	6	7.5%
5	Minnesota	3	3.8%
5	Missouri	3	3.8%
5	Virginia	3	3.8%
5	Wisconsin	3	3.8%
9	Alabama	2	2.5%
9	Arizona	2	2.5%
9	Florida	2	2.5%
9	Georgia	2	2.5%
9	Illinois	2	2.5%
9	Maryland	2	2.5%
9	Massachusetts	2	2.5%
9	Nebraska	2	2.5%
9	New York	2	2.5%
9	Oklahoma	2	2.5%
9	Tennessee	2	2.5%
9	Washington	2	2.5%
21	Arkansas	1	1.3%
21	Colorado	1	1.3%
21	Connecticut	1	1.3%
21	Delaware	1	1.3%
21	Hawaii	1	1.3%
21	Indiana	1	1.3%
21	Kansas	1	1.3%
21	Louisiana	1	1.3%
21	Michigan	1	1.3%
21	New Jersey	1	1.3%
21	New Mexico	1	1.3%
21	Utah	1	1.3%
33	Alaska	0	0.0%
33	Idaho	0	0.0%
33	Iowa	0	0.0%
33	Kentucky	0	0.0%
33	Maine	0	0.0%
33	Mississippi	0	0.0%
33	Montana	0	0.0%
33	Nevada	0	0.0%
33	New Hampshire	0	0.0%
33	North Carolina	0	0.0%
33	North Dakota	0	0.0%
33	Oregon	0	0.0%
33	Rhode Island	0	0.0%
33	South Carolina	0	0.0%
33	South Dakota	0	0.0%
33	Vermont	0	0.0%
33	West Virginia	0	0.0%
33	Wyoming	0	0.0%
	District of Columbia	1	1.3%

Source: U.S. Department of Health and Human Services, Centers for Medicare and Medicaid Services
OSCAR Database (February 5, 2003)
*Certified by CMS to participate in the Medicare/Medicaid programs. National total does not include one facility in U.S. territories. Excludes licensed facilities that do not accept federal funding and facilities managed by the Department of Veterans Affairs.

Beds in Medicare and Medicaid Certified Children's Hospitals in 2003

National Total = 11,839 Beds*

ALPHA ORDER

RANK	STATE	BEDS	% of USA
9	Alabama	384	3.2%
33	Alaska	0	0.0%
32	Arizona	16	0.1%
14	Arkansas	280	2.4%
2	California	1,488	12.6%
17	Colorado	253	2.1%
26	Connecticut	97	0.8%
26	Delaware	97	0.8%
10	Florida	376	3.2%
8	Georgia	400	3.4%
20	Hawaii	201	1.7%
33	Idaho	0	0.0%
11	Illinois	351	3.0%
31	Indiana	20	0.2%
33	Iowa	0	0.0%
29	Kansas	34	0.3%
33	Kentucky	0	0.0%
21	Louisiana	188	1.6%
33	Maine	0	0.0%
23	Maryland	165	1.4%
6	Massachusetts	425	3.6%
19	Michigan	228	1.9%
12	Minnesota	329	2.8%
33	Mississippi	0	0.0%
5	Missouri	432	3.6%
33	Montana	0	0.0%
25	Nebraska	150	1.3%
33	Nevada	0	0.0%
33	New Hampshire	0	0.0%
28	New Jersey	74	0.6%
30	New Mexico	28	0.2%
7	New York	405	3.4%
33	North Carolina	0	0.0%
33	North Dakota	0	0.0%
1	Ohio	1,809	15.3%
24	Oklahoma	160	1.4%
33	Oregon	0	0.0%
4	Pennsylvania	679	5.7%
33	Rhode Island	0	0.0%
33	South Carolina	0	0.0%
33	South Dakota	0	0.0%
22	Tennessee	175	1.5%
3	Texas	1,282	10.8%
18	Utah	232	2.0%
33	Vermont	0	0.0%
13	Virginia	286	2.4%
15	Washington	276	2.3%
33	West Virginia	0	0.0%
15	Wisconsin	276	2.3%
33	Wyoming	0	0.0%

RANK ORDER

RANK	STATE	BEDS	% of USA
1	Ohio	1,809	15.3%
2	California	1,488	12.6%
3	Texas	1,282	10.8%
4	Pennsylvania	679	5.7%
5	Missouri	432	3.6%
6	Massachusetts	425	3.6%
7	New York	405	3.4%
8	Georgia	400	3.4%
9	Alabama	384	3.2%
10	Florida	376	3.2%
11	Illinois	351	3.0%
12	Minnesota	329	2.8%
13	Virginia	286	2.4%
14	Arkansas	280	2.4%
15	Washington	276	2.3%
15	Wisconsin	276	2.3%
17	Colorado	253	2.1%
18	Utah	232	2.0%
19	Michigan	228	1.9%
20	Hawaii	201	1.7%
21	Louisiana	188	1.6%
22	Tennessee	175	1.5%
23	Maryland	165	1.4%
24	Oklahoma	160	1.4%
25	Nebraska	150	1.3%
26	Connecticut	97	0.8%
26	Delaware	97	0.8%
28	New Jersey	74	0.6%
29	Kansas	34	0.3%
30	New Mexico	28	0.2%
31	Indiana	20	0.2%
32	Arizona	16	0.1%
33	Alaska	0	0.0%
33	Idaho	0	0.0%
33	Iowa	0	0.0%
33	Kentucky	0	0.0%
33	Maine	0	0.0%
33	Mississippi	0	0.0%
33	Montana	0	0.0%
33	Nevada	0	0.0%
33	New Hampshire	0	0.0%
33	North Carolina	0	0.0%
33	North Dakota	0	0.0%
33	Oregon	0	0.0%
33	Rhode Island	0	0.0%
33	South Carolina	0	0.0%
33	South Dakota	0	0.0%
33	Vermont	0	0.0%
33	West Virginia	0	0.0%
33	Wyoming	0	0.0%
	District of Columbia	243	2.1%

*Source: U.S. Department of Health and Human Services, Centers for Medicare and Medicaid Services
OSCAR Database (February 5, 2003)*

*Beds in hospitals certified by CMS to participate in the Medicare/Medicaid programs. Excludes licensed facilities that do not accept federal funding and facilities managed by the Department of Veterans Affairs. National total does not include 215 beds in U.S. territories.

Medicare and Medicaid Certified Rehabilitation Hospitals in 2003

National Total = 212 Hospitals*

ALPHA ORDER

RANK	STATE	HOSPITALS	% of USA
8	Alabama	6	2.8%
42	Alaska	0	0.0%
23	Arizona	3	1.4%
8	Arkansas	6	2.8%
6	California	7	3.3%
26	Colorado	2	0.9%
32	Connecticut	1	0.5%
32	Delaware	1	0.5%
4	Florida	13	6.1%
26	Georgia	2	0.9%
32	Hawaii	1	0.5%
32	Idaho	1	0.5%
16	Illinois	4	1.9%
8	Indiana	6	2.8%
42	Iowa	0	0.0%
16	Kansas	4	1.9%
8	Kentucky	6	2.8%
2	Louisiana	25	11.8%
32	Maine	1	0.5%
23	Maryland	3	1.4%
6	Massachusetts	7	3.3%
14	Michigan	5	2.4%
32	Minnesota	1	0.5%
42	Mississippi	0	0.0%
23	Missouri	3	1.4%
42	Montana	0	0.0%
32	Nebraska	1	0.5%
14	Nevada	5	2.4%
26	New Hampshire	2	0.9%
5	New Jersey	8	3.8%
16	New Mexico	4	1.9%
16	New York	4	1.9%
26	North Carolina	2	0.9%
42	North Dakota	0	0.0%
26	Ohio	2	0.9%
16	Oklahoma	4	1.9%
42	Oregon	0	0.0%
3	Pennsylvania	17	8.0%
32	Rhode Island	1	0.5%
16	South Carolina	4	1.9%
42	South Dakota	0	0.0%
8	Tennessee	6	2.8%
1	Texas	29	13.7%
26	Utah	2	0.9%
42	Vermont	0	0.0%
16	Virginia	4	1.9%
32	Washington	1	0.5%
8	West Virginia	6	2.8%
32	Wisconsin	1	0.5%
42	Wyoming	0	0.0%

RANK ORDER

RANK	STATE	HOSPITALS	% of USA
1	Texas	29	13.7%
2	Louisiana	25	11.8%
3	Pennsylvania	17	8.0%
4	Florida	13	6.1%
5	New Jersey	8	3.8%
6	California	7	3.3%
6	Massachusetts	7	3.3%
8	Alabama	6	2.8%
8	Arkansas	6	2.8%
8	Indiana	6	2.8%
8	Kentucky	6	2.8%
8	Tennessee	6	2.8%
8	West Virginia	6	2.8%
14	Michigan	5	2.4%
14	Nevada	5	2.4%
16	Illinois	4	1.9%
16	Kansas	4	1.9%
16	New Mexico	4	1.9%
16	New York	4	1.9%
16	Oklahoma	4	1.9%
16	South Carolina	4	1.9%
16	Virginia	4	1.9%
23	Arizona	3	1.4%
23	Maryland	3	1.4%
23	Missouri	3	1.4%
26	Colorado	2	0.9%
26	Georgia	2	0.9%
26	New Hampshire	2	0.9%
26	North Carolina	2	0.9%
26	Ohio	2	0.9%
26	Utah	2	0.9%
32	Connecticut	1	0.5%
32	Delaware	1	0.5%
32	Hawaii	1	0.5%
32	Idaho	1	0.5%
32	Maine	1	0.5%
32	Minnesota	1	0.5%
32	Nebraska	1	0.5%
32	Rhode Island	1	0.5%
32	Washington	1	0.5%
32	Wisconsin	1	0.5%
42	Alaska	0	0.0%
42	Iowa	0	0.0%
42	Mississippi	0	0.0%
42	Montana	0	0.0%
42	North Dakota	0	0.0%
42	Oregon	0	0.0%
42	South Dakota	0	0.0%
42	Vermont	0	0.0%
42	Wyoming	0	0.0%
	District of Columbia	1	0.5%

Source: U.S. Department of Health and Human Services, Centers for Medicare and Medicaid Services OSCAR Database (February 5, 2003)

Certified by CMS to participate in the Medicare/Medicaid programs. Excludes licensed facilities that do not accept federal funding and facilities managed by the Department of Veterans Affairs. National total does not include one certified hospital in U.S. territories.

Beds in Medicare and Medicaid Certified Rehabilitation Hospitals in 2003

National Total = 13,528 Beds*

ALPHA ORDER

RANK	STATE	BEDS	% of USA
13	Alabama	336	2.5%
42	Alaska	0	0.0%
25	Arizona	168	1.2%
7	Arkansas	459	3.4%
10	California	411	3.0%
24	Colorado	202	1.5%
37	Connecticut	60	0.4%
37	Delaware	60	0.4%
3	Florida	954	7.1%
30	Georgia	116	0.9%
32	Hawaii	100	0.7%
40	Idaho	59	0.4%
11	Illinois	408	3.0%
9	Indiana	418	3.1%
42	Iowa	0	0.0%
16	Kansas	257	1.9%
14	Kentucky	328	2.4%
6	Louisiana	531	3.9%
32	Maine	100	0.7%
29	Maryland	121	0.9%
4	Massachusetts	739	5.5%
15	Michigan	315	2.3%
41	Minnesota	15	0.1%
42	Mississippi	0	0.0%
22	Missouri	220	1.6%
42	Montana	0	0.0%
37	Nebraska	60	0.4%
16	Nevada	257	1.9%
26	New Hampshire	152	1.1%
5	New Jersey	726	5.4%
27	New Mexico	149	1.1%
8	New York	428	3.2%
20	North Carolina	233	1.7%
42	North Dakota	0	0.0%
28	Ohio	145	1.1%
21	Oklahoma	227	1.7%
42	Oregon	0	0.0%
2	Pennsylvania	1,558	11.5%
35	Rhode Island	82	0.6%
19	South Carolina	239	1.8%
42	South Dakota	0	0.0%
12	Tennessee	370	2.7%
1	Texas	1,633	12.1%
34	Utah	98	0.7%
42	Vermont	0	0.0%
23	Virginia	205	1.5%
31	Washington	102	0.8%
18	West Virginia	246	1.8%
36	Wisconsin	81	0.6%
42	Wyoming	0	0.0%

RANK ORDER

RANK	STATE	BEDS	% of USA
1	Texas	1,633	12.1%
2	Pennsylvania	1,558	11.5%
3	Florida	954	7.1%
4	Massachusetts	739	5.5%
5	New Jersey	726	5.4%
6	Louisiana	531	3.9%
7	Arkansas	459	3.4%
8	New York	428	3.2%
9	Indiana	418	3.1%
10	California	411	3.0%
11	Illinois	408	3.0%
12	Tennessee	370	2.7%
13	Alabama	336	2.5%
14	Kentucky	328	2.4%
15	Michigan	315	2.3%
16	Kansas	257	1.9%
16	Nevada	257	1.9%
18	West Virginia	246	1.8%
19	South Carolina	239	1.8%
20	North Carolina	233	1.7%
21	Oklahoma	227	1.7%
22	Missouri	220	1.6%
23	Virginia	205	1.5%
24	Colorado	202	1.5%
25	Arizona	168	1.2%
26	New Hampshire	152	1.1%
27	New Mexico	149	1.1%
28	Ohio	145	1.1%
29	Maryland	121	0.9%
30	Georgia	116	0.9%
31	Washington	102	0.8%
32	Hawaii	100	0.7%
32	Maine	100	0.7%
34	Utah	98	0.7%
35	Rhode Island	82	0.6%
36	Wisconsin	81	0.6%
37	Connecticut	60	0.4%
37	Delaware	60	0.4%
37	Nebraska	60	0.4%
40	Idaho	59	0.4%
41	Minnesota	15	0.1%
42	Alaska	0	0.0%
42	Iowa	0	0.0%
42	Mississippi	0	0.0%
42	Montana	0	0.0%
42	North Dakota	0	0.0%
42	Oregon	0	0.0%
42	South Dakota	0	0.0%
42	Vermont	0	0.0%
42	Wyoming	0	0.0%
	District of Columbia	160	1.2%

Source: U.S. Department of Health and Human Services, Centers for Medicare and Medicaid Services
OSCAR Database (February 5, 2003)
*Beds in hospitals certified by CMS to participate in the Medicare/Medicaid programs. Excludes licensed facilities that do not accept federal funding and facilities managed by the Department of Veterans Affairs. National total does not include 30 beds in U.S. territories.

Medicare and Medicaid Certified Psychiatric Hospitals in 2003

National Total = 478 Psychiatric Hospitals*

<u>ALPHA ORDER</u>

RANK	STATE	HOSPITALS	% of USA
23	Alabama	9	1.9%
43	Alaska	2	0.4%
27	Arizona	6	1.3%
18	Arkansas	10	2.1%
1	California	33	6.9%
27	Colorado	6	1.3%
24	Connecticut	8	1.7%
38	Delaware	3	0.6%
5	Florida	20	4.2%
12	Georgia	14	2.9%
49	Hawaii	1	0.2%
31	Idaho	5	1.0%
8	Illinois	16	3.3%
6	Indiana	19	4.0%
32	Iowa	4	0.8%
32	Kansas	4	0.8%
15	Kentucky	11	2.3%
11	Louisiana	15	3.1%
32	Maine	4	0.8%
18	Maryland	10	2.1%
7	Massachusetts	18	3.8%
18	Michigan	10	2.1%
25	Minnesota	7	1.5%
32	Mississippi	4	0.8%
12	Missouri	14	2.9%
43	Montana	2	0.4%
27	Nebraska	6	1.3%
38	Nevada	3	0.6%
43	New Hampshire	2	0.4%
8	New Jersey	16	3.3%
38	New Mexico	3	0.6%
3	New York	30	6.3%
18	North Carolina	10	2.1%
38	North Dakota	3	0.6%
8	Ohio	16	3.3%
18	Oklahoma	10	2.1%
38	Oregon	3	0.6%
4	Pennsylvania	23	4.8%
43	Rhode Island	2	0.4%
25	South Carolina	7	1.5%
49	South Dakota	1	0.2%
15	Tennessee	11	2.3%
1	Texas	33	6.9%
32	Utah	4	0.8%
43	Vermont	2	0.4%
14	Virginia	12	2.5%
27	Washington	6	1.3%
32	West Virginia	4	0.8%
15	Wisconsin	11	2.3%
43	Wyoming	2	0.4%

<u>RANK ORDER</u>

RANK	STATE	HOSPITALS	% of USA
1	California	33	6.9%
1	Texas	33	6.9%
3	New York	30	6.3%
4	Pennsylvania	23	4.8%
5	Florida	20	4.2%
6	Indiana	19	4.0%
7	Massachusetts	18	3.8%
8	Illinois	16	3.3%
8	New Jersey	16	3.3%
8	Ohio	16	3.3%
11	Louisiana	15	3.1%
12	Georgia	14	2.9%
12	Missouri	14	2.9%
14	Virginia	12	2.5%
15	Kentucky	11	2.3%
15	Tennessee	11	2.3%
15	Wisconsin	11	2.3%
18	Arkansas	10	2.1%
18	Maryland	10	2.1%
18	Michigan	10	2.1%
18	North Carolina	10	2.1%
18	Oklahoma	10	2.1%
23	Alabama	9	1.9%
24	Connecticut	8	1.7%
25	Minnesota	7	1.5%
25	South Carolina	7	1.5%
27	Arizona	6	1.3%
27	Colorado	6	1.3%
27	Nebraska	6	1.3%
27	Washington	6	1.3%
31	Idaho	5	1.0%
32	Iowa	4	0.8%
32	Kansas	4	0.8%
32	Maine	4	0.8%
32	Mississippi	4	0.8%
32	Utah	4	0.8%
32	West Virginia	4	0.8%
38	Delaware	3	0.6%
38	Nevada	3	0.6%
38	New Mexico	3	0.6%
38	North Dakota	3	0.6%
38	Oregon	3	0.6%
43	Alaska	2	0.4%
43	Montana	2	0.4%
43	New Hampshire	2	0.4%
43	Rhode Island	2	0.4%
43	Vermont	2	0.4%
43	Wyoming	2	0.4%
49	Hawaii	1	0.2%
49	South Dakota	1	0.2%
	District of Columbia	3	0.6%

Source: U.S. Department of Health and Human Services, Centers for Medicare and Medicaid Services
        OSCAR Database (February 5, 2003)
*Certified by CMS to participate in the Medicare/Medicaid programs. Excludes licensed facilities that do not accept federal funding and facilities managed by the Department of Veterans Affairs. National total does not include four certified psychiatric hospitals in U.S. territories.

Beds in Medicare and Medicaid Certified Psychiatric Hospitals in 2003

National Total = 58,791 Beds*

ALPHA ORDER

RANK ORDER

RANK	STATE	BEDS	% of USA	RANK	STATE	BEDS	% of USA
28	Alabama	643	1.1%	1	New York	7,212	12.3%
44	Alaska	188	0.3%	2	Pennsylvania	4,746	8.1%
31	Arizona	530	0.9%	3	New Jersey	3,219	5.5%
26	Arkansas	863	1.5%	4	Texas	2,583	4.4%
7	California	2,405	4.1%	5	North Carolina	2,579	4.4%
25	Colorado	890	1.5%	6	Maryland	2,557	4.3%
19	Connecticut	1,220	2.1%	7	California	2,405	4.1%
41	Delaware	237	0.4%	8	Michigan	2,025	3.4%
13	Florida	1,501	2.6%	9	Georgia	1,693	2.9%
9	Georgia	1,693	2.9%	10	Illinois	1,670	2.8%
49	Hawaii	88	0.1%	11	Ohio	1,538	2.6%
48	Idaho	117	0.2%	12	Massachusetts	1,522	2.6%
10	Illinois	1,670	2.8%	13	Florida	1,501	2.6%
18	Indiana	1,258	2.1%	14	Washington	1,492	2.5%
35	Iowa	363	0.6%	15	Louisiana	1,460	2.5%
29	Kansas	561	1.0%	16	Wisconsin	1,409	2.4%
17	Kentucky	1,263	2.1%	17	Kentucky	1,263	2.1%
15	Louisiana	1,460	2.5%	18	Indiana	1,258	2.1%
34	Maine	364	0.6%	19	Connecticut	1,220	2.1%
6	Maryland	2,557	4.3%	20	Virginia	1,177	2.0%
12	Massachusetts	1,522	2.6%	21	Minnesota	1,131	1.9%
8	Michigan	2,025	3.4%	22	Tennessee	1,072	1.8%
21	Minnesota	1,131	1.9%	23	Missouri	1,006	1.7%
38	Mississippi	273	0.5%	24	Nebraska	978	1.7%
23	Missouri	1,006	1.7%	25	Colorado	890	1.5%
45	Montana	182	0.3%	26	Arkansas	863	1.5%
24	Nebraska	978	1.7%	27	South Carolina	802	1.4%
39	Nevada	268	0.5%	28	Alabama	643	1.1%
36	New Hampshire	323	0.5%	29	Kansas	561	1.0%
3	New Jersey	3,219	5.5%	30	Oklahoma	555	0.9%
40	New Mexico	245	0.4%	31	Arizona	530	0.9%
1	New York	7,212	12.3%	32	Utah	485	0.8%
5	North Carolina	2,579	4.4%	32	West Virginia	485	0.8%
42	North Dakota	229	0.4%	34	Maine	364	0.6%
11	Ohio	1,538	2.6%	35	Iowa	363	0.6%
30	Oklahoma	555	0.9%	36	New Hampshire	323	0.5%
37	Oregon	296	0.5%	37	Oregon	296	0.5%
2	Pennsylvania	4,746	8.1%	38	Mississippi	273	0.5%
46	Rhode Island	165	0.3%	39	Nevada	268	0.5%
27	South Carolina	802	1.4%	40	New Mexico	245	0.4%
47	South Dakota	133	0.2%	41	Delaware	237	0.4%
22	Tennessee	1,072	1.8%	42	North Dakota	229	0.4%
4	Texas	2,583	4.4%	43	Vermont	205	0.3%
32	Utah	485	0.8%	44	Alaska	188	0.3%
43	Vermont	205	0.3%	45	Montana	182	0.3%
20	Virginia	1,177	2.0%	46	Rhode Island	165	0.3%
14	Washington	1,492	2.5%	47	South Dakota	133	0.2%
32	West Virginia	485	0.8%	48	Idaho	117	0.2%
16	Wisconsin	1,409	2.4%	49	Hawaii	88	0.1%
50	Wyoming	68	0.1%	50	Wyoming	68	0.1%
					District of Columbia	517	0.9%

Source: U.S. Department of Health and Human Services, Centers for Medicare and Medicaid Services
    OSCAR Database (February 5, 2003)
*Beds in hospitals certified by CMS to participate in the Medicare/Medicaid programs. Excludes licensed facilities
that do not accept federal funding and facilities managed by the Department of Veterans Affairs. National total
does not include 903 beds in U.S. territories.

Medicare and Medicaid Certified Community Mental Health Centers in 2003

National Total = 625 Centers*

ALPHA ORDER

RANK	STATE	CENTERS	% of USA
2	Alabama	72	11.5%
43	Alaska	0	0.0%
30	Arizona	3	0.5%
17	Arkansas	14	2.2%
8	California	20	3.2%
17	Colorado	14	2.2%
29	Connecticut	4	0.6%
43	Delaware	0	0.0%
1	Florida	94	15.0%
23	Georgia	8	1.3%
43	Hawaii	0	0.0%
43	Idaho	0	0.0%
13	Illinois	15	2.4%
22	Indiana	11	1.8%
25	Iowa	7	1.1%
13	Kansas	15	2.4%
19	Kentucky	13	2.1%
5	Louisiana	32	5.1%
40	Maine	1	0.2%
35	Maryland	2	0.3%
13	Massachusetts	15	2.4%
25	Michigan	7	1.1%
19	Minnesota	13	2.1%
27	Mississippi	5	0.8%
11	Missouri	17	2.7%
40	Montana	1	0.2%
40	Nebraska	1	0.2%
35	Nevada	2	0.3%
35	New Hampshire	2	0.3%
4	New Jersey	37	5.9%
13	New Mexico	15	2.4%
27	New York	5	0.8%
7	North Carolina	22	3.5%
43	North Dakota	0	0.0%
10	Ohio	19	3.0%
23	Oklahoma	8	1.3%
21	Oregon	12	1.9%
12	Pennsylvania	16	2.6%
43	Rhode Island	0	0.0%
35	South Carolina	2	0.3%
35	South Dakota	2	0.3%
8	Tennessee	20	3.2%
3	Texas	39	6.2%
30	Utah	3	0.5%
43	Vermont	0	0.0%
30	Virginia	3	0.5%
6	Washington	28	4.5%
30	West Virginia	3	0.5%
43	Wisconsin	0	0.0%
30	Wyoming	3	0.5%

RANK ORDER

RANK	STATE	CENTERS	% of USA
1	Florida	94	15.0%
2	Alabama	72	11.5%
3	Texas	39	6.2%
4	New Jersey	37	5.9%
5	Louisiana	32	5.1%
6	Washington	28	4.5%
7	North Carolina	22	3.5%
8	California	20	3.2%
8	Tennessee	20	3.2%
10	Ohio	19	3.0%
11	Missouri	17	2.7%
12	Pennsylvania	16	2.6%
13	Illinois	15	2.4%
13	Kansas	15	2.4%
13	Massachusetts	15	2.4%
13	New Mexico	15	2.4%
17	Arkansas	14	2.2%
17	Colorado	14	2.2%
19	Kentucky	13	2.1%
19	Minnesota	13	2.1%
21	Oregon	12	1.9%
22	Indiana	11	1.8%
23	Georgia	8	1.3%
23	Oklahoma	8	1.3%
25	Iowa	7	1.1%
25	Michigan	7	1.1%
27	Mississippi	5	0.8%
27	New York	5	0.8%
29	Connecticut	4	0.6%
30	Arizona	3	0.5%
30	Utah	3	0.5%
30	Virginia	3	0.5%
30	West Virginia	3	0.5%
30	Wyoming	3	0.5%
35	Maryland	2	0.3%
35	Nevada	2	0.3%
35	New Hampshire	2	0.3%
35	South Carolina	2	0.3%
35	South Dakota	2	0.3%
40	Maine	1	0.2%
40	Montana	1	0.2%
40	Nebraska	1	0.2%
43	Alaska	0	0.0%
43	Delaware	0	0.0%
43	Hawaii	0	0.0%
43	Idaho	0	0.0%
43	North Dakota	0	0.0%
43	Rhode Island	0	0.0%
43	Vermont	0	0.0%
43	Wisconsin	0	0.0%
	District of Columbia	0	0.0%

Source: U.S. Department of Health and Human Services, Centers for Medicare and Medicaid Services OSCAR Report 10 (February 5, 2003)

Certified by CMS to participate in the Medicare/Medicaid programs. Excludes licensed facilities that do not accept federal funding and facilities managed by the Department of Veterans Affairs. National total does not include nine certified mental health centers in U.S. territories.

Medicare and Medicaid Certified Outpatient Physical Therapy Facilities in 2003

National Total = 2,968 Facilities*

ALPHA ORDER					RANK ORDER			
RANK	STATE	FACILITIES	% of USA		RANK	STATE	FACILITIES	% of USA
33	Alabama	21	0.7%		1	Florida	291	9.8%
37	Alaska	17	0.6%		2	Michigan	235	7.9%
27	Arizona	31	1.0%		3	California	217	7.3%
29	Arkansas	30	1.0%		4	Texas	214	7.2%
3	California	217	7.3%		5	Ohio	136	4.6%
17	Colorado	55	1.9%		6	Pennsylvania	133	4.5%
26	Connecticut	37	1.2%		7	Georgia	132	4.4%
35	Delaware	18	0.6%		8	Virginia	124	4.2%
1	Florida	291	9.8%		9	New Jersey	107	3.6%
7	Georgia	132	4.4%		10	Maryland	94	3.2%
42	Hawaii	9	0.3%		11	Tennessee	91	3.1%
40	Idaho	11	0.4%		12	Illinois	90	3.0%
12	Illinois	90	3.0%		13	Kentucky	79	2.7%
17	Indiana	55	1.9%		14	Missouri	59	2.0%
25	Iowa	40	1.3%		14	Wisconsin	59	2.0%
32	Kansas	22	0.7%		16	South Carolina	56	1.9%
13	Kentucky	79	2.7%		17	Colorado	55	1.9%
19	Louisiana	51	1.7%		17	Indiana	55	1.9%
31	Maine	23	0.8%		19	Louisiana	51	1.7%
10	Maryland	94	3.2%		19	North Carolina	51	1.7%
38	Massachusetts	15	0.5%		21	Minnesota	50	1.7%
2	Michigan	235	7.9%		21	Oklahoma	50	1.7%
21	Minnesota	50	1.7%		23	Mississippi	49	1.7%
23	Mississippi	49	1.7%		23	Washington	49	1.7%
14	Missouri	59	2.0%		25	Iowa	40	1.3%
42	Montana	9	0.3%		26	Connecticut	37	1.2%
45	Nebraska	7	0.2%		27	Arizona	31	1.0%
34	Nevada	20	0.7%		27	New Mexico	31	1.0%
39	New Hampshire	12	0.4%		29	Arkansas	30	1.0%
9	New Jersey	107	3.6%		29	New York	30	1.0%
27	New Mexico	31	1.0%		31	Maine	23	0.8%
29	New York	30	1.0%		32	Kansas	22	0.7%
19	North Carolina	51	1.7%		33	Alabama	21	0.7%
47	North Dakota	5	0.2%		34	Nevada	20	0.7%
5	Ohio	136	4.6%		35	Delaware	18	0.6%
21	Oklahoma	50	1.7%		35	Oregon	18	0.6%
35	Oregon	18	0.6%		37	Alaska	17	0.6%
6	Pennsylvania	133	4.5%		38	Massachusetts	15	0.5%
49	Rhode Island	3	0.1%		39	New Hampshire	12	0.4%
16	South Carolina	56	1.9%		40	Idaho	11	0.4%
46	South Dakota	6	0.2%		41	Utah	10	0.3%
11	Tennessee	91	3.1%		42	Hawaii	9	0.3%
4	Texas	214	7.2%		42	Montana	9	0.3%
41	Utah	10	0.3%		44	West Virginia	8	0.3%
50	Vermont	2	0.1%		45	Nebraska	7	0.2%
8	Virginia	124	4.2%		46	South Dakota	6	0.2%
23	Washington	49	1.7%		47	North Dakota	5	0.2%
44	West Virginia	8	0.3%		48	Wyoming	4	0.1%
14	Wisconsin	59	2.0%		49	Rhode Island	3	0.1%
48	Wyoming	4	0.1%		50	Vermont	2	0.1%
						District of Columbia	2	0.1%

Source: U.S. Department of Health and Human Services, Centers for Medicare and Medicaid Services
   OSCAR Report 10 (February 5, 2003)
*Certified by CMS to participate in the Medicare/Medicaid programs. Excludes licensed facilities that do not accept federal funding and facilities managed by the Department of Veterans Affairs. National total does not include four certified outpatient physical therapy facilities in U.S. territories.

Medicare and Medicaid Certified Rural Health Clinics in 2003

National Total = 3,316 Rural Health Clinics*

ALPHA ORDER

RANK	STATE	CLINICS	% of USA
21	Alabama	58	1.7%
42	Alaska	6	0.2%
41	Arizona	7	0.2%
16	Arkansas	73	2.2%
2	California	245	7.4%
29	Colorado	42	1.3%
45	Connecticut	0	0.0%
45	Delaware	0	0.0%
7	Florida	135	4.1%
11	Georgia	106	3.2%
45	Hawaii	0	0.0%
29	Idaho	42	1.3%
4	Illinois	193	5.8%
24	Indiana	52	1.6%
9	Iowa	125	3.8%
5	Kansas	158	4.8%
12	Kentucky	90	2.7%
26	Louisiana	50	1.5%
27	Maine	48	1.4%
45	Maryland	0	0.0%
45	Massachusetts	0	0.0%
6	Michigan	155	4.7%
18	Minnesota	63	1.9%
8	Mississippi	130	3.9%
3	Missouri	214	6.5%
31	Montana	39	1.2%
16	Nebraska	73	2.2%
42	Nevada	6	0.2%
35	New Hampshire	19	0.6%
45	New Jersey	0	0.0%
39	New Mexico	10	0.3%
40	New York	9	0.3%
10	North Carolina	115	3.5%
15	North Dakota	74	2.2%
36	Ohio	18	0.5%
25	Oklahoma	51	1.5%
33	Oregon	32	1.0%
28	Pennsylvania	47	1.4%
44	Rhode Island	1	0.0%
13	South Carolina	89	2.7%
23	South Dakota	53	1.6%
32	Tennessee	35	1.1%
1	Texas	335	10.1%
38	Utah	15	0.5%
34	Vermont	20	0.6%
22	Virginia	56	1.7%
13	Washington	89	2.7%
19	West Virginia	60	1.8%
19	Wisconsin	60	1.8%
36	Wyoming	18	0.5%

RANK ORDER

RANK	STATE	CLINICS	% of USA
1	Texas	335	10.1%
2	California	245	7.4%
3	Missouri	214	6.5%
4	Illinois	193	5.8%
5	Kansas	158	4.8%
6	Michigan	155	4.7%
7	Florida	135	4.1%
8	Mississippi	130	3.9%
9	Iowa	125	3.8%
10	North Carolina	115	3.5%
11	Georgia	106	3.2%
12	Kentucky	90	2.7%
13	South Carolina	89	2.7%
13	Washington	89	2.7%
15	North Dakota	74	2.2%
16	Arkansas	73	2.2%
16	Nebraska	73	2.2%
18	Minnesota	63	1.9%
19	West Virginia	60	1.8%
19	Wisconsin	60	1.8%
21	Alabama	58	1.7%
22	Virginia	56	1.7%
23	South Dakota	53	1.6%
24	Indiana	52	1.6%
25	Oklahoma	51	1.5%
26	Louisiana	50	1.5%
27	Maine	48	1.4%
28	Pennsylvania	47	1.4%
29	Colorado	42	1.3%
29	Idaho	42	1.3%
31	Montana	39	1.2%
32	Tennessee	35	1.1%
33	Oregon	32	1.0%
34	Vermont	20	0.6%
35	New Hampshire	19	0.6%
36	Ohio	18	0.5%
36	Wyoming	18	0.5%
38	Utah	15	0.5%
39	New Mexico	10	0.3%
40	New York	9	0.3%
41	Arizona	7	0.2%
42	Alaska	6	0.2%
42	Nevada	6	0.2%
44	Rhode Island	1	0.0%
45	Connecticut	0	0.0%
45	Delaware	0	0.0%
45	Hawaii	0	0.0%
45	Maryland	0	0.0%
45	Massachusetts	0	0.0%
45	New Jersey	0	0.0%
	District of Columbia	0	0.0%

Source: U.S. Department of Health and Human Services, Centers for Medicare and Medicaid Services
OSCAR Report 10 (February 5, 2003)

*Certified by CMS to participate in the Medicare/Medicaid programs. Excludes licensed facilities that do not accept federal funding and facilities managed by the Department of Veterans Affairs. There are no certified rural health centers in U.S. territories.

Medicare and Medicaid Certified Home Health Agencies in 2003

National Total = 6,955 Home Health Agencies*

ALPHA ORDER

RANK ORDER

RANK	STATE	AGENCIES	% of USA	RANK	STATE	AGENCIES	% of USA
18	Alabama	141	2.0%	1	Texas	901	13.0%
47	Alaska	16	0.2%	2	California	560	8.1%
29	Arizona	63	0.9%	3	Florida	381	5.5%
13	Arkansas	176	2.5%	4	Ohio	343	4.9%
2	California	560	8.1%	5	Illinois	284	4.1%
21	Colorado	126	1.8%	6	Pennsylvania	283	4.1%
26	Connecticut	83	1.2%	7	Louisiana	236	3.4%
49	Delaware	13	0.2%	8	Minnesota	230	3.3%
3	Florida	381	5.5%	9	New York	205	2.9%
25	Georgia	95	1.4%	10	Michigan	202	2.9%
48	Hawaii	14	0.2%	11	Oklahoma	194	2.8%
37	Idaho	48	0.7%	12	Iowa	183	2.6%
5	Illinois	284	4.1%	13	Arkansas	176	2.5%
15	Indiana	161	2.3%	14	North Carolina	167	2.4%
12	Iowa	183	2.6%	15	Indiana	161	2.3%
20	Kansas	130	1.9%	16	Missouri	160	2.3%
24	Kentucky	110	1.6%	17	Virginia	157	2.3%
7	Louisiana	236	3.4%	18	Alabama	141	2.0%
44	Maine	34	0.5%	19	Tennessee	139	2.0%
35	Maryland	52	0.7%	20	Kansas	130	1.9%
23	Massachusetts	120	1.7%	21	Colorado	126	1.8%
10	Michigan	202	2.9%	22	Wisconsin	122	1.8%
8	Minnesota	230	3.3%	23	Massachusetts	120	1.7%
31	Mississippi	62	0.9%	24	Kentucky	110	1.6%
16	Missouri	160	2.3%	25	Georgia	95	1.4%
37	Montana	48	0.7%	26	Connecticut	83	1.2%
29	Nebraska	63	0.9%	27	South Carolina	72	1.0%
41	Nevada	39	0.6%	28	West Virginia	69	1.0%
43	New Hampshire	35	0.5%	29	Arizona	63	0.9%
35	New Jersey	52	0.7%	29	Nebraska	63	0.9%
32	New Mexico	61	0.9%	31	Mississippi	62	0.9%
9	New York	205	2.9%	32	New Mexico	61	0.9%
14	North Carolina	167	2.4%	32	Washington	61	0.9%
45	North Dakota	30	0.4%	34	Oregon	60	0.9%
4	Ohio	343	4.9%	35	Maryland	52	0.7%
11	Oklahoma	194	2.8%	35	New Jersey	52	0.7%
34	Oregon	60	0.9%	37	Idaho	48	0.7%
6	Pennsylvania	283	4.1%	37	Montana	48	0.7%
46	Rhode Island	22	0.3%	39	South Dakota	47	0.7%
27	South Carolina	72	1.0%	40	Utah	41	0.6%
39	South Dakota	47	0.7%	41	Nevada	39	0.6%
19	Tennessee	139	2.0%	42	Wyoming	38	0.5%
1	Texas	901	13.0%	43	New Hampshire	35	0.5%
40	Utah	41	0.6%	44	Maine	34	0.5%
49	Vermont	13	0.2%	45	North Dakota	30	0.4%
17	Virginia	157	2.3%	46	Rhode Island	22	0.3%
32	Washington	61	0.9%	47	Alaska	16	0.2%
28	West Virginia	69	1.0%	48	Hawaii	14	0.2%
22	Wisconsin	122	1.8%	49	Delaware	13	0.2%
42	Wyoming	38	0.5%	49	Vermont	13	0.2%
					District of Columbia	13	0.2%

Source: U.S. Department of Health and Human Services, Centers for Medicare and Medicaid Services
OSCAR Report 10 (February 5, 2003)

*Certified by CMS to participate in the Medicare/Medicaid programs. Excludes agencies that do not accept federal funding. National total does not include 50 certified home health agencies in U.S. territories. A home health agency provides health services to individuals in their homes for the purpose of promoting, maintaining or restoring health or maximizing the level of independence, while minimizing the effects of disability and illness.

Medicare and Medicaid Certified Hospices in 2003

National Total = 2,299 Hospices*

RANK	STATE	HOSPICES	% of USA
9	Alabama	80	3.5%
50	Alaska	1	0.0%
29	Arizona	36	1.6%
20	Arkansas	46	2.0%
1	California	162	7.0%
28	Colorado	37	1.6%
35	Connecticut	26	1.1%
49	Delaware	5	0.2%
22	Florida	43	1.9%
8	Georgia	83	3.6%
47	Hawaii	7	0.3%
34	Idaho	27	1.2%
5	Illinois	87	3.8%
12	Indiana	64	2.8%
14	Iowa	61	2.7%
26	Kansas	39	1.7%
35	Kentucky	26	1.1%
19	Louisiana	48	2.1%
42	Maine	17	0.7%
31	Maryland	30	1.3%
25	Massachusetts	40	1.7%
7	Michigan	85	3.7%
13	Minnesota	62	2.7%
17	Mississippi	51	2.2%
11	Missouri	69	3.0%
37	Montana	23	1.0%
33	Nebraska	29	1.3%
45	Nevada	10	0.4%
39	New Hampshire	19	0.8%
22	New Jersey	43	1.9%
31	New Mexico	30	1.3%
17	New York	51	2.2%
10	North Carolina	74	3.2%
44	North Dakota	14	0.6%
4	Ohio	88	3.8%
5	Oklahoma	87	3.8%
22	Oregon	43	1.9%
3	Pennsylvania	111	4.8%
47	Rhode Island	7	0.3%
27	South Carolina	38	1.7%
43	South Dakota	15	0.7%
20	Tennessee	46	2.0%
2	Texas	130	5.7%
38	Utah	20	0.9%
46	Vermont	9	0.4%
15	Virginia	55	2.4%
30	Washington	31	1.3%
39	West Virginia	19	0.8%
16	Wisconsin	54	2.3%
41	Wyoming	18	0.8%

RANK	STATE	HOSPICES	% of USA
1	California	162	7.0%
2	Texas	130	5.7%
3	Pennsylvania	111	4.8%
4	Ohio	88	3.8%
5	Illinois	87	3.8%
5	Oklahoma	87	3.8%
7	Michigan	85	3.7%
8	Georgia	83	3.6%
9	Alabama	80	3.5%
10	North Carolina	74	3.2%
11	Missouri	69	3.0%
12	Indiana	64	2.8%
13	Minnesota	62	2.7%
14	Iowa	61	2.7%
15	Virginia	55	2.4%
16	Wisconsin	54	2.3%
17	Mississippi	51	2.2%
17	New York	51	2.2%
19	Louisiana	48	2.1%
20	Arkansas	46	2.0%
20	Tennessee	46	2.0%
22	Florida	43	1.9%
22	New Jersey	43	1.9%
22	Oregon	43	1.9%
25	Massachusetts	40	1.7%
26	Kansas	39	1.7%
27	South Carolina	38	1.7%
28	Colorado	37	1.6%
29	Arizona	36	1.6%
30	Washington	31	1.3%
31	Maryland	30	1.3%
31	New Mexico	30	1.3%
33	Nebraska	29	1.3%
34	Idaho	27	1.2%
35	Connecticut	26	1.1%
35	Kentucky	26	1.1%
37	Montana	23	1.0%
38	Utah	20	0.9%
39	New Hampshire	19	0.8%
39	West Virginia	19	0.8%
41	Wyoming	18	0.8%
42	Maine	17	0.7%
43	South Dakota	15	0.7%
44	North Dakota	14	0.6%
45	Nevada	10	0.4%
46	Vermont	9	0.4%
47	Hawaii	7	0.3%
47	Rhode Island	7	0.3%
49	Delaware	5	0.2%
50	Alaska	1	0.0%
	District of Columbia	3	0.1%

Source: U.S. Department of Health and Human Services, Centers for Medicare and Medicaid Services
OSCAR Report 10 (February 5, 2003)

*Certified by CMS to participate in the Medicare/Medicaid programs. Excludes licensed facilities that do not accept federal funding and facilities managed by the Department of Veterans Affairs. National total does not include 33 certified hospices in U.S. territories. An hospice provides specialized services for terminally ill people and their families.

Hospice Patients in Residential Facilities in 2003

National Total = 30,537 Patients*

ALPHA ORDER				RANK ORDER			
RANK	STATE	PATIENTS	% of USA	RANK	STATE	PATIENTS	% of USA
30	Alabama	204	0.7%	1	Pennsylvania	4,520	14.8%
50	Alaska	0	0.0%	2	Florida	4,037	13.2%
22	Arizona	400	1.3%	3	Texas	2,741	9.0%
32	Arkansas	165	0.5%	4	California	1,661	5.4%
4	California	1,661	5.4%	5	Ohio	1,534	5.0%
17	Colorado	562	1.8%	6	Oklahoma	1,413	4.6%
33	Connecticut	153	0.5%	7	Michigan	1,320	4.3%
46	Delaware	7	0.0%	8	Indiana	929	3.0%
2	Florida	4,037	13.2%	9	Illinois	895	2.9%
14	Georgia	722	2.4%	10	Kentucky	826	2.7%
38	Hawaii	51	0.2%	11	Missouri	767	2.5%
45	Idaho	21	0.1%	12	New York	759	2.5%
9	Illinois	895	2.9%	13	Nebraska	752	2.5%
8	Indiana	929	3.0%	14	Georgia	722	2.4%
21	Iowa	401	1.3%	15	Oregon	691	2.3%
20	Kansas	440	1.4%	16	Minnesota	625	2.0%
10	Kentucky	826	2.7%	17	Colorado	562	1.8%
25	Louisiana	367	1.2%	18	North Carolina	532	1.7%
39	Maine	47	0.2%	19	Washington	462	1.5%
31	Maryland	170	0.6%	20	Kansas	440	1.4%
24	Massachusetts	373	1.2%	21	Iowa	401	1.3%
7	Michigan	1,320	4.3%	22	Arizona	400	1.3%
16	Minnesota	625	2.0%	23	Wisconsin	394	1.3%
36	Mississippi	74	0.2%	24	Massachusetts	373	1.2%
11	Missouri	767	2.5%	25	Louisiana	367	1.2%
43	Montana	30	0.1%	26	New Jersey	345	1.1%
13	Nebraska	752	2.5%	27	South Carolina	265	0.9%
35	Nevada	79	0.3%	28	Tennessee	233	0.8%
40	New Hampshire	43	0.1%	29	Utah	209	0.7%
26	New Jersey	345	1.1%	30	Alabama	204	0.7%
34	New Mexico	84	0.3%	31	Maryland	170	0.6%
12	New York	759	2.5%	32	Arkansas	165	0.5%
18	North Carolina	532	1.7%	33	Connecticut	153	0.5%
37	North Dakota	61	0.2%	34	New Mexico	84	0.3%
5	Ohio	1,534	5.0%	35	Nevada	79	0.3%
6	Oklahoma	1,413	4.6%	36	Mississippi	74	0.2%
15	Oregon	691	2.3%	37	North Dakota	61	0.2%
1	Pennsylvania	4,520	14.8%	38	Hawaii	51	0.2%
49	Rhode Island	1	0.0%	39	Maine	47	0.2%
27	South Carolina	265	0.9%	40	New Hampshire	43	0.1%
46	South Dakota	7	0.0%	40	West Virginia	43	0.1%
28	Tennessee	233	0.8%	42	Vermont	41	0.1%
3	Texas	2,741	9.0%	43	Montana	30	0.1%
29	Utah	209	0.7%	44	Virginia	29	0.1%
42	Vermont	41	0.1%	45	Idaho	21	0.1%
44	Virginia	29	0.1%	46	Delaware	7	0.0%
19	Washington	462	1.5%	46	South Dakota	7	0.0%
40	West Virginia	43	0.1%	48	Wyoming	6	0.0%
23	Wisconsin	394	1.3%	49	Rhode Island	1	0.0%
48	Wyoming	6	0.0%	50	Alaska	0	0.0%
					District of Columbia	46	0.2%

Source: U.S. Department of Health and Human Services, Centers for Medicare and Medicaid Services
    OSCAR Database (February 5, 2003)
*Patients in facilities certified by CMS to participate in the Medicare/Medicaid programs. Excludes licensed facilities that do not accept federal funding and facilities managed by the Department of Veterans Affairs. National total does not include six patients in U.S. territories. An hospice provides specialized services for terminally ill people and their families.

Medicare and Medicaid Certified Nursing Care Facilities in 2003

National Total = 16,478 Nursing Care Facilities*

ALPHA ORDER

RANK ORDER

RANK	STATE	FACILITIES	% of USA		RANK	STATE	FACILITIES	% of USA
28	Alabama	229	1.4%		1	California	1,351	8.2%
50	Alaska	15	0.1%		2	Texas	1,140	6.9%
35	Arizona	134	0.8%		3	Ohio	992	6.0%
27	Arkansas	245	1.5%		4	Illinois	852	5.2%
1	California	1,351	8.2%		5	Pennsylvania	750	4.6%
30	Colorado	222	1.3%		6	Florida	702	4.3%
25	Connecticut	253	1.5%		7	New York	675	4.1%
48	Delaware	42	0.3%		8	Indiana	545	3.3%
6	Florida	702	4.3%		9	Missouri	539	3.3%
18	Georgia	362	2.2%		10	Massachusetts	494	3.0%
45	Hawaii	45	0.3%		11	Iowa	463	2.8%
43	Idaho	82	0.5%		12	Michigan	431	2.6%
4	Illinois	852	5.2%		13	Minnesota	425	2.6%
8	Indiana	545	3.3%		14	North Carolina	415	2.5%
11	Iowa	463	2.8%		15	Wisconsin	407	2.5%
16	Kansas	374	2.3%		16	Kansas	374	2.3%
22	Kentucky	301	1.8%		16	Oklahoma	374	2.3%
21	Louisiana	320	1.9%		18	Georgia	362	2.2%
36	Maine	121	0.7%		19	New Jersey	360	2.2%
26	Maryland	247	1.5%		20	Tennessee	339	2.1%
10	Massachusetts	494	3.0%		21	Louisiana	320	1.9%
12	Michigan	431	2.6%		22	Kentucky	301	1.8%
13	Minnesota	425	2.6%		23	Virginia	277	1.7%
31	Mississippi	203	1.2%		24	Washington	267	1.6%
9	Missouri	539	3.3%		25	Connecticut	253	1.5%
38	Montana	102	0.6%		26	Maryland	247	1.5%
28	Nebraska	229	1.4%		27	Arkansas	245	1.5%
46	Nevada	44	0.3%		28	Alabama	229	1.4%
42	New Hampshire	83	0.5%		28	Nebraska	229	1.4%
19	New Jersey	360	2.2%		30	Colorado	222	1.3%
43	New Mexico	82	0.5%		31	Mississippi	203	1.2%
7	New York	675	4.1%		32	South Carolina	176	1.1%
14	North Carolina	415	2.5%		33	Oregon	145	0.9%
41	North Dakota	84	0.5%		34	West Virginia	137	0.8%
3	Ohio	992	6.0%		35	Arizona	134	0.8%
16	Oklahoma	374	2.3%		36	Maine	121	0.7%
33	Oregon	145	0.9%		37	South Dakota	112	0.7%
5	Pennsylvania	750	4.6%		38	Montana	102	0.6%
39	Rhode Island	97	0.6%		39	Rhode Island	97	0.6%
32	South Carolina	176	1.1%		40	Utah	90	0.5%
37	South Dakota	112	0.7%		41	North Dakota	84	0.5%
20	Tennessee	339	2.1%		42	New Hampshire	83	0.5%
2	Texas	1,140	6.9%		43	Idaho	82	0.5%
40	Utah	90	0.5%		43	New Mexico	82	0.5%
46	Vermont	44	0.3%		45	Hawaii	45	0.3%
23	Virginia	277	1.7%		46	Nevada	44	0.3%
24	Washington	267	1.6%		46	Vermont	44	0.3%
34	West Virginia	137	0.8%		48	Delaware	42	0.3%
15	Wisconsin	407	2.5%		49	Wyoming	39	0.2%
49	Wyoming	39	0.2%		50	Alaska	15	0.1%
						District of Columbia	21	0.1%

Source: U.S. Department of Health and Human Services, Centers for Medicare and Medicaid Services
    OSCAR Database (February 5, 2003)

*Certified by CMS to participate in the Medicare/Medicaid programs. Excludes licensed facilities that do not accept federal funding and facilities managed by the Department of Veterans Affairs. National total does not include nine certified nursing facilities in U.S. territories.

Beds in Medicare and Medicaid Certified Nursing Care Facilities in 2003

National Total = 1,704,448 Beds*

ALPHA ORDER

RANK	STATE	BEDS	% of USA
24	Alabama	26,065	1.5%
50	Alaska	749	0.0%
33	Arizona	15,928	0.9%
26	Arkansas	24,651	1.4%
1	California	125,846	7.4%
29	Colorado	20,281	1.2%
21	Connecticut	30,801	1.8%
46	Delaware	4,301	0.3%
7	Florida	81,492	4.8%
16	Georgia	39,797	2.3%
47	Hawaii	3,983	0.2%
44	Idaho	6,328	0.4%
4	Illinois	100,772	5.9%
9	Indiana	51,983	3.0%
19	Iowa	33,933	2.0%
28	Kansas	24,344	1.4%
25	Kentucky	25,008	1.5%
17	Louisiana	37,770	2.2%
38	Maine	7,561	0.4%
23	Maryland	29,601	1.7%
8	Massachusetts	52,759	3.1%
12	Michigan	47,235	2.8%
15	Minnesota	40,170	2.4%
30	Mississippi	17,953	1.1%
11	Missouri	50,613	3.0%
39	Montana	7,470	0.4%
32	Nebraska	15,944	0.9%
45	Nevada	5,099	0.3%
37	New Hampshire	7,639	0.4%
10	New Jersey	51,242	3.0%
42	New Mexico	7,257	0.4%
2	New York	122,311	7.2%
14	North Carolina	42,013	2.5%
43	North Dakota	6,610	0.4%
5	Ohio	93,405	5.5%
20	Oklahoma	31,904	1.9%
34	Oregon	12,781	0.7%
6	Pennsylvania	90,589	5.3%
36	Rhode Island	9,924	0.6%
31	South Carolina	17,288	1.0%
40	South Dakota	7,464	0.4%
18	Tennessee	37,708	2.2%
3	Texas	111,147	6.5%
41	Utah	7,306	0.4%
48	Vermont	3,622	0.2%
22	Virginia	30,220	1.8%
27	Washington	24,588	1.4%
35	West Virginia	11,247	0.7%
13	Wisconsin	43,571	2.6%
49	Wyoming	3,061	0.2%

RANK ORDER

RANK	STATE	BEDS	% of USA
1	California	125,846	7.4%
2	New York	122,311	7.2%
3	Texas	111,147	6.5%
4	Illinois	100,772	5.9%
5	Ohio	93,405	5.5%
6	Pennsylvania	90,589	5.3%
7	Florida	81,492	4.8%
8	Massachusetts	52,759	3.1%
9	Indiana	51,983	3.0%
10	New Jersey	51,242	3.0%
11	Missouri	50,613	3.0%
12	Michigan	47,235	2.8%
13	Wisconsin	43,571	2.6%
14	North Carolina	42,013	2.5%
15	Minnesota	40,170	2.4%
16	Georgia	39,797	2.3%
17	Louisiana	37,770	2.2%
18	Tennessee	37,708	2.2%
19	Iowa	33,933	2.0%
20	Oklahoma	31,904	1.9%
21	Connecticut	30,801	1.8%
22	Virginia	30,220	1.8%
23	Maryland	29,601	1.7%
24	Alabama	26,065	1.5%
25	Kentucky	25,008	1.5%
26	Arkansas	24,651	1.4%
27	Washington	24,588	1.4%
28	Kansas	24,344	1.4%
29	Colorado	20,281	1.2%
30	Mississippi	17,953	1.1%
31	South Carolina	17,288	1.0%
32	Nebraska	15,944	0.9%
33	Arizona	15,928	0.9%
34	Oregon	12,781	0.7%
35	West Virginia	11,247	0.7%
36	Rhode Island	9,924	0.6%
37	New Hampshire	7,639	0.4%
38	Maine	7,561	0.4%
39	Montana	7,470	0.4%
40	South Dakota	7,464	0.4%
41	Utah	7,306	0.4%
42	New Mexico	7,257	0.4%
43	North Dakota	6,610	0.4%
44	Idaho	6,328	0.4%
45	Nevada	5,099	0.3%
46	Delaware	4,301	0.3%
47	Hawaii	3,983	0.2%
48	Vermont	3,622	0.2%
49	Wyoming	3,061	0.2%
50	Alaska	749	0.0%
	District of Columbia	3,114	0.2%

Source: U.S. Department of Health and Human Services, Centers for Medicare and Medicaid Services
OSCAR Database (February 5, 2003)
*Beds in nursing care facilities certified by CMS to participate in the Medicare/Medicaid programs. National total does not include 357 beds in U.S. territories.

Rate of Beds in Medicare and Medicaid Certified Nursing Care Facilities in 2003

National Rate = 402 Beds per 1,000 Population 85 Years and Older*

ALPHA ORDER

RANK	STATE	RATE
31	Alabama	387
46	Alaska	284
48	Arizona	232
4	Arkansas	530
44	California	296
25	Colorado	421
10	Connecticut	479
28	Delaware	408
47	Florida	246
20	Georgia	453
49	Hawaii	227
36	Idaho	350
6	Illinois	525
2	Indiana	568
7	Iowa	521
12	Kansas	470
24	Kentucky	429
1	Louisiana	644
41	Maine	324
23	Maryland	442
21	Massachusetts	452
40	Michigan	332
14	Minnesota	469
26	Mississippi	419
8	Missouri	513
9	Montana	487
12	Nebraska	470
43	Nevada	300
26	New Hampshire	419
33	New Jersey	377
42	New Mexico	311
30	New York	393
29	North Carolina	398
22	North Dakota	449
5	Ohio	528
3	Oklahoma	558
50	Oregon	223
32	Pennsylvania	381
11	Rhode Island	475
38	South Carolina	344
16	South Dakota	464
17	Tennessee	463
15	Texas	467
39	Utah	336
34	Vermont	362
37	Virginia	346
45	Washington	292
35	West Virginia	354
18	Wisconsin	456
19	Wyoming	454

RANK ORDER

RANK	STATE	RATE
1	Louisiana	644
2	Indiana	568
3	Oklahoma	558
4	Arkansas	530
5	Ohio	528
6	Illinois	525
7	Iowa	521
8	Missouri	513
9	Montana	487
10	Connecticut	479
11	Rhode Island	475
12	Kansas	470
12	Nebraska	470
14	Minnesota	469
15	Texas	467
16	South Dakota	464
17	Tennessee	463
18	Wisconsin	456
19	Wyoming	454
20	Georgia	453
21	Massachusetts	452
22	North Dakota	449
23	Maryland	442
24	Kentucky	429
25	Colorado	421
26	Mississippi	419
26	New Hampshire	419
28	Delaware	408
29	North Carolina	398
30	New York	393
31	Alabama	387
32	Pennsylvania	381
33	New Jersey	377
34	Vermont	362
35	West Virginia	354
36	Idaho	350
37	Virginia	346
38	South Carolina	344
39	Utah	336
40	Michigan	332
41	Maine	324
42	New Mexico	311
43	Nevada	300
44	California	296
45	Washington	292
46	Alaska	284
47	Florida	246
48	Arizona	232
49	Hawaii	227
50	Oregon	223
	District of Columbia	347

Source: MQ Press using data from U.S. Dept of Health & Human Services, Centers for Medicare and Medicaid Services OSCAR Database (February 5, 2003)

*Beds in nursing care facilities certified by CMS to participate in the Medicare/Medicaid programs. National rate does not include beds or population in U.S. territories. Calculated using 2000 Census population count.

Nursing Home Occupancy Rate in 2000

National Rate = 82.4% of Beds in Nursing Homes Occupied

ALPHA ORDER			RANK ORDER		
RANK	STATE	RATE	RANK	STATE	RATE
5	Alabama	91.4	1	New York	93.7
46	Alaska	72.5	2	Mississippi	92.7
39	Arizona	75.9	3	Minnesota	92.1
41	Arkansas	75.1	4	Georgia	91.8
33	California	80.8	5	Alabama	91.4
24	Colorado	84.2	5	Connecticut	91.4
5	Connecticut	91.4	7	New Hampshire	91.3
34	Delaware	79.5	8	North Dakota	91.2
29	Florida	82.8	9	West Virginia	90.5
4	Georgia	91.8	10	South Dakota	90.0
16	Hawaii	88.8	11	Tennessee	89.9
41	Idaho	75.1	12	Kentucky	89.7
40	Illinois	75.5	13	Vermont	89.5
43	Indiana	74.6	14	New Mexico	89.2
35	Iowa	78.9	15	Massachusetts	88.9
30	Kansas	82.1	16	Hawaii	88.8
12	Kentucky	89.7	17	North Carolina	88.6
37	Louisiana	77.9	18	Maine	88.5
18	Maine	88.5	18	Virginia	88.5
32	Maryland	81.4	20	Pennsylvania	88.2
15	Massachusetts	88.9	21	Rhode Island	88.0
25	Michigan	84.1	22	New Jersey	87.8
3	Minnesota	92.1	23	South Carolina	86.9
2	Mississippi	92.7	24	Colorado	84.2
47	Missouri	70.4	25	Michigan	84.1
37	Montana	77.9	26	Wisconsin	83.9
27	Nebraska	83.8	27	Nebraska	83.8
50	Nevada	65.9	28	Wyoming	83.5
7	New Hampshire	91.3	29	Florida	82.8
22	New Jersey	87.8	30	Kansas	82.1
14	New Mexico	89.2	31	Washington	81.7
1	New York	93.7	32	Maryland	81.4
17	North Carolina	88.6	33	California	80.8
8	North Dakota	91.2	34	Delaware	79.5
36	Ohio	78.0	35	Iowa	78.9
48	Oklahoma	70.3	36	Ohio	78.0
45	Oregon	74.0	37	Louisiana	77.9
20	Pennsylvania	88.2	37	Montana	77.9
21	Rhode Island	88.0	39	Arizona	75.9
23	South Carolina	86.9	40	Illinois	75.5
10	South Dakota	90.0	41	Arkansas	75.1
11	Tennessee	89.9	41	Idaho	75.1
49	Texas	68.2	43	Indiana	74.6
44	Utah	74.5	44	Utah	74.5
13	Vermont	89.5	45	Oregon	74.0
18	Virginia	88.5	46	Alaska	72.5
31	Washington	81.7	47	Missouri	70.4
9	West Virginia	90.5	48	Oklahoma	70.3
26	Wisconsin	83.9	49	Texas	68.2
28	Wyoming	83.5	50	Nevada	65.9
				District of Columbia	92.9

*Source: U.S. Department of Health and Human Services, Centers for Medicare and Medicaid Services
"Health, United States, 2002"*

Nursing Home Resident Rate in 2000

National Rate = 349.1 Residents per 1,000 Population Age 85 and Older*

ALPHA ORDER

RANK	STATE	RATE
32	Alabama	343.1
45	Alaska	225.9
49	Arizona	193.4
17	Arkansas	415.5
44	California	250.1
29	Colorado	353.5
4	Connecticut	461.4
25	Delaware	369.7
47	Florida	208.4
16	Georgia	416.1
48	Hawaii	202.6
42	Idaho	257.0
9	Illinois	435.4
3	Indiana	462.3
6	Iowa	448.5
12	Kansas	429.4
21	Kentucky	390.1
1	Louisiana	523.8
37	Maine	313.0
24	Maryland	383.1
13	Massachusetts	426.8
39	Michigan	299.1
5	Minnesota	453.4
26	Mississippi	368.7
20	Missouri	391.5
22	Montana	389.5
7	Nebraska	441.5
46	Nevada	215.3
19	New Hampshire	392.6
33	New Jersey	337.0
40	New Mexico	279.0
27	New York	362.6
31	North Carolina	347.6
11	North Dakota	430.7
2	Ohio	463.5
15	Oklahoma	416.8
50	Oregon	173.9
30	Pennsylvania	353.1
10	Rhode Island	432.6
36	South Carolina	313.1
8	South Dakota	438.8
14	Tennessee	426.1
28	Texas	358.4
41	Utah	262.2
34	Vermont	335.0
38	Virginia	310.4
43	Washington	251.6
35	West Virginia	325.2
18	Wisconsin	406.9
23	Wyoming	386.8

RANK ORDER

RANK	STATE	RATE
1	Louisiana	523.8
2	Ohio	463.5
3	Indiana	462.3
4	Connecticut	461.4
5	Minnesota	453.4
6	Iowa	448.5
7	Nebraska	441.5
8	South Dakota	438.8
9	Illinois	435.4
10	Rhode Island	432.6
11	North Dakota	430.7
12	Kansas	429.4
13	Massachusetts	426.8
14	Tennessee	426.1
15	Oklahoma	416.8
16	Georgia	416.1
17	Arkansas	415.5
18	Wisconsin	406.9
19	New Hampshire	392.6
20	Missouri	391.5
21	Kentucky	390.1
22	Montana	389.5
23	Wyoming	386.8
24	Maryland	383.1
25	Delaware	369.7
26	Mississippi	368.7
27	New York	362.6
28	Texas	358.4
29	Colorado	353.5
30	Pennsylvania	353.1
31	North Carolina	347.6
32	Alabama	343.1
33	New Jersey	337.0
34	Vermont	335.0
35	West Virginia	325.2
36	South Carolina	313.1
37	Maine	313.0
38	Virginia	310.4
39	Michigan	299.1
40	New Mexico	279.0
41	Utah	262.2
42	Idaho	257.0
43	Washington	251.6
44	California	250.1
45	Alaska	225.9
46	Nevada	215.3
47	Florida	208.4
48	Hawaii	202.6
49	Arizona	193.4
50	Oregon	173.9
	District of Columbia	318.4

Source: U.S. Department of Health and Human Services, Centers for Medicare and Medicaid Services "Health, United States, 2002"

*Number of nursing home residents (all ages) per 1,000 resident population 85 years of age and over.

Nursing Home Population 85 Years Old and Older in 2000

National Total = 1,480,000*

ALPHA ORDER

RANK ORDER

RANK	STATE	POPULATION	% of USA	RANK	STATE	POPULATION	% of USA
24	Alabama	23,100	1.6%	1	New York	112,900	7.6%
50	Alaska	600	0.0%	2	California	106,500	7.2%
33	Arizona	13,300	0.9%	3	Texas	85,300	5.8%
28	Arkansas	19,300	1.3%	4	Pennsylvania	83,900	5.7%
2	California	106,500	7.2%	5	Illinois	83,600	5.6%
29	Colorado	17,000	1.1%	6	Ohio	81,900	5.5%
19	Connecticut	29,700	2.0%	7	Florida	69,000	4.7%
45	Delaware	3,900	0.3%	8	Massachusetts	49,800	3.4%
7	Florida	69,000	4.7%	9	New Jersey	45,800	3.1%
16	Georgia	36,600	2.5%	10	Michigan	42,600	2.9%
47	Hawaii	3,600	0.2%	11	Indiana	42,300	2.9%
44	Idaho	4,600	0.3%	12	Wisconsin	38,900	2.6%
5	Illinois	83,600	5.6%	13	Minnesota	38,800	2.6%
11	Indiana	42,300	2.9%	14	Missouri	38,600	2.6%
20	Iowa	29,200	2.0%	15	North Carolina	36,700	2.5%
26	Kansas	22,200	1.5%	16	Georgia	36,600	2.5%
25	Kentucky	22,700	1.5%	17	Tennessee	34,700	2.3%
18	Louisiana	30,700	2.1%	18	Louisiana	30,700	2.1%
37	Maine	7,300	0.5%	19	Connecticut	29,700	2.0%
22	Maryland	25,600	1.7%	20	Iowa	29,200	2.0%
8	Massachusetts	49,800	3.4%	21	Virginia	27,100	1.8%
10	Michigan	42,600	2.9%	22	Maryland	25,600	1.7%
13	Minnesota	38,800	2.6%	23	Oklahoma	23,800	1.6%
30	Mississippi	15,800	1.1%	24	Alabama	23,100	1.6%
14	Missouri	38,600	2.6%	25	Kentucky	22,700	1.5%
42	Montana	6,000	0.4%	26	Kansas	22,200	1.5%
32	Nebraska	15,000	1.0%	27	Washington	21,200	1.4%
46	Nevada	3,700	0.3%	28	Arkansas	19,300	1.3%
38	New Hampshire	7,200	0.5%	29	Colorado	17,000	1.1%
9	New Jersey	45,800	3.1%	30	Mississippi	15,800	1.1%
40	New Mexico	6,500	0.4%	31	South Carolina	15,700	1.1%
1	New York	112,900	7.6%	32	Nebraska	15,000	1.0%
15	North Carolina	36,700	2.5%	33	Arizona	13,300	0.9%
41	North Dakota	6,300	0.4%	34	West Virginia	10,300	0.7%
6	Ohio	81,900	5.5%	35	Oregon	10,000	0.7%
23	Oklahoma	23,800	1.6%	36	Rhode Island	9,000	0.6%
35	Oregon	10,000	0.7%	37	Maine	7,300	0.5%
4	Pennsylvania	83,900	5.7%	38	New Hampshire	7,200	0.5%
36	Rhode Island	9,000	0.6%	39	South Dakota	7,100	0.5%
31	South Carolina	15,700	1.1%	40	New Mexico	6,500	0.4%
39	South Dakota	7,100	0.5%	41	North Dakota	6,300	0.4%
17	Tennessee	34,700	2.3%	42	Montana	6,000	0.4%
3	Texas	85,300	5.8%	43	Utah	5,700	0.4%
43	Utah	5,700	0.4%	44	Idaho	4,600	0.3%
48	Vermont	3,300	0.2%	45	Delaware	3,900	0.3%
21	Virginia	27,100	1.8%	46	Nevada	3,700	0.3%
27	Washington	21,200	1.4%	47	Hawaii	3,600	0.2%
34	West Virginia	10,300	0.7%	48	Vermont	3,300	0.2%
12	Wisconsin	38,900	2.6%	49	Wyoming	2,600	0.2%
49	Wyoming	2,600	0.2%	50	Alaska	600	0.0%
					District of Columbia	2,900	0.2%

Source: MQ Press using data from U.S. Dept of Health & Human Services, Centers for Medicare and Medicaid Services
  "Health, United States, 2002"
*Estimated using nursing home resident rate and population 85 years old and older.

Health Care Establishments in 2000

National Total = 529,506 Establishments*

ALPHA ORDER

RANK	STATE	ESTABLISH'S	% of USA
27	Alabama	6,776	1.3%
48	Alaska	1,234	0.2%
20	Arizona	9,245	1.7%
32	Arkansas	4,619	0.9%
1	California	68,045	12.9%
21	Colorado	8,689	1.6%
25	Connecticut	7,295	1.4%
45	Delaware	1,432	0.3%
4	Florida	34,713	6.6%
10	Georgia	13,186	2.5%
41	Hawaii	2,502	0.5%
40	Idaho	2,534	0.5%
6	Illinois	21,464	4.1%
17	Indiana	9,947	1.9%
30	Iowa	5,335	1.0%
31	Kansas	4,972	0.9%
26	Kentucky	6,855	1.3%
23	Louisiana	7,991	1.5%
39	Maine	2,868	0.5%
15	Maryland	10,832	2.0%
11	Massachusetts	12,870	2.4%
8	Michigan	19,064	3.6%
22	Minnesota	8,380	1.6%
34	Mississippi	3,840	0.7%
16	Missouri	9,952	1.9%
44	Montana	2,012	0.4%
37	Nebraska	2,980	0.6%
36	Nevada	3,469	0.7%
42	New Hampshire	2,271	0.4%
9	New Jersey	18,888	3.6%
38	New Mexico	2,976	0.6%
2	New York	38,374	7.2%
12	North Carolina	12,427	2.3%
49	North Dakota	1,086	0.2%
7	Ohio	20,789	3.9%
28	Oklahoma	6,536	1.2%
24	Oregon	7,524	1.4%
5	Pennsylvania	25,822	4.9%
43	Rhode Island	2,270	0.4%
29	South Carolina	6,021	1.1%
46	South Dakota	1,382	0.3%
18	Tennessee	9,891	1.9%
3	Texas	36,193	6.8%
33	Utah	4,066	0.8%
47	Vermont	1,324	0.3%
14	Virginia	11,491	2.2%
13	Washington	11,621	2.2%
35	West Virginia	3,551	0.7%
19	Wisconsin	9,427	1.8%
50	Wyoming	1,038	0.2%

RANK ORDER

RANK	STATE	ESTABLISH'S	% of USA
1	California	68,045	12.9%
2	New York	38,374	7.2%
3	Texas	36,193	6.8%
4	Florida	34,713	6.6%
5	Pennsylvania	25,822	4.9%
6	Illinois	21,464	4.1%
7	Ohio	20,789	3.9%
8	Michigan	19,064	3.6%
9	New Jersey	18,888	3.6%
10	Georgia	13,186	2.5%
11	Massachusetts	12,870	2.4%
12	North Carolina	12,427	2.3%
13	Washington	11,621	2.2%
14	Virginia	11,491	2.2%
15	Maryland	10,832	2.0%
16	Missouri	9,952	1.9%
17	Indiana	9,947	1.9%
18	Tennessee	9,891	1.9%
19	Wisconsin	9,427	1.8%
20	Arizona	9,245	1.7%
21	Colorado	8,689	1.6%
22	Minnesota	8,380	1.6%
23	Louisiana	7,991	1.5%
24	Oregon	7,524	1.4%
25	Connecticut	7,295	1.4%
26	Kentucky	6,855	1.3%
27	Alabama	6,776	1.3%
28	Oklahoma	6,536	1.2%
29	South Carolina	6,021	1.1%
30	Iowa	5,335	1.0%
31	Kansas	4,972	0.9%
32	Arkansas	4,619	0.9%
33	Utah	4,066	0.8%
34	Mississippi	3,840	0.7%
35	West Virginia	3,551	0.7%
36	Nevada	3,469	0.7%
37	Nebraska	2,980	0.6%
38	New Mexico	2,976	0.6%
39	Maine	2,868	0.5%
40	Idaho	2,534	0.5%
41	Hawaii	2,502	0.5%
42	New Hampshire	2,271	0.4%
43	Rhode Island	2,270	0.4%
44	Montana	2,012	0.4%
45	Delaware	1,432	0.3%
46	South Dakota	1,382	0.3%
47	Vermont	1,324	0.3%
48	Alaska	1,234	0.2%
49	North Dakota	1,086	0.2%
50	Wyoming	1,038	0.2%
	District of Columbia	1,437	0.3%

Source: U.S. Bureau of the Census
   "County Business Patterns 2000 (NAICS)" (http://censtats.census.gov/cbpnaic/cbpnaic.shtml)
*Includes establishments exempt from as well as subject to the federal income tax. Includes those establishments within the North American Industry Classification System (NAICS) classifications 621 (ambulatory health care services), 622 (hospitals) and 623 (nursing and residential care facilities).

IV. FINANCE

IV. FINANCE (Continued)

Persons Not Covered by Health Insurance in 2001

National Total = 41,207,000 Uninsured

ALPHA ORDER

RANK	STATE	UNINSURED	% of USA
21	Alabama	573,000	1.4%
44	Alaska	100,000	0.2%
12	Arizona	950,000	2.3%
28	Arkansas	428,000	1.0%
1	California	6,718,000	16.3%
17	Colorado	687,000	1.7%
32	Connecticut	346,000	0.8%
47	Delaware	73,000	0.2%
4	Florida	2,856,000	6.9%
6	Georgia	1,376,000	3.3%
43	Hawaii	117,000	0.3%
38	Idaho	210,000	0.5%
5	Illinois	1,676,000	4.1%
16	Indiana	714,000	1.7%
37	Iowa	216,000	0.5%
35	Kansas	301,000	0.7%
25	Kentucky	492,000	1.2%
13	Louisiana	845,000	2.1%
40	Maine	132,000	0.3%
18	Maryland	653,000	1.6%
23	Massachusetts	520,000	1.3%
11	Michigan	1,028,000	2.5%
30	Minnesota	392,000	1.0%
26	Mississippi	459,000	1.1%
22	Missouri	565,000	1.4%
41	Montana	121,000	0.3%
39	Nebraska	160,000	0.4%
33	Nevada	344,000	0.8%
42	New Hampshire	119,000	0.3%
10	New Jersey	1,109,000	2.7%
31	New Mexico	373,000	0.9%
3	New York	2,916,000	7.1%
8	North Carolina	1,167,000	2.8%
49	North Dakota	60,000	0.1%
7	Ohio	1,248,000	3.0%
20	Oklahoma	620,000	1.5%
27	Oregon	443,000	1.1%
9	Pennsylvania	1,119,000	2.7%
45	Rhode Island	80,000	0.2%
24	South Carolina	493,000	1.2%
48	South Dakota	69,000	0.2%
19	Tennessee	640,000	1.6%
2	Texas	4,960,000	12.0%
34	Utah	335,000	0.8%
50	Vermont	58,000	0.1%
15	Virginia	774,000	1.9%
14	Washington	780,000	1.9%
36	West Virginia	234,000	0.6%
29	Wisconsin	409,000	1.0%
46	Wyoming	78,000	0.2%

RANK ORDER

RANK	STATE	UNINSURED	% of USA
1	California	6,718,000	16.3%
2	Texas	4,960,000	12.0%
3	New York	2,916,000	7.1%
4	Florida	2,856,000	6.9%
5	Illinois	1,676,000	4.1%
6	Georgia	1,376,000	3.3%
7	Ohio	1,248,000	3.0%
8	North Carolina	1,167,000	2.8%
9	Pennsylvania	1,119,000	2.7%
10	New Jersey	1,109,000	2.7%
11	Michigan	1,028,000	2.5%
12	Arizona	950,000	2.3%
13	Louisiana	845,000	2.1%
14	Washington	780,000	1.9%
15	Virginia	774,000	1.9%
16	Indiana	714,000	1.7%
17	Colorado	687,000	1.7%
18	Maryland	653,000	1.6%
19	Tennessee	640,000	1.6%
20	Oklahoma	620,000	1.5%
21	Alabama	573,000	1.4%
22	Missouri	565,000	1.4%
23	Massachusetts	520,000	1.3%
24	South Carolina	493,000	1.2%
25	Kentucky	492,000	1.2%
26	Mississippi	459,000	1.1%
27	Oregon	443,000	1.1%
28	Arkansas	428,000	1.0%
29	Wisconsin	409,000	1.0%
30	Minnesota	392,000	1.0%
31	New Mexico	373,000	0.9%
32	Connecticut	346,000	0.8%
33	Nevada	344,000	0.8%
34	Utah	335,000	0.8%
35	Kansas	301,000	0.7%
36	West Virginia	234,000	0.6%
37	Iowa	216,000	0.5%
38	Idaho	210,000	0.5%
39	Nebraska	160,000	0.4%
40	Maine	132,000	0.3%
41	Montana	121,000	0.3%
42	New Hampshire	119,000	0.3%
43	Hawaii	117,000	0.3%
44	Alaska	100,000	0.2%
45	Rhode Island	80,000	0.2%
46	Wyoming	78,000	0.2%
47	Delaware	73,000	0.2%
48	South Dakota	69,000	0.2%
49	North Dakota	60,000	0.1%
50	Vermont	58,000	0.1%
	District of Columbia	70,000	0.2%

Source: U.S. Bureau of the Census
"Health Insurance Coverage Status by State for All People: 2001"
(http://ferret.bls.census.gov/macro/032002/health/h06_000.htm)

Percent of Population Not Covered by Health Insurance in 2001

National Percent = 14.6% of Population

ALPHA ORDER

RANK	STATE	PERCENT
22	Alabama	13.1
14	Alaska	15.7
6	Arizona	17.9
10	Arkansas	16.1
3	California	19.5
15	Colorado	15.6
36	Connecticut	10.2
44	Delaware	9.2
7	Florida	17.5
8	Georgia	16.6
38	Hawaii	9.6
12	Idaho	16.0
19	Illinois	13.6
29	Indiana	11.8
50	Iowa	7.5
30	Kansas	11.4
26	Kentucky	12.3
4	Louisiana	19.3
35	Maine	10.3
26	Maryland	12.3
46	Massachusetts	8.2
34	Michigan	10.4
47	Minnesota	8.0
9	Mississippi	16.4
36	Missouri	10.2
19	Montana	13.6
41	Nebraska	9.5
10	Nevada	16.1
42	New Hampshire	9.4
22	New Jersey	13.1
2	New Mexico	20.7
16	New York	15.5
18	North Carolina	14.4
38	North Dakota	9.6
32	Ohio	11.2
5	Oklahoma	18.3
25	Oregon	12.8
44	Pennsylvania	9.2
48	Rhode Island	7.7
26	South Carolina	12.3
43	South Dakota	9.3
31	Tennessee	11.3
1	Texas	23.5
17	Utah	14.8
38	Vermont	9.6
33	Virginia	10.9
22	Washington	13.1
21	West Virginia	13.2
48	Wisconsin	7.7
13	Wyoming	15.9

RANK ORDER

RANK	STATE	PERCENT
1	Texas	23.5
2	New Mexico	20.7
3	California	19.5
4	Louisiana	19.3
5	Oklahoma	18.3
6	Arizona	17.9
7	Florida	17.5
8	Georgia	16.6
9	Mississippi	16.4
10	Arkansas	16.1
10	Nevada	16.1
12	Idaho	16.0
13	Wyoming	15.9
14	Alaska	15.7
15	Colorado	15.6
16	New York	15.5
17	Utah	14.8
18	North Carolina	14.4
19	Illinois	13.6
19	Montana	13.6
21	West Virginia	13.2
22	Alabama	13.1
22	New Jersey	13.1
22	Washington	13.1
25	Oregon	12.8
26	Kentucky	12.3
26	Maryland	12.3
26	South Carolina	12.3
29	Indiana	11.8
30	Kansas	11.4
31	Tennessee	11.3
32	Ohio	11.2
33	Virginia	10.9
34	Michigan	10.4
35	Maine	10.3
36	Connecticut	10.2
36	Missouri	10.2
38	Hawaii	9.6
38	North Dakota	9.6
38	Vermont	9.6
41	Nebraska	9.5
42	New Hampshire	9.4
43	South Dakota	9.3
44	Delaware	9.2
44	Pennsylvania	9.2
46	Massachusetts	8.2
47	Minnesota	8.0
48	Rhode Island	7.7
48	Wisconsin	7.7
50	Iowa	7.5
	District of Columbia	12.7

Source: U.S. Bureau of the Census
   "Health Insurance Coverage Status by State for All People: 2001"
   (http://ferret.bls.census.gov/macro/032002/health/h06_000.htm)

Persons Covered by Health Insurance in 2001

National Total = 240,875,000 Insured

ALPHA ORDER

RANK	STATE	INSURED	% of USA
22	Alabama	3,815,000	1.6%
49	Alaska	534,000	0.2%
21	Arizona	4,365,000	1.8%
33	Arkansas	2,229,000	0.9%
1	California	27,770,000	11.5%
23	Colorado	3,723,000	1.5%
27	Connecticut	3,047,000	1.3%
45	Delaware	719,000	0.3%
4	Florida	13,491,000	5.6%
11	Georgia	6,912,000	2.9%
42	Hawaii	1,096,000	0.5%
41	Idaho	1,105,000	0.5%
6	Illinois	10,655,000	4.4%
14	Indiana	5,322,000	2.2%
30	Iowa	2,645,000	1.1%
31	Kansas	2,341,000	1.0%
26	Kentucky	3,505,000	1.5%
24	Louisiana	3,544,000	1.5%
39	Maine	1,147,000	0.5%
19	Maryland	4,673,000	1.9%
13	Massachusetts	5,802,000	2.4%
8	Michigan	8,864,000	3.7%
20	Minnesota	4,530,000	1.9%
31	Mississippi	2,341,000	1.0%
17	Missouri	4,960,000	2.1%
44	Montana	771,000	0.3%
37	Nebraska	1,523,000	0.6%
35	Nevada	1,791,000	0.7%
40	New Hampshire	1,139,000	0.5%
9	New Jersey	7,361,000	3.1%
38	New Mexico	1,431,000	0.6%
3	New York	15,911,000	6.6%
10	North Carolina	6,932,000	2.9%
47	North Dakota	561,000	0.2%
7	Ohio	9,943,000	4.1%
29	Oklahoma	2,762,000	1.1%
28	Oregon	3,018,000	1.3%
5	Pennsylvania	10,983,000	4.6%
43	Rhode Island	963,000	0.4%
25	South Carolina	3,517,000	1.5%
46	South Dakota	670,000	0.3%
16	Tennessee	5,042,000	2.1%
2	Texas	16,105,000	6.7%
34	Utah	1,927,000	0.8%
48	Vermont	549,000	0.2%
12	Virginia	6,331,000	2.6%
15	Washington	5,151,000	2.1%
36	West Virginia	1,539,000	0.6%
18	Wisconsin	4,927,000	2.0%
50	Wyoming	411,000	0.2%

RANK ORDER

RANK	STATE	INSURED	% of USA
1	California	27,770,000	11.5%
2	Texas	16,105,000	6.7%
3	New York	15,911,000	6.6%
4	Florida	13,491,000	5.6%
5	Pennsylvania	10,983,000	4.6%
6	Illinois	10,655,000	4.4%
7	Ohio	9,943,000	4.1%
8	Michigan	8,864,000	3.7%
9	New Jersey	7,361,000	3.1%
10	North Carolina	6,932,000	2.9%
11	Georgia	6,912,000	2.9%
12	Virginia	6,331,000	2.6%
13	Massachusetts	5,802,000	2.4%
14	Indiana	5,322,000	2.2%
15	Washington	5,151,000	2.1%
16	Tennessee	5,042,000	2.1%
17	Missouri	4,960,000	2.1%
18	Wisconsin	4,927,000	2.0%
19	Maryland	4,673,000	1.9%
20	Minnesota	4,530,000	1.9%
21	Arizona	4,365,000	1.8%
22	Alabama	3,815,000	1.6%
23	Colorado	3,723,000	1.5%
24	Louisiana	3,544,000	1.5%
25	South Carolina	3,517,000	1.5%
26	Kentucky	3,505,000	1.5%
27	Connecticut	3,047,000	1.3%
28	Oregon	3,018,000	1.3%
29	Oklahoma	2,762,000	1.1%
30	Iowa	2,645,000	1.1%
31	Kansas	2,341,000	1.0%
31	Mississippi	2,341,000	1.0%
33	Arkansas	2,229,000	0.9%
34	Utah	1,927,000	0.8%
35	Nevada	1,791,000	0.7%
36	West Virginia	1,539,000	0.6%
37	Nebraska	1,523,000	0.6%
38	New Mexico	1,431,000	0.6%
39	Maine	1,147,000	0.5%
40	New Hampshire	1,139,000	0.5%
41	Idaho	1,105,000	0.5%
42	Hawaii	1,096,000	0.5%
43	Rhode Island	963,000	0.4%
44	Montana	771,000	0.3%
45	Delaware	719,000	0.3%
46	South Dakota	670,000	0.3%
47	North Dakota	561,000	0.2%
48	Vermont	549,000	0.2%
49	Alaska	534,000	0.2%
50	Wyoming	411,000	0.2%
	District of Columbia	484,000	0.2%

Source: U.S. Bureau of the Census
"Health Insurance Coverage Status by State for All People: 2001"
(http://ferret.bls.census.gov/macro/032002/health/h06_000.htm)

Percent of Population Covered by Health Insurance in 2001

National Percent = 85.4% of Population

ALPHA ORDER

RANK	STATE	PERCENT
27	Alabama	86.9
37	Alaska	84.3
45	Arizona	82.1
40	Arkansas	83.9
48	California	80.5
36	Colorado	84.4
14	Connecticut	89.8
6	Delaware	90.8
44	Florida	82.5
43	Georgia	83.4
11	Hawaii	90.4
39	Idaho	84.0
31	Illinois	86.4
22	Indiana	88.2
1	Iowa	92.5
21	Kansas	88.6
23	Kentucky	87.7
47	Louisiana	80.7
16	Maine	89.7
23	Maryland	87.7
5	Massachusetts	91.8
17	Michigan	89.6
4	Minnesota	92.0
42	Mississippi	83.6
14	Missouri	89.8
31	Montana	86.4
10	Nebraska	90.5
40	Nevada	83.9
9	New Hampshire	90.6
27	New Jersey	86.9
49	New Mexico	79.3
35	New York	84.5
33	North Carolina	85.6
11	North Dakota	90.4
19	Ohio	88.8
46	Oklahoma	81.7
26	Oregon	87.2
6	Pennsylvania	90.8
2	Rhode Island	92.3
23	South Carolina	87.7
8	South Dakota	90.7
20	Tennessee	88.7
50	Texas	76.5
34	Utah	85.2
11	Vermont	90.4
18	Virginia	89.1
27	Washington	86.9
30	West Virginia	86.8
2	Wisconsin	92.3
38	Wyoming	84.1

RANK ORDER

RANK	STATE	PERCENT
1	Iowa	92.5
2	Rhode Island	92.3
2	Wisconsin	92.3
4	Minnesota	92.0
5	Massachusetts	91.8
6	Delaware	90.8
6	Pennsylvania	90.8
8	South Dakota	90.7
9	New Hampshire	90.6
10	Nebraska	90.5
11	Hawaii	90.4
11	North Dakota	90.4
11	Vermont	90.4
14	Connecticut	89.8
14	Missouri	89.8
16	Maine	89.7
17	Michigan	89.6
18	Virginia	89.1
19	Ohio	88.8
20	Tennessee	88.7
21	Kansas	88.6
22	Indiana	88.2
23	Kentucky	87.7
23	Maryland	87.7
23	South Carolina	87.7
26	Oregon	87.2
27	Alabama	86.9
27	New Jersey	86.9
27	Washington	86.9
30	West Virginia	86.8
31	Illinois	86.4
31	Montana	86.4
33	North Carolina	85.6
34	Utah	85.2
35	New York	84.5
36	Colorado	84.4
37	Alaska	84.3
38	Wyoming	84.1
39	Idaho	84.0
40	Arkansas	83.9
40	Nevada	83.9
42	Mississippi	83.6
43	Georgia	83.4
44	Florida	82.5
45	Arizona	82.1
46	Oklahoma	81.7
47	Louisiana	80.7
48	California	80.5
49	New Mexico	79.3
50	Texas	76.5
	District of Columbia	87.3

Source: U.S. Bureau of the Census
  "Health Insurance Coverage Status by State for All People: 2001"
  (http://ferret.bls.census.gov/macro/032002/health/h06_000.htm)

Persons Not Covered by Health Insurance in 1997

National Total = 43,448,000 Uninsured

RANK	STATE	UNINSURED	% of USA
20	Alabama	658,000	1.5%
43	Alaska	116,000	0.3%
11	Arizona	1,140,000	2.6%
23	Arkansas	639,000	1.5%
1	California	7,094,000	16.3%
24	Colorado	592,000	1.4%
32	Connecticut	396,000	0.9%
44	Delaware	99,000	0.2%
4	Florida	2,818,000	6.5%
6	Georgia	1,343,000	3.1%
47	Hawaii	89,000	0.2%
38	Idaho	223,000	0.5%
5	Illinois	1,506,000	3.5%
18	Indiana	669,000	1.5%
33	Iowa	340,000	0.8%
34	Kansas	304,000	0.7%
26	Kentucky	587,000	1.4%
14	Louisiana	827,000	1.9%
39	Maine	182,000	0.4%
17	Maryland	677,000	1.6%
16	Massachusetts	755,000	1.7%
12	Michigan	1,133,000	2.6%
29	Minnesota	438,000	1.0%
27	Mississippi	550,000	1.3%
18	Missouri	669,000	1.5%
41	Montana	174,000	0.4%
40	Nebraska	180,000	0.4%
35	Nevada	301,000	0.7%
42	New Hampshire	141,000	0.3%
7	New Jersey	1,320,000	3.0%
30	New Mexico	413,000	1.0%
3	New York	3,174,000	7.3%
10	North Carolina	1,141,000	2.6%
45	North Dakota	97,000	0.2%
8	Ohio	1,297,000	3.0%
24	Oklahoma	592,000	1.4%
28	Oregon	441,000	1.0%
9	Pennsylvania	1,209,000	2.8%
46	Rhode Island	96,000	0.2%
22	South Carolina	641,000	1.5%
48	South Dakota	83,000	0.2%
15	Tennessee	756,000	1.7%
2	Texas	4,835,000	11.1%
37	Utah	280,000	0.6%
50	Vermont	55,000	0.1%
13	Virginia	854,000	2.0%
21	Washington	654,000	1.5%
36	West Virginia	299,000	0.7%
31	Wisconsin	408,000	0.9%
49	Wyoming	77,000	0.2%

RANK	STATE	UNINSURED	% of USA
1	California	7,094,000	16.3%
2	Texas	4,835,000	11.1%
3	New York	3,174,000	7.3%
4	Florida	2,818,000	6.5%
5	Illinois	1,506,000	3.5%
6	Georgia	1,343,000	3.1%
7	New Jersey	1,320,000	3.0%
8	Ohio	1,297,000	3.0%
9	Pennsylvania	1,209,000	2.8%
10	North Carolina	1,141,000	2.6%
11	Arizona	1,140,000	2.6%
12	Michigan	1,133,000	2.6%
13	Virginia	854,000	2.0%
14	Louisiana	827,000	1.9%
15	Tennessee	756,000	1.7%
16	Massachusetts	755,000	1.7%
17	Maryland	677,000	1.6%
18	Indiana	669,000	1.5%
18	Missouri	669,000	1.5%
20	Alabama	658,000	1.5%
21	Washington	654,000	1.5%
22	South Carolina	641,000	1.5%
23	Arkansas	639,000	1.5%
24	Colorado	592,000	1.4%
24	Oklahoma	592,000	1.4%
26	Kentucky	587,000	1.4%
27	Mississippi	550,000	1.3%
28	Oregon	441,000	1.0%
29	Minnesota	438,000	1.0%
30	New Mexico	413,000	1.0%
31	Wisconsin	408,000	0.9%
32	Connecticut	396,000	0.9%
33	Iowa	340,000	0.8%
34	Kansas	304,000	0.7%
35	Nevada	301,000	0.7%
36	West Virginia	299,000	0.7%
37	Utah	280,000	0.6%
38	Idaho	223,000	0.5%
39	Maine	182,000	0.4%
40	Nebraska	180,000	0.4%
41	Montana	174,000	0.4%
42	New Hampshire	141,000	0.3%
43	Alaska	116,000	0.3%
44	Delaware	99,000	0.2%
45	North Dakota	97,000	0.2%
46	Rhode Island	96,000	0.2%
47	Hawaii	89,000	0.2%
48	South Dakota	83,000	0.2%
49	Wyoming	77,000	0.2%
50	Vermont	55,000	0.1%
	District of Columbia	84,000	0.2%

Source: U.S. Bureau of the Census
"Health Insurance Historical Table 4" (http://www.census.gov/hhes/hlthins/historic/hihistt4.html)

Percent of Population Not Covered by Health Insurance in 1997

National Percent = 16.1% of Population

<table>
<tr><td colspan="3">ALPHA ORDER</td><td colspan="3">RANK ORDER</td></tr>
<tr><td>RANK</td><td>STATE</td><td>PERCENT</td><td>RANK</td><td>STATE</td><td>PERCENT</td></tr>
<tr><td>20</td><td>Alabama</td><td>15.5</td><td>1</td><td>Arizona</td><td>24.5</td></tr>
<tr><td>10</td><td>Alaska</td><td>18.1</td><td>1</td><td>Texas</td><td>24.5</td></tr>
<tr><td>1</td><td>Arizona</td><td>24.5</td><td>3</td><td>Arkansas</td><td>24.4</td></tr>
<tr><td>3</td><td>Arkansas</td><td>24.4</td><td>4</td><td>New Mexico</td><td>22.6</td></tr>
<tr><td>5</td><td>California</td><td>21.5</td><td>5</td><td>California</td><td>21.5</td></tr>
<tr><td>23</td><td>Colorado</td><td>15.1</td><td>6</td><td>Mississippi</td><td>20.1</td></tr>
<tr><td>35</td><td>Connecticut</td><td>12.0</td><td>7</td><td>Florida</td><td>19.6</td></tr>
<tr><td>30</td><td>Delaware</td><td>13.1</td><td>8</td><td>Montana</td><td>19.5</td></tr>
<tr><td>7</td><td>Florida</td><td>19.6</td><td>9</td><td>Louisiana</td><td>19.4</td></tr>
<tr><td>13</td><td>Georgia</td><td>17.6</td><td>10</td><td>Alaska</td><td>18.1</td></tr>
<tr><td>50</td><td>Hawaii</td><td>7.5</td><td>11</td><td>Idaho</td><td>17.7</td></tr>
<tr><td>11</td><td>Idaho</td><td>17.7</td><td>11</td><td>Oklahoma</td><td>17.7</td></tr>
<tr><td>34</td><td>Illinois</td><td>12.4</td><td>13</td><td>Georgia</td><td>17.6</td></tr>
<tr><td>42</td><td>Indiana</td><td>11.4</td><td>14</td><td>Nevada</td><td>17.5</td></tr>
<tr><td>35</td><td>Iowa</td><td>12.0</td><td>14</td><td>New York</td><td>17.5</td></tr>
<tr><td>38</td><td>Kansas</td><td>11.7</td><td>16</td><td>West Virginia</td><td>17.1</td></tr>
<tr><td>24</td><td>Kentucky</td><td>15.0</td><td>17</td><td>South Carolina</td><td>16.8</td></tr>
<tr><td>9</td><td>Louisiana</td><td>19.4</td><td>18</td><td>New Jersey</td><td>16.5</td></tr>
<tr><td>25</td><td>Maine</td><td>14.9</td><td>19</td><td>Wyoming</td><td>15.7</td></tr>
<tr><td>27</td><td>Maryland</td><td>13.4</td><td>20</td><td>Alabama</td><td>15.5</td></tr>
<tr><td>31</td><td>Massachusetts</td><td>12.6</td><td>20</td><td>North Carolina</td><td>15.5</td></tr>
<tr><td>40</td><td>Michigan</td><td>11.6</td><td>22</td><td>North Dakota</td><td>15.2</td></tr>
<tr><td>48</td><td>Minnesota</td><td>9.2</td><td>23</td><td>Colorado</td><td>15.1</td></tr>
<tr><td>6</td><td>Mississippi</td><td>20.1</td><td>24</td><td>Kentucky</td><td>15.0</td></tr>
<tr><td>31</td><td>Missouri</td><td>12.6</td><td>25</td><td>Maine</td><td>14.9</td></tr>
<tr><td>8</td><td>Montana</td><td>19.5</td><td>26</td><td>Tennessee</td><td>13.6</td></tr>
<tr><td>44</td><td>Nebraska</td><td>10.8</td><td>27</td><td>Maryland</td><td>13.4</td></tr>
<tr><td>14</td><td>Nevada</td><td>17.5</td><td>27</td><td>Oregon</td><td>13.4</td></tr>
<tr><td>37</td><td>New Hampshire</td><td>11.8</td><td>27</td><td>Utah</td><td>13.4</td></tr>
<tr><td>18</td><td>New Jersey</td><td>16.5</td><td>30</td><td>Delaware</td><td>13.1</td></tr>
<tr><td>4</td><td>New Mexico</td><td>22.6</td><td>31</td><td>Massachusetts</td><td>12.6</td></tr>
<tr><td>14</td><td>New York</td><td>17.5</td><td>31</td><td>Missouri</td><td>12.6</td></tr>
<tr><td>20</td><td>North Carolina</td><td>15.5</td><td>31</td><td>Virginia</td><td>12.6</td></tr>
<tr><td>22</td><td>North Dakota</td><td>15.2</td><td>34</td><td>Illinois</td><td>12.4</td></tr>
<tr><td>41</td><td>Ohio</td><td>11.5</td><td>35</td><td>Connecticut</td><td>12.0</td></tr>
<tr><td>11</td><td>Oklahoma</td><td>17.7</td><td>35</td><td>Iowa</td><td>12.0</td></tr>
<tr><td>27</td><td>Oregon</td><td>13.4</td><td>37</td><td>New Hampshire</td><td>11.8</td></tr>
<tr><td>46</td><td>Pennsylvania</td><td>10.1</td><td>38</td><td>Kansas</td><td>11.7</td></tr>
<tr><td>45</td><td>Rhode Island</td><td>10.2</td><td>38</td><td>South Dakota</td><td>11.7</td></tr>
<tr><td>17</td><td>South Carolina</td><td>16.8</td><td>40</td><td>Michigan</td><td>11.6</td></tr>
<tr><td>38</td><td>South Dakota</td><td>11.7</td><td>41</td><td>Ohio</td><td>11.5</td></tr>
<tr><td>26</td><td>Tennessee</td><td>13.6</td><td>42</td><td>Indiana</td><td>11.4</td></tr>
<tr><td>1</td><td>Texas</td><td>24.5</td><td>42</td><td>Washington</td><td>11.4</td></tr>
<tr><td>27</td><td>Utah</td><td>13.4</td><td>44</td><td>Nebraska</td><td>10.8</td></tr>
<tr><td>47</td><td>Vermont</td><td>9.5</td><td>45</td><td>Rhode Island</td><td>10.2</td></tr>
<tr><td>31</td><td>Virginia</td><td>12.6</td><td>46</td><td>Pennsylvania</td><td>10.1</td></tr>
<tr><td>42</td><td>Washington</td><td>11.4</td><td>47</td><td>Vermont</td><td>9.5</td></tr>
<tr><td>16</td><td>West Virginia</td><td>17.1</td><td>48</td><td>Minnesota</td><td>9.2</td></tr>
<tr><td>49</td><td>Wisconsin</td><td>8.0</td><td>49</td><td>Wisconsin</td><td>8.0</td></tr>
<tr><td>19</td><td>Wyoming</td><td>15.7</td><td>50</td><td>Hawaii</td><td>7.5</td></tr>
<tr><td></td><td></td><td></td><td></td><td>District of Columbia</td><td>16.1</td></tr>
</table>

Source: U.S. Bureau of the Census
"Health Insurance Historical Table 4" (http://www.census.gov/hhes/hlthins/historic/hihistt4.html)

Change in Number of Persons Uninsured: 1997 to 2001

National Change = 2,241,000 Decrease

ALPHA ORDER

RANK	STATE	CHANGE
36	Alabama	(85,000)
21	Alaska	(16,000)
45	Arizona	(190,000)
46	Arkansas	(211,000)
50	California	(376,000)
4	Colorado	95,000
31	Connecticut	(50,000)
26	Delaware	(26,000)
8	Florida	38,000
9	Georgia	33,000
10	Hawaii	28,000
19	Idaho	(13,000)
1	Illinois	170,000
6	Indiana	45,000
43	Iowa	(124,000)
18	Kansas	(3,000)
39	Kentucky	(95,000)
13	Louisiana	18,000
31	Maine	(50,000)
25	Maryland	(24,000)
48	Massachusetts	(235,000)
41	Michigan	(105,000)
29	Minnesota	(46,000)
38	Mississippi	(91,000)
40	Missouri	(104,000)
33	Montana	(53,000)
23	Nebraska	(20,000)
7	Nevada	43,000
24	New Hampshire	(22,000)
46	New Jersey	(211,000)
28	New Mexico	(40,000)
49	New York	(258,000)
12	North Carolina	26,000
27	North Dakota	(37,000)
30	Ohio	(49,000)
10	Oklahoma	28,000
15	Oregon	2,000
37	Pennsylvania	(90,000)
21	Rhode Island	(16,000)
44	South Carolina	(148,000)
20	South Dakota	(14,000)
42	Tennessee	(116,000)
3	Texas	125,000
5	Utah	55,000
14	Vermont	3,000
35	Virginia	(80,000)
2	Washington	126,000
34	West Virginia	(65,000)
16	Wisconsin	1,000
16	Wyoming	1,000

RANK ORDER

RANK	STATE	CHANGE
1	Illinois	170,000
2	Washington	126,000
3	Texas	125,000
4	Colorado	95,000
5	Utah	55,000
6	Indiana	45,000
7	Nevada	43,000
8	Florida	38,000
9	Georgia	33,000
10	Hawaii	28,000
10	Oklahoma	28,000
12	North Carolina	26,000
13	Louisiana	18,000
14	Vermont	3,000
15	Oregon	2,000
16	Wisconsin	1,000
16	Wyoming	1,000
18	Kansas	(3,000)
19	Idaho	(13,000)
20	South Dakota	(14,000)
21	Alaska	(16,000)
21	Rhode Island	(16,000)
23	Nebraska	(20,000)
24	New Hampshire	(22,000)
25	Maryland	(24,000)
26	Delaware	(26,000)
27	North Dakota	(37,000)
28	New Mexico	(40,000)
29	Minnesota	(46,000)
30	Ohio	(49,000)
31	Connecticut	(50,000)
31	Maine	(50,000)
33	Montana	(53,000)
34	West Virginia	(65,000)
35	Virginia	(80,000)
36	Alabama	(85,000)
37	Pennsylvania	(90,000)
38	Mississippi	(91,000)
39	Kentucky	(95,000)
40	Missouri	(104,000)
41	Michigan	(105,000)
42	Tennessee	(116,000)
43	Iowa	(124,000)
44	South Carolina	(148,000)
45	Arizona	(190,000)
46	Arkansas	(211,000)
46	New Jersey	(211,000)
48	Massachusetts	(235,000)
49	New York	(258,000)
50	California	(376,000)
	District of Columbia	(14,000)

Source: Morgan Quitno Press using data from U.S. Bureau of the Census
"Health Insurance Historical Table 4" (http://www.census.gov/hhes/hlthins/historic/hihistt4.html) and
"Health Insurance Coverage Status by State for All People: 2001"
(http://ferret.bls.census.gov/macro/032002/health/h06_000.htm)

Percent Change in Number Uninsured: 1997 to 2001

National Percent Change = 5.2% Decrease*

ALPHA ORDER

RANK	STATE	PERCENT CHANGE
31	Alabama	(12.9)
32	Alaska	(13.8)
39	Arizona	(16.7)
48	Arkansas	(33.0)
21	California	(5.3)
4	Colorado	16.0
30	Connecticut	(12.6)
44	Delaware	(26.3)
14	Florida	1.3
11	Georgia	2.5
1	Hawaii	31.5
22	Idaho	(5.8)
6	Illinois	11.3
7	Indiana	6.7
49	Iowa	(36.5)
18	Kansas	(1.0)
37	Kentucky	(16.2)
13	Louisiana	2.2
45	Maine	(27.5)
19	Maryland	(3.5)
47	Massachusetts	(31.1)
25	Michigan	(9.3)
28	Minnesota	(10.5)
38	Mississippi	(16.5)
34	Missouri	(15.5)
46	Montana	(30.5)
29	Nebraska	(11.1)
5	Nevada	14.3
35	New Hampshire	(15.6)
36	New Jersey	(16.0)
27	New Mexico	(9.7)
24	New York	(8.1)
12	North Carolina	2.3
50	North Dakota	(38.1)
20	Ohio	(3.8)
9	Oklahoma	4.7
16	Oregon	0.5
23	Pennsylvania	(7.4)
39	Rhode Island	(16.7)
43	South Carolina	(23.1)
41	South Dakota	(16.9)
33	Tennessee	(15.3)
10	Texas	2.6
2	Utah	19.6
8	Vermont	5.5
26	Virginia	(9.4)
3	Washington	19.3
42	West Virginia	(21.7)
17	Wisconsin	0.2
14	Wyoming	1.3

RANK ORDER

RANK	STATE	PERCENT CHANGE
1	Hawaii	31.5
2	Utah	19.6
3	Washington	19.3
4	Colorado	16.0
5	Nevada	14.3
6	Illinois	11.3
7	Indiana	6.7
8	Vermont	5.5
9	Oklahoma	4.7
10	Texas	2.6
11	Georgia	2.5
12	North Carolina	2.3
13	Louisiana	2.2
14	Florida	1.3
14	Wyoming	1.3
16	Oregon	0.5
17	Wisconsin	0.2
18	Kansas	(1.0)
19	Maryland	(3.5)
20	Ohio	(3.8)
21	California	(5.3)
22	Idaho	(5.8)
23	Pennsylvania	(7.4)
24	New York	(8.1)
25	Michigan	(9.3)
26	Virginia	(9.4)
27	New Mexico	(9.7)
28	Minnesota	(10.5)
29	Nebraska	(11.1)
30	Connecticut	(12.6)
31	Alabama	(12.9)
32	Alaska	(13.8)
33	Tennessee	(15.3)
34	Missouri	(15.5)
35	New Hampshire	(15.6)
36	New Jersey	(16.0)
37	Kentucky	(16.2)
38	Mississippi	(16.5)
39	Arizona	(16.7)
39	Rhode Island	(16.7)
41	South Dakota	(16.9)
42	West Virginia	(21.7)
43	South Carolina	(23.1)
44	Delaware	(26.3)
45	Maine	(27.5)
46	Montana	(30.5)
47	Massachusetts	(31.1)
48	Arkansas	(33.0)
49	Iowa	(36.5)
50	North Dakota	(38.1)
	District of Columbia	(16.7)

Source: Morgan Quitno Press using data from U.S. Bureau of the Census
    "Health Insurance Historical Table 4" (http://www.census.gov/hhes/hlthins/historic/hihistt4.html) and
    "Health Insurance Coverage Status by State for All People: 2001"
    (http://ferret.bls.census.gov/macro/032002/health/h06_000.htm)

Change in Percent of Population Uninsured: 1997 to 2001

National Percent Change = 9.3% Decrease*

<table>
<tr><td colspan="3">ALPHA ORDER</td><td colspan="3">RANK ORDER</td></tr>
<tr><td>RANK</td><td>STATE</td><td>PERCENT CHANGE</td><td>RANK</td><td>STATE</td><td>PERCENT CHANGE</td></tr>
<tr><td>32</td><td>Alabama</td><td>(15.5)</td><td>1</td><td>Hawaii</td><td>28.0</td></tr>
<tr><td>29</td><td>Alaska</td><td>(13.3)</td><td>2</td><td>Washington</td><td>14.9</td></tr>
<tr><td>43</td><td>Arizona</td><td>(26.9)</td><td>3</td><td>Utah</td><td>10.4</td></tr>
<tr><td>47</td><td>Arkansas</td><td>(34.0)</td><td>4</td><td>Illinois</td><td>9.7</td></tr>
<tr><td>22</td><td>California</td><td>(9.3)</td><td>5</td><td>Indiana</td><td>3.5</td></tr>
<tr><td>7</td><td>Colorado</td><td>3.3</td><td>6</td><td>Oklahoma</td><td>3.4</td></tr>
<tr><td>31</td><td>Connecticut</td><td>(15.0)</td><td>7</td><td>Colorado</td><td>3.3</td></tr>
<tr><td>44</td><td>Delaware</td><td>(29.8)</td><td>8</td><td>Wyoming</td><td>1.3</td></tr>
<tr><td>25</td><td>Florida</td><td>(10.7)</td><td>9</td><td>Vermont</td><td>1.1</td></tr>
<tr><td>16</td><td>Georgia</td><td>(5.7)</td><td>10</td><td>Louisiana</td><td>(0.5)</td></tr>
<tr><td>1</td><td>Hawaii</td><td>28.0</td><td>11</td><td>Kansas</td><td>(2.6)</td></tr>
<tr><td>23</td><td>Idaho</td><td>(9.6)</td><td>11</td><td>Ohio</td><td>(2.6)</td></tr>
<tr><td>4</td><td>Illinois</td><td>9.7</td><td>13</td><td>Wisconsin</td><td>(3.8)</td></tr>
<tr><td>5</td><td>Indiana</td><td>3.5</td><td>14</td><td>Texas</td><td>(4.1)</td></tr>
<tr><td>50</td><td>Iowa</td><td>(37.5)</td><td>15</td><td>Oregon</td><td>(4.5)</td></tr>
<tr><td>11</td><td>Kansas</td><td>(2.6)</td><td>16</td><td>Georgia</td><td>(5.7)</td></tr>
<tr><td>34</td><td>Kentucky</td><td>(18.0)</td><td>17</td><td>North Carolina</td><td>(7.1)</td></tr>
<tr><td>10</td><td>Louisiana</td><td>(0.5)</td><td>18</td><td>Nevada</td><td>(8.0)</td></tr>
<tr><td>46</td><td>Maine</td><td>(30.9)</td><td>19</td><td>Maryland</td><td>(8.2)</td></tr>
<tr><td>19</td><td>Maryland</td><td>(8.2)</td><td>20</td><td>New Mexico</td><td>(8.4)</td></tr>
<tr><td>48</td><td>Massachusetts</td><td>(34.9)</td><td>21</td><td>Pennsylvania</td><td>(8.9)</td></tr>
<tr><td>24</td><td>Michigan</td><td>(10.3)</td><td>22</td><td>California</td><td>(9.3)</td></tr>
<tr><td>28</td><td>Minnesota</td><td>(13.0)</td><td>23</td><td>Idaho</td><td>(9.6)</td></tr>
<tr><td>35</td><td>Mississippi</td><td>(18.4)</td><td>24</td><td>Michigan</td><td>(10.3)</td></tr>
<tr><td>36</td><td>Missouri</td><td>(19.0)</td><td>25</td><td>Florida</td><td>(10.7)</td></tr>
<tr><td>45</td><td>Montana</td><td>(30.3)</td><td>26</td><td>New York</td><td>(11.4)</td></tr>
<tr><td>27</td><td>Nebraska</td><td>(12.0)</td><td>27</td><td>Nebraska</td><td>(12.0)</td></tr>
<tr><td>18</td><td>Nevada</td><td>(8.0)</td><td>28</td><td>Minnesota</td><td>(13.0)</td></tr>
<tr><td>37</td><td>New Hampshire</td><td>(20.3)</td><td>29</td><td>Alaska</td><td>(13.3)</td></tr>
<tr><td>39</td><td>New Jersey</td><td>(20.6)</td><td>30</td><td>Virginia</td><td>(13.5)</td></tr>
<tr><td>20</td><td>New Mexico</td><td>(8.4)</td><td>31</td><td>Connecticut</td><td>(15.0)</td></tr>
<tr><td>26</td><td>New York</td><td>(11.4)</td><td>32</td><td>Alabama</td><td>(15.5)</td></tr>
<tr><td>17</td><td>North Carolina</td><td>(7.1)</td><td>33</td><td>Tennessee</td><td>(16.9)</td></tr>
<tr><td>49</td><td>North Dakota</td><td>(36.8)</td><td>34</td><td>Kentucky</td><td>(18.0)</td></tr>
<tr><td>11</td><td>Ohio</td><td>(2.6)</td><td>35</td><td>Mississippi</td><td>(18.4)</td></tr>
<tr><td>6</td><td>Oklahoma</td><td>3.4</td><td>36</td><td>Missouri</td><td>(19.0)</td></tr>
<tr><td>15</td><td>Oregon</td><td>(4.5)</td><td>37</td><td>New Hampshire</td><td>(20.3)</td></tr>
<tr><td>21</td><td>Pennsylvania</td><td>(8.9)</td><td>38</td><td>South Dakota</td><td>(20.5)</td></tr>
<tr><td>41</td><td>Rhode Island</td><td>(24.5)</td><td>39</td><td>New Jersey</td><td>(20.6)</td></tr>
<tr><td>42</td><td>South Carolina</td><td>(26.8)</td><td>40</td><td>West Virginia</td><td>(22.8)</td></tr>
<tr><td>38</td><td>South Dakota</td><td>(20.5)</td><td>41</td><td>Rhode Island</td><td>(24.5)</td></tr>
<tr><td>33</td><td>Tennessee</td><td>(16.9)</td><td>42</td><td>South Carolina</td><td>(26.8)</td></tr>
<tr><td>14</td><td>Texas</td><td>(4.1)</td><td>43</td><td>Arizona</td><td>(26.9)</td></tr>
<tr><td>3</td><td>Utah</td><td>10.4</td><td>44</td><td>Delaware</td><td>(29.8)</td></tr>
<tr><td>9</td><td>Vermont</td><td>1.1</td><td>45</td><td>Montana</td><td>(30.3)</td></tr>
<tr><td>30</td><td>Virginia</td><td>(13.5)</td><td>46</td><td>Maine</td><td>(30.9)</td></tr>
<tr><td>2</td><td>Washington</td><td>14.9</td><td>47</td><td>Arkansas</td><td>(34.0)</td></tr>
<tr><td>40</td><td>West Virginia</td><td>(22.8)</td><td>48</td><td>Massachusetts</td><td>(34.9)</td></tr>
<tr><td>13</td><td>Wisconsin</td><td>(3.8)</td><td>49</td><td>North Dakota</td><td>(36.8)</td></tr>
<tr><td>8</td><td>Wyoming</td><td>1.3</td><td>50</td><td>Iowa</td><td>(37.5)</td></tr>
<tr><td></td><td></td><td></td><td></td><td>District of Columbia</td><td>(21.1)</td></tr>
</table>

Source: Morgan Quitno Press using data from U.S. Bureau of the Census
"Health Insurance Historical Table 4" (http://www.census.gov/hhes/hlthins/historic/hihistt4.html) and
"Health Insurance Coverage Status by State for All People: 2001"
(http://ferret.bls.census.gov/macro/032002/health/h06_000.htm)

Percent of Children Not Covered by Health Insurance in 2001

National Percent = 11.7% of Children*

ALPHA ORDER

RANK	STATE	PERCENT
29	Alabama	8.9
21	Alaska	10.4
2	Arizona	17.8
12	Arkansas	11.9
5	California	15.1
9	Colorado	13.0
34	Connecticut	7.7
30	Delaware	8.6
3	Florida	15.9
6	Georgia	15.0
26	Hawaii	9.3
12	Idaho	11.9
23	Illinois	10.3
18	Indiana	11.2
46	Iowa	4.7
35	Kansas	7.6
25	Kentucky	9.7
10	Louisiana	12.7
42	Maine	6.2
28	Maryland	9.1
45	Massachusetts	5.3
31	Michigan	8.1
44	Minnesota	5.6
21	Mississippi	10.4
46	Missouri	4.7
11	Montana	12.2
40	Nebraska	7.3
8	Nevada	14.2
41	New Hampshire	7.2
15	New Jersey	11.5
6	New Mexico	15.0
26	New York	9.3
18	North Carolina	11.2
33	North Dakota	7.9
38	Ohio	7.5
4	Oklahoma	15.6
20	Oregon	11.0
32	Pennsylvania	8.0
48	Rhode Island	4.5
24	South Carolina	10.0
35	South Dakota	7.6
42	Tennessee	6.2
1	Texas	21.3
15	Utah	11.5
50	Vermont	3.3
35	Virginia	7.6
17	Washington	11.3
38	West Virginia	7.5
49	Wisconsin	4.2
14	Wyoming	11.7

RANK ORDER

RANK	STATE	PERCENT
1	Texas	21.3
2	Arizona	17.8
3	Florida	15.9
4	Oklahoma	15.6
5	California	15.1
6	Georgia	15.0
6	New Mexico	15.0
8	Nevada	14.2
9	Colorado	13.0
10	Louisiana	12.7
11	Montana	12.2
12	Arkansas	11.9
12	Idaho	11.9
14	Wyoming	11.7
15	New Jersey	11.5
15	Utah	11.5
17	Washington	11.3
18	Indiana	11.2
18	North Carolina	11.2
20	Oregon	11.0
21	Alaska	10.4
21	Mississippi	10.4
23	Illinois	10.3
24	South Carolina	10.0
25	Kentucky	9.7
26	Hawaii	9.3
26	New York	9.3
28	Maryland	9.1
29	Alabama	8.9
30	Delaware	8.6
31	Michigan	8.1
32	Pennsylvania	8.0
33	North Dakota	7.9
34	Connecticut	7.7
35	Kansas	7.6
35	South Dakota	7.6
35	Virginia	7.6
38	Ohio	7.5
38	West Virginia	7.5
40	Nebraska	7.3
41	New Hampshire	7.2
42	Maine	6.2
42	Tennessee	6.2
44	Minnesota	5.6
45	Massachusetts	5.3
46	Iowa	4.7
46	Missouri	4.7
48	Rhode Island	4.5
49	Wisconsin	4.2
50	Vermont	3.3
	District of Columbia	8.6

Source: U.S. Bureau of the Census
  "Health Insurance Historical Table 5" (http://www.census.gov/hhes/hlthins/historic/hihistt5.html)
*Children under 18 years old.

State Children's Health Insurance Program (SCHIP) Enrollment in 2002

National Total = 5,315,229 Children*

ALPHA ORDER

RANK ORDER

RANK	STATE	CHILDREN	% of USA	RANK	STATE	CHILDREN	% of USA
17	Alabama	83,359	1.6%	1	California	856,994	16.1%
33	Alaska	22,291	0.4%	2	New York	807,145	15.2%
14	Arizona	92,705	1.7%	3	Texas	727,452	13.7%
48	Arkansas	1,912	0.0%	4	Florida	368,180	6.9%
1	California	856,994	16.1%	5	Georgia	221,005	4.2%
25	Colorado	51,826	1.0%	6	Ohio	183,034	3.4%
34	Connecticut	21,346	0.4%	7	Pennsylvania	148,689	2.8%
41	Delaware	9,691	0.2%	8	Maryland	125,180	2.4%
4	Florida	368,180	6.9%	9	North Carolina	120,090	2.3%
5	Georgia	221,005	4.2%	10	New Jersey	117,053	2.2%
43	Hawaii	8,474	0.2%	11	Massachusetts	116,699	2.2%
37	Idaho	16,895	0.3%	12	Missouri	112,004	2.1%
20	Illinois	68,032	1.3%	13	Kentucky	93,941	1.8%
22	Indiana	66,225	1.2%	14	Arizona	92,705	1.7%
30	Iowa	34,506	0.6%	15	Louisiana	87,675	1.6%
27	Kansas	40,783	0.8%	16	Oklahoma	84,490	1.6%
13	Kentucky	93,941	1.8%	17	Alabama	83,359	1.6%
15	Louisiana	87,675	1.6%	18	Michigan	71,882	1.4%
32	Maine	22,586	0.4%	19	South Carolina	68,928	1.3%
8	Maryland	125,180	2.4%	20	Illinois	68,032	1.3%
11	Massachusetts	116,699	2.2%	21	Virginia	67,974	1.3%
18	Michigan	71,882	1.4%	22	Indiana	66,225	1.2%
NA	Minnesota**	NA	NA	23	Mississippi	64,805	1.2%
23	Mississippi	64,805	1.2%	24	Wisconsin	62,391	1.2%
12	Missouri	112,004	2.1%	25	Colorado	51,826	1.0%
39	Montana	13,875	0.3%	26	Oregon	42,976	0.8%
38	Nebraska	16,227	0.3%	27	Kansas	40,783	0.8%
28	Nevada	37,878	0.7%	28	Nevada	37,878	0.7%
44	New Hampshire	8,138	0.2%	29	West Virginia	35,949	0.7%
10	New Jersey	117,053	2.2%	30	Iowa	34,506	0.6%
35	New Mexico	19,940	0.4%	31	Utah	33,808	0.6%
2	New York	807,145	15.2%	32	Maine	22,586	0.4%
9	North Carolina	120,090	2.3%	33	Alaska	22,291	0.4%
47	North Dakota	4,463	0.1%	34	Connecticut	21,346	0.4%
6	Ohio	183,034	3.4%	35	New Mexico	19,940	0.4%
16	Oklahoma	84,490	1.6%	36	Rhode Island	19,515	0.4%
26	Oregon	42,976	0.8%	37	Idaho	16,895	0.3%
7	Pennsylvania	148,689	2.8%	38	Nebraska	16,227	0.3%
36	Rhode Island	19,515	0.4%	39	Montana	13,875	0.3%
19	South Carolina	68,928	1.3%	40	South Dakota	11,183	0.2%
40	South Dakota	11,183	0.2%	41	Delaware	9,691	0.2%
NA	Tennessee**	NA	NA	42	Washington	8,754	0.2%
3	Texas	727,452	13.7%	43	Hawaii	8,474	0.2%
31	Utah	33,808	0.6%	44	New Hampshire	8,138	0.2%
45	Vermont	6,162	0.1%	45	Vermont	6,162	0.1%
21	Virginia	67,974	1.3%	46	Wyoming	5,059	0.1%
42	Washington	8,754	0.2%	47	North Dakota	4,463	0.1%
29	West Virginia	35,949	0.7%	48	Arkansas	1,912	0.0%
24	Wisconsin	62,391	1.2%	NA	Minnesota**	NA	NA
46	Wyoming	5,059	0.1%	NA	Tennessee**	NA	NA
					District of Columbia	5,060	0.1%

Source: U.S. Department of Health and Human Services, Centers for Medicare and Medicaid Services
   "Children's Health Insurance Program" (http://www.cms.gov/schip/schip02.pdf)
*Preliminary for fiscal year 2002. The State Children's Health Insurance Program (SCHIP) was created in 1997 to help states expand health insurance to children whose families earn too much to qualify for Medicaid, yet not enough to afford private health insurance.
**Not reported.

Percent Change in State Children's Health Insurance Program (SCHIP) Enrollment: 2001 to 2002
National Percent Change = 15.0% Increase*

ALPHA ORDER

RANK ORDER

RANK	STATE	PERCENT CHANGE		RANK	STATE	PERCENT CHANGE
15	Alabama	22.3		1	Oklahoma	117.4
40	Alaska	2.1		2	New Mexico	92.7
34	Arizona	6.7		3	Delaware	74.1
48	Arkansas	(33.7)		4	Iowa	48.3
14	California	22.9		5	Texas	45.2
27	Colorado	13.2		6	Kentucky	37.6
25	Connecticut	14.6		7	New Hampshire	36.0
3	Delaware	74.1		8	Nevada	35.2
13	Florida	23.3		9	North Dakota	31.1
16	Georgia	20.9		10	Louisiana	26.0
19	Hawaii	18.7		11	South Dakota	23.7
41	Idaho	0.0		12	Mississippi	23.6
47	Illinois	(18.5)		13	Florida	23.3
22	Indiana	16.2		14	California	22.9
4	Iowa	48.3		15	Alabama	22.3
18	Kansas	19.0		16	Georgia	20.9
6	Kentucky	37.6		17	North Carolina	20.1
10	Louisiana	26.0		18	Kansas	19.0
46	Maine	(16.4)		19	Hawaii	18.7
26	Maryland	13.8		20	New Jersey	17.2
33	Massachusetts	7.7		21	Nebraska	16.5
43	Michigan	(5.6)		22	Indiana	16.2
NA	Minnesota**	NA		23	Vermont	15.1
12	Mississippi	23.6		24	Washington	14.9
36	Missouri	4.7		25	Connecticut	14.6
39	Montana	2.6		26	Maryland	13.8
21	Nebraska	16.5		27	Colorado	13.2
8	Nevada	35.2		28	Ohio	12.7
7	New Hampshire	36.0		29	Rhode Island	12.2
20	New Jersey	17.2		30	Wisconsin	9.1
2	New Mexico	92.7		31	Wyoming	8.7
45	New York	(7.5)		32	West Virginia	8.5
17	North Carolina	20.1		33	Massachusetts	7.7
9	North Dakota	31.1		34	Arizona	6.7
28	Ohio	12.7		35	Pennsylvania	5.3
1	Oklahoma	117.4		36	Missouri	4.7
38	Oregon	3.6		37	South Carolina	4.1
35	Pennsylvania	5.3		38	Oregon	3.6
29	Rhode Island	12.2		39	Montana	2.6
37	South Carolina	4.1		40	Alaska	2.1
11	South Dakota	23.7		41	Idaho	0.0
NA	Tennessee**	NA		42	Utah	(2.4)
5	Texas	45.2		43	Michigan	(5.6)
42	Utah	(2.4)		44	Virginia	(7.0)
23	Vermont	15.1		45	New York	(7.5)
44	Virginia	(7.0)		46	Maine	(16.4)
24	Washington	14.9		47	Illinois	(18.5)
32	West Virginia	8.5		48	Arkansas	(33.7)
30	Wisconsin	9.1		NA	Minnesota**	NA
31	Wyoming	8.7		NA	Tennessee**	NA

| | District of Columbia | 80.3 |

Source: MQ Press using data from U.S. Dept of Health & Human Services, Centers for Medicare and Medicaid Services "Children's Health Insurance Program" (http://www.cms.gov/schip/schip02.pdf)

*Preliminary for fiscal year 2002. The State Children's Health Insurance Program (SCHIP) was created in 1997 to help states expand health insurance to children whose families earn too much to qualify for Medicaid, yet not enough to afford private health insurance.

**Not reported.

Percent of Children Enrolled in State Children's
Health Insurance Program (SCHIP) in 2002
National Percent = 7.4% of Children 17 Years and Younger*

ALPHA ORDER

RANK	STATE	PERCENT
16	Alabama	7.4
3	Alaska	11.7
19	Arizona	6.8
48	Arkansas	0.3
8	California	9.3
30	Colorado	4.7
45	Connecticut	2.5
29	Delaware	5.0
5	Florida	10.1
4	Georgia	10.2
41	Hawaii	2.9
33	Idaho	4.6
46	Illinois	2.1
35	Indiana	4.2
30	Iowa	4.7
24	Kansas	5.7
7	Kentucky	9.4
18	Louisiana	7.2
15	Maine	7.5
9	Maryland	9.2
13	Massachusetts	7.8
42	Michigan	2.8
NA	Minnesota**	NA
11	Mississippi	8.4
13	Missouri	7.8
23	Montana	6.0
40	Nebraska	3.6
16	Nevada	7.4
44	New Hampshire	2.6
25	New Jersey	5.6
37	New Mexico	3.9
1	New York	17.2
22	North Carolina	6.1
42	North Dakota	2.8
21	Ohio	6.3
6	Oklahoma	9.5
27	Oregon	5.1
27	Pennsylvania	5.1
12	Rhode Island	7.9
19	South Carolina	6.8
26	South Dakota	5.5
NA	Tennessee**	NA
2	Texas	12.4
30	Utah	4.7
35	Vermont	4.2
37	Virginia	3.9
47	Washington	0.6
10	West Virginia	8.9
33	Wisconsin	4.6
37	Wyoming	3.9

RANK ORDER

RANK	STATE	PERCENT
1	New York	17.2
2	Texas	12.4
3	Alaska	11.7
4	Georgia	10.2
5	Florida	10.1
6	Oklahoma	9.5
7	Kentucky	9.4
8	California	9.3
9	Maryland	9.2
10	West Virginia	8.9
11	Mississippi	8.4
12	Rhode Island	7.9
13	Massachusetts	7.8
13	Missouri	7.8
15	Maine	7.5
16	Alabama	7.4
16	Nevada	7.4
18	Louisiana	7.2
19	Arizona	6.8
19	South Carolina	6.8
21	Ohio	6.3
22	North Carolina	6.1
23	Montana	6.0
24	Kansas	5.7
25	New Jersey	5.6
26	South Dakota	5.5
27	Oregon	5.1
27	Pennsylvania	5.1
29	Delaware	5.0
30	Colorado	4.7
30	Iowa	4.7
30	Utah	4.7
33	Idaho	4.6
33	Wisconsin	4.6
35	Indiana	4.2
35	Vermont	4.2
37	New Mexico	3.9
37	Virginia	3.9
37	Wyoming	3.9
40	Nebraska	3.6
41	Hawaii	2.9
42	Michigan	2.8
42	North Dakota	2.8
44	New Hampshire	2.6
45	Connecticut	2.5
46	Illinois	2.1
47	Washington	0.6
48	Arkansas	0.3
NA	Minnesota**	NA
NA	Tennessee**	NA

District of Columbia   4.4

Source: MQ Press using data from U.S. Dept of Health & Human Services, Centers for Medicare and Medicaid Services
"Children's Health Insurance Program" (http://www.cms.gov/schip/schip02.pdf)
*For fiscal year 2002. The State Children's Health Insurance Program (SCHIP) was created in 1997 to help states
expand health insurance to children whose families earn too much to qualify for Medicaid, yet not enough to afford
private health insurance. Calculated using 2000 Census population counts.

Expenditures for State Children's Health Insurance Program (SCHIP) in 2001

National Total = $3,825,815,526*

ALPHA ORDER

RANK	STATE	EXPENDITURES	% of USA
21	Alabama	$52,726,132	1.4%
26	Alaska	32,703,546	0.9%
16	Arizona	63,107,549	1.6%
49	Arkansas	3,041,237	0.1%
2	California	472,725,298	12.4%
28	Colorado	32,219,993	0.8%
34	Connecticut	20,276,440	0.5%
46	Delaware	3,522,910	0.1%
4	Florida	280,423,871	7.3%
9	Georgia	107,394,549	2.8%
44	Hawaii	4,494,374	0.1%
38	Idaho	16,329,656	0.4%
18	Illinois	60,172,536	1.6%
12	Indiana	81,661,975	2.1%
25	Iowa	33,630,995	0.9%
24	Kansas	34,226,716	0.9%
11	Kentucky	85,961,492	2.2%
22	Louisiana	50,017,975	1.3%
36	Maine	18,534,011	0.5%
6	Maryland	142,892,096	3.7%
13	Massachusetts	77,925,866	2.0%
20	Michigan	54,139,320	1.4%
50	Minnesota	1,050,703	0.0%
19	Mississippi	58,491,668	1.5%
15	Missouri	71,929,237	1.9%
37	Montana	17,078,586	0.4%
39	Nebraska	13,147,172	0.3%
32	Nevada	22,193,839	0.6%
43	New Hampshire	4,549,414	0.1%
5	New Jersey	198,281,030	5.2%
40	New Mexico	9,825,870	0.3%
1	New York	528,852,081	13.8%
10	North Carolina	96,119,888	2.5%
48	North Dakota	3,139,322	0.1%
7	Ohio	140,430,524	3.7%
27	Oklahoma	32,430,733	0.8%
33	Oregon	20,545,897	0.5%
8	Pennsylvania	134,241,636	3.5%
30	Rhode Island	27,115,190	0.7%
17	South Carolina	61,187,513	1.6%
42	South Dakota	6,720,328	0.2%
35	Tennessee	19,341,379	0.5%
3	Texas	364,665,345	9.5%
29	Utah	28,195,260	0.7%
47	Vermont	3,175,394	0.1%
23	Virginia	43,630,115	1.1%
41	Washington	8,447,279	0.2%
31	West Virginia	26,827,504	0.7%
14	Wisconsin	77,751,531	2.0%
45	Wyoming	3,936,548	0.1%

RANK ORDER

RANK	STATE	EXPENDITURES	% of USA
1	New York	$528,852,081	13.8%
2	California	472,725,298	12.4%
3	Texas	364,665,345	9.5%
4	Florida	280,423,871	7.3%
5	New Jersey	198,281,030	5.2%
6	Maryland	142,892,096	3.7%
7	Ohio	140,430,524	3.7%
8	Pennsylvania	134,241,636	3.5%
9	Georgia	107,394,549	2.8%
10	North Carolina	96,119,888	2.5%
11	Kentucky	85,961,492	2.2%
12	Indiana	81,661,975	2.1%
13	Massachusetts	77,925,866	2.0%
14	Wisconsin	77,751,531	2.0%
15	Missouri	71,929,237	1.9%
16	Arizona	63,107,549	1.6%
17	South Carolina	61,187,513	1.6%
18	Illinois	60,172,536	1.6%
19	Mississippi	58,491,668	1.5%
20	Michigan	54,139,320	1.4%
21	Alabama	52,726,132	1.4%
22	Louisiana	50,017,975	1.3%
23	Virginia	43,630,115	1.1%
24	Kansas	34,226,716	0.9%
25	Iowa	33,630,995	0.9%
26	Alaska	32,703,546	0.9%
27	Oklahoma	32,430,733	0.8%
28	Colorado	32,219,993	0.8%
29	Utah	28,195,260	0.7%
30	Rhode Island	27,115,190	0.7%
31	West Virginia	26,827,504	0.7%
32	Nevada	22,193,839	0.6%
33	Oregon	20,545,897	0.5%
34	Connecticut	20,276,440	0.5%
35	Tennessee	19,341,379	0.5%
36	Maine	18,534,011	0.5%
37	Montana	17,078,586	0.4%
38	Idaho	16,329,656	0.4%
39	Nebraska	13,147,172	0.3%
40	New Mexico	9,825,870	0.3%
41	Washington	8,447,279	0.2%
42	South Dakota	6,720,328	0.2%
43	New Hampshire	4,549,414	0.1%
44	Hawaii	4,494,374	0.1%
45	Wyoming	3,936,548	0.1%
46	Delaware	3,522,910	0.1%
47	Vermont	3,175,394	0.1%
48	North Dakota	3,139,322	0.1%
49	Arkansas	3,041,237	0.1%
50	Minnesota	1,050,703	0.0%
	District of Columbia	6,679,004	0.2%

Source: U.S. Department of Health and Human Services, Centers for Medicare and Medicaid Services
"Net Reported Medicaid and SCHIP Expenditures" (http://www.cms.gov/medicaid/mbes/sttotal.pdf)
*For fiscal year 2001. National total includes $67,706,998 spent in U.S. territories. The State Children's Health
Insurance Program (SCHIP) was created in 1997 to help states expand health insurance to children whose families
earn too much to qualify for Medicaid, yet not enough to afford private health insurance.

Per Capita Expenditures for State Children's Health Insurance Program (SCHIP) in 2001
National Per Capita = $13.17*

ALPHA ORDER

RANK ORDER

RANK	STATE	PER CAPITA		RANK	STATE	PER CAPITA
25	Alabama	$11.80		1	Alaska	$51.61
1	Alaska	51.61		2	New York	27.71
24	Arizona	11.89		3	Maryland	26.53
49	Arkansas	1.13		4	Rhode Island	25.59
15	California	13.66		5	New Jersey	23.30
35	Colorado	7.27		6	Kentucky	21.13
38	Connecticut	5.90		7	Mississippi	20.45
44	Delaware	4.42		8	Montana	18.86
9	Florida	17.13		9	Florida	17.13
17	Georgia	12.78		10	Texas	17.06
45	Hawaii	3.66		11	South Carolina	15.06
20	Idaho	12.37		12	West Virginia	14.90
43	Illinois	4.81		13	Maine	14.43
16	Indiana	13.33		14	Wisconsin	14.38
27	Iowa	11.47		15	California	13.66
19	Kansas	12.67		16	Indiana	13.33
6	Kentucky	21.13		17	Georgia	12.78
28	Louisiana	11.19		18	Missouri	12.76
13	Maine	14.43		19	Kansas	12.67
3	Maryland	26.53		20	Idaho	12.37
23	Massachusetts	12.17		20	Utah	12.37
39	Michigan	5.41		22	Ohio	12.33
50	Minnesota	0.21		23	Massachusetts	12.17
7	Mississippi	20.45		24	Arizona	11.89
18	Missouri	12.76		25	Alabama	11.80
8	Montana	18.86		26	North Carolina	11.71
34	Nebraska	7.64		27	Iowa	11.47
30	Nevada	10.58		28	Louisiana	11.19
46	New Hampshire	3.61		29	Pennsylvania	10.91
5	New Jersey	23.30		30	Nevada	10.58
40	New Mexico	5.37		31	Oklahoma	9.35
2	New York	27.71		32	South Dakota	8.86
26	North Carolina	11.71		33	Wyoming	7.97
42	North Dakota	4.93		34	Nebraska	7.64
22	Ohio	12.33		35	Colorado	7.27
31	Oklahoma	9.35		36	Virginia	6.06
37	Oregon	5.92		37	Oregon	5.92
29	Pennsylvania	10.91		38	Connecticut	5.90
4	Rhode Island	25.59		39	Michigan	5.41
11	South Carolina	15.06		40	New Mexico	5.37
32	South Dakota	8.86		41	Vermont	5.18
47	Tennessee	3.36		42	North Dakota	4.93
10	Texas	17.06		43	Illinois	4.81
20	Utah	12.37		44	Delaware	4.42
41	Vermont	5.18		45	Hawaii	3.66
36	Virginia	6.06		46	New Hampshire	3.61
48	Washington	1.41		47	Tennessee	3.36
12	West Virginia	14.90		48	Washington	1.41
14	Wisconsin	14.38		49	Arkansas	1.13
33	Wyoming	7.97		50	Minnesota	0.21
					District of Columbia	11.64

Source: MQ Press using data from U.S. Dept of Health & Human Services, Centers for Medicare and Medicaid Services
"Net Reported Medicaid and SCHIP Expenditures" (http://www.cms.gov/medicaid/mbes/sttotal.pdf)
*For fiscal year 2001. National figure does not include expenditures or population in U.S. territories. The State Children's Health Insurance Program (SCHIP) was created in 1997 to help states expand health insurance to children whose families earn too much to qualify for Medicaid, yet not enough to afford private health insurance.

Expenditures per State Children's Health Insurance Program (SCHIP) Participant in 2001
National Per Participant = $813*

ALPHA ORDER

RANK ORDER

RANK	STATE	PER PARTICIPANT
31	Alabama	$773
5	Alaska	1,498
35	Arizona	727
15	Arkansas	1,055
42	California	678
40	Colorado	704
14	Connecticut	1,088
44	Delaware	633
22	Florida	939
49	Georgia	588
45	Hawaii	630
17	Idaho	966
36	Illinois	721
7	Indiana	1,433
6	Iowa	1,445
16	Kansas	998
11	Kentucky	1,259
37	Louisiana	719
41	Maine	686
9	Maryland	1,299
37	Massachusetts	719
39	Michigan	711
1	Minnesota	21,443
12	Mississippi	1,115
43	Missouri	673
10	Montana	1,263
21	Nebraska	944
30	Nevada	792
32	New Hampshire	761
3	New Jersey	1,986
20	New Mexico	950
46	New York	606
18	North Carolina	961
24	North Dakota	922
25	Ohio	864
27	Oklahoma	835
50	Oregon	495
19	Pennsylvania	951
4	Rhode Island	1,559
23	South Carolina	925
33	South Dakota	743
2	Tennessee	2,245
34	Texas	728
28	Utah	814
48	Vermont	593
47	Virginia	597
13	Washington	1,108
29	West Virginia	809
8	Wisconsin	1,360
26	Wyoming	846

RANK	STATE	PER PARTICIPANT
1	Minnesota	$21,443
2	Tennessee	2,245
3	New Jersey	1,986
4	Rhode Island	1,559
5	Alaska	1,498
6	Iowa	1,445
7	Indiana	1,433
8	Wisconsin	1,360
9	Maryland	1,299
10	Montana	1,263
11	Kentucky	1,259
12	Mississippi	1,115
13	Washington	1,108
14	Connecticut	1,088
15	Arkansas	1,055
16	Kansas	998
17	Idaho	966
18	North Carolina	961
19	Pennsylvania	951
20	New Mexico	950
21	Nebraska	944
22	Florida	939
23	South Carolina	925
24	North Dakota	922
25	Ohio	864
26	Wyoming	846
27	Oklahoma	835
28	Utah	814
29	West Virginia	809
30	Nevada	792
31	Alabama	773
32	New Hampshire	761
33	South Dakota	743
34	Texas	728
35	Arizona	727
36	Illinois	721
37	Louisiana	719
37	Massachusetts	719
39	Michigan	711
40	Colorado	704
41	Maine	686
42	California	678
43	Missouri	673
44	Delaware	633
45	Hawaii	630
46	New York	606
47	Virginia	597
48	Vermont	593
49	Georgia	588
50	Oregon	495
	District of Columbia	2,379

Source: MQ Press using data from U.S. Dept of Health & Human Services, Centers for Medicare and Medicaid Services
"Net Reported Medicaid and SCHIP Expenditures" (http://www.cms.gov/medicaid/mbes/sttotal.pdf)
*For fiscal year 2001. National figure does not include expenditures or participants in U.S. territories. The State Children's Health Insurance Program (SCHIP) was created in 1997 to help states expand health insurance to children whose families earn too much to qualify for Medicaid, yet not enough to afford private health insurance.

Percent of Population Covered by Private Health Insurance in 2001

National Percent = 70.9% of Population

ALPHA ORDER

RANK	STATE	PERCENT
33	Alabama	70.4
41	Alaska	66.1
39	Arizona	66.8
45	Arkansas	63.6
45	California	63.6
23	Colorado	73.8
9	Connecticut	79.0
6	Delaware	79.6
43	Florida	65.7
36	Georgia	68.9
26	Hawaii	73.2
31	Idaho	70.8
24	Illinois	73.5
10	Indiana	78.3
1	Iowa	85.1
17	Kansas	75.6
33	Kentucky	70.4
48	Louisiana	62.7
30	Maine	71.4
8	Maryland	79.1
20	Massachusetts	74.4
11	Michigan	78.2
2	Minnesota	83.7
49	Mississippi	60.5
14	Missouri	76.5
32	Montana	70.7
12	Nebraska	78.0
27	Nevada	72.8
4	New Hampshire	80.9
19	New Jersey	75.4
50	New Mexico	56.7
40	New York	66.7
37	North Carolina	68.5
16	North Dakota	75.9
13	Ohio	76.9
42	Oklahoma	65.8
27	Oregon	72.8
7	Pennsylvania	79.2
15	Rhode Island	76.2
29	South Carolina	72.4
5	South Dakota	79.9
37	Tennessee	68.5
47	Texas	63.0
18	Utah	75.5
24	Vermont	73.5
21	Virginia	74.3
22	Washington	74.1
44	West Virginia	65.3
3	Wisconsin	81.4
35	Wyoming	70.1

RANK ORDER

RANK	STATE	PERCENT
1	Iowa	85.1
2	Minnesota	83.7
3	Wisconsin	81.4
4	New Hampshire	80.9
5	South Dakota	79.9
6	Delaware	79.6
7	Pennsylvania	79.2
8	Maryland	79.1
9	Connecticut	79.0
10	Indiana	78.3
11	Michigan	78.2
12	Nebraska	78.0
13	Ohio	76.9
14	Missouri	76.5
15	Rhode Island	76.2
16	North Dakota	75.9
17	Kansas	75.6
18	Utah	75.5
19	New Jersey	75.4
20	Massachusetts	74.4
21	Virginia	74.3
22	Washington	74.1
23	Colorado	73.8
24	Illinois	73.5
24	Vermont	73.5
26	Hawaii	73.2
27	Nevada	72.8
27	Oregon	72.8
29	South Carolina	72.4
30	Maine	71.4
31	Idaho	70.8
32	Montana	70.7
33	Alabama	70.4
33	Kentucky	70.4
35	Wyoming	70.1
36	Georgia	68.9
37	North Carolina	68.5
37	Tennessee	68.5
39	Arizona	66.8
40	New York	66.7
41	Alaska	66.1
42	Oklahoma	65.8
43	Florida	65.7
44	West Virginia	65.3
45	Arkansas	63.6
45	California	63.6
47	Texas	63.0
48	Louisiana	62.7
49	Mississippi	60.5
50	New Mexico	56.7
	District of Columbia	68.0

Source: U.S. Bureau of the Census
   "Health Insurance Historical Table 4" (http://www.census.gov/hhes/hlthins/historic/hihistt4.html)

Percent of Population Covered by Employment-Based Private Health Insurance in 2001
National Percent = 62.6% of Population

ALPHA ORDER

RANK	STATE	PERCENT
27	Alabama	62.8
32	Alaska	61.2
41	Arizona	58.1
48	Arkansas	53.7
43	California	55.9
21	Colorado	65.3
7	Connecticut	70.7
2	Delaware	73.0
43	Florida	55.9
31	Georgia	61.9
18	Hawaii	66.1
33	Idaho	61.1
22	Illinois	65.2
11	Indiana	68.7
9	Iowa	69.0
28	Kansas	62.5
24	Kentucky	63.4
46	Louisiana	54.9
25	Maine	63.2
5	Maryland	71.9
14	Massachusetts	67.2
4	Michigan	72.3
3	Minnesota	72.9
49	Mississippi	53.3
19	Missouri	65.7
47	Montana	54.0
29	Nebraska	62.4
15	Nevada	67.1
1	New Hampshire	73.5
10	New Jersey	68.9
50	New Mexico	49.7
33	New York	61.1
36	North Carolina	60.6
40	North Dakota	58.4
8	Ohio	69.9
42	Oklahoma	57.0
37	Oregon	60.4
11	Pennsylvania	68.7
17	Rhode Island	66.2
23	South Carolina	64.2
30	South Dakota	62.1
35	Tennessee	60.8
43	Texas	55.9
13	Utah	68.4
19	Vermont	65.7
16	Virginia	66.5
26	Washington	63.1
39	West Virginia	58.9
6	Wisconsin	71.1
37	Wyoming	60.4

RANK ORDER

RANK	STATE	PERCENT
1	New Hampshire	73.5
2	Delaware	73.0
3	Minnesota	72.9
4	Michigan	72.3
5	Maryland	71.9
6	Wisconsin	71.1
7	Connecticut	70.7
8	Ohio	69.9
9	Iowa	69.0
10	New Jersey	68.9
11	Indiana	68.7
11	Pennsylvania	68.7
13	Utah	68.4
14	Massachusetts	67.2
15	Nevada	67.1
16	Virginia	66.5
17	Rhode Island	66.2
18	Hawaii	66.1
19	Missouri	65.7
19	Vermont	65.7
21	Colorado	65.3
22	Illinois	65.2
23	South Carolina	64.2
24	Kentucky	63.4
25	Maine	63.2
26	Washington	63.1
27	Alabama	62.8
28	Kansas	62.5
29	Nebraska	62.4
30	South Dakota	62.1
31	Georgia	61.9
32	Alaska	61.2
33	Idaho	61.1
33	New York	61.1
35	Tennessee	60.8
36	North Carolina	60.6
37	Oregon	60.4
37	Wyoming	60.4
39	West Virginia	58.9
40	North Dakota	58.4
41	Arizona	58.1
42	Oklahoma	57.0
43	California	55.9
43	Florida	55.9
43	Texas	55.9
46	Louisiana	54.9
47	Montana	54.0
48	Arkansas	53.7
49	Mississippi	53.3
50	New Mexico	49.7
	District of Columbia	60.4

Source: U.S. Bureau of the Census
"Health Insurance Historical Table 4" (http://www.census.gov/hhes/hlthins/historic/hihistt4.html)

Percent of Population Covered by Government Health Insurance in 2001

National Percent = 28.1% of Population*

ALPHA ORDER

RANK	STATE	PERCENT
12	Alabama	32.9
6	Alaska	36.0
29	Arizona	28.6
4	Arkansas	37.2
33	California	27.0
47	Colorado	21.9
42	Connecticut	24.5
34	Delaware	26.1
14	Florida	32.6
39	Georgia	25.0
7	Hawaii	35.9
27	Idaho	29.0
43	Illinois	24.0
45	Indiana	23.2
40	Iowa	24.8
19	Kansas	31.1
9	Kentucky	35.3
21	Louisiana	31.0
5	Maine	36.6
47	Maryland	21.9
26	Massachusetts	29.1
37	Michigan	25.3
49	Minnesota	19.4
1	Mississippi	39.7
30	Missouri	28.2
11	Montana	33.3
28	Nebraska	28.7
46	Nevada	22.2
41	New Hampshire	24.7
37	New Jersey	25.3
3	New Mexico	37.8
18	New York	31.2
15	North Carolina	32.5
17	North Dakota	31.4
36	Ohio	25.6
22	Oklahoma	30.6
31	Oregon	27.7
32	Pennsylvania	27.2
13	Rhode Island	32.7
10	South Carolina	33.9
23	South Dakota	30.2
8	Tennessee	35.8
44	Texas	23.9
50	Utah	18.5
16	Vermont	31.7
19	Virginia	31.1
25	Washington	29.6
2	West Virginia	38.6
34	Wisconsin	26.1
24	Wyoming	30.0

RANK ORDER

RANK	STATE	PERCENT
1	Mississippi	39.7
2	West Virginia	38.6
3	New Mexico	37.8
4	Arkansas	37.2
5	Maine	36.6
6	Alaska	36.0
7	Hawaii	35.9
8	Tennessee	35.8
9	Kentucky	35.3
10	South Carolina	33.9
11	Montana	33.3
12	Alabama	32.9
13	Rhode Island	32.7
14	Florida	32.6
15	North Carolina	32.5
16	Vermont	31.7
17	North Dakota	31.4
18	New York	31.2
19	Kansas	31.1
19	Virginia	31.1
21	Louisiana	31.0
22	Oklahoma	30.6
23	South Dakota	30.2
24	Wyoming	30.0
25	Washington	29.6
26	Massachusetts	29.1
27	Idaho	29.0
28	Nebraska	28.7
29	Arizona	28.6
30	Missouri	28.2
31	Oregon	27.7
32	Pennsylvania	27.2
33	California	27.0
34	Delaware	26.1
34	Wisconsin	26.1
36	Ohio	25.6
37	Michigan	25.3
37	New Jersey	25.3
39	Georgia	25.0
40	Iowa	24.8
41	New Hampshire	24.7
42	Connecticut	24.5
43	Illinois	24.0
44	Texas	23.9
45	Indiana	23.2
46	Nevada	22.2
47	Colorado	21.9
47	Maryland	21.9
49	Minnesota	19.4
50	Utah	18.5
	District of Columbia	31.2

Source: Morgan Quitno Press using data from U.S. Bureau of the Census
  "Health Insurance Historical Table 4" (http://www.census.gov/hhes/hlthins/historic/hihistt4.html)
*Includes Medicaid, Medicare and Military health care.

Percent of Population Covered by Military Health Insurance in 2001

National Percent = 3.4% of Population*

ALPHA ORDER

RANK	STATE	PERCENT
22	Alabama	4.3
1	Alaska	15.0
13	Arizona	5.4
16	Arkansas	5.0
33	California	2.9
15	Colorado	5.1
37	Connecticut	2.1
28	Delaware	3.8
27	Florida	4.0
24	Georgia	4.2
3	Hawaii	10.0
22	Idaho	4.3
48	Illinois	1.4
42	Indiana	1.9
40	Iowa	2.0
11	Kansas	6.2
5	Kentucky	6.9
12	Louisiana	6.0
20	Maine	4.5
31	Maryland	3.1
37	Massachusetts	2.1
49	Michigan	1.2
46	Minnesota	1.6
18	Mississippi	4.7
32	Missouri	3.0
8	Montana	6.5
8	Nebraska	6.5
26	Nevada	4.1
29	New Hampshire	3.4
49	New Jersey	1.2
24	New Mexico	4.2
43	New York	1.8
10	North Carolina	6.4
4	North Dakota	7.9
46	Ohio	1.6
14	Oklahoma	5.3
35	Oregon	2.6
43	Pennsylvania	1.8
36	Rhode Island	2.5
17	South Carolina	4.9
5	South Dakota	6.9
21	Tennessee	4.4
33	Texas	2.9
37	Utah	2.1
40	Vermont	2.0
2	Virginia	10.6
19	Washington	4.6
30	West Virginia	3.2
45	Wisconsin	1.7
7	Wyoming	6.7

RANK ORDER

RANK	STATE	PERCENT
1	Alaska	15.0
2	Virginia	10.6
3	Hawaii	10.0
4	North Dakota	7.9
5	Kentucky	6.9
5	South Dakota	6.9
7	Wyoming	6.7
8	Montana	6.5
8	Nebraska	6.5
10	North Carolina	6.4
11	Kansas	6.2
12	Louisiana	6.0
13	Arizona	5.4
14	Oklahoma	5.3
15	Colorado	5.1
16	Arkansas	5.0
17	South Carolina	4.9
18	Mississippi	4.7
19	Washington	4.6
20	Maine	4.5
21	Tennessee	4.4
22	Alabama	4.3
22	Idaho	4.3
24	Georgia	4.2
24	New Mexico	4.2
26	Nevada	4.1
27	Florida	4.0
28	Delaware	3.8
29	New Hampshire	3.4
30	West Virginia	3.2
31	Maryland	3.1
32	Missouri	3.0
33	California	2.9
33	Texas	2.9
35	Oregon	2.6
36	Rhode Island	2.5
37	Connecticut	2.1
37	Massachusetts	2.1
37	Utah	2.1
40	Iowa	2.0
40	Vermont	2.0
42	Indiana	1.9
43	New York	1.8
43	Pennsylvania	1.8
45	Wisconsin	1.7
46	Minnesota	1.6
46	Ohio	1.6
48	Illinois	1.4
49	Michigan	1.2
49	New Jersey	1.2
	District of Columbia	2.1

Source: U.S. Bureau of the Census
   "Health Insurance Historical Table 4" (http://www.census.gov/hhes/hlthins/historic/hihistt4.html)
*Includes CHAMPUS (Comprehensive Health and Medical Plan for Uniformed Services)/Tricare, Veterans
and military health care.

Health Maintenance Organizations (HMOs) in 2002

National Total = 496 HMOs*

ALPHA ORDER					RANK ORDER				
RANK	STATE		HMOs	% of USA	RANK	STATE		HMOs	% of USA
33	Alabama		4	0.8%	1	California		32	6.5%
50	Alaska		0	0.0%	2	Florida		31	6.3%
17	Arizona		10	2.0%	2	Texas		31	6.3%
33	Arkansas		4	0.8%	4	New York		28	5.6%
1	California		32	6.5%	4	Ohio		28	5.6%
13	Colorado		13	2.6%	6	Michigan		22	4.4%
23	Connecticut		8	1.6%	7	Missouri		19	3.8%
33	Delaware		4	0.8%	8	Wisconsin		18	3.6%
2	Florida		31	6.3%	9	Pennsylvania		17	3.4%
16	Georgia		11	2.2%	10	Tennessee		16	3.2%
29	Hawaii		5	1.0%	11	Illinois		15	3.0%
39	Idaho		3	0.6%	11	North Carolina		15	3.0%
11	Illinois		15	3.0%	13	Colorado		13	2.6%
15	Indiana		12	2.4%	13	New Jersey		13	2.6%
39	Iowa		3	0.6%	15	Indiana		12	2.4%
26	Kansas		7	1.4%	16	Georgia		11	2.2%
27	Kentucky		6	1.2%	17	Arizona		10	2.0%
17	Louisiana		10	2.0%	17	Louisiana		10	2.0%
33	Maine		4	0.8%	17	Oklahoma		10	2.0%
20	Maryland		9	1.8%	20	Maryland		9	1.8%
20	Massachusetts		9	1.8%	20	Massachusetts		9	1.8%
6	Michigan		22	4.4%	20	Virginia		9	1.8%
23	Minnesota		8	1.6%	23	Connecticut		8	1.6%
44	Mississippi		2	0.4%	23	Minnesota		8	1.6%
7	Missouri		19	3.8%	23	Utah		8	1.6%
44	Montana		2	0.4%	26	Kansas		7	1.4%
33	Nebraska		4	0.8%	27	Kentucky		6	1.2%
27	Nevada		6	1.2%	27	Nevada		6	1.2%
39	New Hampshire		3	0.6%	29	Hawaii		5	1.0%
13	New Jersey		13	2.6%	29	Oregon		5	1.0%
33	New Mexico		4	0.8%	29	South Carolina		5	1.0%
4	New York		28	5.6%	29	Washington		5	1.0%
11	North Carolina		15	3.0%	33	Alabama		4	0.8%
48	North Dakota		1	0.2%	33	Arkansas		4	0.8%
4	Ohio		28	5.6%	33	Delaware		4	0.8%
17	Oklahoma		10	2.0%	33	Maine		4	0.8%
29	Oregon		5	1.0%	33	Nebraska		4	0.8%
9	Pennsylvania		17	3.4%	33	New Mexico		4	0.8%
39	Rhode Island		3	0.6%	39	Idaho		3	0.6%
29	South Carolina		5	1.0%	39	Iowa		3	0.6%
39	South Dakota		3	0.6%	39	New Hampshire		3	0.6%
10	Tennessee		16	3.2%	39	Rhode Island		3	0.6%
2	Texas		31	6.3%	39	South Dakota		3	0.6%
23	Utah		8	1.6%	44	Mississippi		2	0.4%
44	Vermont		2	0.4%	44	Montana		2	0.4%
20	Virginia		9	1.8%	44	Vermont		2	0.4%
29	Washington		5	1.0%	44	West Virginia		2	0.4%
44	West Virginia		2	0.4%	48	North Dakota		1	0.2%
8	Wisconsin		18	3.6%	48	Wyoming		1	0.2%
48	Wyoming		1	0.2%	50	Alaska		0	0.0%
						District of Columbia		6	1.2%

Source: InterStudy Publications (Minneapolis, MN)
"HMO Industry Report 12.2"
As of January 1, 2002. Total does not include one HMO in Guam and three in Puerto Rico. Health plans are allocated to states based upon their primary service areas. This means each plan is counted once. However, many plans serve more than one state.

Enrollees in Health Maintenance Organizations (HMOs) in 2002

National Total = 74,261,470 Enrollees*

RANK	STATE	ENROLLEES	% of USA
37	Alabama	208,691	0.3%
50	Alaska	0	0.0%
15	Arizona	1,366,827	1.8%
38	Arkansas	207,784	0.3%
1	California	17,420,190	23.5%
14	Colorado	1,454,677	2.0%
17	Connecticut	1,311,275	1.8%
39	Delaware	182,776	0.2%
3	Florida	4,886,056	6.6%
19	Georgia	1,275,066	1.7%
31	Hawaii	401,843	0.5%
47	Idaho	38,919	0.1%
10	Illinois	2,245,624	3.0%
26	Indiana	653,848	0.9%
41	Iowa	149,519	0.2%
34	Kansas	356,221	0.5%
18	Kentucky	1,294,372	1.7%
27	Louisiana	626,780	0.8%
36	Maine	307,996	0.4%
11	Maryland**	1,865,493	2.5%
6	Massachusetts	2,701,835	3.6%
8	Michigan	2,550,675	3.4%
16	Minnesota	1,335,686	1.8%
46	Mississippi	40,232	0.1%
12	Missouri	1,757,908	2.4%
45	Montana	52,065	0.1%
42	Nebraska	148,800	0.2%
30	Nevada	472,006	0.6%
32	New Hampshire	381,334	0.5%
7	New Jersey	2,621,756	3.5%
28	New Mexico	531,180	0.7%
2	New York	6,390,207	8.6%
20	North Carolina	1,210,061	1.6%
49	North Dakota	2,298	0.0%
9	Ohio	2,461,064	3.3%
29	Oklahoma	512,735	0.7%
23	Oregon	1,046,426	1.4%
4	Pennsylvania	3,838,124	5.2%
33	Rhode Island	368,895	0.5%
35	South Carolina	323,748	0.4%
43	South Dakota	86,727	0.1%
22	Tennessee	1,065,683	1.4%
5	Texas	3,179,663	4.3%
25	Utah	726,338	1.0%
44	Vermont	64,071	0.1%
21	Virginia**	1,141,778	1.5%
24	Washington	1,042,069	1.4%
40	West Virginia**	180,414	0.2%
13	Wisconsin	1,585,227	2.1%
48	Wyoming	10,100	0.0%

RANK	STATE	ENROLLEES	% of USA
1	California	17,420,190	23.5%
2	New York	6,390,207	8.6%
3	Florida	4,886,056	6.6%
4	Pennsylvania	3,838,124	5.2%
5	Texas	3,179,663	4.3%
6	Massachusetts	2,701,835	3.6%
7	New Jersey	2,621,756	3.5%
8	Michigan	2,550,675	3.4%
9	Ohio	2,461,064	3.3%
10	Illinois	2,245,624	3.0%
11	Maryland**	1,865,493	2.5%
12	Missouri	1,757,908	2.4%
13	Wisconsin	1,585,227	2.1%
14	Colorado	1,454,677	2.0%
15	Arizona	1,366,827	1.8%
16	Minnesota	1,335,686	1.8%
17	Connecticut	1,311,275	1.8%
18	Kentucky	1,294,372	1.7%
19	Georgia	1,275,066	1.7%
20	North Carolina	1,210,061	1.6%
21	Virginia**	1,141,778	1.5%
22	Tennessee	1,065,683	1.4%
23	Oregon	1,046,426	1.4%
24	Washington	1,042,069	1.4%
25	Utah	726,338	1.0%
26	Indiana	653,848	0.9%
27	Louisiana	626,780	0.8%
28	New Mexico	531,180	0.7%
29	Oklahoma	512,735	0.7%
30	Nevada	472,006	0.6%
31	Hawaii	401,843	0.5%
32	New Hampshire	381,334	0.5%
33	Rhode Island	368,895	0.5%
34	Kansas	356,221	0.5%
35	South Carolina	323,748	0.4%
36	Maine	307,996	0.4%
37	Alabama	208,691	0.3%
38	Arkansas	207,784	0.3%
39	Delaware	182,776	0.2%
40	West Virginia**	180,414	0.2%
41	Iowa	149,519	0.2%
42	Nebraska	148,800	0.2%
43	South Dakota	86,727	0.1%
44	Vermont	64,071	0.1%
45	Montana	52,065	0.1%
46	Mississippi	40,232	0.1%
47	Idaho	38,919	0.1%
48	Wyoming	10,100	0.0%
49	North Dakota	2,298	0.0%
50	Alaska	0	0.0%
	District of Columbia	178,408	0.2%

Source: InterStudy Publications (Minneapolis, MN)
   "HMO Industry Report 12.2"
*As of January 1, 2002. Total does not include 1,859,118 enrollees in U.S. territories.
**Maryland, Virginia and West Virginia include partial enrollment from six HMOs serving the Washington, DC metropolitan area.

Percent Change in Enrollees in Health Maintenance Organizations (HMOs): 2001 to 2002
National Percent Change = 4.8% Decrease*

ALPHA ORDER

RANK	STATE	PERCENT CHANGE
46	Alabama	(27.7)
NA	Alaska**	NA
41	Arizona	(17.7)
45	Arkansas	(26.2)
17	California	(0.7)
27	Colorado	(7.1)
20	Connecticut	(3.1)
12	Delaware	2.5
11	Florida	2.7
19	Georgia	(2.2)
10	Hawaii	4.2
47	Idaho	(29.8)
24	Illinois	(5.9)
30	Indiana	(8.2)
43	Iowa	(21.6)
40	Kansas	(17.6)
8	Kentucky	5.4
34	Louisiana	(9.9)
37	Maine	(13.5)
30	Maryland	(8.2)
25	Massachusetts	(6.0)
23	Michigan	(3.8)
21	Minnesota	(3.6)
2	Mississippi	59.4
13	Missouri	1.4
44	Montana	(25.4)
35	Nebraska	(12.5)
6	Nevada	15.6
42	New Hampshire	(21.4)
18	New Jersey	(1.6)
9	New Mexico	4.8
22	New York	(3.7)
29	North Carolina	(7.7)
49	North Dakota	(71.9)
28	Ohio	(7.2)
7	Oklahoma	6.9
38	Oregon	(13.8)
26	Pennsylvania	(6.4)
14	Rhode Island	0.6
39	South Carolina	(15.4)
3	South Dakota	18.8
48	Tennessee	(43.3)
36	Texas	(13.0)
32	Utah	(8.4)
1	Vermont	149.3
16	Virginia	(0.2)
5	Washington	15.7
33	West Virginia	(8.5)
15	Wisconsin	(0.1)
4	Wyoming	17.4

RANK ORDER

RANK	STATE	PERCENT CHANGE
1	Vermont	149.3
2	Mississippi	59.4
3	South Dakota	18.8
4	Wyoming	17.4
5	Washington	15.7
6	Nevada	15.6
7	Oklahoma	6.9
8	Kentucky	5.4
9	New Mexico	4.8
10	Hawaii	4.2
11	Florida	2.7
12	Delaware	2.5
13	Missouri	1.4
14	Rhode Island	0.6
15	Wisconsin	(0.1)
16	Virginia	(0.2)
17	California	(0.7)
18	New Jersey	(1.6)
19	Georgia	(2.2)
20	Connecticut	(3.1)
21	Minnesota	(3.6)
22	New York	(3.7)
23	Michigan	(3.8)
24	Illinois	(5.9)
25	Massachusetts	(6.0)
26	Pennsylvania	(6.4)
27	Colorado	(7.1)
28	Ohio	(7.2)
29	North Carolina	(7.7)
30	Indiana	(8.2)
30	Maryland	(8.2)
32	Utah	(8.4)
33	West Virginia	(8.5)
34	Louisiana	(9.9)
35	Nebraska	(12.5)
36	Texas	(13.0)
37	Maine	(13.5)
38	Oregon	(13.8)
39	South Carolina	(15.4)
40	Kansas	(17.6)
41	Arizona	(17.7)
42	New Hampshire	(21.4)
43	Iowa	(21.6)
44	Montana	(25.4)
45	Arkansas	(26.2)
46	Alabama	(27.7)
47	Idaho	(29.8)
48	Tennessee	(43.3)
49	North Dakota	(71.9)
NA	Alaska**	NA

District of Columbia   0.6

Source: InterStudy Publications (Minneapolis, MN)
      "HMO Industry Report 12.2"
*As of January 1, 2002. National rate does not include enrollees in U.S. territories.
**Not applicable.

Percent of Population Enrolled in Health Maintenance Organizations (HMOs) in 2002
National Percent = 25.8% Enrolled in HMOs*

RANK	STATE	PERCENT
45	Alabama	4.7
50	Alaska	0.0
21	Arizona	25.0
42	Arkansas	7.7
1	California	49.6
7	Colorado	32.3
3	Connecticut	37.9
23	Delaware	22.6
16	Florida	29.2
30	Georgia	14.9
7	Hawaii	32.3
46	Idaho	2.9
27	Illinois	17.8
37	Indiana	10.6
44	Iowa	5.1
35	Kansas	13.1
9	Kentucky	31.6
34	Louisiana	14.0
22	Maine	23.8
5	Maryland	34.2
2	Massachusetts	42.0
20	Michigan	25.4
19	Minnesota	26.6
48	Mississippi	1.4
12	Missouri	31.0
43	Montana	5.7
40	Nebraska	8.6
24	Nevada	21.7
14	New Hampshire	29.9
13	New Jersey	30.5
18	New Mexico	28.6
6	New York	33.4
33	North Carolina	14.5
49	North Dakota	0.4
25	Ohio	21.5
31	Oklahoma	14.7
15	Oregon	29.7
11	Pennsylvania	31.1
4	Rhode Island	34.5
41	South Carolina	7.9
36	South Dakota	11.4
26	Tennessee	18.4
32	Texas	14.6
10	Utah	31.4
38	Vermont	10.4
29	Virginia	15.7
28	Washington	17.2
39	West Virginia	10.0
17	Wisconsin	29.1
47	Wyoming	2.0

RANK	STATE	PERCENT
1	California	49.6
2	Massachusetts	42.0
3	Connecticut	37.9
4	Rhode Island	34.5
5	Maryland	34.2
6	New York	33.4
7	Colorado	32.3
7	Hawaii	32.3
9	Kentucky	31.6
10	Utah	31.4
11	Pennsylvania	31.1
12	Missouri	31.0
13	New Jersey	30.5
14	New Hampshire	29.9
15	Oregon	29.7
16	Florida	29.2
17	Wisconsin	29.1
18	New Mexico	28.6
19	Minnesota	26.6
20	Michigan	25.4
21	Arizona	25.0
22	Maine	23.8
23	Delaware	22.6
24	Nevada	21.7
25	Ohio	21.5
26	Tennessee	18.4
27	Illinois	17.8
28	Washington	17.2
29	Virginia	15.7
30	Georgia	14.9
31	Oklahoma	14.7
32	Texas	14.6
33	North Carolina	14.5
34	Louisiana	14.0
35	Kansas	13.1
36	South Dakota	11.4
37	Indiana	10.6
38	Vermont	10.4
39	West Virginia	10.0
40	Nebraska	8.6
41	South Carolina	7.9
42	Arkansas	7.7
43	Montana	5.7
44	Iowa	5.1
45	Alabama	4.7
46	Idaho	2.9
47	Wyoming	2.0
48	Mississippi	1.4
49	North Dakota	0.4
50	Alaska	0.0
	District of Columbia	31.3

Source: Morgan Quitno Press using data from InterStudy Publications (Minneapolis, MN)
"HMO Industry Report 12.2"
*As of January 1, 2002. National percent does not include enrollees or population in U.S. territories.

Percent of Insured Population Enrolled in Health Maintenance Organizations (HMOs) in 2002
National Percent = 30.8% of Insured are Enrolled in HMOs*

ALPHA ORDER

RANK ORDER

RANK	STATE	PERCENT
45	Alabama	5.5
50	Alaska	0.0
19	Arizona	31.3
41	Arkansas	9.3
1	California	62.7
6	Colorado	39.1
3	Connecticut	43.0
24	Delaware	25.4
12	Florida	36.2
31	Georgia	18.4
11	Hawaii	36.7
46	Idaho	3.5
26	Illinois	21.1
37	Indiana	12.3
44	Iowa	5.7
35	Kansas	15.2
10	Kentucky	36.9
33	Louisiana	17.7
22	Maine	26.9
5	Maryland	39.9
2	Massachusetts	46.6
21	Michigan	28.8
20	Minnesota	29.5
48	Mississippi	1.7
14	Missouri	35.4
43	Montana	6.8
40	Nebraska	9.8
23	Nevada	26.4
17	New Hampshire	33.5
13	New Jersey	35.6
9	New Mexico	37.1
4	New York	40.2
34	North Carolina	17.5
49	North Dakota	0.4
25	Ohio	24.8
30	Oklahoma	18.6
16	Oregon	34.7
15	Pennsylvania	34.9
7	Rhode Island	38.3
42	South Carolina	9.2
36	South Dakota	12.9
26	Tennessee	21.1
29	Texas	19.7
8	Utah	37.7
38	Vermont	11.7
32	Virginia	18.0
28	Washington	20.2
38	West Virginia	11.7
18	Wisconsin	32.2
47	Wyoming	2.5

RANK	STATE	PERCENT
1	California	62.7
2	Massachusetts	46.6
3	Connecticut	43.0
4	New York	40.2
5	Maryland	39.9
6	Colorado	39.1
7	Rhode Island	38.3
8	Utah	37.7
9	New Mexico	37.1
10	Kentucky	36.9
11	Hawaii	36.7
12	Florida	36.2
13	New Jersey	35.6
14	Missouri	35.4
15	Pennsylvania	34.9
16	Oregon	34.7
17	New Hampshire	33.5
18	Wisconsin	32.2
19	Arizona	31.3
20	Minnesota	29.5
21	Michigan	28.8
22	Maine	26.9
23	Nevada	26.4
24	Delaware	25.4
25	Ohio	24.8
26	Illinois	21.1
26	Tennessee	21.1
28	Washington	20.2
29	Texas	19.7
30	Oklahoma	18.6
31	Georgia	18.4
32	Virginia	18.0
33	Louisiana	17.7
34	North Carolina	17.5
35	Kansas	15.2
36	South Dakota	12.9
37	Indiana	12.3
38	Vermont	11.7
38	West Virginia	11.7
40	Nebraska	9.8
41	Arkansas	9.3
42	South Carolina	9.2
43	Montana	6.8
44	Iowa	5.7
45	Alabama	5.5
46	Idaho	3.5
47	Wyoming	2.5
48	Mississippi	1.7
49	North Dakota	0.4
50	Alaska	0.0

| | District of Columbia | 36.9 |

Source: Morgan Quitno Press using data from InterStudy Publications (Minneapolis, MN) "HMO Industry Report 12.2"
As of January 1, 2002. Calculated using estimated number of insured as of 2001 from the U.S. Census Bureau.

Medicare Enrollees in 2001

National Total = 40,025,724 Enrollees*

RANK	STATE	ENROLLEES	% of USA		RANK	STATE	ENROLLEES	% of USA
19	Alabama	695,195	1.7%		1	California	3,954,996	9.9%
50	Alaska	43,815	0.1%		2	Florida	2,838,345	7.1%
20	Arizona	690,628	1.7%		3	New York	2,728,967	6.8%
31	Arkansas	441,863	1.1%		4	Texas	2,299,599	5.7%
1	California	3,954,996	9.9%		5	Pennsylvania	2,095,453	5.2%
30	Colorado	475,616	1.2%		6	Ohio	1,705,333	4.3%
26	Connecticut	516,359	1.3%		7	Illinois	1,639,986	4.1%
46	Delaware	113,967	0.3%		8	Michigan	1,414,054	3.5%
2	Florida	2,838,345	7.1%		9	New Jersey	1,207,663	3.0%
12	Georgia	932,965	2.3%		10	North Carolina	1,154,864	2.9%
43	Hawaii	168,296	0.4%		11	Massachusetts	961,409	2.4%
42	Idaho	168,550	0.4%		12	Georgia	932,965	2.3%
7	Illinois	1,639,986	4.1%		13	Virginia	909,536	2.3%
15	Indiana	858,150	2.1%		14	Missouri	866,815	2.2%
29	Iowa	478,063	1.2%		15	Indiana	858,150	2.1%
33	Kansas	391,076	1.0%		16	Tennessee	842,264	2.1%
23	Kentucky	629,709	1.6%		17	Wisconsin	787,442	2.0%
24	Louisiana	605,395	1.5%		18	Washington	745,859	1.9%
38	Maine	219,310	0.5%		19	Alabama	695,195	1.7%
22	Maryland	654,607	1.6%		20	Arizona	690,628	1.7%
11	Massachusetts	961,409	2.4%		21	Minnesota	660,399	1.6%
8	Michigan	1,414,054	3.5%		22	Maryland	654,607	1.6%
21	Minnesota	660,399	1.6%		23	Kentucky	629,709	1.6%
32	Mississippi	423,436	1.1%		24	Louisiana	605,395	1.5%
14	Missouri	866,815	2.2%		25	South Carolina	579,597	1.4%
44	Montana	138,266	0.3%		26	Connecticut	516,359	1.3%
35	Nebraska	254,680	0.6%		27	Oklahoma	510,582	1.3%
36	Nevada	250,543	0.6%		28	Oregon	495,704	1.2%
40	New Hampshire	172,704	0.4%		29	Iowa	478,063	1.2%
9	New Jersey	1,207,663	3.0%		30	Colorado	475,616	1.2%
37	New Mexico	238,418	0.6%		31	Arkansas	441,863	1.1%
3	New York	2,728,967	6.8%		32	Mississippi	423,436	1.1%
10	North Carolina	1,154,864	2.9%		33	Kansas	391,076	1.0%
47	North Dakota	103,126	0.3%		34	West Virginia	339,853	0.8%
6	Ohio	1,705,333	4.3%		35	Nebraska	254,680	0.6%
27	Oklahoma	510,582	1.3%		36	Nevada	250,543	0.6%
28	Oregon	495,704	1.2%		37	New Mexico	238,418	0.6%
5	Pennsylvania	2,095,453	5.2%		38	Maine	219,310	0.5%
41	Rhode Island	171,822	0.4%		39	Utah	210,400	0.5%
25	South Carolina	579,597	1.4%		40	New Hampshire	172,704	0.4%
45	South Dakota	120,019	0.3%		41	Rhode Island	171,822	0.4%
16	Tennessee	842,264	2.1%		42	Idaho	168,550	0.4%
4	Texas	2,299,599	5.7%		43	Hawaii	168,296	0.4%
39	Utah	210,400	0.5%		44	Montana	138,266	0.3%
48	Vermont	90,049	0.2%		45	South Dakota	120,019	0.3%
13	Virginia	909,536	2.3%		46	Delaware	113,967	0.3%
18	Washington	745,859	1.9%		47	North Dakota	103,126	0.3%
34	West Virginia	339,853	0.8%		48	Vermont	90,049	0.2%
17	Wisconsin	787,442	2.0%		49	Wyoming	66,439	0.2%
49	Wyoming	66,439	0.2%		50	Alaska	43,815	0.1%
						District of Columbia	74,701	0.2%

Source: U.S. Department of Health and Human Services, Centers for Medicare and Medicaid Services "Medicare Enrollment" (http://www.cms.gov/statistics/enrollment/st01all.asp)
As of July 2001. Includes aged and disabled enrollees. Total includes 549,746 enrollees in Puerto Rico and 339,091 enrollees in other outlying areas, foreign or whose address is unknown.

Percent Change in Medicare Enrollees: 2000 to 2001

National Percent Change = 1.0% Increase

ALPHA ORDER				RANK ORDER		
RANK	STATE	PERCENT CHANGE		RANK	STATE	PERCENT CHANGE
18	Alabama	1.4		1	Nevada	4.5
2	Alaska	4.3		2	Alaska	4.3
3	Arizona	2.3		3	Arizona	2.3
33	Arkansas	0.6		4	Idaho	2.1
18	California	1.4		4	South Carolina	2.1
11	Colorado	1.7		4	Utah	2.1
44	Connecticut	0.2		7	North Carolina	1.9
11	Delaware	1.7		8	Georgia	1.8
24	Florida	1.2		8	Hawaii	1.8
8	Georgia	1.8		8	Virginia	1.8
8	Hawaii	1.8		11	Colorado	1.7
4	Idaho	2.1		11	Delaware	1.7
42	Illinois	0.3		11	New Mexico	1.7
31	Indiana	0.7		14	Tennessee	1.6
42	Iowa	0.3		15	New Hampshire	1.5
44	Kansas	0.2		15	Texas	1.5
26	Kentucky	1.1		15	Wyoming	1.5
33	Louisiana	0.6		18	Alabama	1.4
22	Maine	1.3		18	California	1.4
18	Maryland	1.4		18	Maryland	1.4
47	Massachusetts	0.1		18	Washington	1.4
30	Michigan	0.8		22	Maine	1.3
29	Minnesota	0.9		22	Oregon	1.3
24	Mississippi	1.2		24	Florida	1.2
31	Missouri	0.7		24	Mississippi	1.2
26	Montana	1.1		26	Kentucky	1.1
40	Nebraska	0.4		26	Montana	1.1
1	Nevada	4.5		26	Vermont	1.1
15	New Hampshire	1.5		29	Minnesota	0.9
40	New Jersey	0.4		30	Michigan	0.8
11	New Mexico	1.7		31	Indiana	0.7
37	New York	0.5		31	Missouri	0.7
7	North Carolina	1.9		33	Arkansas	0.6
50	North Dakota	(0.1)		33	Louisiana	0.6
44	Ohio	0.2		33	West Virginia	0.6
37	Oklahoma	0.5		33	Wisconsin	0.6
22	Oregon	1.3		37	New York	0.5
49	Pennsylvania	0.0		37	Oklahoma	0.5
47	Rhode Island	0.1		37	South Dakota	0.5
4	South Carolina	2.1		40	Nebraska	0.4
37	South Dakota	0.5		40	New Jersey	0.4
14	Tennessee	1.6		42	Illinois	0.3
15	Texas	1.5		42	Iowa	0.3
4	Utah	2.1		44	Connecticut	0.2
26	Vermont	1.1		44	Kansas	0.2
8	Virginia	1.8		44	Ohio	0.2
18	Washington	1.4		47	Massachusetts	0.1
33	West Virginia	0.6		47	Rhode Island	0.1
33	Wisconsin	0.6		49	Pennsylvania	0.0
15	Wyoming	1.5		50	North Dakota	(0.1)
					District of Columbia	(0.8)

Source: U.S. Department of Health and Human Services, Centers for Medicare and Medicaid Services
"Medicare Beneficiaries Enrolled by State" (http://www.cms.gov/statistics/enrollment/stenrtrend99_01.asp)

Medicare Benefit Payments in 2001

National Total = $236,492,552,000*

ALPHA ORDER					RANK ORDER			

RANK	STATE	BENEFITS	% of USA		RANK	STATE	BENEFITS	% of USA
18	Alabama	$4,270,957,000	1.8%		1	California	$24,858,719,000	10.5%
50	Alaska	169,288,000	0.1%		2	Florida	21,580,488,000	9.1%
23	Arizona	3,322,292,000	1.4%		3	New York	20,436,630,000	8.6%
28	Arkansas	2,420,406,000	1.0%		4	Texas	16,336,061,000	6.9%
1	California	24,858,719,000	10.5%		5	Pennsylvania	15,141,847,000	6.4%
27	Colorado	2,698,488,000	1.1%		6	Ohio	10,685,164,000	4.5%
26	Connecticut	3,117,052,000	1.3%		7	Illinois	8,001,947,000	3.4%
47	Delaware	500,000,000	0.2%		8	Michigan	7,012,604,000	3.0%
2	Florida	21,580,488,000	9.1%		9	New Jersey	6,885,642,000	2.9%
17	Georgia	4,397,178,000	1.9%		10	North Carolina	6,797,677,000	2.9%
42	Hawaii	717,998,000	0.3%		11	Massachusetts	5,963,041,000	2.5%
41	Idaho	741,441,000	0.3%		12	Tennessee	5,545,549,000	2.3%
7	Illinois	8,001,947,000	3.4%		13	Indiana	4,999,250,000	2.1%
13	Indiana	4,999,250,000	2.1%		14	Louisiana	4,902,926,000	2.1%
34	Iowa	1,632,032,000	0.7%		15	Missouri	4,755,402,000	2.0%
31	Kansas	2,141,312,000	0.9%		16	Maryland	4,611,432,000	1.9%
21	Kentucky	3,640,057,000	1.5%		17	Georgia	4,397,178,000	1.9%
14	Louisiana	4,902,926,000	2.1%		18	Alabama	4,270,957,000	1.8%
40	Maine	875,798,000	0.4%		19	Wisconsin	3,961,455,000	1.7%
16	Maryland	4,611,432,000	1.9%		20	Virginia	3,897,031,000	1.6%
11	Massachusetts	5,963,041,000	2.5%		21	Kentucky	3,640,057,000	1.5%
8	Michigan	7,012,604,000	3.0%		22	South Carolina	3,356,574,000	1.4%
25	Minnesota	3,136,907,000	1.3%		23	Arizona	3,322,292,000	1.4%
32	Mississippi	2,140,391,000	0.9%		24	Washington	3,209,406,000	1.4%
15	Missouri	4,755,402,000	2.0%		25	Minnesota	3,136,907,000	1.3%
44	Montana	663,416,000	0.3%		26	Connecticut	3,117,052,000	1.3%
35	Nebraska	1,366,977,000	0.6%		27	Colorado	2,698,488,000	1.1%
36	Nevada	1,272,774,000	0.5%		28	Arkansas	2,420,406,000	1.0%
43	New Hampshire	714,188,000	0.3%		29	Oklahoma	2,343,403,000	1.0%
9	New Jersey	6,885,642,000	2.9%		30	Oregon	2,181,557,000	0.9%
39	New Mexico	879,540,000	0.4%		31	Kansas	2,141,312,000	0.9%
3	New York	20,436,630,000	8.6%		32	Mississippi	2,140,391,000	0.9%
10	North Carolina	6,797,677,000	2.9%		33	West Virginia	1,822,039,000	0.8%
46	North Dakota	562,654,000	0.2%		34	Iowa	1,632,032,000	0.7%
6	Ohio	10,685,164,000	4.5%		35	Nebraska	1,366,977,000	0.6%
29	Oklahoma	2,343,403,000	1.0%		36	Nevada	1,272,774,000	0.5%
30	Oregon	2,181,557,000	0.9%		37	Rhode Island	1,146,888,000	0.5%
5	Pennsylvania	15,141,847,000	6.4%		38	Utah	1,077,334,000	0.5%
37	Rhode Island	1,146,888,000	0.5%		39	New Mexico	879,540,000	0.4%
22	South Carolina	3,356,574,000	1.4%		40	Maine	875,798,000	0.4%
45	South Dakota	622,092,000	0.3%		41	Idaho	741,441,000	0.3%
12	Tennessee	5,545,549,000	2.3%		42	Hawaii	717,998,000	0.3%
4	Texas	16,336,061,000	6.9%		43	New Hampshire	714,188,000	0.3%
38	Utah	1,077,334,000	0.5%		44	Montana	663,416,000	0.3%
48	Vermont	361,871,000	0.2%		45	South Dakota	622,092,000	0.3%
20	Virginia	3,897,031,000	1.6%		46	North Dakota	562,654,000	0.2%
24	Washington	3,209,406,000	1.4%		47	Delaware	500,000,000	0.2%
33	West Virginia	1,822,039,000	0.8%		48	Vermont	361,871,000	0.2%
19	Wisconsin	3,961,455,000	1.7%		49	Wyoming	281,639,000	0.1%
49	Wyoming	281,639,000	0.1%		50	Alaska	169,288,000	0.1%
						District of Columbia	792,265,000	0.3%

Source: U.S. Department of Health and Human Services, Centers for Medicare and Medicaid Services
"Medicare Estimated Benefit Payments by State" (www.cms.gov/statistics/feeforservice/BenefitPayments01.pdf)
For fiscal year 2001. Includes payments to aged and disabled enrollees. Total includes $1,454,823,000 in payments to enrollees in Puerto Rico and $88,652,000 to enrollees in "other outlying areas."

Per Capita Medicare Benefit Payments in 2001

National Per Capita = $823*

ALPHA ORDER				RANK ORDER		
RANK	STATE	PER CAPITA		RANK	STATE	PER CAPITA
8	Alabama	$956		1	Florida	$1,318
50	Alaska	267		2	Pennsylvania	1,231
36	Arizona	626		3	Louisiana	1,097
12	Arkansas	898		4	Rhode Island	1,082
28	California	718		5	New York	1,071
37	Colorado	609		6	West Virginia	1,012
11	Connecticut	908		7	Tennessee	965
34	Delaware	628		8	Alabama	956
1	Florida	1,318		9	Ohio	938
47	Georgia	523		10	Massachusetts	932
40	Hawaii	585		11	Connecticut	908
43	Idaho	561		12	Arkansas	898
32	Illinois	639		13	Kentucky	895
20	Indiana	816		14	North Dakota	884
44	Iowa	557		15	Maryland	856
23	Kansas	792		16	Missouri	844
13	Kentucky	895		17	North Carolina	828
3	Louisiana	1,097		18	South Carolina	826
30	Maine	682		19	South Dakota	820
15	Maryland	856		20	Indiana	816
10	Massachusetts	932		21	New Jersey	809
29	Michigan	701		22	Nebraska	795
33	Minnesota	629		23	Kansas	792
25	Mississippi	748		24	Texas	764
16	Missouri	844		25	Mississippi	748
26	Montana	733		26	Montana	733
22	Nebraska	795		26	Wisconsin	733
38	Nevada	607		28	California	718
42	New Hampshire	567		29	Michigan	701
21	New Jersey	809		30	Maine	682
48	New Mexico	480		31	Oklahoma	675
5	New York	1,071		32	Illinois	639
17	North Carolina	828		33	Minnesota	629
14	North Dakota	884		34	Delaware	628
9	Ohio	938		34	Oregon	628
31	Oklahoma	675		36	Arizona	626
34	Oregon	628		37	Colorado	609
2	Pennsylvania	1,231		38	Nevada	607
4	Rhode Island	1,082		39	Vermont	590
18	South Carolina	826		40	Hawaii	585
19	South Dakota	820		41	Wyoming	570
7	Tennessee	965		42	New Hampshire	567
24	Texas	764		43	Idaho	561
49	Utah	473		44	Iowa	557
39	Vermont	590		45	Virginia	541
45	Virginia	541		46	Washington	535
46	Washington	535		47	Georgia	523
6	West Virginia	1,012		48	New Mexico	480
26	Wisconsin	733		49	Utah	473
41	Wyoming	570		50	Alaska	267
					District of Columbia	1,381

Source: MQ Press using data from U.S. Dept of Health & Human Services, Centers for Medicare and Medicaid Services
"Medicare Estimated Benefit Payments by State" (www.cms.gov/statistics/feeforservice/BenefitPayments01.pdf)
*For fiscal year 2001. Includes aged and disabled enrollees. National rate does not include payments or enrollees
in Puerto Rico and in "other outlying areas." Payments are based on the state of the provider or plan. Thus data
showing payments per capita should be viewed as estimates and interpreted with caution.

Medicare Payments per Enrollee in 2001

National Rate = $6,003*

RANK	STATE	PER ENROLLEE
12	Alabama	$6,144
48	Alaska	3,864
33	Arizona	4,811
21	Arkansas	5,478
9	California	6,285
19	Colorado	5,674
13	Connecticut	6,037
40	Delaware	4,387
2	Florida	7,603
36	Georgia	4,713
43	Hawaii	4,266
39	Idaho	4,399
32	Illinois	4,879
15	Indiana	5,826
50	Iowa	3,414
22	Kansas	5,475
17	Kentucky	5,781
1	Louisiana	8,099
47	Maine	3,993
6	Maryland	7,045
11	Massachusetts	6,202
31	Michigan	4,959
35	Minnesota	4,750
29	Mississippi	5,055
20	Missouri	5,486
34	Montana	4,798
24	Nebraska	5,367
28	Nevada	5,080
45	New Hampshire	4,135
18	New Jersey	5,702
49	New Mexico	3,689
3	New York	7,489
14	North Carolina	5,886
23	North Dakota	5,456
10	Ohio	6,266
37	Oklahoma	4,590
38	Oregon	4,401
4	Pennsylvania	7,226
7	Rhode Island	6,675
16	South Carolina	5,791
26	South Dakota	5,183
8	Tennessee	6,584
5	Texas	7,104
27	Utah	5,120
46	Vermont	4,019
42	Virginia	4,285
41	Washington	4,303
25	West Virginia	5,361
30	Wisconsin	5,031
44	Wyoming	4,239

RANK	STATE	PER ENROLLEE
1	Louisiana	$8,099
2	Florida	7,603
3	New York	7,489
4	Pennsylvania	7,226
5	Texas	7,104
6	Maryland	7,045
7	Rhode Island	6,675
8	Tennessee	6,584
9	California	6,285
10	Ohio	6,266
11	Massachusetts	6,202
12	Alabama	6,144
13	Connecticut	6,037
14	North Carolina	5,886
15	Indiana	5,826
16	South Carolina	5,791
17	Kentucky	5,781
18	New Jersey	5,702
19	Colorado	5,674
20	Missouri	5,486
21	Arkansas	5,478
22	Kansas	5,475
23	North Dakota	5,456
24	Nebraska	5,367
25	West Virginia	5,361
26	South Dakota	5,183
27	Utah	5,120
28	Nevada	5,080
29	Mississippi	5,055
30	Wisconsin	5,031
31	Michigan	4,959
32	Illinois	4,879
33	Arizona	4,811
34	Montana	4,798
35	Minnesota	4,750
36	Georgia	4,713
37	Oklahoma	4,590
38	Oregon	4,401
39	Idaho	4,399
40	Delaware	4,387
41	Washington	4,303
42	Virginia	4,285
43	Hawaii	4,266
44	Wyoming	4,239
45	New Hampshire	4,135
46	Vermont	4,019
47	Maine	3,993
48	Alaska	3,864
49	New Mexico	3,689
50	Iowa	3,414
	District of Columbia	10,606

Source: MQ Press using data from U.S. Dept of Health & Human Services, Centers for Medicare and Medicaid Services "Medicare Estimated Benefit Payments by State" (www.cms.gov/statistics/feeforservice/BenefitPayments01.pdf)
*For fiscal year 2001. Includes aged and disabled enrollees. National rate does not include payments or enrollees in Puerto Rico and in "other outlying areas." Payments are based on the state of the provider or plan. Thus data showing payments per beneficiary should be viewed as estimates and interpreted with caution.

Percent of Population Enrolled in Medicare in 2001

National Percent = 13.7% of Population*

ALPHA ORDER

RANK	STATE	PERCENT
10	Alabama	15.6
50	Alaska	6.9
38	Arizona	13.0
5	Arkansas	16.4
45	California	11.4
48	Colorado	10.7
14	Connecticut	15.0
24	Delaware	14.3
2	Florida	17.3
46	Georgia	11.1
32	Hawaii	13.7
40	Idaho	12.8
37	Illinois	13.1
31	Indiana	14.0
6	Iowa	16.3
23	Kansas	14.5
11	Kentucky	15.5
34	Louisiana	13.5
3	Maine	17.1
43	Maryland	12.2
14	Massachusetts	15.0
29	Michigan	14.1
36	Minnesota	13.2
17	Mississippi	14.8
12	Missouri	15.4
13	Montana	15.3
17	Nebraska	14.8
44	Nevada	11.9
32	New Hampshire	13.7
28	New Jersey	14.2
38	New Mexico	13.0
24	New York	14.3
29	North Carolina	14.1
7	North Dakota	16.2
14	Ohio	15.0
19	Oklahoma	14.7
24	Oregon	14.3
4	Pennsylvania	17.0
7	Rhode Island	16.2
24	South Carolina	14.3
9	South Dakota	15.8
21	Tennessee	14.6
47	Texas	10.8
49	Utah	9.2
19	Vermont	14.7
41	Virginia	12.6
42	Washington	12.4
1	West Virginia	18.9
21	Wisconsin	14.6
34	Wyoming	13.5

RANK ORDER

RANK	STATE	PERCENT
1	West Virginia	18.9
2	Florida	17.3
3	Maine	17.1
4	Pennsylvania	17.0
5	Arkansas	16.4
6	Iowa	16.3
7	North Dakota	16.2
7	Rhode Island	16.2
9	South Dakota	15.8
10	Alabama	15.6
11	Kentucky	15.5
12	Missouri	15.4
13	Montana	15.3
14	Connecticut	15.0
14	Massachusetts	15.0
14	Ohio	15.0
17	Mississippi	14.8
17	Nebraska	14.8
19	Oklahoma	14.7
19	Vermont	14.7
21	Tennessee	14.6
21	Wisconsin	14.6
23	Kansas	14.5
24	Delaware	14.3
24	New York	14.3
24	Oregon	14.3
24	South Carolina	14.3
28	New Jersey	14.2
29	Michigan	14.1
29	North Carolina	14.1
31	Indiana	14.0
32	Hawaii	13.7
32	New Hampshire	13.7
34	Louisiana	13.5
34	Wyoming	13.5
36	Minnesota	13.2
37	Illinois	13.1
38	Arizona	13.0
38	New Mexico	13.0
40	Idaho	12.8
41	Virginia	12.6
42	Washington	12.4
43	Maryland	12.2
44	Nevada	11.9
45	California	11.4
46	Georgia	11.1
47	Texas	10.8
48	Colorado	10.7
49	Utah	9.2
50	Alaska	6.9
	District of Columbia	13.0

Source: MQ Press using data from U.S. Dept of Health & Human Services, Centers for Medicare and Medicaid Services "Medicare Estimated Benefit Payments by State" (www.cms.gov/statistics/feeforservice/BenefitPayments01.pdf)
*For fiscal year 2001. Includes aged and disabled enrollees. National rate includes only residents of the 50 states and the District of Columbia.

Medicare Managed Care Enrollees in 2002

National Total = 5,525,427 Enrollees*

ALPHA ORDER

RANK	STATE	ENROLLEES	% of USA
22	Alabama	44,723	0.8%
42	Alaska	0	0.0%
6	Arizona	215,551	3.9%
42	Arkansas	0	0.0%
1	California	1,415,579	25.6%
12	Colorado	136,918	2.5%
28	Connecticut	31,020	0.6%
41	Delaware	456	0.0%
2	Florida	580,816	10.5%
24	Georgia	37,018	0.7%
18	Hawaii	59,195	1.1%
32	Idaho	13,180	0.2%
14	Illinois	99,418	1.8%
30	Indiana	18,507	0.3%
34	Iowa	7,609	0.1%
42	Kansas	0	0.0%
42	Kentucky	0	0.0%
17	Louisiana	68,273	1.2%
42	Maine	0	0.0%
26	Maryland	34,375	0.6%
7	Massachusetts	212,247	3.8%
27	Michigan	31,868	0.6%
15	Minnesota	85,455	1.5%
39	Mississippi	1,044	0.0%
10	Missouri	159,051	2.9%
42	Montana	0	0.0%
33	Nebraska	9,227	0.2%
16	Nevada	81,518	1.5%
38	New Hampshire	1,120	0.0%
13	New Jersey	105,112	1.9%
25	New Mexico	35,843	0.6%
4	New York	470,962	8.5%
20	North Carolina	49,712	0.9%
40	North Dakota	651	0.0%
5	Ohio	253,148	4.6%
23	Oklahoma	41,173	0.7%
9	Oregon	184,037	3.3%
3	Pennsylvania	500,327	9.1%
19	Rhode Island	57,888	1.0%
42	South Carolina	0	0.0%
37	South Dakota	1,911	0.0%
21	Tennessee	48,976	0.9%
8	Texas	187,700	3.4%
31	Utah	17,985	0.3%
42	Vermont	0	0.0%
35	Virginia	2,994	0.1%
11	Washington	138,114	2.5%
36	West Virginia	2,014	0.0%
29	Wisconsin	20,758	0.4%
42	Wyoming	0	0.0%

RANK ORDER

RANK	STATE	ENROLLEES	% of USA
1	California	1,415,579	25.6%
2	Florida	580,816	10.5%
3	Pennsylvania	500,327	9.1%
4	New York	470,962	8.5%
5	Ohio	253,148	4.6%
6	Arizona	215,551	3.9%
7	Massachusetts	212,247	3.8%
8	Texas	187,700	3.4%
9	Oregon	184,037	3.3%
10	Missouri	159,051	2.9%
11	Washington	138,114	2.5%
12	Colorado	136,918	2.5%
13	New Jersey	105,112	1.9%
14	Illinois	99,418	1.8%
15	Minnesota	85,455	1.5%
16	Nevada	81,518	1.5%
17	Louisiana	68,273	1.2%
18	Hawaii	59,195	1.1%
19	Rhode Island	57,888	1.0%
20	North Carolina	49,712	0.9%
21	Tennessee	48,976	0.9%
22	Alabama	44,723	0.8%
23	Oklahoma	41,173	0.7%
24	Georgia	37,018	0.7%
25	New Mexico	35,843	0.6%
26	Maryland	34,375	0.6%
27	Michigan	31,868	0.6%
28	Connecticut	31,020	0.6%
29	Wisconsin	20,758	0.4%
30	Indiana	18,507	0.3%
31	Utah	17,985	0.3%
32	Idaho	13,180	0.2%
33	Nebraska	9,227	0.2%
34	Iowa	7,609	0.1%
35	Virginia	2,994	0.1%
36	West Virginia	2,014	0.0%
37	South Dakota	1,911	0.0%
38	New Hampshire	1,120	0.0%
39	Mississippi	1,044	0.0%
40	North Dakota	651	0.0%
41	Delaware	456	0.0%
42	Alaska	0	0.0%
42	Arkansas	0	0.0%
42	Kansas	0	0.0%
42	Kentucky	0	0.0%
42	Maine	0	0.0%
42	Montana	0	0.0%
42	South Carolina	0	0.0%
42	Vermont	0	0.0%
42	Wyoming	0	0.0%
	District of Columbia	0	0.0%

Source: U.S. Department of Health and Human Services, Centers for Medicare and Medicaid Services
   "2002 Data Compendium" (http://www.cms.gov/researchers/pubs/datacompendium/)
*As of July 2002. Includes TEFRA, Cost, and Health Care Prepayment Plans (HCPP) and other demo plans.
National total includes 52,371 enrollees in the United Mine Workers' plan not shown separately by state.

Percent of Medicare Enrollees in Managed Care Programs in 2002

National Percent = 14% of Medicare Enrollees*

ALPHA ORDER

RANK	STATE	PERCENT
23	Alabama	7
39	Alaska	0
6	Arizona	32
39	Arkansas	0
2	California	36
7	Colorado	29
24	Connecticut	6
39	Delaware	0
10	Florida	21
28	Georgia	4
3	Hawaii	35
20	Idaho	8
24	Illinois	6
32	Indiana	2
32	Iowa	2
39	Kansas	0
39	Kentucky	0
17	Louisiana	11
39	Maine	0
27	Maryland	5
9	Massachusetts	22
32	Michigan	2
16	Minnesota	13
39	Mississippi	0
11	Missouri	19
39	Montana	0
28	Nebraska	4
5	Nevada	33
36	New Hampshire	1
18	New Jersey	9
14	New Mexico	15
13	New York	17
28	North Carolina	4
36	North Dakota	1
14	Ohio	15
20	Oklahoma	8
1	Oregon	37
8	Pennsylvania	24
4	Rhode Island	34
39	South Carolina	0
32	South Dakota	2
24	Tennessee	6
20	Texas	8
18	Utah	9
39	Vermont	0
39	Virginia	0
11	Washington	19
36	West Virginia	1
31	Wisconsin	3
39	Wyoming	0

RANK ORDER

RANK	STATE	PERCENT
1	Oregon	37
2	California	36
3	Hawaii	35
4	Rhode Island	34
5	Nevada	33
6	Arizona	32
7	Colorado	29
8	Pennsylvania	24
9	Massachusetts	22
10	Florida	21
11	Missouri	19
11	Washington	19
13	New York	17
14	New Mexico	15
14	Ohio	15
16	Minnesota	13
17	Louisiana	11
18	New Jersey	9
18	Utah	9
20	Idaho	8
20	Oklahoma	8
20	Texas	8
23	Alabama	7
24	Connecticut	6
24	Illinois	6
24	Tennessee	6
27	Maryland	5
28	Georgia	4
28	Nebraska	4
28	North Carolina	4
31	Wisconsin	3
32	Indiana	2
32	Iowa	2
32	Michigan	2
32	South Dakota	2
36	New Hampshire	1
36	North Dakota	1
36	West Virginia	1
39	Alaska	0
39	Arkansas	0
39	Delaware	0
39	Kansas	0
39	Kentucky	0
39	Maine	0
39	Mississippi	0
39	Montana	0
39	South Carolina	0
39	Vermont	0
39	Virginia	0
39	Wyoming	0
	District of Columbia	0

Source: U.S. Department of Health and Human Services, Centers for Medicare and Medicaid Services
"2002 Data Compendium" (http://www.cms.gov/researchers/pubs/datacompendium/)
*As of July 2002. Includes TEFRA, Cost, and Health Care Prepayment Plans (HCPP) and other demo plans.
National figure includes enrollees in the United Mine Workers' plan not shown separately by state.

Medicare Physicians in 2002

National Total = 888,061 Physicians*

ALPHA ORDER

RANK	STATE	PHYSICIANS	% of USA
29	Alabama	10,021	1.1%
49	Alaska	1,816	0.2%
23	Arizona	13,860	1.6%
31	Arkansas	8,331	0.9%
1	California	93,909	10.6%
22	Colorado	13,969	1.6%
24	Connecticut	12,749	1.4%
48	Delaware	2,496	0.3%
5	Florida	46,697	5.3%
12	Georgia	22,157	2.5%
41	Hawaii**	4,192	0.5%
43	Idaho	3,385	0.4%
8	Illinois	33,797	3.8%
20	Indiana	17,237	1.9%
28	Iowa	10,230	1.2%
30	Kansas	8,526	1.0%
25	Kentucky	11,530	1.3%
21	Louisiana	15,238	1.7%
34	Maine	5,904	0.7%
14	Maryland	20,486	2.3%
6	Massachusetts	35,160	4.0%
9	Michigan	30,658	3.5%
19	Minnesota	17,433	2.0%
35	Mississippi	5,787	0.7%
15	Missouri	18,907	2.1%
44	Montana	3,080	0.3%
38	Nebraska	5,431	0.6%
40	Nevada	4,650	0.5%
37	New Hampshire	5,433	0.6%
10	New Jersey	30,251	3.4%
39	New Mexico	4,757	0.5%
2	New York	71,535	8.1%
11	North Carolina	23,932	2.7%
46	North Dakota	2,732	0.3%
7	Ohio	35,040	3.9%
32	Oklahoma	8,258	0.9%
26	Oregon	11,398	1.3%
4	Pennsylvania	46,953	5.3%
42	Rhode Island	3,632	0.4%
27	South Carolina	11,106	1.3%
47	South Dakota	2,559	0.3%
16	Tennessee	18,322	2.1%
3	Texas	50,291	5.7%
33	Utah	6,041	0.7%
45	Vermont	2,830	0.3%
17	Virginia	18,211	2.1%
13	Washington	21,306	2.4%
36	West Virginia	5,534	0.6%
18	Wisconsin	17,944	2.0%
50	Wyoming	1,554	0.2%

RANK ORDER

RANK	STATE	PHYSICIANS	% of USA
1	California	93,909	10.6%
2	New York	71,535	8.1%
3	Texas	50,291	5.7%
4	Pennsylvania	46,953	5.3%
5	Florida	46,697	5.3%
6	Massachusetts	35,160	4.0%
7	Ohio	35,040	3.9%
8	Illinois	33,797	3.8%
9	Michigan	30,658	3.5%
10	New Jersey	30,251	3.4%
11	North Carolina	23,932	2.7%
12	Georgia	22,157	2.5%
13	Washington	21,306	2.4%
14	Maryland	20,486	2.3%
15	Missouri	18,907	2.1%
16	Tennessee	18,322	2.1%
17	Virginia	18,211	2.1%
18	Wisconsin	17,944	2.0%
19	Minnesota	17,433	2.0%
20	Indiana	17,237	1.9%
21	Louisiana	15,238	1.7%
22	Colorado	13,969	1.6%
23	Arizona	13,860	1.6%
24	Connecticut	12,749	1.4%
25	Kentucky	11,530	1.3%
26	Oregon	11,398	1.3%
27	South Carolina	11,106	1.3%
28	Iowa	10,230	1.2%
29	Alabama	10,021	1.1%
30	Kansas	8,526	1.0%
31	Arkansas	8,331	0.9%
32	Oklahoma	8,258	0.9%
33	Utah	6,041	0.7%
34	Maine	5,904	0.7%
35	Mississippi	5,787	0.7%
36	West Virginia	5,534	0.6%
37	New Hampshire	5,433	0.6%
38	Nebraska	5,431	0.6%
39	New Mexico	4,757	0.5%
40	Nevada	4,650	0.5%
41	Hawaii**	4,192	0.5%
42	Rhode Island	3,632	0.4%
43	Idaho	3,385	0.4%
44	Montana	3,080	0.3%
45	Vermont	2,830	0.3%
46	North Dakota	2,732	0.3%
47	South Dakota	2,559	0.3%
48	Delaware	2,496	0.3%
49	Alaska	1,816	0.2%
50	Wyoming	1,554	0.2%
	District of Columbia	4,402	0.5%

Source: U.S. Department of Health and Human Services, Centers for Medicare and Medicaid Services
"2002 Data Compendium" (http://www.cms.gov/researchers/pubs/datacompendium/)
*Medicare Part B. "Physicians" include MD, DO, DDM, DDS, DPM, OD and CH. National total includes 6,214 physicians in Puerto Rico and the Virgin Islands.
**Physicians for Guam are included in Hawaii's total.*

Percent of Physicians Participating in Medicare in 2002

National Percent = 89.3% of Physicians Participate in Medicare*

ALPHA ORDER

RANK	STATE	PERCENT
6	Alabama	96.1
43	Alaska	86.1
34	Arizona	90.6
9	Arkansas	95.5
49	California	78.6
37	Colorado	89.5
35	Connecticut	90.5
30	Delaware	92.0
22	Florida	92.9
33	Georgia	90.8
15	Hawaii	94.3
47	Idaho	80.8
24	Illinois	92.6
45	Indiana	85.5
16	Iowa	94.2
13	Kansas	94.6
20	Kentucky	93.7
26	Louisiana	92.3
20	Maine	93.7
17	Maryland	94.1
28	Massachusetts	92.1
2	Michigan	96.9
48	Minnesota	80.4
44	Mississippi	85.6
8	Missouri	95.6
36	Montana	89.9
19	Nebraska	93.8
3	Nevada	96.2
31	New Hampshire	91.1
42	New Jersey	87.4
24	New Mexico	92.6
46	New York	81.2
31	North Carolina	91.1
1	North Dakota	97.2
9	Ohio	95.5
18	Oklahoma	93.9
23	Oregon	92.8
7	Pennsylvania	95.8
50	Rhode Island	75.6
28	South Carolina	92.1
38	South Dakota	89.3
27	Tennessee	92.2
40	Texas	88.0
3	Utah	96.2
11	Vermont	94.9
39	Virginia	88.6
3	Washington	96.2
12	West Virginia	94.8
14	Wisconsin	94.5
41	Wyoming	87.7

RANK ORDER

RANK	STATE	PERCENT
1	North Dakota	97.2
2	Michigan	96.9
3	Nevada	96.2
3	Utah	96.2
3	Washington	96.2
6	Alabama	96.1
7	Pennsylvania	95.8
8	Missouri	95.6
9	Arkansas	95.5
9	Ohio	95.5
11	Vermont	94.9
12	West Virginia	94.8
13	Kansas	94.6
14	Wisconsin	94.5
15	Hawaii	94.3
16	Iowa	94.2
17	Maryland	94.1
18	Oklahoma	93.9
19	Nebraska	93.8
20	Kentucky	93.7
20	Maine	93.7
22	Florida	92.9
23	Oregon	92.8
24	Illinois	92.6
24	New Mexico	92.6
26	Louisiana	92.3
27	Tennessee	92.2
28	Massachusetts	92.1
28	South Carolina	92.1
30	Delaware	92.0
31	New Hampshire	91.1
31	North Carolina	91.1
33	Georgia	90.8
34	Arizona	90.6
35	Connecticut	90.5
36	Montana	89.9
37	Colorado	89.5
38	South Dakota	89.3
39	Virginia	88.6
40	Texas	88.0
41	Wyoming	87.7
42	New Jersey	87.4
43	Alaska	86.1
44	Mississippi	85.6
45	Indiana	85.5
46	New York	81.2
47	Idaho	80.8
48	Minnesota	80.4
49	California	78.6
50	Rhode Island	75.6
	District of Columbia	90.8

Source: U.S. Department of Health and Human Services, Centers for Medicare and Medicaid Services
"2002 Data Compendium" (http://www.cms.gov/researchers/pubs/datacompendium/)
*As of January 1, 2002. Refers to Medicare Part B. Physicians include MD's, DO's, limited license practitioners and non-physician practitioners.

Average Medicare Reimbursement Per Day for Nursing Home Care: 2000

National Average = $236 Per Day*

ALPHA ORDER

RANK	STATE	PER DAY
45	Alabama	$193
8	Alaska	262
6	Arizona	269
48	Arkansas	185
1	California	311
4	Colorado	270
20	Connecticut	232
22	Delaware	231
11	Florida	255
40	Georgia	207
9	Hawaii	261
31	Idaho	217
15	Illinois	239
28	Indiana	225
35	Iowa	213
25	Kansas	228
42	Kentucky	203
19	Louisiana	233
29	Maine	222
17	Maryland	237
12	Massachusetts	254
36	Michigan	212
41	Minnesota	205
46	Mississippi	187
24	Missouri	229
38	Montana	209
30	Nebraska	218
4	Nevada	270
14	New Hampshire	240
7	New Jersey	264
25	New Mexico	228
13	New York	252
47	North Carolina	186
49	North Dakota	174
18	Ohio	235
27	Oklahoma	226
2	Oregon	276
23	Pennsylvania	230
20	Rhode Island	232
43	South Carolina	198
49	South Dakota	174
38	Tennessee	209
16	Texas	238
10	Utah	259
44	Vermont	197
31	Virginia	217
3	Washington	275
37	West Virginia	211
33	Wisconsin	216
33	Wyoming	216

RANK ORDER

RANK	STATE	PER DAY
1	California	$311
2	Oregon	276
3	Washington	275
4	Colorado	270
4	Nevada	270
6	Arizona	269
7	New Jersey	264
8	Alaska	262
9	Hawaii	261
10	Utah	259
11	Florida	255
12	Massachusetts	254
13	New York	252
14	New Hampshire	240
15	Illinois	239
16	Texas	238
17	Maryland	237
18	Ohio	235
19	Louisiana	233
20	Connecticut	232
20	Rhode Island	232
22	Delaware	231
23	Pennsylvania	230
24	Missouri	229
25	Kansas	228
25	New Mexico	228
27	Oklahoma	226
28	Indiana	225
29	Maine	222
30	Nebraska	218
31	Idaho	217
31	Virginia	217
33	Wisconsin	216
33	Wyoming	216
35	Iowa	213
36	Michigan	212
37	West Virginia	211
38	Montana	209
38	Tennessee	209
40	Georgia	207
41	Minnesota	205
42	Kentucky	203
43	South Carolina	198
44	Vermont	197
45	Alabama	193
46	Mississippi	187
47	North Carolina	186
48	Arkansas	185
49	North Dakota	174
49	South Dakota	174
	District of Columbia	254

Source: U.S. Department of Health and Human Services, Centers for Medicare and Medicaid Services
"2002 Data Compendium" (http://www.cms.gov/researchers/pubs/datacompendium/)
*In Medicare skilled nursing facilities.

Medicaid Enrollment in 2001

National Total = 36,562,567 Enrollees*

ALPHA ORDER

RANK ORDER

RANK	STATE	ENROLLEES	% of USA
17	Alabama	652,408	1.8%
44	Alaska	115,639	0.3%
23	Arizona	549,318	1.5%
27	Arkansas	443,647	1.2%
1	California	5,487,094	15.0%
32	Colorado	268,674	0.7%
31	Connecticut	331,307	0.9%
45	Delaware	102,000	0.3%
3	Florida	1,923,121	5.3%
10	Georgia	1,040,566	2.8%
38	Hawaii	163,197	0.4%
41	Idaho	133,745	0.4%
5	Illinois	1,455,621	4.0%
19	Indiana	616,752	1.7%
34	Iowa	233,240	0.6%
36	Kansas	205,337	0.6%
21	Kentucky	607,702	1.7%
14	Louisiana	825,959	2.3%
35	Maine	222,348	0.6%
20	Maryland	616,696	1.7%
12	Massachusetts	954,841	2.6%
8	Michigan	1,137,599	3.1%
25	Minnesota	501,798	1.4%
22	Mississippi	586,026	1.6%
13	Missouri	839,563	2.3%
48	Montana	73,153	0.2%
37	Nebraska	201,543	0.6%
43	Nevada	124,289	0.3%
47	New Hampshire	78,589	0.2%
16	New Jersey	759,206	2.1%
30	New Mexico	331,798	0.9%
2	New York	2,803,470	7.7%
11	North Carolina	959,085	2.6%
49	North Dakota	43,819	0.1%
7	Ohio	1,293,390	3.5%
28	Oklahoma	442,387	1.2%
29	Oregon	412,983	1.1%
9	Pennsylvania	1,048,922	2.9%
39	Rhode Island	163,024	0.4%
18	South Carolina	644,346	1.8%
46	South Dakota	81,784	0.2%
6	Tennessee	1,426,622	3.9%
4	Texas	1,821,570	5.0%
40	Utah	138,616	0.4%
42	Vermont	128,594	0.4%
26	Virginia	475,714	1.3%
15	Washington	766,366	2.1%
33	West Virginia	264,087	0.7%
24	Wisconsin	514,658	1.4%
50	Wyoming	39,657	0.1%

RANK	STATE	ENROLLEES	% of USA
1	California	5,487,094	15.0%
2	New York	2,803,470	7.7%
3	Florida	1,923,121	5.3%
4	Texas	1,821,570	5.0%
5	Illinois	1,455,621	4.0%
6	Tennessee	1,426,622	3.9%
7	Ohio	1,293,390	3.5%
8	Michigan	1,137,599	3.1%
9	Pennsylvania	1,048,922	2.9%
10	Georgia	1,040,566	2.8%
11	North Carolina	959,085	2.6%
12	Massachusetts	954,841	2.6%
13	Missouri	839,563	2.3%
14	Louisiana	825,959	2.3%
15	Washington	766,366	2.1%
16	New Jersey	759,206	2.1%
17	Alabama	652,408	1.8%
18	South Carolina	644,346	1.8%
19	Indiana	616,752	1.7%
20	Maryland	616,696	1.7%
21	Kentucky	607,702	1.7%
22	Mississippi	586,026	1.6%
23	Arizona	549,318	1.5%
24	Wisconsin	514,658	1.4%
25	Minnesota	501,798	1.4%
26	Virginia	475,714	1.3%
27	Arkansas	443,647	1.2%
28	Oklahoma	442,387	1.2%
29	Oregon	412,983	1.1%
30	New Mexico	331,798	0.9%
31	Connecticut	331,307	0.9%
32	Colorado	268,674	0.7%
33	West Virginia	264,087	0.7%
34	Iowa	233,240	0.6%
35	Maine	222,348	0.6%
36	Kansas	205,337	0.6%
37	Nebraska	201,543	0.6%
38	Hawaii	163,197	0.4%
39	Rhode Island	163,024	0.4%
40	Utah	138,616	0.4%
41	Idaho	133,745	0.4%
42	Vermont	128,594	0.4%
43	Nevada	124,289	0.3%
44	Alaska	115,639	0.3%
45	Delaware	102,000	0.3%
46	South Dakota	81,784	0.2%
47	New Hampshire	78,589	0.2%
48	Montana	73,153	0.2%
49	North Dakota	43,819	0.1%
50	Wyoming	39,657	0.1%
	District of Columbia	123,745	0.3%

Source: U.S. Department of Health and Human Services, Centers for Medicare and Medicaid Services
   "Medicaid Managed Care State Enrollment" (http://www.cms.gov/medicaid/managedcare/mcsten01.pdf)
*As of June 30, 2001. National total includes 1,386,952 Medicaid enrollees in Puerto Rico and the Virgin Islands

Percent of Population Enrolled in Medicaid in 2001

National Percent = 12.3% of Population*

ALPHA ORDER				RANK ORDER		
RANK	STATE	PERCENT		RANK	STATE	PERCENT
17	Alabama	14.6		1	Tennessee	24.8
5	Alaska	18.3		2	Vermont	21.0
32	Arizona	10.4		3	Mississippi	20.5
8	Arkansas	16.5		4	Louisiana	18.5
9	California	15.9		5	Alaska	18.3
48	Colorado	6.1		6	New Mexico	18.1
36	Connecticut	9.6		7	Maine	17.3
19	Delaware	12.8		8	Arkansas	16.5
24	Florida	11.7		9	California	15.9
22	Georgia	12.4		9	South Carolina	15.9
18	Hawaii	13.3		11	Rhode Island	15.4
33	Idaho	10.1		12	Kentucky	14.9
27	Illinois	11.6		12	Massachusetts	14.9
33	Indiana	10.1		12	Missouri	14.9
42	Iowa	8.0		15	New York	14.7
44	Kansas	7.6		15	West Virginia	14.7
12	Kentucky	14.9		17	Alabama	14.6
4	Louisiana	18.5		18	Hawaii	13.3
7	Maine	17.3		19	Delaware	12.8
28	Maryland	11.4		19	Oklahoma	12.8
12	Massachusetts	14.9		19	Washington	12.8
28	Michigan	11.4		22	Georgia	12.4
33	Minnesota	10.1		23	Oregon	11.9
3	Mississippi	20.5		24	Florida	11.7
12	Missouri	14.9		24	Nebraska	11.7
41	Montana	8.1		24	North Carolina	11.7
24	Nebraska	11.7		27	Illinois	11.6
50	Nevada	5.9		28	Maryland	11.4
47	New Hampshire	6.2		28	Michigan	11.4
38	New Jersey	8.9		28	Ohio	11.4
6	New Mexico	18.1		31	South Dakota	10.8
15	New York	14.7		32	Arizona	10.4
24	North Carolina	11.7		33	Idaho	10.1
45	North Dakota	6.9		33	Indiana	10.1
28	Ohio	11.4		33	Minnesota	10.1
19	Oklahoma	12.8		36	Connecticut	9.6
23	Oregon	11.9		37	Wisconsin	9.5
39	Pennsylvania	8.5		38	New Jersey	8.9
11	Rhode Island	15.4		39	Pennsylvania	8.5
9	South Carolina	15.9		39	Texas	8.5
31	South Dakota	10.8		41	Montana	8.1
1	Tennessee	24.8		42	Iowa	8.0
39	Texas	8.5		42	Wyoming	8.0
48	Utah	6.1		44	Kansas	7.6
2	Vermont	21.0		45	North Dakota	6.9
46	Virginia	6.6		46	Virginia	6.6
19	Washington	12.8		47	New Hampshire	6.2
15	West Virginia	14.7		48	Colorado	6.1
37	Wisconsin	9.5		48	Utah	6.1
42	Wyoming	8.0		50	Nevada	5.9
					District of Columbia	21.6

Source: MQ Press using data from U.S. Dept of Health & Human Services, Centers for Medicare and Medicaid Services
"Medicaid Managed Care State Enrollment" (http://www.cms.gov/medicaid/managedcare/mcsten01.pdf)
*As of June 30, 2001. National percent does not include recipients or population in U.S. territories.

Percent of Children Covered by Medicaid in 2001

National Percent = 22.7% of Children*

RANK	STATE	PERCENT
12	Alabama	26.2
11	Alaska	26.4
27	Arizona	21.8
5	Arkansas	34.1
13	California	25.8
50	Colorado	10.3
45	Connecticut	14.1
44	Delaware	14.2
19	Florida	24.3
21	Georgia	24.1
26	Hawaii	22.0
16	Idaho	25.1
35	Illinois	19.3
39	Indiana	15.3
38	Iowa	16.0
35	Kansas	19.3
14	Kentucky	25.4
9	Louisiana	27.6
8	Maine	29.0
49	Maryland	11.8
18	Massachusetts	24.6
32	Michigan	20.3
42	Minnesota	14.4
1	Mississippi	42.0
22	Missouri	23.9
30	Montana	20.9
28	Nebraska	21.3
47	Nevada	12.8
41	New Hampshire	15.2
46	New Jersey	13.9
2	New Mexico	41.1
7	New York	29.7
14	North Carolina	25.4
31	North Dakota	20.8
29	Ohio	21.2
10	Oklahoma	26.7
24	Oregon	22.5
33	Pennsylvania	19.7
17	Rhode Island	24.7
19	South Carolina	24.3
43	South Dakota	14.3
6	Tennessee	31.7
24	Texas	22.5
39	Utah	15.3
3	Vermont	35.4
48	Virginia	12.2
23	Washington	22.7
4	West Virginia	35.0
37	Wisconsin	18.5
34	Wyoming	19.4

RANK	STATE	PERCENT
1	Mississippi	42.0
2	New Mexico	41.1
3	Vermont	35.4
4	West Virginia	35.0
5	Arkansas	34.1
6	Tennessee	31.7
7	New York	29.7
8	Maine	29.0
9	Louisiana	27.6
10	Oklahoma	26.7
11	Alaska	26.4
12	Alabama	26.2
13	California	25.8
14	Kentucky	25.4
14	North Carolina	25.4
16	Idaho	25.1
17	Rhode Island	24.7
18	Massachusetts	24.6
19	Florida	24.3
19	South Carolina	24.3
21	Georgia	24.1
22	Missouri	23.9
23	Washington	22.7
24	Oregon	22.5
24	Texas	22.5
26	Hawaii	22.0
27	Arizona	21.8
28	Nebraska	21.3
29	Ohio	21.2
30	Montana	20.9
31	North Dakota	20.8
32	Michigan	20.3
33	Pennsylvania	19.7
34	Wyoming	19.4
35	Illinois	19.3
35	Kansas	19.3
37	Wisconsin	18.5
38	Iowa	16.0
39	Indiana	15.3
39	Utah	15.3
41	New Hampshire	15.2
42	Minnesota	14.4
43	South Dakota	14.3
44	Delaware	14.2
45	Connecticut	14.1
46	New Jersey	13.9
47	Nevada	12.8
48	Virginia	12.2
49	Maryland	11.8
50	Colorado	10.3
	District of Columbia	42.3

Source: U.S. Bureau of the Census
   "Health Insurance Historical Table 5" (http://www.census.gov/hhes/hlthins/historic/hihistt5.html)
Children under 18 years old.

Medicaid Expenditures in 2001

National Total = 228,038,957,366*

RANK	STATE	EXPENDITURES	% of USA
25	Alabama	$2,987,666,155	1.3%
46	Alaska	623,849,658	0.3%
27	Arizona	2,823,781,986	1.2%
31	Arkansas	1,947,374,774	0.9%
2	California	25,783,182,157	11.3%
29	Colorado	2,246,846,225	1.0%
22	Connecticut	3,379,452,846	1.5%
45	Delaware	634,627,717	0.3%
5	Florida	9,046,039,737	4.0%
13	Georgia	5,314,515,759	2.3%
43	Hawaii	675,387,513	0.3%
41	Idaho	745,855,247	0.3%
7	Illinois	8,421,128,340	3.7%
17	Indiana	4,199,897,954	1.8%
33	Iowa	1,750,634,100	0.8%
32	Kansas	1,774,905,778	0.8%
21	Kentucky	3,398,140,533	1.5%
16	Louisiana	4,309,670,892	1.9%
36	Maine	1,387,289,958	0.6%
20	Maryland	3,494,364,509	1.5%
10	Massachusetts	6,935,485,066	3.0%
8	Michigan	7,891,425,058	3.5%
19	Minnesota	4,076,897,096	1.8%
28	Mississippi	2,516,554,645	1.1%
14	Missouri	4,963,312,151	2.2%
47	Montana	522,262,125	0.2%
38	Nebraska	1,252,239,800	0.5%
42	Nevada	715,657,410	0.3%
39	New Hampshire	922,260,770	0.4%
9	New Jersey	7,361,441,113	3.2%
35	New Mexico	1,544,568,698	0.7%
1	New York	32,467,565,342	14.2%
11	North Carolina	6,429,406,966	2.8%
49	North Dakota	429,684,824	0.2%
6	Ohio	8,857,117,272	3.9%
30	Oklahoma	2,170,592,307	1.0%
26	Oregon	2,877,746,620	1.3%
4	Pennsylvania	11,386,112,560	5.0%
37	Rhode Island	1,255,255,995	0.6%
24	South Carolina	3,120,234,851	1.4%
48	South Dakota	477,246,104	0.2%
12	Tennessee	5,666,154,206	2.5%
3	Texas	12,240,275,240	5.4%
40	Utah	905,205,923	0.4%
44	Vermont	647,676,351	0.3%
23	Virginia	3,201,548,208	1.4%
15	Washington	4,769,737,694	2.1%
34	West Virginia	1,617,888,766	0.7%
18	Wisconsin	4,178,643,338	1.8%
50	Wyoming	264,187,162	0.1%

RANK	STATE	EXPENDITURES	% of USA
1	New York	$32,467,565,342	14.2%
2	California	25,783,182,157	11.3%
3	Texas	12,240,275,240	5.4%
4	Pennsylvania	11,386,112,560	5.0%
5	Florida	9,046,039,737	4.0%
6	Ohio	8,857,117,272	3.9%
7	Illinois	8,421,128,340	3.7%
8	Michigan	7,891,425,058	3.5%
9	New Jersey	7,361,441,113	3.2%
10	Massachusetts	6,935,485,066	3.0%
11	North Carolina	6,429,406,966	2.8%
12	Tennessee	5,666,154,206	2.5%
13	Georgia	5,314,515,759	2.3%
14	Missouri	4,963,312,151	2.2%
15	Washington	4,769,737,694	2.1%
16	Louisiana	4,309,670,892	1.9%
17	Indiana	4,199,897,954	1.8%
18	Wisconsin	4,178,643,338	1.8%
19	Minnesota	4,076,897,096	1.8%
20	Maryland	3,494,364,509	1.5%
21	Kentucky	3,398,140,533	1.5%
22	Connecticut	3,379,452,846	1.5%
23	Virginia	3,201,548,208	1.4%
24	South Carolina	3,120,234,851	1.4%
25	Alabama	2,987,666,155	1.3%
26	Oregon	2,877,746,620	1.3%
27	Arizona	2,823,781,986	1.2%
28	Mississippi	2,516,554,645	1.1%
29	Colorado	2,246,846,225	1.0%
30	Oklahoma	2,170,592,307	1.0%
31	Arkansas	1,947,374,774	0.9%
32	Kansas	1,774,905,778	0.8%
33	Iowa	1,750,634,100	0.8%
34	West Virginia	1,617,888,766	0.7%
35	New Mexico	1,544,568,698	0.7%
36	Maine	1,387,289,958	0.6%
37	Rhode Island	1,255,255,995	0.6%
38	Nebraska	1,252,239,800	0.5%
39	New Hampshire	922,260,770	0.4%
40	Utah	905,205,923	0.4%
41	Idaho	745,855,247	0.3%
42	Nevada	715,657,410	0.3%
43	Hawaii	675,387,513	0.3%
44	Vermont	647,676,351	0.3%
45	Delaware	634,627,717	0.3%
46	Alaska	623,849,658	0.3%
47	Montana	522,262,125	0.2%
48	South Dakota	477,246,104	0.2%
49	North Dakota	429,684,824	0.2%
50	Wyoming	264,187,162	0.1%
	District of Columbia	1,019,107,672	0.4%

Source: U.S. Department of Health and Human Services, Centers for Medicare and Medicaid Services
"Medicaid Financial Statistics Tables (HCFA-64 Report)" (http://www.cms.gov/medicaid/mbes/sttotal.pdf)
For fiscal year 2001. National total includes $410,854,195 in expenditures in U.S. territories. Includes Medical Assistance Payments ($216 billion) and Administrative Costs ($12 billion).

Per Capita Medicaid Expenditures in 2001

National Per Capita = $723*

<table>
<tr><td colspan="3">ALPHA ORDER</td><td colspan="3">RANK ORDER</td></tr>
<tr><td>RANK</td><td>STATE</td><td>PER CAPITA</td><td>RANK</td><td>STATE</td><td>PER CAPITA</td></tr>
<tr><td>33</td><td>Alabama</td><td>$669</td><td>1</td><td>New York</td><td>$1,701</td></tr>
<tr><td>7</td><td>Alaska</td><td>985</td><td>2</td><td>Rhode Island</td><td>1,185</td></tr>
<tr><td>46</td><td>Arizona</td><td>532</td><td>3</td><td>Massachusetts</td><td>1,083</td></tr>
<tr><td>29</td><td>Arkansas</td><td>723</td><td>4</td><td>Maine</td><td>1,080</td></tr>
<tr><td>26</td><td>California</td><td>745</td><td>5</td><td>Vermont</td><td>1,057</td></tr>
<tr><td>47</td><td>Colorado</td><td>507</td><td>6</td><td>Tennessee</td><td>986</td></tr>
<tr><td>8</td><td>Connecticut</td><td>984</td><td>7</td><td>Alaska</td><td>985</td></tr>
<tr><td>19</td><td>Delaware</td><td>797</td><td>8</td><td>Connecticut</td><td>984</td></tr>
<tr><td>43</td><td>Florida</td><td>552</td><td>9</td><td>Louisiana</td><td>964</td></tr>
<tr><td>36</td><td>Georgia</td><td>632</td><td>10</td><td>Pennsylvania</td><td>925</td></tr>
<tr><td>44</td><td>Hawaii</td><td>550</td><td>11</td><td>West Virginia</td><td>898</td></tr>
<tr><td>42</td><td>Idaho</td><td>565</td><td>12</td><td>Mississippi</td><td>880</td></tr>
<tr><td>32</td><td>Illinois</td><td>673</td><td>12</td><td>Missouri</td><td>880</td></tr>
<tr><td>30</td><td>Indiana</td><td>686</td><td>14</td><td>New Jersey</td><td>865</td></tr>
<tr><td>39</td><td>Iowa</td><td>597</td><td>15</td><td>New Mexico</td><td>844</td></tr>
<tr><td>34</td><td>Kansas</td><td>657</td><td>16</td><td>Kentucky</td><td>835</td></tr>
<tr><td>16</td><td>Kentucky</td><td>835</td><td>17</td><td>Oregon</td><td>829</td></tr>
<tr><td>9</td><td>Louisiana</td><td>964</td><td>18</td><td>Minnesota</td><td>818</td></tr>
<tr><td>4</td><td>Maine</td><td>1,080</td><td>19</td><td>Delaware</td><td>797</td></tr>
<tr><td>35</td><td>Maryland</td><td>649</td><td>20</td><td>Washington</td><td>796</td></tr>
<tr><td>3</td><td>Massachusetts</td><td>1,083</td><td>21</td><td>Michigan</td><td>789</td></tr>
<tr><td>21</td><td>Michigan</td><td>789</td><td>22</td><td>North Carolina</td><td>783</td></tr>
<tr><td>18</td><td>Minnesota</td><td>818</td><td>23</td><td>Ohio</td><td>778</td></tr>
<tr><td>12</td><td>Mississippi</td><td>880</td><td>24</td><td>Wisconsin</td><td>773</td></tr>
<tr><td>12</td><td>Missouri</td><td>880</td><td>25</td><td>South Carolina</td><td>768</td></tr>
<tr><td>40</td><td>Montana</td><td>577</td><td>26</td><td>California</td><td>745</td></tr>
<tr><td>28</td><td>Nebraska</td><td>728</td><td>27</td><td>New Hampshire</td><td>732</td></tr>
<tr><td>50</td><td>Nevada</td><td>341</td><td>28</td><td>Nebraska</td><td>728</td></tr>
<tr><td>27</td><td>New Hampshire</td><td>732</td><td>29</td><td>Arkansas</td><td>723</td></tr>
<tr><td>14</td><td>New Jersey</td><td>865</td><td>30</td><td>Indiana</td><td>686</td></tr>
<tr><td>15</td><td>New Mexico</td><td>844</td><td>31</td><td>North Dakota</td><td>675</td></tr>
<tr><td>1</td><td>New York</td><td>1,701</td><td>32</td><td>Illinois</td><td>673</td></tr>
<tr><td>22</td><td>North Carolina</td><td>783</td><td>33</td><td>Alabama</td><td>669</td></tr>
<tr><td>31</td><td>North Dakota</td><td>675</td><td>34</td><td>Kansas</td><td>657</td></tr>
<tr><td>23</td><td>Ohio</td><td>778</td><td>35</td><td>Maryland</td><td>649</td></tr>
<tr><td>38</td><td>Oklahoma</td><td>626</td><td>36</td><td>Georgia</td><td>632</td></tr>
<tr><td>17</td><td>Oregon</td><td>829</td><td>37</td><td>South Dakota</td><td>629</td></tr>
<tr><td>10</td><td>Pennsylvania</td><td>925</td><td>38</td><td>Oklahoma</td><td>626</td></tr>
<tr><td>2</td><td>Rhode Island</td><td>1,185</td><td>39</td><td>Iowa</td><td>597</td></tr>
<tr><td>25</td><td>South Carolina</td><td>768</td><td>40</td><td>Montana</td><td>577</td></tr>
<tr><td>37</td><td>South Dakota</td><td>629</td><td>41</td><td>Texas</td><td>573</td></tr>
<tr><td>6</td><td>Tennessee</td><td>986</td><td>42</td><td>Idaho</td><td>565</td></tr>
<tr><td>41</td><td>Texas</td><td>573</td><td>43</td><td>Florida</td><td>552</td></tr>
<tr><td>49</td><td>Utah</td><td>397</td><td>44</td><td>Hawaii</td><td>550</td></tr>
<tr><td>5</td><td>Vermont</td><td>1,057</td><td>45</td><td>Wyoming</td><td>535</td></tr>
<tr><td>48</td><td>Virginia</td><td>445</td><td>46</td><td>Arizona</td><td>532</td></tr>
<tr><td>20</td><td>Washington</td><td>796</td><td>47</td><td>Colorado</td><td>507</td></tr>
<tr><td>11</td><td>West Virginia</td><td>898</td><td>48</td><td>Virginia</td><td>445</td></tr>
<tr><td>24</td><td>Wisconsin</td><td>773</td><td>49</td><td>Utah</td><td>397</td></tr>
<tr><td>45</td><td>Wyoming</td><td>535</td><td>50</td><td>Nevada</td><td>341</td></tr>
<tr><td></td><td></td><td></td><td></td><td>District of Columbia</td><td>1,776</td></tr>
</table>

Source: MQ Press using data from U.S. Dept of Health & Human Services, Centers for Medicare and Medicaid Services
"Medicaid Financial Statistics Tables (HCFA-64 Report)" (http://www.cms.gov/medicaid/mbes/sttotal.pdf)
*For fiscal year 2001. National figure does not include expenditures or enrollees in U.S. territories. Includes
Medical Assistance Payments and Administrative Costs.

Percent Change in Medicaid Expenditures: 1997 to 2001

National Percent Change = 37.4% Increase*

ALPHA ORDER

RANK	STATE	PERCENT CHANGE
35	Alabama	33.3
8	Alaska	57.5
13	Arizona	50.5
24	Arkansas	41.0
12	California	53.0
19	Colorado	42.8
46	Connecticut	21.6
15	Delaware	47.0
25	Florida	39.6
17	Georgia	45.0
50	Hawaii	16.4
4	Idaho	66.0
48	Illinois	19.8
6	Indiana	63.8
28	Iowa	37.9
2	Kansas	67.2
37	Kentucky	30.2
27	Louisiana	38.3
42	Maine	26.9
47	Maryland	21.2
29	Massachusetts	36.9
40	Michigan	28.6
23	Minnesota	41.7
16	Mississippi	46.0
10	Missouri	54.5
36	Montana	30.9
7	Nebraska	59.2
18	Nevada	42.9
45	New Hampshire	21.7
38	New Jersey	29.8
9	New Mexico	55.5
39	New York	28.8
21	North Carolina	41.9
41	North Dakota	27.2
34	Ohio	33.6
3	Oklahoma	67.0
1	Oregon	79.4
32	Pennsylvania	35.9
33	Rhode Island	33.8
20	South Carolina	42.7
22	South Dakota	41.8
11	Tennessee	53.2
44	Texas	22.4
30	Utah	36.5
5	Vermont	64.8
31	Virginia	36.1
26	Washington	39.1
43	West Virginia	24.0
14	Wisconsin	49.1
49	Wyoming	19.2

RANK ORDER

RANK	STATE	PERCENT CHANGE
1	Oregon	79.4
2	Kansas	67.2
3	Oklahoma	67.0
4	Idaho	66.0
5	Vermont	64.8
6	Indiana	63.8
7	Nebraska	59.2
8	Alaska	57.5
9	New Mexico	55.5
10	Missouri	54.5
11	Tennessee	53.2
12	California	53.0
13	Arizona	50.5
14	Wisconsin	49.1
15	Delaware	47.0
16	Mississippi	46.0
17	Georgia	45.0
18	Nevada	42.9
19	Colorado	42.8
20	South Carolina	42.7
21	North Carolina	41.9
22	South Dakota	41.8
23	Minnesota	41.7
24	Arkansas	41.0
25	Florida	39.6
26	Washington	39.1
27	Louisiana	38.3
28	Iowa	37.9
29	Massachusetts	36.9
30	Utah	36.5
31	Virginia	36.1
32	Pennsylvania	35.9
33	Rhode Island	33.8
34	Ohio	33.6
35	Alabama	33.3
36	Montana	30.9
37	Kentucky	30.2
38	New Jersey	29.8
39	New York	28.8
40	Michigan	28.6
41	North Dakota	27.2
42	Maine	26.9
43	West Virginia	24.0
44	Texas	22.4
45	New Hampshire	21.7
46	Connecticut	21.6
47	Maryland	21.2
48	Illinois	19.8
49	Wyoming	19.2
50	Hawaii	16.4

| | District of Columbia | 16.4 |

Source: MQ Press using data from U.S. Dept of Health & Human Services, Centers for Medicare and Medicaid Services
"Medicaid Financial Statistics Tables (HCFA-64 Report)" (http://www.cms.gov/medicaid/mbes/sttotal.pdf)
*For fiscal years 2001 and 1997. National figure includes expenditures in U.S. territories.

Medicaid Expenditures per Enrollee in 2001

National Rate = $6,237 per Enrollee*

ALPHA ORDER			RANK ORDER		
RANK	STATE	PER ENROLLEE	RANK	STATE	PER ENROLLEE
46	Alabama	$4,579	1	New Hampshire	$11,735
36	Alaska	5,395	2	New York	11,581
38	Arizona	5,141	3	Pennsylvania	10,855
47	Arkansas	4,389	4	Connecticut	10,200
44	California	4,699	5	North Dakota	9,806
8	Colorado	8,363	6	New Jersey	9,696
4	Connecticut	10,200	7	Kansas	8,644
26	Delaware	6,222	8	Colorado	8,363
43	Florida	4,704	9	Minnesota	8,125
39	Georgia	5,107	10	Wisconsin	8,119
49	Hawaii	4,138	11	Rhode Island	7,700
35	Idaho	5,577	12	Iowa	7,506
31	Illinois	5,785	13	Massachusetts	7,263
18	Indiana	6,810	14	Montana	7,139
12	Iowa	7,506	15	Oregon	6,968
7	Kansas	8,644	16	Michigan	6,937
34	Kentucky	5,592	17	Ohio	6,848
37	Louisiana	5,218	18	Indiana	6,810
24	Maine	6,239	19	Virginia	6,730
33	Maryland	5,666	20	Texas	6,720
13	Massachusetts	7,263	21	North Carolina	6,704
16	Michigan	6,937	22	Wyoming	6,662
9	Minnesota	8,125	23	Utah	6,530
48	Mississippi	4,294	24	Maine	6,239
29	Missouri	5,912	25	Washington	6,224
14	Montana	7,139	26	Delaware	6,222
27	Nebraska	6,213	27	Nebraska	6,213
32	Nevada	5,758	28	West Virginia	6,126
1	New Hampshire	11,735	29	Missouri	5,912
6	New Jersey	9,696	30	South Dakota	5,835
45	New Mexico	4,655	31	Illinois	5,785
2	New York	11,581	32	Nevada	5,758
21	North Carolina	6,704	33	Maryland	5,666
5	North Dakota	9,806	34	Kentucky	5,592
17	Ohio	6,848	35	Idaho	5,577
41	Oklahoma	4,907	36	Alaska	5,395
15	Oregon	6,968	37	Louisiana	5,218
3	Pennsylvania	10,855	38	Arizona	5,141
11	Rhode Island	7,700	39	Georgia	5,107
42	South Carolina	4,842	40	Vermont	5,037
30	South Dakota	5,835	41	Oklahoma	4,907
50	Tennessee	3,972	42	South Carolina	4,842
20	Texas	6,720	43	Florida	4,704
23	Utah	6,530	44	California	4,699
40	Vermont	5,037	45	New Mexico	4,655
19	Virginia	6,730	46	Alabama	4,579
25	Washington	6,224	47	Arkansas	4,389
28	West Virginia	6,126	48	Mississippi	4,294
10	Wisconsin	8,119	49	Hawaii	4,138
22	Wyoming	6,662	50	Tennessee	3,972
				District of Columbia	8,236

Source: MQ Press using data from U.S. Dept of Health & Human Services, Centers for Medicare and Medicaid Services "Medicaid Financial Statistics Tables (HCFA-64 Report)" (http://www.cms.gov/medicaid/mbes/sttotal.pdf)
*For fiscal year 2001. National figure includes expenditures and enrollees in U.S. territories. Includes Medical Assistance Payments and Administrative Costs.

Percent Change in Expenditures per Medicaid Enrollee: 1997 to 2001

National Percent Change = 20.6% Increase*

ALPHA ORDER			RANK ORDER		
RANK	STATE	PERCENT CHANGE	RANK	STATE	PERCENT CHANGE
44	Alabama	1.6	1	Pennsylvania	105.5
23	Alaska	19.2	2	Oklahoma	65.1
25	Arizona	18.3	3	Oregon	63.5
50	Arkansas	(15.0)	4	Kansas	50.9
10	California	33.6	5	Virginia	49.3
22	Colorado	21.5	6	West Virginia	45.8
12	Connecticut	32.2	7	Wyoming	45.4
28	Delaware	16.1	8	Texas	39.7
42	Florida	2.4	9	Mississippi	35.4
19	Georgia	22.9	10	California	33.6
24	Hawaii	18.9	11	Washington	32.5
45	Idaho	0.0	12	Connecticut	32.2
35	Illinois	12.7	13	North Dakota	31.5
37	Indiana	7.6	14	Iowa	28.7
14	Iowa	28.7	15	Tennessee	27.7
4	Kansas	50.9	16	Montana	26.7
34	Kentucky	13.0	17	Michigan	26.1
38	Louisiana	6.4	18	Vermont	24.3
48	Maine	(11.2)	19	Georgia	22.9
47	Maryland	(8.6)	20	Wisconsin	22.5
41	Massachusetts	2.7	21	North Carolina	22.1
17	Michigan	26.1	22	Colorado	21.5
30	Minnesota	13.7	23	Alaska	19.2
9	Mississippi	35.4	24	Hawaii	18.9
32	Missouri	13.2	25	Arizona	18.3
16	Montana	26.7	26	New Jersey	17.1
29	Nebraska	13.9	27	Utah	16.6
43	Nevada	1.7	28	Delaware	16.1
36	New Hampshire	9.8	29	Nebraska	13.9
26	New Jersey	17.1	30	Minnesota	13.7
31	New Mexico	13.6	31	New Mexico	13.6
39	New York	5.5	32	Missouri	13.2
21	North Carolina	22.1	33	Ohio	13.1
13	North Dakota	31.5	34	Kentucky	13.0
33	Ohio	13.1	35	Illinois	12.7
2	Oklahoma	65.1	36	New Hampshire	9.8
3	Oregon	63.5	37	Indiana	7.6
1	Pennsylvania	105.5	38	Louisiana	6.4
46	Rhode Island	(6.3)	39	New York	5.5
49	South Carolina	(12.9)	40	South Dakota	4.7
40	South Dakota	4.7	41	Massachusetts	2.7
15	Tennessee	27.7	42	Florida	2.4
8	Texas	39.7	43	Nevada	1.7
27	Utah	16.6	44	Alabama	1.6
18	Vermont	24.3	45	Idaho	0.0
5	Virginia	49.3	46	Rhode Island	(6.3)
11	Washington	32.5	47	Maryland	(8.6)
6	West Virginia	45.8	48	Maine	(11.2)
20	Wisconsin	22.5	49	South Carolina	(12.9)
7	Wyoming	45.4	50	Arkansas	(15.0)
				District of Columbia	17.6

Source: MQ Press using data from U.S. Dept of Health & Human Services, Centers for Medicare and Medicaid Services
"Medicaid Financial Statistics Tables (HCFA-64 Report)" (http://www.cms.gov/medicaid/mbes/sttotal.pdf)
*For fiscal years 2001 and 1997. National figure includes expenditures and enrollees in U.S. territories.

Medicaid Managed Care Enrollment in 2001

National Total = 20,773,813 Enrollees*

ALPHA ORDER

RANK	STATE	ENROLLEES	% of USA
19	Alabama	350,485	1.7%
49	Alaska	0	0.0%
12	Arizona	527,674	2.5%
26	Arkansas	257,662	1.2%
1	California	2,870,514	13.8%
27	Colorado	247,181	1.2%
28	Connecticut	239,829	1.2%
39	Delaware	83,422	0.4%
3	Florida	1,184,506	5.7%
6	Georgia	878,140	4.2%
34	Hawaii	127,779	0.6%
46	Idaho	37,913	0.2%
32	Illinois	136,497	0.7%
15	Indiana	433,014	2.1%
30	Iowa	206,751	1.0%
36	Kansas	118,209	0.6%
13	Kentucky	489,711	2.4%
42	Louisiana	56,542	0.3%
38	Maine	96,051	0.5%
16	Maryland	421,355	2.0%
11	Massachusetts	616,241	3.0%
4	Michigan	1,023,264	4.9%
20	Minnesota	322,640	1.6%
22	Mississippi	297,916	1.4%
17	Missouri	378,771	1.8%
44	Montana	46,995	0.2%
31	Nebraska	150,840	0.7%
43	Nevada	47,518	0.2%
48	New Hampshire	6,200	0.0%
14	New Jersey	459,087	2.2%
29	New Mexico	212,456	1.0%
9	New York	728,709	3.5%
10	North Carolina	674,133	3.2%
47	North Dakota	25,540	0.1%
24	Ohio	277,617	1.3%
21	Oklahoma	299,272	1.4%
18	Oregon	360,926	1.7%
5	Pennsylvania	898,171	4.3%
37	Rhode Island	111,624	0.5%
45	South Carolina	41,716	0.2%
40	South Dakota	79,641	0.4%
2	Tennessee	1,426,622	6.9%
8	Texas	753,613	3.6%
33	Utah	128,898	0.6%
41	Vermont	78,181	0.4%
23	Virginia	291,767	1.4%
7	Washington	766,366	3.7%
35	West Virginia	122,230	0.6%
25	Wisconsin	266,577	1.3%
49	Wyoming	0	0.0%

RANK ORDER

RANK	STATE	ENROLLEES	% of USA
1	California	2,870,514	13.8%
2	Tennessee	1,426,622	6.9%
3	Florida	1,184,506	5.7%
4	Michigan	1,023,264	4.9%
5	Pennsylvania	898,171	4.3%
6	Georgia	878,140	4.2%
7	Washington	766,366	3.7%
8	Texas	753,613	3.6%
9	New York	728,709	3.5%
10	North Carolina	674,133	3.2%
11	Massachusetts	616,241	3.0%
12	Arizona	527,674	2.5%
13	Kentucky	489,711	2.4%
14	New Jersey	459,087	2.2%
15	Indiana	433,014	2.1%
16	Maryland	421,355	2.0%
17	Missouri	378,771	1.8%
18	Oregon	360,926	1.7%
19	Alabama	350,485	1.7%
20	Minnesota	322,640	1.6%
21	Oklahoma	299,272	1.4%
22	Mississippi	297,916	1.4%
23	Virginia	291,767	1.4%
24	Ohio	277,617	1.3%
25	Wisconsin	266,577	1.3%
26	Arkansas	257,662	1.2%
27	Colorado	247,181	1.2%
28	Connecticut	239,829	1.2%
29	New Mexico	212,456	1.0%
30	Iowa	206,751	1.0%
31	Nebraska	150,840	0.7%
32	Illinois	136,497	0.7%
33	Utah	128,898	0.6%
34	Hawaii	127,779	0.6%
35	West Virginia	122,230	0.6%
36	Kansas	118,209	0.6%
37	Rhode Island	111,624	0.5%
38	Maine	96,051	0.5%
39	Delaware	83,422	0.4%
40	South Dakota	79,641	0.4%
41	Vermont	78,181	0.4%
42	Louisiana	56,542	0.3%
43	Nevada	47,518	0.2%
44	Montana	46,995	0.2%
45	South Carolina	41,716	0.2%
46	Idaho	37,913	0.2%
47	North Dakota	25,540	0.1%
48	New Hampshire	6,200	0.0%
49	Alaska	0	0.0%
49	Wyoming	0	0.0%
	District of Columbia	79,673	0.4%

Source: U.S. Department of Health and Human Services, Centers for Medicare and Medicaid Services
"Medicaid Managed Care State Enrollment" (http://www.cms.gov/medicaid/managedcare/mcsten01.pdf)
*As of June 30, 2001. Enrollment in state health care reform programs that expand eligibility beyond traditional
Medicaid standards. National total includes 1,037,374 Medicaid managed care enrollees in Puerto Rico.

Percent of Medicaid Enrollees in Managed Care in 2001

National Percent = 56.8% of Medicaid Enrollees*

ALPHA ORDER

RANK	STATE	PERCENT
33	Alabama	53.7
49	Alaska	0.0
4	Arizona	96.1
31	Arkansas	58.1
34	California	52.3
6	Colorado	92.0
16	Connecticut	72.4
12	Delaware	81.8
26	Florida	61.6
11	Georgia	84.4
14	Hawaii	78.3
42	Idaho	28.4
45	Illinois	9.4
18	Indiana	70.2
8	Iowa	88.6
32	Kansas	57.6
13	Kentucky	80.6
47	Louisiana	6.9
39	Maine	43.2
20	Maryland	68.3
22	Massachusetts	64.5
7	Michigan	90.0
23	Minnesota	64.3
36	Mississippi	50.8
38	Missouri	45.1
24	Montana	64.2
15	Nebraska	74.8
41	Nevada	38.2
46	New Hampshire	7.9
29	New Jersey	60.5
25	New Mexico	64.0
43	New York	26.0
17	North Carolina	70.3
30	North Dakota	58.3
44	Ohio	21.5
21	Oklahoma	67.7
9	Oregon	87.4
10	Pennsylvania	85.6
19	Rhode Island	68.5
48	South Carolina	6.5
3	South Dakota	97.4
1	Tennessee	100.0
40	Texas	41.4
5	Utah	93.0
28	Vermont	60.8
27	Virginia	61.3
1	Washington	100.0
37	West Virginia	46.3
35	Wisconsin	51.8
49	Wyoming	0.0

RANK ORDER

RANK	STATE	PERCENT
1	Tennessee	100.0
1	Washington	100.0
3	South Dakota	97.4
4	Arizona	96.1
5	Utah	93.0
6	Colorado	92.0
7	Michigan	90.0
8	Iowa	88.6
9	Oregon	87.4
10	Pennsylvania	85.6
11	Georgia	84.4
12	Delaware	81.8
13	Kentucky	80.6
14	Hawaii	78.3
15	Nebraska	74.8
16	Connecticut	72.4
17	North Carolina	70.3
18	Indiana	70.2
19	Rhode Island	68.5
20	Maryland	68.3
21	Oklahoma	67.7
22	Massachusetts	64.5
23	Minnesota	64.3
24	Montana	64.2
25	New Mexico	64.0
26	Florida	61.6
27	Virginia	61.3
28	Vermont	60.8
29	New Jersey	60.5
30	North Dakota	58.3
31	Arkansas	58.1
32	Kansas	57.6
33	Alabama	53.7
34	California	52.3
35	Wisconsin	51.8
36	Mississippi	50.8
37	West Virginia	46.3
38	Missouri	45.1
39	Maine	43.2
40	Texas	41.4
41	Nevada	38.2
42	Idaho	28.4
43	New York	26.0
44	Ohio	21.5
45	Illinois	9.4
46	New Hampshire	7.9
47	Louisiana	6.9
48	South Carolina	6.5
49	Alaska	0.0
49	Wyoming	0.0
	District of Columbia	64.4

Source: U.S. Department of Health and Human Services, Centers for Medicare and Medicaid Services
   "Medicaid Managed Care State Enrollment" (http://www.cms.gov/medicaid/managedcare/mcsten01.pdf)
*As of June 30, 2001. Enrollment in state health care reform programs that expand eligibility beyond traditional
Medicaid standards. National percent includes Medicaid enrollees in Puerto Rico and the Virgin Islands.

Federal Medicaid Matching Fund Rate for 2003

National Average = 72.60% of States' Funds Matched by Federal Government*

ALPHA ORDER

RANK ORDER

RANK	STATE	RATE		RANK	STATE	RATE
9	Alabama	79.42		1	Mississippi	83.63
33	Alaska	70.79		2	West Virginia	82.53
14	Arizona	77.08		3	New Mexico	82.19
4	Arkansas	82.00		4	Arkansas	82.00
39	California	65.00		5	Montana	81.07
39	Colorado	65.00		6	Louisiana	79.90
39	Connecticut	65.00		7	Utah	79.87
39	Delaware	65.00		8	Idaho	79.67
29	Florida	71.18		9	Alabama	79.42
27	Georgia	71.72		10	Oklahoma	79.39
31	Hawaii	71.14		11	Kentucky	78.92
8	Idaho	79.67		12	South Carolina	78.87
39	Illinois	65.00		13	North Dakota	77.85
21	Indiana	73.38		14	Arizona	77.08
18	Iowa	74.45		15	Maine	76.35
24	Kansas	72.11		16	South Dakota	75.70
11	Kentucky	78.92		17	Tennessee	75.21
6	Louisiana	79.90		18	Iowa	74.45
15	Maine	76.35		19	North Carolina	73.79
39	Maryland	65.00		20	Vermont	73.69
39	Massachusetts	65.00		21	Indiana	73.38
34	Michigan	68.79		22	Wyoming	72.92
39	Minnesota	65.00		23	Missouri	72.86
1	Mississippi	83.63		24	Kansas	72.11
23	Missouri	72.86		24	Oregon	72.11
5	Montana	81.07		26	Texas	71.99
28	Nebraska	71.66		27	Georgia	71.72
37	Nevada	66.67		28	Nebraska	71.66
39	New Hampshire	65.00		29	Florida	71.18
39	New Jersey	65.00		29	Ohio	71.18
3	New Mexico	82.19		31	Hawaii	71.14
39	New York	65.00		32	Wisconsin	70.90
19	North Carolina	73.79		33	Alaska	70.79
13	North Dakota	77.85		34	Michigan	68.79
29	Ohio	71.18		35	Rhode Island	68.78
10	Oklahoma	79.39		36	Pennsylvania	68.28
24	Oregon	72.11		37	Nevada	66.67
36	Pennsylvania	68.28		38	Virginia	65.37
35	Rhode Island	68.78		39	California	65.00
12	South Carolina	78.87		39	Colorado	65.00
16	South Dakota	75.70		39	Connecticut	65.00
17	Tennessee	75.21		39	Delaware	65.00
26	Texas	71.99		39	Illinois	65.00
7	Utah	79.87		39	Maryland	65.00
20	Vermont	73.69		39	Massachusetts	65.00
38	Virginia	65.37		39	Minnesota	65.00
39	Washington	65.00		39	New Hampshire	65.00
2	West Virginia	82.53		39	New Jersey	65.00
32	Wisconsin	70.90		39	New York	65.00
22	Wyoming	72.92		39	Washington	65.00
					District of Columbia	79.00

Source: U.S. Department of Health and Human Services, Centers for Medicare and Medicaid Services "Enhanced Federal Medical Assistance Percentages" (http://aspe.os.dhhs.gov/health/fmap03.htm)
For fiscal year 2003. These are "enhanced" matching rates established by the Children's Health Insurance Program, signed into law in August 1997. Sixty-five percent is the minimum. National average is a simple average of the 51 individual rates and is not weighted for population or funds.

Projected National Health Care Expenditures in 2003

Total Health Care Expenditures = $1,653,400,000,000*

The 1998 health care expenditures broken down to the state level and shown in this book were released in August of 2000. The Centers for Medicare and Medicaid (CMS) are committed to updating these numbers and hope to have new estimates available later this year.

Given the high level of interest in health care finance data, we have assembled a table showing the most recent national level health care expenditure projections. We will continue to monitor CMS data releases and will include the state expenditure updates in forthcoming editions.

	PROJECTED EXPENDITURES IN 2003	PROJECTED PERCENT CHANGE: 2002 TO 2003
Total Health Care Expenditures	$1,653,400,000,000	7.0
Per Capita Total Health Care Expenditures	$5,734	
Personal Health Care Expenditures	$1,425,000,000,000	7.0
Per Capita Personal Health Care Expenditures	$4,942	
Hospital Care Expenditures	$501,600,000,000	5.3
Per Capita Hospital Care Expenditures	$1,739	
Physician Services Expenditures	$361,200,000,000	7.5
Per Capita Physician Services Expenditures	$1,253	
Dental Services Expenditures	$71,800,000,000	5.3
Per Capita Dental Services Expenditures	$249	
Other Professional Services	$50,400,000,000	8.2
Per Capita Other Professional Services	$175	
Home Health Care Expenditures	$42,800,000,000	7.3
Per Capita Home Health Care Expenditures	$148	
Prescription Drugs	$181,500,000,000	12.8
Per Capita Prescription Drugs	$629	
Nursing Home Care	$107,100,000,000	3.2
Per Capita Nursing Home Care	$371	
Other Personal Care Expenditures	$49,900,000,000	10.8
Per Capita Other Personal Care Expenditures	$173	

Source: U.S. Department of Health and Human Services, Centers for Medicare and Medicaid Services
  "National Health Expenditure Amounts and Average Annual Percent Change, by Type of Expenditure"
  http://www.cms.hhs.gov/statistics/nhe/projections-2001/t2.asp
*Per Capita figures calculated by Morgan Quitno Press using 2002 Census population estimates.
For definitions see the corresponding 1998 state tables in this chapter.

Personal Health Care Expenditures in 1998

National Total = $1,016,383,000,000*

ALPHA ORDER

RANK	STATE	EXPENDITURES	% of USA
22	Alabama	$16,056,000,000	1.6%
48	Alaska	2,299,000,000	0.2%
24	Arizona	14,782,000,000	1.5%
33	Arkansas	8,463,000,000	0.8%
1	California	110,057,000,000	10.8%
26	Colorado	13,669,000,000	1.3%
23	Connecticut	15,221,000,000	1.5%
44	Delaware	3,106,000,000	0.3%
4	Florida	59,724,000,000	5.9%
12	Georgia	27,219,000,000	2.7%
40	Hawaii	4,658,000,000	0.5%
43	Idaho	3,397,000,000	0.3%
6	Illinois	44,305,000,000	4.4%
15	Indiana	21,259,000,000	2.1%
30	Iowa	10,198,000,000	1.0%
31	Kansas	9,394,000,000	0.9%
25	Kentucky	14,414,000,000	1.4%
21	Louisiana	16,500,000,000	1.6%
39	Maine	4,925,000,000	0.5%
19	Maryland	19,646,000,000	1.9%
10	Massachusetts	30,039,000,000	3.0%
8	Michigan	35,647,000,000	3.5%
17	Minnesota	20,313,000,000	2.0%
32	Mississippi	8,882,000,000	0.9%
16	Missouri	20,911,000,000	2.1%
46	Montana	2,838,000,000	0.3%
35	Nebraska	6,095,000,000	0.6%
37	Nevada	5,606,000,000	0.6%
40	New Hampshire	4,658,000,000	0.5%
9	New Jersey	32,695,000,000	3.2%
38	New Mexico	5,344,000,000	0.5%
2	New York	85,785,000,000	8.4%
11	North Carolina	27,327,000,000	2.7%
47	North Dakota	2,680,000,000	0.3%
7	Ohio	42,581,000,000	4.2%
28	Oklahoma	10,988,000,000	1.1%
29	Oregon	10,840,000,000	1.1%
5	Pennsylvania	51,322,000,000	5.0%
42	Rhode Island	4,515,000,000	0.4%
27	South Carolina	13,204,000,000	1.3%
45	South Dakota	2,842,000,000	0.3%
14	Tennessee	22,021,000,000	2.2%
3	Texas	67,750,000,000	6.7%
36	Utah	5,944,000,000	0.6%
49	Vermont	2,066,000,000	0.2%
13	Virginia	22,261,000,000	2.2%
20	Washington	19,292,000,000	1.9%
34	West Virginia	7,037,000,000	0.7%
18	Wisconsin	19,945,000,000	2.0%
50	Wyoming	1,407,000,000	0.1%

RANK ORDER

RANK	STATE	EXPENDITURES	% of USA
1	California	$110,057,000,000	10.8%
2	New York	85,785,000,000	8.4%
3	Texas	67,750,000,000	6.7%
4	Florida	59,724,000,000	5.9%
5	Pennsylvania	51,322,000,000	5.0%
6	Illinois	44,305,000,000	4.4%
7	Ohio	42,581,000,000	4.2%
8	Michigan	35,647,000,000	3.5%
9	New Jersey	32,695,000,000	3.2%
10	Massachusetts	30,039,000,000	3.0%
11	North Carolina	27,327,000,000	2.7%
12	Georgia	27,219,000,000	2.7%
13	Virginia	22,261,000,000	2.2%
14	Tennessee	22,021,000,000	2.2%
15	Indiana	21,259,000,000	2.1%
16	Missouri	20,911,000,000	2.1%
17	Minnesota	20,313,000,000	2.0%
18	Wisconsin	19,945,000,000	2.0%
19	Maryland	19,646,000,000	1.9%
20	Washington	19,292,000,000	1.9%
21	Louisiana	16,500,000,000	1.6%
22	Alabama	16,056,000,000	1.6%
23	Connecticut	15,221,000,000	1.5%
24	Arizona	14,782,000,000	1.5%
25	Kentucky	14,414,000,000	1.4%
26	Colorado	13,669,000,000	1.3%
27	South Carolina	13,204,000,000	1.3%
28	Oklahoma	10,988,000,000	1.1%
29	Oregon	10,840,000,000	1.1%
30	Iowa	10,198,000,000	1.0%
31	Kansas	9,394,000,000	0.9%
32	Mississippi	8,882,000,000	0.9%
33	Arkansas	8,463,000,000	0.8%
34	West Virginia	7,037,000,000	0.7%
35	Nebraska	6,095,000,000	0.6%
36	Utah	5,944,000,000	0.6%
37	Nevada	5,606,000,000	0.6%
38	New Mexico	5,344,000,000	0.5%
39	Maine	4,925,000,000	0.5%
40	Hawaii	4,658,000,000	0.5%
40	New Hampshire	4,658,000,000	0.5%
42	Rhode Island	4,515,000,000	0.4%
43	Idaho	3,397,000,000	0.3%
44	Delaware	3,106,000,000	0.3%
45	South Dakota	2,842,000,000	0.3%
46	Montana	2,838,000,000	0.3%
47	North Dakota	2,680,000,000	0.3%
48	Alaska	2,299,000,000	0.2%
49	Vermont	2,066,000,000	0.2%
50	Wyoming	1,407,000,000	0.1%
	District of Columbia	4,258,000,000	0.4%

Source: U.S. Department of Health and Human Services, Centers for Medicare and Medicaid Services
   "State Health Care Expenditures" (http://www.hcfa.gov/stats/nhe-oact/stateestimates/)
*By state of provider. Includes hospital care, physician services, dental services, home health care, drugs, vision products, nursing home care and other personal health care services and products.

Health Care Expenditures as a Percent of Gross State Product in 1998

National Percent = 11.6% of Total Gross State Product*

ALPHA ORDER

RANK	STATE	PERCENT
5	Alabama	14.6
47	Alaska	9.5
34	Arizona	11.0
11	Arkansas	13.7
44	California	9.8
45	Colorado	9.6
36	Connecticut	10.7
48	Delaware	9.2
6	Florida	14.3
36	Georgia	10.7
30	Hawaii	11.7
34	Idaho	11.0
39	Illinois	10.4
23	Indiana	12.2
25	Iowa	12.1
23	Kansas	12.2
12	Kentucky	13.5
16	Louisiana	12.8
3	Maine	15.2
28	Maryland	11.9
21	Massachusetts	12.5
25	Michigan	12.1
19	Minnesota	12.6
6	Mississippi	14.3
16	Missouri	12.8
6	Montana	14.3
29	Nebraska	11.8
49	Nevada	8.9
32	New Hampshire	11.3
41	New Jersey	10.2
33	New Mexico	11.2
25	New York	12.1
31	North Carolina	11.6
2	North Dakota	15.6
21	Ohio	12.5
12	Oklahoma	13.5
40	Oregon	10.3
9	Pennsylvania	14.1
4	Rhode Island	14.8
15	South Carolina	13.2
14	South Dakota	13.4
10	Tennessee	13.8
38	Texas	10.5
42	Utah	10.0
18	Vermont	12.7
45	Virginia	9.6
42	Washington	10.0
1	West Virginia	17.6
19	Wisconsin	12.6
50	Wyoming	8.0

RANK ORDER

RANK	STATE	PERCENT
1	West Virginia	17.6
2	North Dakota	15.6
3	Maine	15.2
4	Rhode Island	14.8
5	Alabama	14.6
6	Florida	14.3
6	Mississippi	14.3
6	Montana	14.3
9	Pennsylvania	14.1
10	Tennessee	13.8
11	Arkansas	13.7
12	Kentucky	13.5
12	Oklahoma	13.5
14	South Dakota	13.4
15	South Carolina	13.2
16	Louisiana	12.8
16	Missouri	12.8
18	Vermont	12.7
19	Minnesota	12.6
19	Wisconsin	12.6
21	Massachusetts	12.5
21	Ohio	12.5
23	Indiana	12.2
23	Kansas	12.2
25	Iowa	12.1
25	Michigan	12.1
25	New York	12.1
28	Maryland	11.9
29	Nebraska	11.8
30	Hawaii	11.7
31	North Carolina	11.6
32	New Hampshire	11.3
33	New Mexico	11.2
34	Arizona	11.0
34	Idaho	11.0
36	Connecticut	10.7
36	Georgia	10.7
38	Texas	10.5
39	Illinois	10.4
40	Oregon	10.3
41	New Jersey	10.2
42	Utah	10.0
42	Washington	10.0
44	California	9.8
45	Colorado	9.6
45	Virginia	9.6
47	Alaska	9.5
48	Delaware	9.2
49	Nevada	8.9
50	Wyoming	8.0
	District of Columbia	7.9

Source: MQ Press using data from U.S. Dept of Health & Human Services, Centers for Medicare and Medicaid Services "State Health Care Expenditures" (http://www.hcfa.gov/stats/nhe-oact/stateestimates/)
*By state of provider. Includes hospital care, physician services, dental services, home health care, drugs, vision products, nursing home care and other personal health care services and products.

Percent Change in Personal Health Care Expenditures: 1990 to 1998

National Percent Change = 66.0% Increase*

ALPHA ORDER

RANK ORDER

RANK	STATE	PERCENT CHANGE		RANK	STATE	PERCENT CHANGE
21	Alabama	75.2		1	Idaho	100.2
30	Alaska	70.7		2	Nevada	99.8
26	Arizona	72.6		3	North Carolina	98.8
28	Arkansas	71.8		4	South Carolina	94.0
50	California	48.0		5	Mississippi	87.8
19	Colorado	76.6		5	South Dakota	87.8
49	Connecticut	52.0		7	Kentucky	84.3
14	Delaware	79.7		8	Utah	83.9
37	Florida	66.9		9	New Mexico	83.2
16	Georgia	77.9		10	Maine	82.7
31	Hawaii	69.7		11	New Hampshire	82.1
1	Idaho	100.2		12	Tennessee	80.3
44	Illinois	60.4		13	Texas	79.8
35	Indiana	67.5		14	Delaware	79.7
33	Iowa	68.1		15	West Virginia	79.1
32	Kansas	69.6		16	Georgia	77.9
7	Kentucky	84.3		17	Wyoming	77.4
39	Louisiana	65.4		18	Minnesota	77.2
10	Maine	82.7		19	Colorado	76.6
36	Maryland	67.1		20	Vermont	76.3
47	Massachusetts	57.9		21	Alabama	75.2
43	Michigan	61.1		22	Montana	74.3
18	Minnesota	77.2		22	Wisconsin	74.3
5	Mississippi	87.8		24	Oregon	73.5
40	Missouri	64.8		25	Oklahoma	72.8
22	Montana	74.3		26	Arizona	72.6
26	Nebraska	72.6		26	Nebraska	72.6
2	Nevada	99.8		28	Arkansas	71.8
11	New Hampshire	82.1		29	Washington	71.1
42	New Jersey	62.1		30	Alaska	70.7
9	New Mexico	83.2		31	Hawaii	69.7
45	New York	59.1		32	Kansas	69.6
3	North Carolina	98.8		33	Iowa	68.1
41	North Dakota	63.5		34	Virginia	68.0
46	Ohio	58.3		35	Indiana	67.5
25	Oklahoma	72.8		36	Maryland	67.1
24	Oregon	73.5		37	Florida	66.9
48	Pennsylvania	57.3		38	Rhode Island	65.5
38	Rhode Island	65.5		39	Louisiana	65.4
4	South Carolina	94.0		40	Missouri	64.8
5	South Dakota	87.8		41	North Dakota	63.5
12	Tennessee	80.3		42	New Jersey	62.1
13	Texas	79.8		43	Michigan	61.1
8	Utah	83.9		44	Illinois	60.4
20	Vermont	76.3		45	New York	59.1
34	Virginia	68.0		46	Ohio	58.3
29	Washington	71.1		47	Massachusetts	57.9
15	West Virginia	79.1		48	Pennsylvania	57.3
22	Wisconsin	74.3		49	Connecticut	52.0
17	Wyoming	77.4		50	California	48.0
					District of Columbia	19.5

Source: MQ Press using data from U.S. Dept of Health & Human Services, Centers for Medicare and Medicaid Services "State Health Care Expenditures" (http://www.hcfa.gov/stats/nhe-oact/stateestimates/)
*By state of provider. Includes hospital care, physician services, dental services, home health care, drugs, vision products, nursing home care and other personal health care services and products.

Average Annual Change in Expenditures for Personal Health Care: 1990 to 1998
National Percent Change = 13.9% Average Annual Increase*

Source: U.S. Department of Health and Human Services, Centers for Medicare and Medicaid Services
"State Health Care Expenditures" (http://www.hcfa.gov/stats/nhe-oact/stateestimates/)
*By state of provider. Includes hospital care, physician services, dental services, home health care, drugs, vision products, nursing home care and other personal health care services and products.

Per Capita Personal Health Care Expenditures in 1998

National Per Capita = $3,761*

ALPHA ORDER

RANK	STATE	PER CAPITA
23	Alabama	$3,690
22	Alaska	3,737
46	Arizona	3,167
39	Arkansas	3,334
38	California	3,367
34	Colorado	3,444
3	Connecticut	4,651
8	Delaware	4,174
11	Florida	4,006
30	Georgia	3,564
14	Hawaii	3,913
50	Idaho	2,760
24	Illinois	3,671
29	Indiana	3,599
30	Iowa	3,564
32	Kansas	3,560
26	Kentucky	3,664
21	Louisiana	3,782
12	Maine	3,948
18	Maryland	3,830
1	Massachusetts	4,889
27	Michigan	3,630
5	Minnesota	4,298
43	Mississippi	3,228
17	Missouri	3,846
44	Montana	3,227
25	Nebraska	3,670
45	Nevada	3,215
13	New Hampshire	3,928
10	New Jersey	4,039
47	New Mexico	3,083
2	New York	4,724
28	North Carolina	3,621
7	North Dakota	4,202
20	Ohio	3,789
41	Oklahoma	3,290
40	Oregon	3,303
6	Pennsylvania	4,276
4	Rhode Island	4,571
35	South Carolina	3,439
15	South Dakota	3,889
9	Tennessee	4,053
36	Texas	3,437
49	Utah	2,830
33	Vermont	3,498
42	Virginia	3,279
37	Washington	3,392
16	West Virginia	3,884
19	Wisconsin	3,819
48	Wyoming	2,931

RANK ORDER

RANK	STATE	PER CAPITA
1	Massachusetts	$4,889
2	New York	4,724
3	Connecticut	4,651
4	Rhode Island	4,571
5	Minnesota	4,298
6	Pennsylvania	4,276
7	North Dakota	4,202
8	Delaware	4,174
9	Tennessee	4,053
10	New Jersey	4,039
11	Florida	4,006
12	Maine	3,948
13	New Hampshire	3,928
14	Hawaii	3,913
15	South Dakota	3,889
16	West Virginia	3,884
17	Missouri	3,846
18	Maryland	3,830
19	Wisconsin	3,819
20	Ohio	3,789
21	Louisiana	3,782
22	Alaska	3,737
23	Alabama	3,690
24	Illinois	3,671
25	Nebraska	3,670
26	Kentucky	3,664
27	Michigan	3,630
28	North Carolina	3,621
29	Indiana	3,599
30	Georgia	3,564
30	Iowa	3,564
32	Kansas	3,560
33	Vermont	3,498
34	Colorado	3,444
35	South Carolina	3,439
36	Texas	3,437
37	Washington	3,392
38	California	3,367
39	Arkansas	3,334
40	Oregon	3,303
41	Oklahoma	3,290
42	Virginia	3,279
43	Mississippi	3,228
44	Montana	3,227
45	Nevada	3,215
46	Arizona	3,167
47	New Mexico	3,083
48	Wyoming	2,931
49	Utah	2,830
50	Idaho	2,760
	District of Columbia	8,166

Source: MQ Press using data from U.S. Dept of Health & Human Services, Centers for Medicare and Medicaid Services
"State Health Care Expenditures" (http://www.hcfa.gov/stats/nhe-oact/stateestimates/)
*By state of provider. Per capita calculated using resident population. These figures may be skewed due to residents crossing state borders for care. Includes hospital care, physician services, dental services, home health care, drugs, vision products, nursing home care and other personal health care services and products.

Percent Change in Per Capita Expenditures for Personal Health Care: 1990 to 1998
National Percent Change = 53.3% Increase*

ALPHA ORDER

RANK	STATE	PERCENT CHANGE
18	Alabama	63.1
37	Alaska	53.5
49	Arizona	36.1
24	Arkansas	59.4
50	California	35.6
46	Colorado	47.0
39	Connecticut	52.8
21	Delaware	61.6
47	Florida	45.7
42	Georgia	51.5
26	Hawaii	58.6
12	Idaho	64.6
41	Illinois	52.1
29	Indiana	57.5
17	Iowa	63.3
24	Kansas	59.4
7	Kentucky	73.0
23	Louisiana	60.0
1	Maine	80.4
30	Maryland	56.3
35	Massachusetts	54.7
40	Michigan	52.7
13	Minnesota	64.5
5	Mississippi	75.9
33	Missouri	55.4
26	Montana	58.6
14	Nebraska	64.3
48	Nevada	39.6
8	New Hampshire	70.7
34	New Jersey	55.3
22	New Mexico	60.7
28	New York	57.7
6	North Carolina	75.4
16	North Dakota	63.4
38	Ohio	53.0
19	Oklahoma	62.9
44	Oregon	51.2
31	Pennsylvania	55.9
10	Rhode Island	68.4
4	South Carolina	76.8
2	South Dakota	79.1
20	Tennessee	62.3
32	Texas	55.5
43	Utah	51.4
9	Vermont	68.5
36	Virginia	53.7
45	Washington	47.4
3	West Virginia	77.2
15	Wisconsin	63.6
11	Wyoming	67.6

RANK ORDER

RANK	STATE	PERCENT CHANGE
1	Maine	80.4
2	South Dakota	79.1
3	West Virginia	77.2
4	South Carolina	76.8
5	Mississippi	75.9
6	North Carolina	75.4
7	Kentucky	73.0
8	New Hampshire	70.7
9	Vermont	68.5
10	Rhode Island	68.4
11	Wyoming	67.6
12	Idaho	64.6
13	Minnesota	64.5
14	Nebraska	64.3
15	Wisconsin	63.6
16	North Dakota	63.4
17	Iowa	63.3
18	Alabama	63.1
19	Oklahoma	62.9
20	Tennessee	62.3
21	Delaware	61.6
22	New Mexico	60.7
23	Louisiana	60.0
24	Arkansas	59.4
24	Kansas	59.4
26	Hawaii	58.6
26	Montana	58.6
28	New York	57.7
29	Indiana	57.5
30	Maryland	56.3
31	Pennsylvania	55.9
32	Texas	55.5
33	Missouri	55.4
34	New Jersey	55.3
35	Massachusetts	54.7
36	Virginia	53.7
37	Alaska	53.5
38	Ohio	53.0
39	Connecticut	52.8
40	Michigan	52.7
41	Illinois	52.1
42	Georgia	51.5
43	Utah	51.4
44	Oregon	51.2
45	Washington	47.4
46	Colorado	47.0
47	Florida	45.7
48	Nevada	39.6
49	Arizona	36.1
50	California	35.6
	District of Columbia	38.4

Source: MQ Press using data from U.S. Dept of Health & Human Services, Centers for Medicare and Medicaid Services "State Health Care Expenditures" (http://www.hcfa.gov/stats/nhe-oact/stateestimates/)
*By state of provider. Per capita calculated using resident population. These figures may be skewed due to residents crossing state borders for care. Includes hospital care, physician services, dental services, home health care, drugs, vision products, nursing home care and other personal health care services and products.

Average Annual Change in Per Capita Expenditures
For Personal Health Care: 1990 to 1998
National Percent Change = 5.5% Average Annual Increase*

ALPHA ORDER

RANK	STATE	PERCENT CHANGE
15	Alabama	6.3
36	Alaska	5.5
49	Arizona	3.9
23	Arkansas	6.0
49	California	3.9
46	Colorado	4.9
39	Connecticut	5.4
20	Delaware	6.2
47	Florida	4.8
42	Georgia	5.3
26	Hawaii	5.9
12	Idaho	6.4
39	Illinois	5.4
29	Indiana	5.8
15	Iowa	6.3
23	Kansas	6.0
7	Kentucky	7.1
23	Louisiana	6.0
1	Maine	7.7
30	Maryland	5.7
35	Massachusetts	5.6
39	Michigan	5.4
12	Minnesota	6.4
5	Mississippi	7.3
30	Missouri	5.7
26	Montana	5.9
12	Nebraska	6.4
48	Nevada	4.3
8	New Hampshire	6.9
30	New Jersey	5.7
22	New Mexico	6.1
26	New York	5.9
5	North Carolina	7.3
15	North Dakota	6.3
36	Ohio	5.5
15	Oklahoma	6.3
42	Oregon	5.3
30	Pennsylvania	5.7
9	Rhode Island	6.7
3	South Carolina	7.4
2	South Dakota	7.6
20	Tennessee	6.2
30	Texas	5.7
42	Utah	5.3
9	Vermont	6.7
36	Virginia	5.5
45	Washington	5.0
3	West Virginia	7.4
15	Wisconsin	6.3
9	Wyoming	6.7

RANK ORDER

RANK	STATE	PERCENT CHANGE
1	Maine	7.7
2	South Dakota	7.6
3	South Carolina	7.4
3	West Virginia	7.4
5	Mississippi	7.3
5	North Carolina	7.3
7	Kentucky	7.1
8	New Hampshire	6.9
9	Rhode Island	6.7
9	Vermont	6.7
9	Wyoming	6.7
12	Idaho	6.4
12	Minnesota	6.4
12	Nebraska	6.4
15	Alabama	6.3
15	Iowa	6.3
15	North Dakota	6.3
15	Oklahoma	6.3
15	Wisconsin	6.3
20	Delaware	6.2
20	Tennessee	6.2
22	New Mexico	6.1
23	Arkansas	6.0
23	Kansas	6.0
23	Louisiana	6.0
26	Hawaii	5.9
26	Montana	5.9
26	New York	5.9
29	Indiana	5.8
30	Maryland	5.7
30	Missouri	5.7
30	New Jersey	5.7
30	Pennsylvania	5.7
30	Texas	5.7
35	Massachusetts	5.6
36	Alaska	5.5
36	Ohio	5.5
36	Virginia	5.5
39	Connecticut	5.4
39	Illinois	5.4
39	Michigan	5.4
42	Georgia	5.3
42	Oregon	5.3
42	Utah	5.3
45	Washington	5.0
46	Colorado	4.9
47	Florida	4.8
48	Nevada	4.3
49	Arizona	3.9
49	California	3.9
	District of Columbia	4.1

Source: MQ Press using data from U.S. Dept of Health & Human Services, Centers for Medicare and Medicaid Services
"State Health Care Expenditures" (http://www.hcfa.gov/stats/nhe-oact/stateestimates/)
*By state of provider. Per capita calculated using resident population. These figures may be skewed due to residents crossing state borders for care. Includes hospital care, physician services, dental services, home health care, drugs, vision products, nursing home care and other personal health care services and products.

Expenditures for Hospital Care in 1998

National Total = $380,050,000,000*

<table>
<tr><td colspan="4">ALPHA ORDER</td><td colspan="4">RANK ORDER</td></tr>
<tr><td>RANK</td><td>STATE</td><td>EXPENDITURES</td><td>% of USA</td><td>RANK</td><td>STATE</td><td>EXPENDITURES</td><td>% of USA</td></tr>
<tr><td>20</td><td>Alabama</td><td>$6,618,000,000</td><td>1.7%</td><td>1</td><td>California</td><td>$34,948,000,000</td><td>9.2%</td></tr>
<tr><td>48</td><td>Alaska</td><td>986,000,000</td><td>0.3%</td><td>2</td><td>New York</td><td>32,636,000,000</td><td>8.6%</td></tr>
<tr><td>25</td><td>Arizona</td><td>4,977,000,000</td><td>1.3%</td><td>3</td><td>Texas</td><td>25,322,000,000</td><td>6.7%</td></tr>
<tr><td>33</td><td>Arkansas</td><td>3,324,000,000</td><td>0.9%</td><td>4</td><td>Pennsylvania</td><td>20,213,000,000</td><td>5.3%</td></tr>
<tr><td>1</td><td>California</td><td>34,948,000,000</td><td>9.2%</td><td>5</td><td>Florida</td><td>19,742,000,000</td><td>5.2%</td></tr>
<tr><td>26</td><td>Colorado</td><td>4,850,000,000</td><td>1.3%</td><td>6</td><td>Illinois</td><td>17,996,000,000</td><td>4.7%</td></tr>
<tr><td>27</td><td>Connecticut</td><td>4,686,000,000</td><td>1.2%</td><td>7</td><td>Ohio</td><td>16,763,000,000</td><td>4.4%</td></tr>
<tr><td>47</td><td>Delaware</td><td>1,166,000,000</td><td>0.3%</td><td>8</td><td>Michigan</td><td>14,641,000,000</td><td>3.9%</td></tr>
<tr><td>5</td><td>Florida</td><td>19,742,000,000</td><td>5.2%</td><td>9</td><td>Massachusetts</td><td>11,305,000,000</td><td>3.0%</td></tr>
<tr><td>12</td><td>Georgia</td><td>10,396,000,000</td><td>2.7%</td><td>10</td><td>New Jersey</td><td>11,191,000,000</td><td>2.9%</td></tr>
<tr><td>40</td><td>Hawaii</td><td>1,775,000,000</td><td>0.5%</td><td>11</td><td>North Carolina</td><td>10,987,000,000</td><td>2.9%</td></tr>
<tr><td>45</td><td>Idaho</td><td>1,236,000,000</td><td>0.3%</td><td>12</td><td>Georgia</td><td>10,396,000,000</td><td>2.7%</td></tr>
<tr><td>6</td><td>Illinois</td><td>17,996,000,000</td><td>4.7%</td><td>13</td><td>Missouri</td><td>8,828,000,000</td><td>2.3%</td></tr>
<tr><td>15</td><td>Indiana</td><td>8,515,000,000</td><td>2.2%</td><td>14</td><td>Virginia</td><td>8,689,000,000</td><td>2.3%</td></tr>
<tr><td>29</td><td>Iowa</td><td>4,084,000,000</td><td>1.1%</td><td>15</td><td>Indiana</td><td>8,515,000,000</td><td>2.2%</td></tr>
<tr><td>31</td><td>Kansas</td><td>3,580,000,000</td><td>0.9%</td><td>16</td><td>Tennessee</td><td>8,276,000,000</td><td>2.2%</td></tr>
<tr><td>23</td><td>Kentucky</td><td>5,731,000,000</td><td>1.5%</td><td>17</td><td>Maryland</td><td>7,313,000,000</td><td>1.9%</td></tr>
<tr><td>19</td><td>Louisiana</td><td>7,139,000,000</td><td>1.9%</td><td>18</td><td>Wisconsin</td><td>7,252,000,000</td><td>1.9%</td></tr>
<tr><td>39</td><td>Maine</td><td>1,846,000,000</td><td>0.5%</td><td>19</td><td>Louisiana</td><td>7,139,000,000</td><td>1.9%</td></tr>
<tr><td>17</td><td>Maryland</td><td>7,313,000,000</td><td>1.9%</td><td>20</td><td>Alabama</td><td>6,618,000,000</td><td>1.7%</td></tr>
<tr><td>9</td><td>Massachusetts</td><td>11,305,000,000</td><td>3.0%</td><td>21</td><td>Minnesota</td><td>6,540,000,000</td><td>1.7%</td></tr>
<tr><td>8</td><td>Michigan</td><td>14,641,000,000</td><td>3.9%</td><td>22</td><td>Washington</td><td>6,362,000,000</td><td>1.7%</td></tr>
<tr><td>21</td><td>Minnesota</td><td>6,540,000,000</td><td>1.7%</td><td>23</td><td>Kentucky</td><td>5,731,000,000</td><td>1.5%</td></tr>
<tr><td>30</td><td>Mississippi</td><td>3,848,000,000</td><td>1.0%</td><td>24</td><td>South Carolina</td><td>5,597,000,000</td><td>1.5%</td></tr>
<tr><td>13</td><td>Missouri</td><td>8,828,000,000</td><td>2.3%</td><td>25</td><td>Arizona</td><td>4,977,000,000</td><td>1.3%</td></tr>
<tr><td>46</td><td>Montana</td><td>1,224,000,000</td><td>0.3%</td><td>26</td><td>Colorado</td><td>4,850,000,000</td><td>1.3%</td></tr>
<tr><td>35</td><td>Nebraska</td><td>2,597,000,000</td><td>0.7%</td><td>27</td><td>Connecticut</td><td>4,686,000,000</td><td>1.2%</td></tr>
<tr><td>38</td><td>Nevada</td><td>1,865,000,000</td><td>0.5%</td><td>28</td><td>Oklahoma</td><td>4,218,000,000</td><td>1.1%</td></tr>
<tr><td>42</td><td>New Hampshire</td><td>1,559,000,000</td><td>0.4%</td><td>29</td><td>Iowa</td><td>4,084,000,000</td><td>1.1%</td></tr>
<tr><td>10</td><td>New Jersey</td><td>11,191,000,000</td><td>2.9%</td><td>30</td><td>Mississippi</td><td>3,848,000,000</td><td>1.0%</td></tr>
<tr><td>36</td><td>New Mexico</td><td>2,317,000,000</td><td>0.6%</td><td>31</td><td>Kansas</td><td>3,580,000,000</td><td>0.9%</td></tr>
<tr><td>2</td><td>New York</td><td>32,636,000,000</td><td>8.6%</td><td>32</td><td>Oregon</td><td>3,545,000,000</td><td>0.9%</td></tr>
<tr><td>11</td><td>North Carolina</td><td>10,987,000,000</td><td>2.9%</td><td>33</td><td>Arkansas</td><td>3,324,000,000</td><td>0.9%</td></tr>
<tr><td>43</td><td>North Dakota</td><td>1,282,000,000</td><td>0.3%</td><td>34</td><td>West Virginia</td><td>2,955,000,000</td><td>0.8%</td></tr>
<tr><td>7</td><td>Ohio</td><td>16,763,000,000</td><td>4.4%</td><td>35</td><td>Nebraska</td><td>2,597,000,000</td><td>0.7%</td></tr>
<tr><td>28</td><td>Oklahoma</td><td>4,218,000,000</td><td>1.1%</td><td>36</td><td>New Mexico</td><td>2,317,000,000</td><td>0.6%</td></tr>
<tr><td>32</td><td>Oregon</td><td>3,545,000,000</td><td>0.9%</td><td>37</td><td>Utah</td><td>2,290,000,000</td><td>0.6%</td></tr>
<tr><td>4</td><td>Pennsylvania</td><td>20,213,000,000</td><td>5.3%</td><td>38</td><td>Nevada</td><td>1,865,000,000</td><td>0.5%</td></tr>
<tr><td>41</td><td>Rhode Island</td><td>1,702,000,000</td><td>0.4%</td><td>39</td><td>Maine</td><td>1,846,000,000</td><td>0.5%</td></tr>
<tr><td>24</td><td>South Carolina</td><td>5,597,000,000</td><td>1.5%</td><td>40</td><td>Hawaii</td><td>1,775,000,000</td><td>0.5%</td></tr>
<tr><td>44</td><td>South Dakota</td><td>1,257,000,000</td><td>0.3%</td><td>41</td><td>Rhode Island</td><td>1,702,000,000</td><td>0.4%</td></tr>
<tr><td>16</td><td>Tennessee</td><td>8,276,000,000</td><td>2.2%</td><td>42</td><td>New Hampshire</td><td>1,559,000,000</td><td>0.4%</td></tr>
<tr><td>3</td><td>Texas</td><td>25,322,000,000</td><td>6.7%</td><td>43</td><td>North Dakota</td><td>1,282,000,000</td><td>0.3%</td></tr>
<tr><td>37</td><td>Utah</td><td>2,290,000,000</td><td>0.6%</td><td>44</td><td>South Dakota</td><td>1,257,000,000</td><td>0.3%</td></tr>
<tr><td>49</td><td>Vermont</td><td>712,000,000</td><td>0.2%</td><td>45</td><td>Idaho</td><td>1,236,000,000</td><td>0.3%</td></tr>
<tr><td>14</td><td>Virginia</td><td>8,689,000,000</td><td>2.3%</td><td>46</td><td>Montana</td><td>1,224,000,000</td><td>0.3%</td></tr>
<tr><td>22</td><td>Washington</td><td>6,362,000,000</td><td>1.7%</td><td>47</td><td>Delaware</td><td>1,166,000,000</td><td>0.3%</td></tr>
<tr><td>34</td><td>West Virginia</td><td>2,955,000,000</td><td>0.8%</td><td>48</td><td>Alaska</td><td>986,000,000</td><td>0.3%</td></tr>
<tr><td>18</td><td>Wisconsin</td><td>7,252,000,000</td><td>1.9%</td><td>49</td><td>Vermont</td><td>712,000,000</td><td>0.2%</td></tr>
<tr><td>50</td><td>Wyoming</td><td>582,000,000</td><td>0.2%</td><td>50</td><td>Wyoming</td><td>582,000,000</td><td>0.2%</td></tr>
<tr><td></td><td></td><td></td><td></td><td></td><td>District of Columbia</td><td>2,585,000,000</td><td>0.7%</td></tr>
</table>

*Source: U.S. Department of Health and Human Services, Centers for Medicare and Medicaid Services
"State Health Care Expenditures" (http://www.hcfa.gov/stats/nhe-oact/stateestimates/)*
*By state of provider.

Percent of Total Personal Health Care Expenditures
Spent on Hospital Care in 1998
National Percent = 37.4%*

ALPHA ORDER

RANK	STATE	PERCENT
13	Alabama	41.2
7	Alaska	42.9
42	Arizona	33.7
22	Arkansas	39.3
49	California	31.8
39	Colorado	35.5
50	Connecticut	30.8
33	Delaware	37.5
45	Florida	33.1
26	Georgia	38.2
27	Hawaii	38.1
37	Idaho	36.4
15	Illinois	40.6
17	Indiana	40.1
18	Iowa	40.0
27	Kansas	38.1
19	Kentucky	39.8
4	Louisiana	43.3
33	Maine	37.5
36	Maryland	37.2
31	Massachusetts	37.6
14	Michigan	41.1
48	Minnesota	32.2
4	Mississippi	43.3
10	Missouri	42.2
6	Montana	43.1
8	Nebraska	42.6
44	Nevada	33.3
43	New Hampshire	33.5
41	New Jersey	34.2
3	New Mexico	43.4
29	New York	38.0
16	North Carolina	40.2
1	North Dakota	47.8
20	Ohio	39.4
25	Oklahoma	38.4
47	Oregon	32.7
20	Pennsylvania	39.4
30	Rhode Island	37.7
9	South Carolina	42.4
2	South Dakota	44.2
31	Tennessee	37.6
35	Texas	37.4
24	Utah	38.5
40	Vermont	34.5
23	Virginia	39.0
46	Washington	33.0
11	West Virginia	42.0
37	Wisconsin	36.4
12	Wyoming	41.4

RANK ORDER

RANK	STATE	PERCENT
1	North Dakota	47.8
2	South Dakota	44.2
3	New Mexico	43.4
4	Louisiana	43.3
4	Mississippi	43.3
6	Montana	43.1
7	Alaska	42.9
8	Nebraska	42.6
9	South Carolina	42.4
10	Missouri	42.2
11	West Virginia	42.0
12	Wyoming	41.4
13	Alabama	41.2
14	Michigan	41.1
15	Illinois	40.6
16	North Carolina	40.2
17	Indiana	40.1
18	Iowa	40.0
19	Kentucky	39.8
20	Ohio	39.4
20	Pennsylvania	39.4
22	Arkansas	39.3
23	Virginia	39.0
24	Utah	38.5
25	Oklahoma	38.4
26	Georgia	38.2
27	Hawaii	38.1
27	Kansas	38.1
29	New York	38.0
30	Rhode Island	37.7
31	Massachusetts	37.6
31	Tennessee	37.6
33	Delaware	37.5
33	Maine	37.5
35	Texas	37.4
36	Maryland	37.2
37	Idaho	36.4
37	Wisconsin	36.4
39	Colorado	35.5
40	Vermont	34.5
41	New Jersey	34.2
42	Arizona	33.7
43	New Hampshire	33.5
44	Nevada	33.3
45	Florida	33.1
46	Washington	33.0
47	Oregon	32.7
48	Minnesota	32.2
49	California	31.8
50	Connecticut	30.8
	District of Columbia	60.7

Source: MQ Press using data from U.S. Dept of Health & Human Services, Centers for Medicare and Medicaid Services
"State Health Care Expenditures" (http://www.hcfa.gov/stats/nhe-oact/stateestimates/)
*By state of provider.

Percent Change in Expenditures for Hospital Care: 1990 to 1998

National Percent Change = 49.6% Increase*

ALPHA ORDER				RANK ORDER		
RANK	STATE	PERCENT CHANGE		RANK	STATE	PERCENT CHANGE
16	Alabama	64.9		1	North Carolina	86.3
8	Alaska	76.7		2	Idaho	86.1
33	Arizona	54.7		3	South Dakota	81.1
26	Arkansas	57.7		4	Montana	80.5
50	California	25.0		5	South Carolina	80.0
28	Colorado	56.3		6	Nevada	78.8
49	Connecticut	28.1		6	North Dakota	78.8
18	Delaware	64.7		8	Alaska	76.7
43	Florida	46.7		9	Mississippi	75.9
30	Georgia	55.6		10	Utah	72.8
37	Hawaii	54.1		11	New Mexico	69.9
2	Idaho	86.1		12	West Virginia	67.8
44	Illinois	45.2		13	Kentucky	67.0
20	Indiana	61.2		14	Wisconsin	65.7
32	Iowa	55.2		15	Maine	65.3
29	Kansas	55.8		16	Alabama	64.9
13	Kentucky	67.0		16	Wyoming	64.9
35	Louisiana	54.4		18	Delaware	64.7
15	Maine	65.3		19	Nebraska	63.7
27	Maryland	57.0		20	Indiana	61.2
47	Massachusetts	38.7		21	Washington	60.5
36	Michigan	54.2		22	Minnesota	60.2
22	Minnesota	60.2		23	Vermont	59.3
9	Mississippi	75.9		24	Texas	58.9
40	Missouri	47.8		25	Oklahoma	57.8
4	Montana	80.5		26	Arkansas	57.7
19	Nebraska	63.7		27	Maryland	57.0
6	Nevada	78.8		28	Colorado	56.3
40	New Hampshire	47.8		29	Kansas	55.8
46	New Jersey	42.5		30	Georgia	55.6
11	New Mexico	69.9		31	Rhode Island	55.4
45	New York	43.7		32	Iowa	55.2
1	North Carolina	86.3		33	Arizona	54.7
6	North Dakota	78.8		34	Oregon	54.5
42	Ohio	46.9		35	Louisiana	54.4
25	Oklahoma	57.8		36	Michigan	54.2
34	Oregon	54.5		37	Hawaii	54.1
48	Pennsylvania	36.0		38	Virginia	53.4
31	Rhode Island	55.4		39	Tennessee	50.3
5	South Carolina	80.0		40	Missouri	47.8
3	South Dakota	81.1		40	New Hampshire	47.8
39	Tennessee	50.3		42	Ohio	46.9
24	Texas	58.9		43	Florida	46.7
10	Utah	72.8		44	Illinois	45.2
23	Vermont	59.3		45	New York	43.7
38	Virginia	53.4		46	New Jersey	42.5
21	Washington	60.5		47	Massachusetts	38.7
12	West Virginia	67.8		48	Pennsylvania	36.0
14	Wisconsin	65.7		49	Connecticut	28.1
16	Wyoming	64.9		50	California	25.0
					District of Columbia	21.0

Source: MQ Press using data from U.S. Dept of Health & Human Services, Centers for Medicare and Medicaid Services "State Health Care Expenditures" (http://www.hcfa.gov/stats/nhe-oact/stateestimates/)
*By state of provider.

Average Annual Change in Expenditures for Hospital Care: 1990 to 1998

National Percent Change = 5.2% Average Annual Increase*

ALPHA ORDER				RANK ORDER		
RANK	STATE	PERCENT CHANGE		RANK	STATE	PERCENT CHANGE
16	Alabama	6.4		1	Idaho	8.1
8	Alaska	7.4		1	North Carolina	8.1
32	Arizona	5.6		3	Montana	7.7
25	Arkansas	5.9		3	South Dakota	7.7
50	California	2.8		5	South Carolina	7.6
28	Colorado	5.7		6	Nevada	7.5
49	Connecticut	3.1		6	North Dakota	7.5
16	Delaware	6.4		8	Alaska	7.4
42	Florida	4.9		9	Mississippi	7.3
28	Georgia	5.7		10	Utah	7.1
32	Hawaii	5.6		11	New Mexico	6.8
1	Idaho	8.1		12	West Virginia	6.7
44	Illinois	4.8		13	Kentucky	6.6
20	Indiana	6.1		14	Maine	6.5
32	Iowa	5.6		14	Wisconsin	6.5
28	Kansas	5.7		16	Alabama	6.4
13	Kentucky	6.6		16	Delaware	6.4
32	Louisiana	5.6		16	Nebraska	6.4
14	Maine	6.5		16	Wyoming	6.4
27	Maryland	5.8		20	Indiana	6.1
47	Massachusetts	4.2		20	Minnesota	6.1
32	Michigan	5.6		20	Washington	6.1
20	Minnesota	6.1		23	Texas	6.0
9	Mississippi	7.3		23	Vermont	6.0
40	Missouri	5.0		25	Arkansas	5.9
3	Montana	7.7		25	Oklahoma	5.9
16	Nebraska	6.4		27	Maryland	5.8
6	Nevada	7.5		28	Colorado	5.7
40	New Hampshire	5.0		28	Georgia	5.7
46	New Jersey	4.5		28	Kansas	5.7
11	New Mexico	6.8		28	Rhode Island	5.7
45	New York	4.6		32	Arizona	5.6
1	North Carolina	8.1		32	Hawaii	5.6
6	North Dakota	7.5		32	Iowa	5.6
42	Ohio	4.9		32	Louisiana	5.6
25	Oklahoma	5.9		32	Michigan	5.6
32	Oregon	5.6		32	Oregon	5.6
48	Pennsylvania	3.9		38	Virginia	5.5
28	Rhode Island	5.7		39	Tennessee	5.2
5	South Carolina	7.6		40	Missouri	5.0
3	South Dakota	7.7		40	New Hampshire	5.0
39	Tennessee	5.2		42	Florida	4.9
23	Texas	6.0		42	Ohio	4.9
10	Utah	7.1		44	Illinois	4.8
23	Vermont	6.0		45	New York	4.6
38	Virginia	5.5		46	New Jersey	4.5
20	Washington	6.1		47	Massachusetts	4.2
12	West Virginia	6.7		48	Pennsylvania	3.9
14	Wisconsin	6.5		49	Connecticut	3.1
16	Wyoming	6.4		50	California	2.8
					District of Columbia	2.4

Source: U.S. Department of Health and Human Services, Centers for Medicare and Medicaid Services
    "State Health Care Expenditures" (http://www.hcfa.gov/stats/nhe-oact/stateestimates/)
*By state of provider.

Per Capita Expenditures for Hospital Care in 1998

National Per Capita = $1,406*

ALPHA ORDER

ALPHA ORDER

RANK	STATE	PER CAPITA
14	Alabama	$1,521
10	Alaska	1,603
49	Arizona	1,066
37	Arkansas	1,310
48	California	1,069
41	Colorado	1,222
24	Connecticut	1,432
11	Delaware	1,567
35	Florida	1,324
32	Georgia	1,361
16	Hawaii	1,491
50	Idaho	1,004
16	Illinois	1,491
23	Indiana	1,441
25	Iowa	1,427
33	Kansas	1,357
21	Kentucky	1,457
7	Louisiana	1,636
19	Maine	1,480
26	Maryland	1,426
2	Massachusetts	1,840
16	Michigan	1,491
30	Minnesota	1,384
27	Mississippi	1,399
9	Missouri	1,624
28	Montana	1,392
12	Nebraska	1,564
47	Nevada	1,070
36	New Hampshire	1,315
31	New Jersey	1,382
34	New Mexico	1,337
3	New York	1,797
22	North Carolina	1,456
1	North Dakota	2,010
15	Ohio	1,492
40	Oklahoma	1,263
46	Oregon	1,080
6	Pennsylvania	1,684
4	Rhode Island	1,723
20	South Carolina	1,458
5	South Dakota	1,720
13	Tennessee	1,523
38	Texas	1,285
45	Utah	1,090
43	Vermont	1,206
39	Virginia	1,280
44	Washington	1,119
8	West Virginia	1,631
29	Wisconsin	1,389
42	Wyoming	1,212

RANK ORDER

RANK	STATE	PER CAPITA
1	North Dakota	$2,010
2	Massachusetts	1,840
3	New York	1,797
4	Rhode Island	1,723
5	South Dakota	1,720
6	Pennsylvania	1,684
7	Louisiana	1,636
8	West Virginia	1,631
9	Missouri	1,624
10	Alaska	1,603
11	Delaware	1,567
12	Nebraska	1,564
13	Tennessee	1,523
14	Alabama	1,521
15	Ohio	1,492
16	Hawaii	1,491
16	Illinois	1,491
16	Michigan	1,491
19	Maine	1,480
20	South Carolina	1,458
21	Kentucky	1,457
22	North Carolina	1,456
23	Indiana	1,441
24	Connecticut	1,432
25	Iowa	1,427
26	Maryland	1,426
27	Mississippi	1,399
28	Montana	1,392
29	Wisconsin	1,389
30	Minnesota	1,384
31	New Jersey	1,382
32	Georgia	1,361
33	Kansas	1,357
34	New Mexico	1,337
35	Florida	1,324
36	New Hampshire	1,315
37	Arkansas	1,310
38	Texas	1,285
39	Virginia	1,280
40	Oklahoma	1,263
41	Colorado	1,222
42	Wyoming	1,212
43	Vermont	1,206
44	Washington	1,119
45	Utah	1,090
46	Oregon	1,080
47	Nevada	1,070
48	California	1,069
49	Arizona	1,066
50	Idaho	1,004

| | District of Columbia | 4,958 |

Source: MQ Press using data from U.S. Dept of Health & Human Services, Centers for Medicare and Medicaid Services "State Health Care Expenditures" (http://www.hcfa.gov/stats/nhe-oact/stateestimates/)
*By state of provider. Per capita calculated using resident population. These figures may be skewed due to residents crossing state borders for care.

Percent Change in Per Capita Expenditures for Hospital Care: 1990 to 1998

National Percent Change = 38.0% Increase*

ALPHA ORDER

RANK	STATE	PERCENT CHANGE
15	Alabama	53.5
9	Alaska	58.9
49	Arizona	22.0
27	Arkansas	46.4
50	California	14.6
45	Colorado	30.1
46	Connecticut	28.8
24	Delaware	48.1
47	Florida	28.0
44	Georgia	32.5
29	Hawaii	44.1
16	Idaho	53.0
37	Illinois	37.8
18	Indiana	51.5
19	Iowa	50.7
26	Kansas	46.5
11	Kentucky	56.8
20	Louisiana	49.3
8	Maine	63.2
25	Maryland	46.9
40	Massachusetts	35.8
28	Michigan	46.2
23	Minnesota	48.7
4	Mississippi	64.8
34	Missouri	39.4
6	Montana	64.2
12	Nebraska	55.9
48	Nevada	25.0
35	New Hampshire	38.6
39	New Jersey	36.6
21	New Mexico	49.1
30	New York	42.4
5	North Carolina	64.3
1	North Dakota	78.7
32	Ohio	42.0
22	Oklahoma	48.8
43	Oregon	34.5
42	Pennsylvania	34.8
10	Rhode Island	58.1
7	South Carolina	64.0
2	South Dakota	72.7
41	Tennessee	35.3
38	Texas	37.4
31	Utah	42.3
17	Vermont	52.3
33	Virginia	40.5
36	Washington	38.3
3	West Virginia	66.1
14	Wisconsin	55.5
13	Wyoming	55.6

RANK ORDER

RANK	STATE	PERCENT CHANGE
1	North Dakota	78.7
2	South Dakota	72.7
3	West Virginia	66.1
4	Mississippi	64.8
5	North Carolina	64.3
6	Montana	64.2
7	South Carolina	64.0
8	Maine	63.2
9	Alaska	58.9
10	Rhode Island	58.1
11	Kentucky	56.8
12	Nebraska	55.9
13	Wyoming	55.6
14	Wisconsin	55.5
15	Alabama	53.5
16	Idaho	53.0
17	Vermont	52.3
18	Indiana	51.5
19	Iowa	50.7
20	Louisiana	49.3
21	New Mexico	49.1
22	Oklahoma	48.8
23	Minnesota	48.7
24	Delaware	48.1
25	Maryland	46.9
26	Kansas	46.5
27	Arkansas	46.4
28	Michigan	46.2
29	Hawaii	44.1
30	New York	42.4
31	Utah	42.3
32	Ohio	42.0
33	Virginia	40.5
34	Missouri	39.4
35	New Hampshire	38.6
36	Washington	38.3
37	Illinois	37.8
38	Texas	37.4
39	New Jersey	36.6
40	Massachusetts	35.8
41	Tennessee	35.3
42	Pennsylvania	34.8
43	Oregon	34.5
44	Georgia	32.5
45	Colorado	30.1
46	Connecticut	28.8
47	Florida	28.0
48	Nevada	25.0
49	Arizona	22.0
50	California	14.6
	District of Columbia	40.1

Source: MQ Press using data from U.S. Dept of Health & Human Services, Centers for Medicare and Medicaid Services
"State Health Care Expenditures" (http://www.hcfa.gov/stats/nhe-oact/stateestimates/)
*By state of provider. Per capita calculated using resident population. These figures may be skewed due to residents crossing state borders for care.

Average Annual Change in Per Capita Expenditures
For Hospital Care: 1990 to 1998
National Percent Change = 4.1% Average Annual Increase*

ALPHA ORDER

RANK ORDER

RANK	STATE	PERCENT CHANGE	RANK	STATE	PERCENT CHANGE
15	Alabama	5.5	1	North Dakota	7.5
9	Alaska	6.0	2	South Dakota	7.1
49	Arizona	2.5	3	West Virginia	6.5
25	Arkansas	4.9	4	Mississippi	6.4
50	California	1.7	4	Montana	6.4
45	Colorado	3.3	4	North Carolina	6.4
46	Connecticut	3.2	4	South Carolina	6.4
24	Delaware	5.0	8	Maine	6.3
47	Florida	3.1	9	Alaska	6.0
44	Georgia	3.6	10	Rhode Island	5.9
29	Hawaii	4.7	11	Kentucky	5.8
15	Idaho	5.5	12	Nebraska	5.7
36	Illinois	4.1	12	Wisconsin	5.7
18	Indiana	5.3	12	Wyoming	5.7
18	Iowa	5.3	15	Alabama	5.5
25	Kansas	4.9	15	Idaho	5.5
11	Kentucky	5.8	17	Vermont	5.4
20	Louisiana	5.1	18	Indiana	5.3
8	Maine	6.3	18	Iowa	5.3
25	Maryland	4.9	20	Louisiana	5.1
40	Massachusetts	3.9	20	Minnesota	5.1
25	Michigan	4.9	20	New Mexico	5.1
20	Minnesota	5.1	20	Oklahoma	5.1
4	Mississippi	6.4	24	Delaware	5.0
34	Missouri	4.2	25	Arkansas	4.9
4	Montana	6.4	25	Kansas	4.9
12	Nebraska	5.7	25	Maryland	4.9
48	Nevada	2.8	25	Michigan	4.9
34	New Hampshire	4.2	29	Hawaii	4.7
39	New Jersey	4.0	30	New York	4.5
20	New Mexico	5.1	30	Ohio	4.5
30	New York	4.5	30	Utah	4.5
4	North Carolina	6.4	33	Virginia	4.3
1	North Dakota	7.5	34	Missouri	4.2
30	Ohio	4.5	34	New Hampshire	4.2
20	Oklahoma	5.1	36	Illinois	4.1
41	Oregon	3.8	36	Texas	4.1
41	Pennsylvania	3.8	36	Washington	4.1
10	Rhode Island	5.9	39	New Jersey	4.0
4	South Carolina	6.4	40	Massachusetts	3.9
2	South Dakota	7.1	41	Oregon	3.8
41	Tennessee	3.8	41	Pennsylvania	3.8
36	Texas	4.1	41	Tennessee	3.8
30	Utah	4.5	44	Georgia	3.6
17	Vermont	5.4	45	Colorado	3.3
33	Virginia	4.3	46	Connecticut	3.2
36	Washington	4.1	47	Florida	3.1
3	West Virginia	6.5	48	Nevada	2.8
12	Wisconsin	5.7	49	Arizona	2.5
12	Wyoming	5.7	50	California	1.7
				District of Columbia	4.3

Source: MQ Press using data from U.S. Dept of Health & Human Services, Centers for Medicare and Medicaid Services "State Health Care Expenditures" (http://www.hcfa.gov/stats/nhe-oact/stateestimates/)

*By state of provider. Per capita calculated using resident population. These figures may be skewed due to residents crossing state borders for care.

Expenditures for Physician and Other Professional Services in 1998

National Total = $296,102,000,000*

ALPHA ORDER

RANK	STATE	EXPENDITURES	% of USA	RANK	STATE	EXPENDITURES	% of USA
22	Alabama	$4,609,000,000	1.6%	1	California	$44,239,000,000	14.9%
48	Alaska	568,000,000	0.2%	2	New York	20,103,000,000	6.8%
21	Arizona	5,135,000,000	1.7%	3	Texas	20,071,000,000	6.8%
32	Arkansas	2,225,000,000	0.8%	4	Florida	18,985,000,000	6.4%
1	California	44,239,000,000	14.9%	5	Pennsylvania	13,434,000,000	4.5%
23	Colorado	4,314,000,000	1.5%	6	Illinois	11,975,000,000	4.0%
24	Connecticut	4,292,000,000	1.4%	7	Ohio	11,024,000,000	3.7%
44	Delaware	792,000,000	0.3%	8	New Jersey	9,506,000,000	3.2%
4	Florida	18,985,000,000	6.4%	9	Michigan	9,186,000,000	3.1%
10	Georgia	8,510,000,000	2.9%	10	Georgia	8,510,000,000	2.9%
37	Hawaii	1,594,000,000	0.5%	11	Massachusetts	8,322,000,000	2.8%
43	Idaho	935,000,000	0.3%	12	Minnesota	7,183,000,000	2.4%
6	Illinois	11,975,000,000	4.0%	13	North Carolina	7,106,000,000	2.4%
19	Indiana	5,613,000,000	1.9%	14	Tennessee	6,719,000,000	2.3%
31	Iowa	2,457,000,000	0.8%	15	Virginia	6,265,000,000	2.1%
30	Kansas	2,538,000,000	0.9%	16	Maryland	5,978,000,000	2.0%
26	Kentucky	3,785,000,000	1.3%	17	Washington	5,908,000,000	2.0%
25	Louisiana	4,249,000,000	1.4%	18	Wisconsin	5,844,000,000	2.0%
41	Maine	1,219,000,000	0.4%	19	Indiana	5,613,000,000	1.9%
16	Maryland	5,978,000,000	2.0%	20	Missouri	5,310,000,000	1.8%
11	Massachusetts	8,322,000,000	2.8%	21	Arizona	5,135,000,000	1.7%
9	Michigan	9,186,000,000	3.1%	22	Alabama	4,609,000,000	1.6%
12	Minnesota	7,183,000,000	2.4%	23	Colorado	4,314,000,000	1.5%
33	Mississippi	2,212,000,000	0.7%	24	Connecticut	4,292,000,000	1.4%
20	Missouri	5,310,000,000	1.8%	25	Louisiana	4,249,000,000	1.4%
46	Montana	695,000,000	0.2%	26	Kentucky	3,785,000,000	1.3%
40	Nebraska	1,367,000,000	0.5%	27	Oregon	3,285,000,000	1.1%
34	Nevada	1,918,000,000	0.6%	28	South Carolina	3,254,000,000	1.1%
39	New Hampshire	1,405,000,000	0.5%	29	Oklahoma	2,978,000,000	1.0%
8	New Jersey	9,506,000,000	3.2%	30	Kansas	2,538,000,000	0.9%
38	New Mexico	1,415,000,000	0.5%	31	Iowa	2,457,000,000	0.8%
2	New York	20,103,000,000	6.8%	32	Arkansas	2,225,000,000	0.8%
13	North Carolina	7,106,000,000	2.4%	33	Mississippi	2,212,000,000	0.7%
47	North Dakota	612,000,000	0.2%	34	Nevada	1,918,000,000	0.6%
7	Ohio	11,024,000,000	3.7%	35	West Virginia	1,793,000,000	0.6%
29	Oklahoma	2,978,000,000	1.0%	36	Utah	1,648,000,000	0.6%
27	Oregon	3,285,000,000	1.1%	37	Hawaii	1,594,000,000	0.5%
5	Pennsylvania	13,434,000,000	4.5%	38	New Mexico	1,415,000,000	0.5%
42	Rhode Island	1,095,000,000	0.4%	39	New Hampshire	1,405,000,000	0.5%
28	South Carolina	3,254,000,000	1.1%	40	Nebraska	1,367,000,000	0.5%
45	South Dakota	747,000,000	0.3%	41	Maine	1,219,000,000	0.4%
14	Tennessee	6,719,000,000	2.3%	42	Rhode Island	1,095,000,000	0.4%
3	Texas	20,071,000,000	6.8%	43	Idaho	935,000,000	0.3%
36	Utah	1,648,000,000	0.6%	44	Delaware	792,000,000	0.3%
49	Vermont	563,000,000	0.2%	45	South Dakota	747,000,000	0.3%
15	Virginia	6,265,000,000	2.1%	46	Montana	695,000,000	0.2%
17	Washington	5,908,000,000	2.0%	47	North Dakota	612,000,000	0.2%
35	West Virginia	1,793,000,000	0.6%	48	Alaska	568,000,000	0.2%
18	Wisconsin	5,844,000,000	2.0%	49	Vermont	563,000,000	0.2%
50	Wyoming	343,000,000	0.1%	50	Wyoming	343,000,000	0.1%
					District of Columbia	781,000,000	0.3%

Source: U.S. Department of Health and Human Services, Centers for Medicare and Medicaid Services
"State Health Care Expenditures" (http://www.hcfa.gov/stats/nhe-oact/stateestimates/)
*By state of provider. Includes "other professional services" previously listed as a separate category. These include services of licensed professionals such as chiropractors, optometrists, podiatrists and independently practicing nurses. Also includes specialty clinics, independently billing laboratories and Medicare ambulance services.

Percent of Total Personal Health Care Expenditures Spent on Physician and Other Professional Services in 1998
National Percent = 29.1%*

ALPHA ORDER

RANK	STATE	PERCENT
17	Alabama	28.7
42	Alaska	24.7
3	Arizona	34.7
29	Arkansas	26.3
1	California	40.2
7	Colorado	31.6
18	Connecticut	28.2
37	Delaware	25.5
6	Florida	31.8
8	Georgia	31.3
4	Hawaii	34.2
22	Idaho	27.5
25	Illinois	27.0
28	Indiana	26.4
47	Iowa	24.1
25	Kansas	27.0
29	Kentucky	26.3
35	Louisiana	25.8
41	Maine	24.8
11	Maryland	30.4
20	Massachusetts	27.7
35	Michigan	25.8
2	Minnesota	35.4
40	Mississippi	24.9
39	Missouri	25.4
44	Montana	24.5
50	Nebraska	22.4
4	Nevada	34.2
13	New Hampshire	30.2
16	New Jersey	29.1
27	New Mexico	26.5
48	New York	23.4
33	North Carolina	26.0
49	North Dakota	22.8
34	Ohio	25.9
24	Oklahoma	27.1
12	Oregon	30.3
32	Pennsylvania	26.2
46	Rhode Island	24.3
43	South Carolina	24.6
29	South Dakota	26.3
10	Tennessee	30.5
14	Texas	29.6
20	Utah	27.7
23	Vermont	27.3
19	Virginia	28.1
9	Washington	30.6
37	West Virginia	25.5
15	Wisconsin	29.3
45	Wyoming	24.4

RANK ORDER

RANK	STATE	PERCENT
1	California	40.2
2	Minnesota	35.4
3	Arizona	34.7
4	Hawaii	34.2
4	Nevada	34.2
6	Florida	31.8
7	Colorado	31.6
8	Georgia	31.3
9	Washington	30.6
10	Tennessee	30.5
11	Maryland	30.4
12	Oregon	30.3
13	New Hampshire	30.2
14	Texas	29.6
15	Wisconsin	29.3
16	New Jersey	29.1
17	Alabama	28.7
18	Connecticut	28.2
19	Virginia	28.1
20	Massachusetts	27.7
20	Utah	27.7
22	Idaho	27.5
23	Vermont	27.3
24	Oklahoma	27.1
25	Illinois	27.0
25	Kansas	27.0
27	New Mexico	26.5
28	Indiana	26.4
29	Arkansas	26.3
29	Kentucky	26.3
29	South Dakota	26.3
32	Pennsylvania	26.2
33	North Carolina	26.0
34	Ohio	25.9
35	Louisiana	25.8
35	Michigan	25.8
37	Delaware	25.5
37	West Virginia	25.5
39	Missouri	25.4
40	Mississippi	24.9
41	Maine	24.8
42	Alaska	24.7
43	South Carolina	24.6
44	Montana	24.5
45	Wyoming	24.4
46	Rhode Island	24.3
47	Iowa	24.1
48	New York	23.4
49	North Dakota	22.8
50	Nebraska	22.4

	District of Columbia	18.3

Source: MQ Press using data from U.S. Dept of Health & Human Services, Centers for Medicare and Medicaid Services "State Health Care Expenditures" (http://www.hcfa.gov/stats/nhe-oact/stateestimates/)

*By state of provider. Includes "other professional services" previously listed as a separate category. These include services of licensed professionals such as chiropractors, optometrists, podiatrists and independently practicing nurses. Also includes specialty clinics, independently billing laboratories and Medicare ambulance services.

Percent Change in Expenditures for Physician and Other Professional Services: 1990 to 1998
National Percent Change = 63.6% Increase*

RANK	STATE	PERCENT CHANGE
22	Alabama	67.1
42	Alaska	57.8
26	Arizona	62.6
42	Arkansas	57.8
44	California	56.6
18	Colorado	75.1
46	Connecticut	52.3
31	Delaware	61.0
48	Florida	48.9
11	Georgia	84.2
2	Hawaii	102.0
6	Idaho	95.6
37	Illinois	59.9
33	Indiana	60.7
28	Iowa	62.3
35	Kansas	60.6
16	Kentucky	79.1
45	Louisiana	55.9
9	Maine	86.1
27	Maryland	62.4
21	Massachusetts	69.6
47	Michigan	51.8
5	Minnesota	95.9
8	Mississippi	88.7
30	Missouri	61.1
25	Montana	62.8
39	Nebraska	59.0
13	Nevada	82.7
3	New Hampshire	100.1
33	New Jersey	60.7
12	New Mexico	83.1
35	New York	60.6
9	North Carolina	86.1
50	North Dakota	36.9
49	Ohio	44.6
23	Oklahoma	67.0
29	Oregon	61.9
38	Pennsylvania	59.4
41	Rhode Island	58.0
7	South Carolina	92.9
1	South Dakota	102.4
4	Tennessee	96.8
19	Texas	74.2
17	Utah	77.8
14	Vermont	81.0
40	Virginia	58.8
32	Washington	60.8
24	West Virginia	63.7
15	Wisconsin	79.4
20	Wyoming	71.5

RANK	STATE	PERCENT CHANGE
1	South Dakota	102.4
2	Hawaii	102.0
3	New Hampshire	100.1
4	Tennessee	96.8
5	Minnesota	95.9
6	Idaho	95.6
7	South Carolina	92.9
8	Mississippi	88.7
9	Maine	86.1
9	North Carolina	86.1
11	Georgia	84.2
12	New Mexico	83.1
13	Nevada	82.7
14	Vermont	81.0
15	Wisconsin	79.4
16	Kentucky	79.1
17	Utah	77.8
18	Colorado	75.1
19	Texas	74.2
20	Wyoming	71.5
21	Massachusetts	69.6
22	Alabama	67.1
23	Oklahoma	67.0
24	West Virginia	63.7
25	Montana	62.8
26	Arizona	62.6
27	Maryland	62.4
28	Iowa	62.3
29	Oregon	61.9
30	Missouri	61.1
31	Delaware	61.0
32	Washington	60.8
33	Indiana	60.7
33	New Jersey	60.7
35	Kansas	60.6
35	New York	60.6
37	Illinois	59.9
38	Pennsylvania	59.4
39	Nebraska	59.0
40	Virginia	58.8
41	Rhode Island	58.0
42	Alaska	57.8
42	Arkansas	57.8
44	California	56.6
45	Louisiana	55.9
46	Connecticut	52.3
47	Michigan	51.8
48	Florida	48.9
49	Ohio	44.6
50	North Dakota	36.9

| | District of Columbia | (11.5) |

Source: MQ Press using data from U.S. Dept of Health & Human Services, Centers for Medicare and Medicaid Services "State Health Care Expenditures" (http://www.hcfa.gov/stats/nhe-oact/stateestimates/)

*By state of provider. Includes "other professional services" previously listed as a separate category. These include services of licensed professionals such as chiropractors, optometrists, podiatrists and independently practicing nurses. Also includes specialty clinics, independently billing laboratories and Medicare ambulance services.

Average Annual Change in Expenditures for Physician and Other Professional Services: 1990 to 1998
National Percent Change = 6.3% Average Annual Increase*

ALPHA ORDER

RANK	STATE	PERCENT CHANGE
22	Alabama	6.6
41	Alaska	5.9
25	Arizona	6.3
41	Arkansas	5.9
44	California	5.8
18	Colorado	7.3
46	Connecticut	5.4
30	Delaware	6.1
48	Florida	5.1
11	Georgia	7.9
1	Hawaii	9.2
6	Idaho	8.7
37	Illinois	6.0
30	Indiana	6.1
27	Iowa	6.2
30	Kansas	6.1
15	Kentucky	7.6
45	Louisiana	5.7
9	Maine	8.1
27	Maryland	6.2
21	Massachusetts	6.8
46	Michigan	5.4
4	Minnesota	8.8
8	Mississippi	8.3
30	Missouri	6.1
25	Montana	6.3
37	Nebraska	6.0
13	Nevada	7.8
3	New Hampshire	9.1
30	New Jersey	6.1
11	New Mexico	7.9
30	New York	6.1
9	North Carolina	8.1
50	North Dakota	4.0
49	Ohio	4.7
22	Oklahoma	6.6
27	Oregon	6.2
37	Pennsylvania	6.0
41	Rhode Island	5.9
7	South Carolina	8.6
1	South Dakota	9.2
4	Tennessee	8.8
19	Texas	7.2
17	Utah	7.5
14	Vermont	7.7
37	Virginia	6.0
30	Washington	6.1
24	West Virginia	6.4
15	Wisconsin	7.6
20	Wyoming	7.0

RANK ORDER

RANK	STATE	PERCENT CHANGE
1	Hawaii	9.2
1	South Dakota	9.2
3	New Hampshire	9.1
4	Minnesota	8.8
4	Tennessee	8.8
6	Idaho	8.7
7	South Carolina	8.6
8	Mississippi	8.3
9	Maine	8.1
9	North Carolina	8.1
11	Georgia	7.9
11	New Mexico	7.9
13	Nevada	7.8
14	Vermont	7.7
15	Kentucky	7.6
15	Wisconsin	7.6
17	Utah	7.5
18	Colorado	7.3
19	Texas	7.2
20	Wyoming	7.0
21	Massachusetts	6.8
22	Alabama	6.6
22	Oklahoma	6.6
24	West Virginia	6.4
25	Arizona	6.3
25	Montana	6.3
27	Iowa	6.2
27	Maryland	6.2
27	Oregon	6.2
30	Delaware	6.1
30	Indiana	6.1
30	Kansas	6.1
30	Missouri	6.1
30	New Jersey	6.1
30	New York	6.1
30	Washington	6.1
37	Illinois	6.0
37	Nebraska	6.0
37	Pennsylvania	6.0
37	Virginia	6.0
41	Alaska	5.9
41	Arkansas	5.9
41	Rhode Island	5.9
44	California	5.8
45	Louisiana	5.7
46	Connecticut	5.4
46	Michigan	5.4
48	Florida	5.1
49	Ohio	4.7
50	North Dakota	4.0

District of Columbia   (1.5)

Source: U.S. Department of Health and Human Services, Centers for Medicare and Medicaid Services
     "State Health Care Expenditures" (http://www.hcfa.gov/stats/nhe-oact/stateestimates/)
*By state of provider. Includes "other professional services" previously listed as a separate category. These include services of licensed professionals such as chiropractors, optometrists, podiatrists and independently practicing nurses. Also includes specialty clinics, independently billing laboratories and Medicare ambulance services.

Per Capita Expenditures for Physician and Other Professional Services in 1998

National Per Capita = $1,096*

ALPHA ORDER

RANK ORDER

RANK	STATE	PER CAPITA
20	Alabama	$1,059
38	Alaska	923
16	Arizona	1,100
41	Arkansas	877
2	California	1,354
18	Colorado	1,087
5	Connecticut	1,312
19	Delaware	1,064
6	Florida	1,273
13	Georgia	1,114
4	Hawaii	1,339
49	Idaho	760
25	Illinois	992
35	Indiana	950
42	Iowa	859
31	Kansas	962
31	Kentucky	962
30	Louisiana	974
28	Maine	977
10	Maryland	1,165
2	Massachusetts	1,354
37	Michigan	935
1	Minnesota	1,520
46	Mississippi	804
28	Missouri	977
47	Montana	790
44	Nebraska	823
16	Nevada	1,100
8	New Hampshire	1,185
9	New Jersey	1,174
45	New Mexico	816
15	New York	1,107
36	North Carolina	942
33	North Dakota	960
27	Ohio	981
40	Oklahoma	892
24	Oregon	1,001
11	Pennsylvania	1,119
14	Rhode Island	1,109
43	South Carolina	847
22	South Dakota	1,022
7	Tennessee	1,237
23	Texas	1,018
48	Utah	785
34	Vermont	953
38	Virginia	923
21	Washington	1,039
26	West Virginia	990
11	Wisconsin	1,119
50	Wyoming	715

RANK	STATE	PER CAPITA
1	Minnesota	$1,520
2	California	1,354
2	Massachusetts	1,354
4	Hawaii	1,339
5	Connecticut	1,312
6	Florida	1,273
7	Tennessee	1,237
8	New Hampshire	1,185
9	New Jersey	1,174
10	Maryland	1,165
11	Pennsylvania	1,119
11	Wisconsin	1,119
13	Georgia	1,114
14	Rhode Island	1,109
15	New York	1,107
16	Arizona	1,100
16	Nevada	1,100
18	Colorado	1,087
19	Delaware	1,064
20	Alabama	1,059
21	Washington	1,039
22	South Dakota	1,022
23	Texas	1,018
24	Oregon	1,001
25	Illinois	992
26	West Virginia	990
27	Ohio	981
28	Maine	977
28	Missouri	977
30	Louisiana	974
31	Kansas	962
31	Kentucky	962
33	North Dakota	960
34	Vermont	953
35	Indiana	950
36	North Carolina	942
37	Michigan	935
38	Alaska	923
38	Virginia	923
40	Oklahoma	892
41	Arkansas	877
42	Iowa	859
43	South Carolina	847
44	Nebraska	823
45	New Mexico	816
46	Mississippi	804
47	Montana	790
48	Utah	785
49	Idaho	760
50	Wyoming	715

District of Columbia	1,498

Source: MQ Press using data from U.S. Dept of Health & Human Services, Centers for Medicare and Medicaid Services
"State Health Care Expenditures" (http://www.hcfa.gov/stats/nhe-oact/stateestimates/)
*By state of provider. Per capita calculated using resident population. These figures may be skewed due to residents
crossing state borders for care. Includes "other professional services" previously listed as a separate category.
Services include licensed professionals such as chiropractors, optometrists, podiatrists and independently
practicing nurses. Includes specialty clinics, independently billing laboratories and Medicare ambulance services.

Percent Change in Per Capita Expenditures for Physician and Other Professional Services: 1990 to 1998
National Percent Change = 51.0% Increase*

ALPHA ORDER

RANK	STATE	PERCENT CHANGE
24	Alabama	55.5
43	Alaska	41.8
49	Arizona	28.2
37	Arkansas	46.4
42	California	43.6
38	Colorado	45.7
26	Connecticut	53.1
40	Delaware	44.8
48	Florida	30.0
23	Georgia	56.9
2	Hawaii	88.9
16	Idaho	61.0
29	Illinois	51.7
31	Indiana	51.0
21	Iowa	57.6
31	Kansas	51.0
11	Kentucky	68.2
33	Louisiana	50.8
4	Maine	83.6
27	Maryland	51.9
12	Massachusetts	66.1
41	Michigan	43.8
5	Minnesota	81.8
7	Mississippi	76.7
27	Missouri	51.9
35	Montana	47.9
30	Nebraska	51.3
50	Nevada	27.6
3	New Hampshire	87.8
25	New Jersey	53.9
18	New Mexico	60.3
19	New York	59.3
13	North Carolina	64.1
47	North Dakota	36.9
45	Ohio	39.7
22	Oklahoma	57.3
44	Oregon	41.0
20	Pennsylvania	57.8
17	Rhode Island	60.7
8	South Carolina	75.7
1	South Dakota	92.8
6	Tennessee	77.2
34	Texas	50.6
36	Utah	46.5
9	Vermont	73.0
39	Virginia	45.4
46	Washington	38.5
15	West Virginia	62.0
10	Wisconsin	68.3
14	Wyoming	62.1

RANK ORDER

RANK	STATE	PERCENT CHANGE
1	South Dakota	92.8
2	Hawaii	88.9
3	New Hampshire	87.8
4	Maine	83.6
5	Minnesota	81.8
6	Tennessee	77.2
7	Mississippi	76.7
8	South Carolina	75.7
9	Vermont	73.0
10	Wisconsin	68.3
11	Kentucky	68.2
12	Massachusetts	66.1
13	North Carolina	64.1
14	Wyoming	62.1
15	West Virginia	62.0
16	Idaho	61.0
17	Rhode Island	60.7
18	New Mexico	60.3
19	New York	59.3
20	Pennsylvania	57.8
21	Iowa	57.6
22	Oklahoma	57.3
23	Georgia	56.9
24	Alabama	55.5
25	New Jersey	53.9
26	Connecticut	53.1
27	Maryland	51.9
27	Missouri	51.9
29	Illinois	51.7
30	Nebraska	51.3
31	Indiana	51.0
31	Kansas	51.0
33	Louisiana	50.8
34	Texas	50.6
35	Montana	47.9
36	Utah	46.5
37	Arkansas	46.4
38	Colorado	45.7
39	Virginia	45.4
40	Delaware	44.8
41	Michigan	43.8
42	California	43.6
43	Alaska	41.8
44	Oregon	41.0
45	Ohio	39.7
46	Washington	38.5
47	North Dakota	36.9
48	Florida	30.0
49	Arizona	28.2
50	Nevada	27.6
	District of Columbia	2.5

Source: MQ Press using data from U.S. Dept of Health & Human Services, Centers for Medicare and Medicaid Services "State Health Care Expenditures" (http://www.hcfa.gov/stats/nhe-oact/stateestimates/)

*By state of provider. Per capita calculated using resident population. These figures may be skewed due to residents crossing state borders for care. Includes "other professional services" previously listed as a separate category. Services include licensed professionals such as chiropractors, optometrists, podiatrists and independently practicing nurses. Includes specialty clinics, independently billing laboratories and Medicare ambulance services.

Average Annual Change in Per Capita Expenditures
For Physician Services: 1990 to 1998
National Percent Change = 5.3% Average Annual Increase*

ALPHA ORDER

RANK	STATE	PERCENT CHANGE
24	Alabama	5.7
43	Alaska	4.5
49	Arizona	3.2
36	Arkansas	4.9
41	California	4.6
38	Colorado	4.8
25	Connecticut	5.5
40	Delaware	4.7
48	Florida	3.3
22	Georgia	5.8
2	Hawaii	8.3
16	Idaho	6.1
29	Illinois	5.3
29	Indiana	5.3
20	Iowa	5.9
29	Kansas	5.3
10	Kentucky	6.7
29	Louisiana	5.3
4	Maine	7.9
27	Maryland	5.4
12	Massachusetts	6.6
41	Michigan	4.6
5	Minnesota	7.8
6	Mississippi	7.4
27	Missouri	5.4
35	Montana	5.0
29	Nebraska	5.3
50	Nevada	3.1
3	New Hampshire	8.2
25	New Jersey	5.5
16	New Mexico	6.1
19	New York	6.0
13	North Carolina	6.4
47	North Dakota	4.0
45	Ohio	4.3
22	Oklahoma	5.8
44	Oregon	4.4
20	Pennsylvania	5.9
16	Rhode Island	6.1
8	South Carolina	7.3
1	South Dakota	8.6
6	Tennessee	7.4
29	Texas	5.3
36	Utah	4.9
9	Vermont	7.1
38	Virginia	4.8
46	Washington	4.2
14	West Virginia	6.2
10	Wisconsin	6.7
14	Wyoming	6.2

RANK ORDER

RANK	STATE	PERCENT CHANGE
1	South Dakota	8.6
2	Hawaii	8.3
3	New Hampshire	8.2
4	Maine	7.9
5	Minnesota	7.8
6	Mississippi	7.4
6	Tennessee	7.4
8	South Carolina	7.3
9	Vermont	7.1
10	Kentucky	6.7
10	Wisconsin	6.7
12	Massachusetts	6.6
13	North Carolina	6.4
14	West Virginia	6.2
14	Wyoming	6.2
16	Idaho	6.1
16	New Mexico	6.1
16	Rhode Island	6.1
19	New York	6.0
20	Iowa	5.9
20	Pennsylvania	5.9
22	Georgia	5.8
22	Oklahoma	5.8
24	Alabama	5.7
25	Connecticut	5.5
25	New Jersey	5.5
27	Maryland	5.4
27	Missouri	5.4
29	Illinois	5.3
29	Indiana	5.3
29	Kansas	5.3
29	Louisiana	5.3
29	Nebraska	5.3
29	Texas	5.3
35	Montana	5.0
36	Arkansas	4.9
36	Utah	4.9
38	Colorado	4.8
38	Virginia	4.8
40	Delaware	4.7
41	California	4.6
41	Michigan	4.6
43	Alaska	4.5
44	Oregon	4.4
45	Ohio	4.3
46	Washington	4.2
47	North Dakota	4.0
48	Florida	3.3
49	Arizona	3.2
50	Nevada	3.1
	District of Columbia	0.3

Source: MQ Press using data from U.S. Dept of Health & Human Services, Centers for Medicare and Medicaid Services
"State Health Care Expenditures" (http://www.hcfa.gov/stats/nhe-oact/stateestimates/)
*By state of provider. Per capita calculated using resident population. These figures may be skewed due to residents
crossing state borders for care. Includes "other professional services" previously listed as a separate category.
Services include licensed professionals such as chiropractors, optometrists, podiatrists and independently
practicing nurses. Includes specialty clinics, independently billing laboratories and Medicare ambulance services.

Expenditures for Prescription Drugs in 1998

National Total = $90,648,000,000*

ALPHA ORDER

RANK	STATE	EXPENDITURES	% of USA
21	Alabama	$1,552,000,000	1.7%
49	Alaska	133,000,000	0.1%
24	Arizona	1,397,000,000	1.5%
32	Arkansas	903,000,000	1.0%
1	California	7,537,000,000	8.3%
28	Colorado	970,000,000	1.1%
25	Connecticut	1,354,000,000	1.5%
44	Delaware	300,000,000	0.3%
3	Florida	6,204,000,000	6.8%
11	Georgia	2,460,000,000	2.7%
43	Hawaii	311,000,000	0.3%
42	Idaho	334,000,000	0.4%
6	Illinois	3,964,000,000	4.4%
15	Indiana	2,058,000,000	2.3%
30	Iowa	945,000,000	1.0%
33	Kansas	854,000,000	0.9%
20	Kentucky	1,564,000,000	1.7%
22	Louisiana	1,507,000,000	1.7%
38	Maine	456,000,000	0.5%
18	Maryland	1,678,000,000	1.9%
12	Massachusetts	2,172,000,000	2.4%
8	Michigan	3,885,000,000	4.3%
23	Minnesota	1,491,000,000	1.6%
29	Mississippi	962,000,000	1.1%
16	Missouri	1,814,000,000	2.0%
45	Montana	234,000,000	0.3%
35	Nebraska	626,000,000	0.7%
37	Nevada	478,000,000	0.5%
41	New Hampshire	391,000,000	0.4%
9	New Jersey	3,545,000,000	3.9%
39	New Mexico	402,000,000	0.4%
2	New York	7,122,000,000	7.9%
10	North Carolina	2,566,000,000	2.8%
47	North Dakota	192,000,000	0.2%
7	Ohio	3,898,000,000	4.3%
27	Oklahoma	1,056,000,000	1.2%
31	Oregon	918,000,000	1.0%
5	Pennsylvania	5,035,000,000	5.6%
40	Rhode Island	400,000,000	0.4%
26	South Carolina	1,315,000,000	1.5%
46	South Dakota	201,000,000	0.2%
14	Tennessee	2,129,000,000	2.3%
4	Texas	6,023,000,000	6.6%
36	Utah	564,000,000	0.6%
48	Vermont	183,000,000	0.2%
13	Virginia	2,130,000,000	2.3%
19	Washington	1,603,000,000	1.8%
34	West Virginia	776,000,000	0.9%
17	Wisconsin	1,745,000,000	1.9%
49	Wyoming	133,000,000	0.1%

RANK ORDER

RANK	STATE	EXPENDITURES	% of USA
1	California	$7,537,000,000	8.3%
2	New York	7,122,000,000	7.9%
3	Florida	6,204,000,000	6.8%
4	Texas	6,023,000,000	6.6%
5	Pennsylvania	5,035,000,000	5.6%
6	Illinois	3,964,000,000	4.4%
7	Ohio	3,898,000,000	4.3%
8	Michigan	3,885,000,000	4.3%
9	New Jersey	3,545,000,000	3.9%
10	North Carolina	2,566,000,000	2.8%
11	Georgia	2,460,000,000	2.7%
12	Massachusetts	2,172,000,000	2.4%
13	Virginia	2,130,000,000	2.3%
14	Tennessee	2,129,000,000	2.3%
15	Indiana	2,058,000,000	2.3%
16	Missouri	1,814,000,000	2.0%
17	Wisconsin	1,745,000,000	1.9%
18	Maryland	1,678,000,000	1.9%
19	Washington	1,603,000,000	1.8%
20	Kentucky	1,564,000,000	1.7%
21	Alabama	1,552,000,000	1.7%
22	Louisiana	1,507,000,000	1.7%
23	Minnesota	1,491,000,000	1.6%
24	Arizona	1,397,000,000	1.5%
25	Connecticut	1,354,000,000	1.5%
26	South Carolina	1,315,000,000	1.5%
27	Oklahoma	1,056,000,000	1.2%
28	Colorado	970,000,000	1.1%
29	Mississippi	962,000,000	1.1%
30	Iowa	945,000,000	1.0%
31	Oregon	918,000,000	1.0%
32	Arkansas	903,000,000	1.0%
33	Kansas	854,000,000	0,9%
34	West Virginia	776,000,000	0.9%
35	Nebraska	626,000,000	0.7%
36	Utah	564,000,000	0.6%
37	Nevada	478,000,000	0.5%
38	Maine	456,000,000	0.5%
39	New Mexico	402,000,000	0.4%
40	Rhode Island	400,000,000	0.4%
41	New Hampshire	391,000,000	0.4%
42	Idaho	334,000,000	0.4%
43	Hawaii	311,000,000	0.3%
44	Delaware	300,000,000	0.3%
45	Montana	234,000,000	0.3%
46	South Dakota	201,000,000	0.2%
47	North Dakota	192,000,000	0.2%
48	Vermont	183,000,000	0.2%
49	Alaska	133,000,000	0.1%
49	Wyoming	133,000,000	0.1%
	District of Columbia	180,000,000	0.2%

Source: U.S. Department of Health and Human Services, Centers for Medicare and Medicaid Services
    "State Health Care Expenditures" (http://www.hcfa.gov/stats/nhe-oact/stateestimates/)
*Purchases in retail outlets. By state of outlet.

Percent of Total Personal Health Care Expenditures
Spent on Prescription Drugs in 1998
National Percent = 8.9%*

ALPHA ORDER

RANK	STATE	PERCENT
12	Alabama	9.7
50	Alaska	5.8
18	Arizona	9.5
6	Arkansas	10.7
48	California	6.8
46	Colorado	7.1
28	Connecticut	8.9
12	Delaware	9.7
7	Florida	10.4
27	Georgia	9.0
49	Hawaii	6.7
10	Idaho	9.8
28	Illinois	8.9
12	Indiana	9.7
22	Iowa	9.3
25	Kansas	9.1
2	Kentucky	10.9
25	Louisiana	9.1
22	Maine	9.3
35	Maryland	8.5
44	Massachusetts	7.2
2	Michigan	10.9
43	Minnesota	7.3
4	Mississippi	10.8
33	Missouri	8.7
41	Montana	8.2
8	Nebraska	10.3
35	Nevada	8.5
38	New Hampshire	8.4
4	New Jersey	10.8
42	New Mexico	7.5
39	New York	8.3
21	North Carolina	9.4
44	North Dakota	7.2
24	Ohio	9.2
16	Oklahoma	9.6
35	Oregon	8.5
10	Pennsylvania	9.8
28	Rhode Island	8.9
9	South Carolina	10.0
46	South Dakota	7.1
12	Tennessee	9.7
28	Texas	8.9
18	Utah	9.5
28	Vermont	8.9
16	Virginia	9.6
39	Washington	8.3
1	West Virginia	11.0
33	Wisconsin	8.7
18	Wyoming	9.5

RANK ORDER

RANK	STATE	PERCENT
1	West Virginia	11.0
2	Kentucky	10.9
2	Michigan	10.9
4	Mississippi	10.8
4	New Jersey	10.8
6	Arkansas	10.7
7	Florida	10.4
8	Nebraska	10.3
9	South Carolina	10.0
10	Idaho	9.8
10	Pennsylvania	9.8
12	Alabama	9.7
12	Delaware	9.7
12	Indiana	9.7
12	Tennessee	9.7
16	Oklahoma	9.6
16	Virginia	9.6
18	Arizona	9.5
18	Utah	9.5
18	Wyoming	9.5
21	North Carolina	9.4
22	Iowa	9.3
22	Maine	9.3
24	Ohio	9.2
25	Kansas	9.1
25	Louisiana	9.1
27	Georgia	9.0
28	Connecticut	8.9
28	Illinois	8.9
28	Rhode Island	8.9
28	Texas	8.9
28	Vermont	8.9
33	Missouri	8.7
33	Wisconsin	8.7
35	Maryland	8.5
35	Nevada	8.5
35	Oregon	8.5
38	New Hampshire	8.4
39	New York	8.3
39	Washington	8.3
41	Montana	8.2
42	New Mexico	7.5
43	Minnesota	7.3
44	Massachusetts	7.2
44	North Dakota	7.2
46	Colorado	7.1
46	South Dakota	7.1
48	California	6.8
49	Hawaii	6.7
50	Alaska	5.8
	District of Columbia	4.2

Source: MQ Press using data from U.S. Dept of Health & Human Services, Centers for Medicare and Medicaid Services
"State Health Care Expenditures" (http://www.hcfa.gov/stats/nhe-oact/stateestimates/)
*Purchases in retail outlets. By state of outlet.

Percent Change in Expenditures for Prescription Drugs: 1990 to 1998

National Percent Change = 140.6% Increase*

ALPHA ORDER

RANK	STATE	PERCENT CHANGE
37	Alabama	129.6
25	Alaska	141.8
4	Arizona	180.0
30	Arkansas	134.5
49	California	98.2
8	Colorado	161.5
19	Connecticut	144.8
2	Delaware	200.0
3	Florida	198.1
15	Georgia	152.6
50	Hawaii	84.0
9	Idaho	160.9
46	Illinois	122.9
40	Indiana	127.7
34	Iowa	131.6
43	Kansas	124.7
23	Kentucky	142.1
47	Louisiana	120.3
7	Maine	165.1
42	Maryland	125.5
28	Massachusetts	136.6
27	Michigan	137.0
10	Minnesota	158.9
29	Mississippi	135.2
45	Missouri	124.0
17	Montana	148.9
16	Nebraska	152.4
1	Nevada	236.6
21	New Hampshire	144.4
13	New Jersey	155.6
44	New Mexico	124.6
14	New York	152.8
12	North Carolina	156.9
48	North Dakota	111.0
36	Ohio	129.8
31	Oklahoma	134.1
5	Oregon	179.9
18	Pennsylvania	146.6
33	Rhode Island	132.6
6	South Carolina	166.7
41	South Dakota	125.8
20	Tennessee	144.7
22	Texas	142.5
11	Utah	157.5
39	Vermont	128.8
32	Virginia	133.6
23	Washington	142.1
35	West Virginia	131.0
26	Wisconsin	141.0
38	Wyoming	129.3

RANK ORDER

RANK	STATE	PERCENT CHANGE
1	Nevada	236.6
2	Delaware	200.0
3	Florida	198.1
4	Arizona	180.0
5	Oregon	179.9
6	South Carolina	166.7
7	Maine	165.1
8	Colorado	161.5
9	Idaho	160.9
10	Minnesota	158.9
11	Utah	157.5
12	North Carolina	156.9
13	New Jersey	155.6
14	New York	152.8
15	Georgia	152.6
16	Nebraska	152.4
17	Montana	148.9
18	Pennsylvania	146.6
19	Connecticut	144.8
20	Tennessee	144.7
21	New Hampshire	144.4
22	Texas	142.5
23	Kentucky	142.1
23	Washington	142.1
25	Alaska	141.8
26	Wisconsin	141.0
27	Michigan	137.0
28	Massachusetts	136.6
29	Mississippi	135.2
30	Arkansas	134.5
31	Oklahoma	134.1
32	Virginia	133.6
33	Rhode Island	132.6
34	Iowa	131.6
35	West Virginia	131.0
36	Ohio	129.8
37	Alabama	129.6
38	Wyoming	129.3
39	Vermont	128.8
40	Indiana	127.7
41	South Dakota	125.8
42	Maryland	125.5
43	Kansas	124.7
44	New Mexico	124.6
45	Missouri	124.0
46	Illinois	122.9
47	Louisiana	120.3
48	North Dakota	111.0
49	California	98.2
50	Hawaii	84.0

District of Columbia	125.0

Source: MQ Press using data from U.S. Dept of Health & Human Services, Centers for Medicare and Medicaid Services "State Health Care Expenditures" (http://www.hcfa.gov/stats/nhe-oact/stateestimates/)
*Purchases in retail outlets. By state of outlet.

Average Annual Change in Expenditures for Prescription Drugs: 1990 to 1998

National Percent Change = 11.6% Average Annual Increase*

ALPHA ORDER			RANK ORDER		
RANK	STATE	PERCENT CHANGE	RANK	STATE	PERCENT CHANGE
37	Alabama	10.9	1	Nevada	16.4
22	Alaska	11.7	2	Delaware	14.7
4	Arizona	13.7	3	Florida	14.6
30	Arkansas	11.2	4	Arizona	13.7
49	California	8.9	4	Oregon	13.7
8	Colorado	12.8	6	Maine	13.0
19	Connecticut	11.8	6	South Carolina	13.0
2	Delaware	14.7	8	Colorado	12.8
3	Florida	14.6	9	Idaho	12.7
14	Georgia	12.3	10	Minnesota	12.6
50	Hawaii	7.9	10	Utah	12.6
9	Idaho	12.7	12	North Carolina	12.5
46	Illinois	10.5	13	New Jersey	12.4
40	Indiana	10.8	14	Georgia	12.3
33	Iowa	11.1	14	Nebraska	12.3
41	Kansas	10.7	14	New York	12.3
22	Kentucky	11.7	17	Montana	12.1
47	Louisiana	10.4	18	Pennsylvania	11.9
6	Maine	13.0	19	Connecticut	11.8
41	Maryland	10.7	19	New Hampshire	11.8
27	Massachusetts	11.4	19	Tennessee	11.8
27	Michigan	11.4	22	Alaska	11.7
10	Minnesota	12.6	22	Kentucky	11.7
29	Mississippi	11.3	22	Texas	11.7
44	Missouri	10.6	22	Washington	11.7
17	Montana	12.1	26	Wisconsin	11.6
14	Nebraska	12.3	27	Massachusetts	11.4
1	Nevada	16.4	27	Michigan	11.4
19	New Hampshire	11.8	29	Mississippi	11.3
13	New Jersey	12.4	30	Arkansas	11.2
44	New Mexico	10.6	30	Oklahoma	11.2
14	New York	12.3	30	Virginia	11.2
12	North Carolina	12.5	33	Iowa	11.1
48	North Dakota	9.8	33	Rhode Island	11.1
35	Ohio	11.0	35	Ohio	11.0
30	Oklahoma	11.2	35	West Virginia	11.0
4	Oregon	13.7	37	Alabama	10.9
18	Pennsylvania	11.9	37	Vermont	10.9
33	Rhode Island	11.1	37	Wyoming	10.9
6	South Carolina	13.0	40	Indiana	10.8
41	South Dakota	10.7	41	Kansas	10.7
19	Tennessee	11.8	41	Maryland	10.7
22	Texas	11.7	41	South Dakota	10.7
10	Utah	12.6	44	Missouri	10.6
37	Vermont	10.9	44	New Mexico	10.6
30	Virginia	11.2	46	Illinois	10.5
22	Washington	11.7	47	Louisiana	10.4
35	West Virginia	11.0	48	North Dakota	9.8
26	Wisconsin	11.6	49	California	8.9
37	Wyoming	10.9	50	Hawaii	7.9
				District of Columbia	10.7

Source: U.S. Department of Health and Human Services, Centers for Medicare and Medicaid Services
    "State Health Care Expenditures" (http://www.hcfa.gov/stats/nhe-oact/stateestimates/)
*Purchases in retail outlets. By state of outlet.

Per Capita Expenditures for Prescription Drugs in 1998

National Per Capita = $335*

<u>ALPHA ORDER</u>

RANK	STATE	PER CAPITA
14	Alabama	$357
50	Alaska	216
37	Arizona	299
15	Arkansas	356
49	California	231
47	Colorado	244
5	Connecticut	414
7	Delaware	403
4	Florida	416
30	Georgia	322
46	Hawaii	261
43	Idaho	271
27	Illinois	328
18	Indiana	348
25	Iowa	330
29	Kansas	324
8	Kentucky	398
20	Louisiana	345
13	Maine	366
28	Maryland	327
16	Massachusetts	353
9	Michigan	396
32	Minnesota	315
17	Mississippi	350
23	Missouri	334
45	Montana	266
12	Nebraska	377
42	Nevada	274
25	New Hampshire	330
1	New Jersey	438
48	New Mexico	232
10	New York	392
22	North Carolina	340
36	North Dakota	301
19	Ohio	347
31	Oklahoma	316
39	Oregon	280
3	Pennsylvania	420
6	Rhode Island	405
21	South Carolina	342
41	South Dakota	275
10	Tennessee	392
35	Texas	306
44	Utah	268
34	Vermont	310
33	Virginia	314
38	Washington	282
2	West Virginia	428
23	Wisconsin	334
40	Wyoming	277

<u>RANK ORDER</u>

RANK	STATE	PER CAPITA
1	New Jersey	$438
2	West Virginia	428
3	Pennsylvania	420
4	Florida	416
5	Connecticut	414
6	Rhode Island	405
7	Delaware	403
8	Kentucky	398
9	Michigan	396
10	New York	392
10	Tennessee	392
12	Nebraska	377
13	Maine	366
14	Alabama	357
15	Arkansas	356
16	Massachusetts	353
17	Mississippi	350
18	Indiana	348
19	Ohio	347
20	Louisiana	345
21	South Carolina	342
22	North Carolina	340
23	Missouri	334
23	Wisconsin	334
25	Iowa	330
25	New Hampshire	330
27	Illinois	328
28	Maryland	327
29	Kansas	324
30	Georgia	322
31	Oklahoma	316
32	Minnesota	315
33	Virginia	314
34	Vermont	310
35	Texas	306
36	North Dakota	301
37	Arizona	299
38	Washington	282
39	Oregon	280
40	Wyoming	277
41	South Dakota	275
42	Nevada	274
43	Idaho	271
44	Utah	268
45	Montana	266
46	Hawaii	261
47	Colorado	244
48	New Mexico	232
49	California	231
50	Alaska	216
	District of Columbia	345

Source: MQ Press using data from U.S. Dept of Health & Human Services, Centers for Medicare and Medicaid Services "State Health Care Expenditures" (http://www.hcfa.gov/stats/nhe-oact/stateestimates/)
Purchases in retail outlets. By state of outlet.

Percent Change in Per Capita Expenditures for Prescription Drugs: 1990 to 1998

National Percent Change = 121.9% Increase*

ALPHA ORDER

RANK ORDER

RANK	STATE	PERCENT CHANGE	RANK	STATE	PERCENT CHANGE
36	Alabama	113.8	1	Delaware	170.5
29	Alaska	118.2	2	Maine	161.4
27	Arizona	119.9	3	Florida	160.0
31	Arkansas	117.1	4	New York	151.3
49	California	81.9	5	Connecticut	146.4
30	Colorado	117.9	6	New Jersey	144.7
5	Connecticut	146.4	7	Pennsylvania	144.2
1	Delaware	170.5	8	Oregon	143.5
3	Florida	160.0	9	South Carolina	142.6
35	Georgia	114.7	10	Minnesota	140.5
50	Hawaii	71.7	11	Nebraska	140.1
33	Idaho	115.1	12	Rhode Island	136.8
41	Illinois	111.6	13	Nevada	134.2
38	Indiana	113.5	14	Massachusetts	130.7
22	Iowa	124.5	15	New Hampshire	129.2
40	Kansas	111.8	16	West Virginia	128.9
17	Kentucky	127.4	17	Kentucky	127.4
39	Louisiana	113.0	18	North Carolina	126.7
2	Maine	161.4	19	Wisconsin	125.7
43	Maryland	111.0	20	Montana	125.4
14	Massachusetts	130.7	21	Michigan	125.0
21	Michigan	125.0	22	Iowa	124.5
10	Minnesota	140.5	23	Ohio	122.4
26	Mississippi	120.1	24	Oklahoma	121.0
42	Missouri	111.4	25	Tennessee	120.2
20	Montana	125.4	26	Mississippi	120.1
11	Nebraska	140.1	27	Arizona	119.9
13	Nevada	134.2	28	Vermont	118.3
15	New Hampshire	129.2	29	Alaska	118.2
6	New Jersey	144.7	30	Colorado	117.9
48	New Mexico	96.6	31	Arkansas	117.1
4	New York	151.3	32	Wyoming	116.4
18	North Carolina	126.7	33	Idaho	115.1
45	North Dakota	110.5	34	South Dakota	114.8
23	Ohio	122.4	35	Georgia	114.7
24	Oklahoma	121.0	36	Alabama	113.8
8	Oregon	143.5	37	Virginia	113.6
7	Pennsylvania	144.2	38	Indiana	113.5
12	Rhode Island	136.8	39	Louisiana	113.0
9	South Carolina	142.6	40	Kansas	111.8
34	South Dakota	114.8	41	Illinois	111.6
25	Tennessee	120.2	42	Missouri	111.4
46	Texas	109.6	43	Maryland	111.0
43	Utah	111.0	43	Utah	111.0
28	Vermont	118.3	45	North Dakota	110.5
37	Virginia	113.6	46	Texas	109.6
47	Washington	108.9	47	Washington	108.9
16	West Virginia	128.9	48	New Mexico	96.6
19	Wisconsin	125.7	49	California	81.9
32	Wyoming	116.4	50	Hawaii	71.7

District of Columbia 161.4

Source: MQ Press using data from U.S. Dept of Health & Human Services, Centers for Medicare and Medicaid Services
"State Health Care Expenditures" (http://www.hcfa.gov/stats/nhe-oact/stateestimates/)
*Purchases in retail outlets. By state of outlet.

Average Annual Change in Per Capita Expenditures
For Prescription Drugs: 1990 to 1998
National Percent Change = 10.5% Average Annual Increase*

ALPHA ORDER

RANK	STATE	PERCENT CHANGE
33	Alabama	10.0
29	Alaska	10.2
27	Arizona	10.3
29	Arkansas	10.2
49	California	7.8
29	Colorado	10.2
5	Connecticut	11.9
1	Delaware	13.2
3	Florida	12.7
33	Georgia	10.0
50	Hawaii	7.0
33	Idaho	10.0
40	Illinois	9.8
38	Indiana	9.9
22	Iowa	10.6
40	Kansas	9.8
17	Kentucky	10.8
38	Louisiana	9.9
2	Maine	12.8
40	Maryland	9.8
14	Massachusetts	11.0
19	Michigan	10.7
10	Minnesota	11.6
24	Mississippi	10.4
40	Missouri	9.8
19	Montana	10.7
10	Nebraska	11.6
13	Nevada	11.2
15	New Hampshire	10.9
6	New Jersey	11.8
48	New Mexico	8.8
4	New York	12.2
17	North Carolina	10.8
45	North Dakota	9.7
23	Ohio	10.5
24	Oklahoma	10.4
6	Oregon	11.8
6	Pennsylvania	11.8
12	Rhode Island	11.4
9	South Carolina	11.7
33	South Dakota	10.0
24	Tennessee	10.4
45	Texas	9.7
40	Utah	9.8
27	Vermont	10.3
33	Virginia	10.0
47	Washington	9.6
15	West Virginia	10.9
19	Wisconsin	10.7
32	Wyoming	10.1

RANK ORDER

RANK	STATE	PERCENT CHANGE
1	Delaware	13.2
2	Maine	12.8
3	Florida	12.7
4	New York	12.2
5	Connecticut	11.9
6	New Jersey	11.8
6	Oregon	11.8
6	Pennsylvania	11.8
9	South Carolina	11.7
10	Minnesota	11.6
10	Nebraska	11.6
12	Rhode Island	11.4
13	Nevada	11.2
14	Massachusetts	11.0
15	New Hampshire	10.9
15	West Virginia	10.9
17	Kentucky	10.8
17	North Carolina	10.8
19	Michigan	10.7
19	Montana	10.7
19	Wisconsin	10.7
22	Iowa	10.6
23	Ohio	10.5
24	Mississippi	10.4
24	Oklahoma	10.4
24	Tennessee	10.4
27	Arizona	10.3
27	Vermont	10.3
29	Alaska	10.2
29	Arkansas	10.2
29	Colorado	10.2
32	Wyoming	10.1
33	Alabama	10.0
33	Georgia	10.0
33	Idaho	10.0
33	South Dakota	10.0
33	Virginia	10.0
38	Indiana	9.9
38	Louisiana	9.9
40	Illinois	9.8
40	Kansas	9.8
40	Maryland	9.8
40	Missouri	9.8
40	Utah	9.8
45	North Dakota	9.7
45	Texas	9.7
47	Washington	9.6
48	New Mexico	8.8
49	California	7.8
50	Hawaii	7.0
	District of Columbia	12.8

Source: MQ Press using data from U.S. Dept of Health & Human Services, Centers for Medicare and Medicaid Services
"State Health Care Expenditures" (http://www.hcfa.gov/stats/nhe-oact/stateestimates/)
*Purchases in retail outlets. By state of outlet.

Expenditures for Dental Services in 1998

National Total = $53,829,000,000*

ALPHA ORDER

RANK	STATE	EXPENDITURES	% of USA
26	Alabama	$652,000,000	1.2%
44	Alaska	173,000,000	0.3%
24	Arizona	867,000,000	1.6%
33	Arkansas	392,000,000	0.7%
1	California	7,999,000,000	14.9%
19	Colorado	944,000,000	1.8%
22	Connecticut	896,000,000	1.7%
45	Delaware	155,000,000	0.3%
4	Florida	2,957,000,000	5.5%
12	Georgia	1,381,000,000	2.6%
36	Hawaii	284,000,000	0.5%
40	Idaho	253,000,000	0.5%
5	Illinois	2,283,000,000	4.2%
18	Indiana	1,021,000,000	1.9%
31	Iowa	482,000,000	0.9%
30	Kansas	484,000,000	0.9%
28	Kentucky	533,000,000	1.0%
25	Louisiana	703,000,000	1.3%
41	Maine	233,000,000	0.4%
17	Maryland	1,047,000,000	1.9%
11	Massachusetts	1,472,000,000	2.7%
7	Michigan	2,141,000,000	4.0%
16	Minnesota	1,052,000,000	2.0%
35	Mississippi	317,000,000	0.6%
23	Missouri	877,000,000	1.6%
46	Montana	151,000,000	0.3%
38	Nebraska	274,000,000	0.5%
34	Nevada	391,000,000	0.7%
37	New Hampshire	283,000,000	0.5%
9	New Jersey	1,917,000,000	3.6%
39	New Mexico	268,000,000	0.5%
2	New York	3,698,000,000	6.9%
13	North Carolina	1,323,000,000	2.5%
49	North Dakota	110,000,000	0.2%
8	Ohio	1,978,000,000	3.7%
29	Oklahoma	505,000,000	0.9%
21	Oregon	902,000,000	1.7%
6	Pennsylvania	2,237,000,000	4.2%
43	Rhode Island	217,000,000	0.4%
27	South Carolina	591,000,000	1.1%
48	South Dakota	121,000,000	0.2%
20	Tennessee	927,000,000	1.7%
3	Texas	3,218,000,000	6.0%
32	Utah	461,000,000	0.9%
47	Vermont	127,000,000	0.2%
14	Virginia	1,272,000,000	2.4%
10	Washington	1,722,000,000	3.2%
42	West Virginia	221,000,000	0.4%
15	Wisconsin	1,089,000,000	2.0%
50	Wyoming	76,000,000	0.1%

RANK ORDER

RANK	STATE	EXPENDITURES	% of USA
1	California	$7,999,000,000	14.9%
2	New York	3,698,000,000	6.9%
3	Texas	3,218,000,000	6.0%
4	Florida	2,957,000,000	5.5%
5	Illinois	2,283,000,000	4.2%
6	Pennsylvania	2,237,000,000	4.2%
7	Michigan	2,141,000,000	4.0%
8	Ohio	1,978,000,000	3.7%
9	New Jersey	1,917,000,000	3.6%
10	Washington	1,722,000,000	3.2%
11	Massachusetts	1,472,000,000	2.7%
12	Georgia	1,381,000,000	2.6%
13	North Carolina	1,323,000,000	2.5%
14	Virginia	1,272,000,000	2.4%
15	Wisconsin	1,089,000,000	2.0%
16	Minnesota	1,052,000,000	2.0%
17	Maryland	1,047,000,000	1.9%
18	Indiana	1,021,000,000	1.9%
19	Colorado	944,000,000	1.8%
20	Tennessee	927,000,000	1.7%
21	Oregon	902,000,000	1.7%
22	Connecticut	896,000,000	1.7%
23	Missouri	877,000,000	1.6%
24	Arizona	867,000,000	1.6%
25	Louisiana	703,000,000	1.3%
26	Alabama	652,000,000	1.2%
27	South Carolina	591,000,000	1.1%
28	Kentucky	533,000,000	1.0%
29	Oklahoma	505,000,000	0.9%
30	Kansas	484,000,000	0.9%
31	Iowa	482,000,000	0.9%
32	Utah	461,000,000	0.9%
33	Arkansas	392,000,000	0.7%
34	Nevada	391,000,000	0.7%
35	Mississippi	317,000,000	0.6%
36	Hawaii	284,000,000	0.5%
37	New Hampshire	283,000,000	0.5%
38	Nebraska	274,000,000	0.5%
39	New Mexico	268,000,000	0.5%
40	Idaho	253,000,000	0.5%
41	Maine	233,000,000	0.4%
42	West Virginia	221,000,000	0.4%
43	Rhode Island	217,000,000	0.4%
44	Alaska	173,000,000	0.3%
45	Delaware	155,000,000	0.3%
46	Montana	151,000,000	0.3%
47	Vermont	127,000,000	0.2%
48	South Dakota	121,000,000	0.2%
49	North Dakota	110,000,000	0.2%
50	Wyoming	76,000,000	0.1%
	District of Columbia	151,000,000	0.3%

Source: U.S. Department of Health and Human Services, Centers for Medicare and Medicaid Services
    "State Health Care Expenditures" (http://www.hcfa.gov/stats/nhe-oact/stateestimates/)
*By state of provider.

Percent of Total Personal Health Care Expenditures
Spent on Dental Services in 1998
National Percent = 5.3%*

ALPHA ORDER

RANK	STATE	PERCENT
46	Alabama	4.1
4	Alaska	7.5
13	Arizona	5.9
35	Arkansas	4.6
6	California	7.3
8	Colorado	6.9
13	Connecticut	5.9
25	Delaware	5.0
25	Florida	5.0
24	Georgia	5.1
9	Hawaii	6.1
5	Idaho	7.4
21	Illinois	5.2
29	Indiana	4.8
32	Iowa	4.7
21	Kansas	5.2
48	Kentucky	3.7
41	Louisiana	4.3
32	Maine	4.7
19	Maryland	5.3
28	Massachusetts	4.9
12	Michigan	6.0
21	Minnesota	5.2
49	Mississippi	3.6
44	Missouri	4.2
19	Montana	5.3
38	Nebraska	4.5
7	Nevada	7.0
9	New Hampshire	6.1
13	New Jersey	5.9
25	New Mexico	5.0
41	New York	4.3
29	North Carolina	4.8
46	North Dakota	4.1
35	Ohio	4.6
35	Oklahoma	4.6
2	Oregon	8.3
40	Pennsylvania	4.4
29	Rhode Island	4.8
38	South Carolina	4.5
41	South Dakota	4.3
44	Tennessee	4.2
32	Texas	4.7
3	Utah	7.8
9	Vermont	6.1
16	Virginia	5.7
1	Washington	8.9
50	West Virginia	3.1
17	Wisconsin	5.5
18	Wyoming	5.4

RANK ORDER

RANK	STATE	PERCENT
1	Washington	8.9
2	Oregon	8.3
3	Utah	7.8
4	Alaska	7.5
5	Idaho	7.4
6	California	7.3
7	Nevada	7.0
8	Colorado	6.9
9	Hawaii	6.1
9	New Hampshire	6.1
9	Vermont	6.1
12	Michigan	6.0
13	Arizona	5.9
13	Connecticut	5.9
13	New Jersey	5.9
16	Virginia	5.7
17	Wisconsin	5.5
18	Wyoming	5.4
19	Maryland	5.3
19	Montana	5.3
21	Illinois	5.2
21	Kansas	5.2
21	Minnesota	5.2
24	Georgia	5.1
25	Delaware	5.0
25	Florida	5.0
25	New Mexico	5.0
28	Massachusetts	4.9
29	Indiana	4.8
29	North Carolina	4.8
29	Rhode Island	4.8
32	Iowa	4.7
32	Maine	4.7
32	Texas	4.7
35	Arkansas	4.6
35	Ohio	4.6
35	Oklahoma	4.6
38	Nebraska	4.5
38	South Carolina	4.5
40	Pennsylvania	4.4
41	Louisiana	4.3
41	New York	4.3
41	South Dakota	4.3
44	Missouri	4.2
44	Tennessee	4.2
46	Alabama	4.1
46	North Dakota	4.1
48	Kentucky	3.7
49	Mississippi	3.6
50	West Virginia	3.1

| | District of Columbia | 3.5 |

Source: MQ Press using data from U.S. Dept of Health & Human Services, Centers for Medicare and Medicaid Services "State Health Care Expenditures" (http://www.hcfa.gov/stats/nhe-oact/stateestimates/)
*By state of provider.

Average Annual Change in Expenditures for Dental Services: 1990 to 1998

National Percent Change = 6.9% Average Annual Increase*

ALPHA ORDER			RANK ORDER		
RANK	STATE	PERCENT CHANGE	RANK	STATE	PERCENT CHANGE
26	Alabama	7.4	1	Nevada	11.1
20	Alaska	7.8	2	Idaho	9.3
6	Arizona	8.6	3	North Carolina	9.0
11	Arkansas	8.4	3	Utah	9.0
39	California	6.5	5	Louisiana	8.8
6	Colorado	8.6	6	Arizona	8.6
50	Connecticut	4.3	6	Colorado	8.6
12	Delaware	8.3	6	Oregon	8.6
28	Florida	7.3	6	Texas	8.6
17	Georgia	7.9	10	New Mexico	8.5
49	Hawaii	4.8	11	Arkansas	8.4
2	Idaho	9.3	12	Delaware	8.3
39	Illinois	6.5	12	Kentucky	8.3
14	Indiana	8.2	14	Indiana	8.2
28	Iowa	7.3	15	Washington	8.1
24	Kansas	7.5	16	South Carolina	8.0
12	Kentucky	8.3	17	Georgia	7.9
5	Louisiana	8.8	17	Mississippi	7.9
31	Maine	7.2	17	Tennessee	7.9
37	Maryland	6.6	20	Alaska	7.8
42	Massachusetts	6.3	20	Montana	7.8
43	Michigan	6.1	20	New Hampshire	7.8
37	Minnesota	6.6	23	South Dakota	7.7
17	Mississippi	7.9	24	Kansas	7.5
35	Missouri	6.9	24	Vermont	7.5
20	Montana	7.8	26	Alabama	7.4
33	Nebraska	7.0	26	Virginia	7.4
1	Nevada	11.1	28	Florida	7.3
20	New Hampshire	7.8	28	Iowa	7.3
45	New Jersey	5.4	28	Wisconsin	7.3
10	New Mexico	8.5	31	Maine	7.2
47	New York	5.0	31	North Dakota	7.2
3	North Carolina	9.0	33	Nebraska	7.0
31	North Dakota	7.2	33	West Virginia	7.0
39	Ohio	6.5	35	Missouri	6.9
36	Oklahoma	6.8	36	Oklahoma	6.8
6	Oregon	8.6	37	Maryland	6.6
48	Pennsylvania	4.9	37	Minnesota	6.6
46	Rhode Island	5.1	39	California	6.5
16	South Carolina	8.0	39	Illinois	6.5
23	South Dakota	7.7	39	Ohio	6.5
17	Tennessee	7.9	42	Massachusetts	6.3
6	Texas	8.6	43	Michigan	6.1
3	Utah	9.0	44	Wyoming	5.6
24	Vermont	7.5	45	New Jersey	5.4
26	Virginia	7.4	46	Rhode Island	5.1
15	Washington	8.1	47	New York	5.0
33	West Virginia	7.0	48	Pennsylvania	4.9
28	Wisconsin	7.3	49	Hawaii	4.8
44	Wyoming	5.6	50	Connecticut	4.3
				District of Columbia	5.3

Source: U.S. Department of Health and Human Services, Centers for Medicare and Medicaid Services
    "State Health Care Expenditures" (http://www.hcfa.gov/stats/nhe-oact/stateestimates/)
*Purchases in retail outlets. By state of outlet. Includes over-the-counter drugs and sundries.

Per Capita Expenditures for Dental Services in 1998

National Per Capita = $199*

ALPHA ORDER				RANK ORDER		
RANK	STATE	PER CAPITA		RANK	STATE	PER CAPITA
47	Alabama	$150		1	Washington	$303
2	Alaska	281		2	Alaska	281
26	Arizona	186		3	Oregon	275
44	Arkansas	154		4	Connecticut	274
5	California	245		5	California	245
9	Colorado	238		6	Massachusetts	240
4	Connecticut	274		7	Hawaii	239
18	Delaware	208		7	New Hampshire	239
22	Florida	198		9	Colorado	238
29	Georgia	181		10	New Jersey	237
7	Hawaii	239		11	Nevada	224
19	Idaho	206		12	Minnesota	223
23	Illinois	189		13	Rhode Island	220
32	Indiana	173		14	Utah	219
36	Iowa	168		15	Michigan	218
28	Kansas	183		16	Vermont	215
48	Kentucky	135		17	Wisconsin	209
40	Louisiana	161		18	Delaware	208
24	Maine	187		19	Idaho	206
20	Maryland	204		20	Maryland	204
6	Massachusetts	240		20	New York	204
15	Michigan	218		22	Florida	198
12	Minnesota	223		23	Illinois	189
50	Mississippi	115		24	Maine	187
40	Missouri	161		24	Virginia	187
33	Montana	172		26	Arizona	186
38	Nebraska	165		26	Pennsylvania	186
11	Nevada	224		28	Kansas	183
7	New Hampshire	239		29	Georgia	181
10	New Jersey	237		30	Ohio	176
43	New Mexico	155		31	North Carolina	175
20	New York	204		32	Indiana	173
31	North Carolina	175		33	Montana	172
33	North Dakota	172		33	North Dakota	172
30	Ohio	176		35	Tennessee	171
46	Oklahoma	151		36	Iowa	168
3	Oregon	275		37	South Dakota	166
26	Pennsylvania	186		38	Nebraska	165
13	Rhode Island	220		39	Texas	163
44	South Carolina	154		40	Louisiana	161
37	South Dakota	166		40	Missouri	161
35	Tennessee	171		42	Wyoming	158
39	Texas	163		43	New Mexico	155
14	Utah	219		44	Arkansas	154
16	Vermont	215		44	South Carolina	154
24	Virginia	187		46	Oklahoma	151
1	Washington	303		47	Alabama	150
49	West Virginia	122		48	Kentucky	135
17	Wisconsin	209		49	West Virginia	122
42	Wyoming	158		50	Mississippi	115
					District of Columbia	290

Source: MQ Press using data from U.S. Dept of Health & Human Services, Centers for Medicare and Medicaid Services
"State Health Care Expenditures" (http://www.hcfa.gov/stats/nhe-oact/stateestimates/)
*By state of provider. Per capita calculated using resident population. These figures may be skewed due to residents crossing state borders for care.

Per Capita Medicaid Expenditures for Dental Services in 1998

National Per Capita = $7.37*

ALPHA ORDER				RANK ORDER		
RANK	STATE	PER CAPITA		RANK	STATE	PER CAPITA
40	Alabama	$2.99		1	California	$20.47
5	Alaska	13.00		2	Washington	20.22
6	Arizona	12.43		3	Massachusetts	14.00
31	Arkansas	4.33		4	Vermont	13.55
1	California	20.47		5	Alaska	13.00
39	Colorado	3.02		6	Arizona	12.43
42	Connecticut	2.75		7	Rhode Island	12.15
35	Delaware	4.03		8	West Virginia	11.59
25	Florida	4.96		9	Iowa	9.44
29	Georgia	4.58		10	Kentucky	8.64
49	Hawaii	0.84		11	Utah	8.57
12	Idaho	8.12		12	Idaho	8.12
41	Illinois	2.90		13	Nevada	8.03
30	Indiana	4.57		14	Montana	7.96
9	Iowa	9.44		15	Nebraska	7.83
37	Kansas	3.79		16	Texas	6.90
10	Kentucky	8.64		17	New York	6.61
34	Louisiana	4.13		18	Maine	6.41
18	Maine	6.41		19	North Dakota	6.27
50	Maryland	0.39		20	North Carolina	5.96
3	Massachusetts	14.00		21	Tennessee	5.89
22	Michigan	5.50		22	Michigan	5.50
27	Minnesota	4.65		23	South Dakota	5.47
48	Mississippi	1.09		24	Pennsylvania	5.17
43	Missouri	2.39		25	Florida	4.96
14	Montana	7.96		26	South Carolina	4.69
15	Nebraska	7.83		27	Minnesota	4.65
13	Nevada	8.03		28	New Mexico	4.61
32	New Hampshire	4.22		29	Georgia	4.58
44	New Jersey	2.22		30	Indiana	4.57
28	New Mexico	4.61		31	Arkansas	4.33
17	New York	6.61		32	New Hampshire	4.22
20	North Carolina	5.96		33	Wyoming	4.17
19	North Dakota	6.27		34	Louisiana	4.13
36	Ohio	3.83		35	Delaware	4.03
45	Oklahoma	2.10		36	Ohio	3.83
47	Oregon	1.52		37	Kansas	3.79
24	Pennsylvania	5.17		38	Wisconsin	3.64
7	Rhode Island	12.15		39	Colorado	3.02
26	South Carolina	4.69		40	Alabama	2.99
23	South Dakota	5.47		41	Illinois	2.90
21	Tennessee	5.89		42	Connecticut	2.75
16	Texas	6.90		43	Missouri	2.39
11	Utah	8.57		44	New Jersey	2.22
4	Vermont	13.55		45	Oklahoma	2.10
46	Virginia	1.91		46	Virginia	1.91
2	Washington	20.22		47	Oregon	1.52
8	West Virginia	11.59		48	Mississippi	1.09
38	Wisconsin	3.64		49	Hawaii	0.84
33	Wyoming	4.17		50	Maryland	0.39
					District of Columbia	3.84

Source: MQ Press using data from U.S. Dept of Health & Human Services, Centers for Medicare and Medicaid Services "State Health Care Expenditures" (http://www.hcfa.gov/stats/nhe-oact/stateestimates/)
By state of provider. Per capita calculated using resident population. These figures may be skewed due to residents crossing state borders for care.

Expenditures for Other Personal Health Care Services in 1998

National Total = $31,917,000,000*

ALPHA ORDER				RANK ORDER			
RANK	STATE	EXPENDITURES	% of USA	RANK	STATE	EXPENDITURES	% of USA
26	Alabama	$407,000,000	1.3%	1	New York	$4,431,000,000	13.9%
35	Alaska	262,000,000	0.8%	2	Texas	2,083,000,000	6.5%
34	Arizona	300,000,000	0.9%	3	California	2,033,000,000	6.4%
36	Arkansas	240,000,000	0.8%	4	Pennsylvania	1,596,000,000	5.0%
3	California	2,033,000,000	6.4%	5	Florida	1,525,000,000	4.8%
22	Colorado	464,000,000	1.5%	6	Illinois	1,320,000,000	4.1%
21	Connecticut	548,000,000	1.7%	7	Massachusetts	1,144,000,000	3.6%
43	Delaware	153,000,000	0.5%	8	Ohio	940,000,000	2.9%
5	Florida	1,525,000,000	4.8%	9	North Carolina	880,000,000	2.8%
13	Georgia	778,000,000	2.4%	10	Michigan	868,000,000	2.7%
44	Hawaii	149,000,000	0.5%	11	Minnesota	808,000,000	2.5%
46	Idaho	116,000,000	0.4%	12	New Jersey	793,000,000	2.5%
6	Illinois	1,320,000,000	4.1%	13	Georgia	778,000,000	2.4%
28	Indiana	381,000,000	1.2%	14	Washington	732,000,000	2.3%
31	Iowa	344,000,000	1.1%	15	Virginia	666,000,000	2.1%
24	Kansas	437,000,000	1.4%	16	Wisconsin	656,000,000	2.1%
25	Kentucky	425,000,000	1.3%	17	Missouri	644,000,000	2.0%
32	Louisiana	342,000,000	1.1%	18	Maryland	598,000,000	1.9%
30	Maine	345,000,000	1.1%	19	South Carolina	576,000,000	1.8%
18	Maryland	598,000,000	1.9%	20	Oregon	563,000,000	1.8%
7	Massachusetts	1,144,000,000	3.6%	21	Connecticut	548,000,000	1.7%
10	Michigan	868,000,000	2.7%	22	Colorado	464,000,000	1.5%
11	Minnesota	808,000,000	2.5%	23	Tennessee	459,000,000	1.4%
39	Mississippi	211,000,000	0.7%	24	Kansas	437,000,000	1.4%
17	Missouri	644,000,000	2.0%	25	Kentucky	425,000,000	1.3%
48	Montana	99,000,000	0.3%	26	Alabama	407,000,000	1.3%
40	Nebraska	179,000,000	0.6%	27	Oklahoma	383,000,000	1.2%
45	Nevada	140,000,000	0.4%	28	Indiana	381,000,000	1.2%
38	New Hampshire	234,000,000	0.7%	29	Rhode Island	358,000,000	1.1%
12	New Jersey	793,000,000	2.5%	30	Maine	345,000,000	1.1%
37	New Mexico	238,000,000	0.7%	31	Iowa	344,000,000	1.1%
1	New York	4,431,000,000	13.9%	32	Louisiana	342,000,000	1.1%
9	North Carolina	880,000,000	2.8%	33	West Virginia	331,000,000	1.0%
49	North Dakota	83,000,000	0.3%	34	Arizona	300,000,000	0.9%
8	Ohio	940,000,000	2.9%	35	Alaska	262,000,000	0.8%
27	Oklahoma	383,000,000	1.2%	36	Arkansas	240,000,000	0.8%
20	Oregon	563,000,000	1.8%	37	New Mexico	238,000,000	0.7%
4	Pennsylvania	1,596,000,000	5.0%	38	New Hampshire	234,000,000	0.7%
29	Rhode Island	358,000,000	1.1%	39	Mississippi	211,000,000	0.7%
19	South Carolina	576,000,000	1.8%	40	Nebraska	179,000,000	0.6%
47	South Dakota	113,000,000	0.4%	41	Utah	160,000,000	0.5%
23	Tennessee	459,000,000	1.4%	42	Vermont	155,000,000	0.5%
2	Texas	2,083,000,000	6.5%	43	Delaware	153,000,000	0.5%
41	Utah	160,000,000	0.5%	44	Hawaii	149,000,000	0.5%
42	Vermont	155,000,000	0.5%	45	Nevada	140,000,000	0.4%
15	Virginia	666,000,000	2.1%	46	Idaho	116,000,000	0.4%
14	Washington	732,000,000	2.3%	47	South Dakota	113,000,000	0.4%
33	West Virginia	331,000,000	1.0%	48	Montana	99,000,000	0.3%
16	Wisconsin	656,000,000	2.1%	49	North Dakota	83,000,000	0.3%
50	Wyoming	69,000,000	0.2%	50	Wyoming	69,000,000	0.2%
					District of Columbia	161,000,000	0.5%

Source: U.S. Department of Health and Human Services, Centers for Medicare and Medicaid Services
"State Health Care Expenditures" (http://www.hcfa.gov/stats/nhe-oact/stateestimates/)
By state of provider. Includes on-site services provided by employers for the health care needs of their employees.
Also includes shipboard facilities and field stations operated by the U.S. Department of Defense; certain state and
local maternal and child health programs; school health programs and federal agency programs targeting veterans,
military personnel, Native Americans and persons with dependency and mental-health-related problems.

Percent of Total Personal Health Care Expenditures
Spent on Other Personal Health Care Services in 1998
National Percent = 3.1%*

ALPHA ORDER				RANK ORDER		
RANK	STATE	PERCENT		RANK	STATE	PERCENT
40	Alabama	2.5		1	Alaska	11.4
1	Alaska	11.4		2	Rhode Island	7.9
48	Arizona	2.0		3	Vermont	7.5
37	Arkansas	2.8		4	Maine	7.0
49	California	1.8		5	New York	5.2
21	Colorado	3.4		5	Oregon	5.2
18	Connecticut	3.6		7	New Hampshire	5.0
8	Delaware	4.9		8	Delaware	4.9
39	Florida	2.6		8	Wyoming	4.9
34	Georgia	2.9		10	Kansas	4.7
25	Hawaii	3.2		10	West Virginia	4.7
21	Idaho	3.4		12	New Mexico	4.5
31	Illinois	3.0		13	South Carolina	4.4
49	Indiana	1.8		14	Minnesota	4.0
21	Iowa	3.4		14	South Dakota	4.0
10	Kansas	4.7		16	Massachusetts	3.8
34	Kentucky	2.9		16	Washington	3.8
46	Louisiana	2.1		18	Connecticut	3.6
4	Maine	7.0		19	Montana	3.5
31	Maryland	3.0		19	Oklahoma	3.5
16	Massachusetts	3.8		21	Colorado	3.4
42	Michigan	2.4		21	Idaho	3.4
14	Minnesota	4.0		21	Iowa	3.4
42	Mississippi	2.4		24	Wisconsin	3.3
27	Missouri	3.1		25	Hawaii	3.2
19	Montana	3.5		25	North Carolina	3.2
34	Nebraska	2.9		27	Missouri	3.1
40	Nevada	2.5		27	North Dakota	3.1
7	New Hampshire	5.0		27	Pennsylvania	3.1
42	New Jersey	2.4		27	Texas	3.1
12	New Mexico	4.5		31	Illinois	3.0
5	New York	5.2		31	Maryland	3.0
25	North Carolina	3.2		31	Virginia	3.0
27	North Dakota	3.1		34	Georgia	2.9
45	Ohio	2.2		34	Kentucky	2.9
19	Oklahoma	3.5		34	Nebraska	2.9
5	Oregon	5.2		37	Arkansas	2.8
27	Pennsylvania	3.1		38	Utah	2.7
2	Rhode Island	7.9		39	Florida	2.6
13	South Carolina	4.4		40	Alabama	2.5
14	South Dakota	4.0		40	Nevada	2.5
46	Tennessee	2.1		42	Michigan	2.4
27	Texas	3.1		42	Mississippi	2.4
38	Utah	2.7		42	New Jersey	2.4
3	Vermont	7.5		45	Ohio	2.2
31	Virginia	3.0		46	Louisiana	2.1
16	Washington	3.8		46	Tennessee	2.1
10	West Virginia	4.7		48	Arizona	2.0
24	Wisconsin	3.3		49	California	1.8
8	Wyoming	4.9		49	Indiana	1.8
					District of Columbia	3.8

Source: MQ Press using data from U.S. Dept of Health & Human Services, Centers for Medicare and Medicaid Services
"State Health Care Expenditures" (http://www.hcfa.gov/stats/nhe-oact/stateestimates/)
*By state of provider. Includes on-site services provided by employers for the health care needs of their employees.
Also includes shipboard facilities and field stations operated by the U.S. Department of Defense; certain state and
local maternal and child health programs; school health programs and federal agency programs targeting veterans,
military personnel, Native Americans and persons with dependency and mental-health-related problems.

Average Annual Change in Expenditures for
Other Personal Health Care Services: 1990 to 1998
National Percent Change = 14.1% Average Annual Increase*

ALPHA ORDER

RANK	STATE	PERCENT CHANGE
44	Alabama	10.1
48	Alaska	7.9
42	Arizona	11.1
11	Arkansas	17.5
50	California	6.9
34	Colorado	12.7
31	Connecticut	12.9
15	Delaware	16.5
29	Florida	13.1
40	Georgia	11.6
45	Hawaii	9.3
26	Idaho	14.2
20	Illinois	15.0
46	Indiana	9.1
7	Iowa	19.4
1	Kansas	22.7
25	Kentucky	14.4
43	Louisiana	10.8
2	Maine	22.3
34	Maryland	12.7
24	Massachusetts	14.8
37	Michigan	12.1
14	Minnesota	16.9
41	Mississippi	11.2
13	Missouri	17.0
48	Montana	7.9
28	Nebraska	13.3
16	Nevada	15.9
16	New Hampshire	15.9
47	New Jersey	8.2
19	New Mexico	15.3
5	New York	20.2
9	North Carolina	18.1
38	North Dakota	11.8
39	Ohio	11.7
8	Oklahoma	19.2
11	Oregon	17.5
20	Pennsylvania	15.0
3	Rhode Island	21.8
23	South Carolina	14.9
32	South Dakota	12.8
27	Tennessee	13.6
18	Texas	15.7
32	Utah	12.8
9	Vermont	18.1
30	Virginia	13.0
20	Washington	15.0
4	West Virginia	20.4
36	Wisconsin	12.2
6	Wyoming	20.0

RANK ORDER

RANK	STATE	PERCENT CHANGE
1	Kansas	22.7
2	Maine	22.3
3	Rhode Island	21.8
4	West Virginia	20.4
5	New York	20.2
6	Wyoming	20.0
7	Iowa	19.4
8	Oklahoma	19.2
9	North Carolina	18.1
9	Vermont	18.1
11	Arkansas	17.5
11	Oregon	17.5
13	Missouri	17.0
14	Minnesota	16.9
15	Delaware	16.5
16	Nevada	15.9
16	New Hampshire	15.9
18	Texas	15.7
19	New Mexico	15.3
20	Illinois	15.0
20	Pennsylvania	15.0
20	Washington	15.0
23	South Carolina	14.9
24	Massachusetts	14.8
25	Kentucky	14.4
26	Idaho	14.2
27	Tennessee	13.6
28	Nebraska	13.3
29	Florida	13.1
30	Virginia	13.0
31	Connecticut	12.9
32	South Dakota	12.8
32	Utah	12.8
34	Colorado	12.7
34	Maryland	12.7
36	Wisconsin	12.2
37	Michigan	12.1
38	North Dakota	11.8
39	Ohio	11.7
40	Georgia	11.6
41	Mississippi	11.2
42	Arizona	11.1
43	Louisiana	10.8
44	Alabama	10.1
45	Hawaii	9.3
46	Indiana	9.1
47	New Jersey	8.2
48	Alaska	7.9
48	Montana	7.9
50	California	6.9
	District of Columbia	7.1

Source: U.S. Department of Health and Human Services, Centers for Medicare and Medicaid Services
"State Health Care Expenditures" (http://www.hcfa.gov/stats/nhe-oact/stateestimates/)
*By state of provider. Includes on-site services provided by employers for the health care needs of their employees.
Also includes shipboard facilities and field stations operated by the U.S. Department of Defense; certain state and
local maternal and child health programs; school health programs and federal agency programs targeting veterans,
military personnel, Native Americans and persons with dependency and mental-health-related problems.

Per Capita Expenditures for Other Personal Health Care Services in 1998

National Per Capita = $118*

ALPHA ORDER				RANK ORDER		
RANK	STATE	PER CAPITA		RANK	STATE	PER CAPITA
39	Alabama	$94		1	Alaska	$426
1	Alaska	426		2	Rhode Island	362
48	Arizona	64		3	Maine	277
38	Arkansas	95		4	Vermont	262
50	California	62		5	New York	244
25	Colorado	117		6	Delaware	206
12	Connecticut	167		7	New Hampshire	197
6	Delaware	206		8	Massachusetts	186
34	Florida	102		9	West Virginia	183
34	Georgia	102		10	Oregon	172
22	Hawaii	125		11	Minnesota	171
39	Idaho	94		12	Connecticut	167
30	Illinois	109		13	Kansas	166
48	Indiana	64		14	South Dakota	155
23	Iowa	120		15	South Carolina	150
13	Kansas	166		16	Wyoming	144
31	Kentucky	108		17	New Mexico	137
45	Louisiana	78		18	Pennsylvania	133
3	Maine	277		19	North Dakota	130
25	Maryland	117		20	Washington	129
8	Massachusetts	186		21	Wisconsin	126
41	Michigan	88		22	Hawaii	125
11	Minnesota	171		23	Iowa	120
46	Mississippi	77		24	Missouri	118
24	Missouri	118		25	Colorado	117
29	Montana	113		25	Maryland	117
31	Nebraska	108		25	North Carolina	117
44	Nevada	80		28	Oklahoma	115
7	New Hampshire	197		29	Montana	113
36	New Jersey	98		30	Illinois	109
17	New Mexico	137		31	Kentucky	108
5	New York	244		31	Nebraska	108
25	North Carolina	117		33	Texas	106
19	North Dakota	130		34	Florida	102
42	Ohio	84		34	Georgia	102
28	Oklahoma	115		36	New Jersey	98
10	Oregon	172		36	Virginia	98
18	Pennsylvania	133		38	Arkansas	95
2	Rhode Island	362		39	Alabama	94
15	South Carolina	150		39	Idaho	94
14	South Dakota	155		41	Michigan	88
42	Tennessee	84		42	Ohio	84
33	Texas	106		42	Tennessee	84
47	Utah	76		44	Nevada	80
4	Vermont	262		45	Louisiana	78
36	Virginia	98		46	Mississippi	77
20	Washington	129		47	Utah	76
9	West Virginia	183		48	Arizona	64
21	Wisconsin	126		48	Indiana	64
16	Wyoming	144		50	California	62
					District of Columbia	309

Source: MQ Press using data from U.S. Dept of Health & Human Services, Centers for Medicare and Medicaid Services
"State Health Care Expenditures" (http://www.hcfa.gov/stats/nhe-oact/stateestimates/)
*By state of provider. Includes on-site services provided by employers for the health care needs of their employees.
Also includes shipboard facilities and field stations operated by the U.S. Department of Defense; certain state and
local maternal and child health programs; school health programs and federal agency programs targeting veterans,
military personnel, Native Americans and persons with dependency and mental-health-related problems.

Expenditures for Home Health Care in 1998

National Total = $29,255,000,000*

ALPHA ORDER

RANK	STATE	EXPENDITURES	% of USA
19	Alabama	$470,000,000	1.6%
50	Alaska	9,000,000	0.0%
27	Arizona	331,000,000	1.1%
31	Arkansas	242,000,000	0.8%
4	California	1,951,000,000	6.7%
28	Colorado	324,000,000	1.1%
15	Connecticut	599,000,000	2.0%
41	Delaware	110,000,000	0.4%
3	Florida	2,225,000,000	7.6%
12	Georgia	810,000,000	2.8%
44	Hawaii	60,000,000	0.2%
44	Idaho	60,000,000	0.2%
8	Illinois	972,000,000	3.3%
21	Indiana	415,000,000	1.4%
30	Iowa	248,000,000	0.8%
32	Kansas	220,000,000	0.8%
17	Kentucky	506,000,000	1.7%
13	Louisiana	629,000,000	2.2%
33	Maine	188,000,000	0.6%
25	Maryland	390,000,000	1.3%
7	Massachusetts	999,000,000	3.4%
11	Michigan	841,000,000	2.9%
20	Minnesota	419,000,000	1.4%
29	Mississippi	293,000,000	1.0%
16	Missouri	567,000,000	1.9%
46	Montana	56,000,000	0.2%
42	Nebraska	71,000,000	0.2%
35	Nevada	180,000,000	0.6%
37	New Hampshire	145,000,000	0.5%
9	New Jersey	938,000,000	3.2%
38	New Mexico	143,000,000	0.5%
1	New York	4,292,000,000	14.7%
10	North Carolina	934,000,000	3.2%
48	North Dakota	20,000,000	0.1%
5	Ohio	1,224,000,000	4.2%
23	Oklahoma	391,000,000	1.3%
36	Oregon	151,000,000	0.5%
6	Pennsylvania	1,109,000,000	3.8%
40	Rhode Island	134,000,000	0.5%
23	South Carolina	391,000,000	1.3%
49	South Dakota	11,000,000	0.0%
14	Tennessee	617,000,000	2.1%
2	Texas	2,862,000,000	9.8%
39	Utah	136,000,000	0.5%
43	Vermont	68,000,000	0.2%
18	Virginia	484,000,000	1.7%
26	Washington	365,000,000	1.2%
34	West Virginia	187,000,000	0.6%
22	Wisconsin	393,000,000	1.3%
47	Wyoming	24,000,000	0.1%

RANK ORDER

RANK	STATE	EXPENDITURES	% of USA
1	New York	$4,292,000,000	14.7%
2	Texas	2,862,000,000	9.8%
3	Florida	2,225,000,000	7.6%
4	California	1,951,000,000	6.7%
5	Ohio	1,224,000,000	4.2%
6	Pennsylvania	1,109,000,000	3.8%
7	Massachusetts	999,000,000	3.4%
8	Illinois	972,000,000	3.3%
9	New Jersey	938,000,000	3.2%
10	North Carolina	934,000,000	3.2%
11	Michigan	841,000,000	2.9%
12	Georgia	810,000,000	2.8%
13	Louisiana	629,000,000	2.2%
14	Tennessee	617,000,000	2.1%
15	Connecticut	599,000,000	2.0%
16	Missouri	567,000,000	1.9%
17	Kentucky	506,000,000	1.7%
18	Virginia	484,000,000	1.7%
19	Alabama	470,000,000	1.6%
20	Minnesota	419,000,000	1.4%
21	Indiana	415,000,000	1.4%
22	Wisconsin	393,000,000	1.3%
23	Oklahoma	391,000,000	1.3%
23	South Carolina	391,000,000	1.3%
25	Maryland	390,000,000	1.3%
26	Washington	365,000,000	1.2%
27	Arizona	331,000,000	1.1%
28	Colorado	324,000,000	1.1%
29	Mississippi	293,000,000	1.0%
30	Iowa	248,000,000	0.8%
31	Arkansas	242,000,000	0.8%
32	Kansas	220,000,000	0.8%
33	Maine	188,000,000	0.6%
34	West Virginia	187,000,000	0.6%
35	Nevada	180,000,000	0.6%
36	Oregon	151,000,000	0.5%
37	New Hampshire	145,000,000	0.5%
38	New Mexico	143,000,000	0.5%
39	Utah	136,000,000	0.5%
40	Rhode Island	134,000,000	0.5%
41	Delaware	110,000,000	0.4%
42	Nebraska	71,000,000	0.2%
43	Vermont	68,000,000	0.2%
44	Hawaii	60,000,000	0.2%
44	Idaho	60,000,000	0.2%
46	Montana	56,000,000	0.2%
47	Wyoming	24,000,000	0.1%
48	North Dakota	20,000,000	0.1%
49	South Dakota	11,000,000	0.0%
50	Alaska	9,000,000	0.0%
	District of Columbia	54,000,000	0.2%

Source: U.S. Department of Health and Human Services, Centers for Medicare and Medicaid Services
"State Health Care Expenditures" (http://www.hcfa.gov/stats/nhe-oact/stateestimates/)
*By state of provider. Includes spending for services and products by public and private freestanding home health agencies. Excludes home health care services provided by hospital-based agencies which are included in hospital expenditures.

Percent of Total Personal Health Care Expenditures
Spent on Home Health Care in 1998
National Percent = 2.9%*

ALPHA ORDER

RANK	STATE	PERCENT
19	Alabama	2.9
49	Alaska	0.4
32	Arizona	2.2
19	Arkansas	2.9
42	California	1.8
27	Colorado	2.4
3	Connecticut	3.9
8	Delaware	3.5
6	Florida	3.7
16	Georgia	3.0
46	Hawaii	1.3
42	Idaho	1.8
32	Illinois	2.2
37	Indiana	2.0
27	Iowa	2.4
30	Kansas	2.3
8	Kentucky	3.5
4	Louisiana	3.8
4	Maine	3.8
37	Maryland	2.0
11	Massachusetts	3.3
27	Michigan	2.4
36	Minnesota	2.1
11	Mississippi	3.3
24	Missouri	2.7
37	Montana	2.0
47	Nebraska	1.2
14	Nevada	3.2
15	New Hampshire	3.1
19	New Jersey	2.9
24	New Mexico	2.7
1	New York	5.0
10	North Carolina	3.4
48	North Dakota	0.7
19	Ohio	2.9
7	Oklahoma	3.6
45	Oregon	1.4
32	Pennsylvania	2.2
16	Rhode Island	3.0
16	South Carolina	3.0
49	South Dakota	0.4
23	Tennessee	2.8
2	Texas	4.2
30	Utah	2.3
11	Vermont	3.3
32	Virginia	2.2
41	Washington	1.9
24	West Virginia	2.7
37	Wisconsin	2.0
44	Wyoming	1.7

RANK ORDER

RANK	STATE	PERCENT
1	New York	5.0
2	Texas	4.2
3	Connecticut	3.9
4	Louisiana	3.8
4	Maine	3.8
6	Florida	3.7
7	Oklahoma	3.6
8	Delaware	3.5
8	Kentucky	3.5
10	North Carolina	3.4
11	Massachusetts	3.3
11	Mississippi	3.3
11	Vermont	3.3
14	Nevada	3.2
15	New Hampshire	3.1
16	Georgia	3.0
16	Rhode Island	3.0
16	South Carolina	3.0
19	Alabama	2.9
19	Arkansas	2.9
19	New Jersey	2.9
19	Ohio	2.9
23	Tennessee	2.8
24	Missouri	2.7
24	New Mexico	2.7
24	West Virginia	2.7
27	Colorado	2.4
27	Iowa	2.4
27	Michigan	2.4
30	Kansas	2.3
30	Utah	2.3
32	Arizona	2.2
32	Illinois	2.2
32	Pennsylvania	2.2
32	Virginia	2.2
36	Minnesota	2.1
37	Indiana	2.0
37	Maryland	2.0
37	Montana	2.0
37	Wisconsin	2.0
41	Washington	1.9
42	California	1.8
42	Idaho	1.8
44	Wyoming	1.7
45	Oregon	1.4
46	Hawaii	1.3
47	Nebraska	1.2
48	North Dakota	0.7
49	Alaska	0.4
49	South Dakota	0.4
	District of Columbia	1.3

Source: MQ Press using data from U.S. Dept of Health & Human Services, Centers for Medicare and Medicaid Services "State Health Care Expenditures" (http://www.hcfa.gov/stats/nhe-oact/stateestimates/)
*By state of provider. Includes spending for services and products by public and private freestanding home health agencies. Excludes home health care services provided by hospital-based agencies which are included in hospital expenditures.

Average Annual Change in Expenditures for Home Health Care: 1990 to 1998

National Percent Change = 10.5% Average Annual Increase*

ALPHA ORDER

RANK	STATE	PERCENT CHANGE
31	Alabama	10.8
4	Alaska	20.7
25	Arizona	12.3
14	Arkansas	15.0
33	California	10.5
17	Colorado	14.3
32	Connecticut	10.7
10	Delaware	17.2
30	Florida	11.3
28	Georgia	11.5
1	Hawaii	25.1
6	Idaho	18.9
34	Illinois	10.4
21	Indiana	13.8
20	Iowa	14.0
21	Kansas	13.8
13	Kentucky	15.2
2	Louisiana	21.3
16	Maine	14.4
39	Maryland	9.5
43	Massachusetts	8.5
50	Michigan	4.6
42	Minnesota	9.2
41	Mississippi	9.4
23	Missouri	13.6
46	Montana	7.7
36	Nebraska	10.1
7	Nevada	18.6
15	New Hampshire	14.5
38	New Jersey	9.6
5	New Mexico	20.1
49	New York	4.7
12	North Carolina	15.3
45	North Dakota	7.8
11	Ohio	15.7
8	Oklahoma	18.1
24	Oregon	13.2
37	Pennsylvania	9.9
28	Rhode Island	11.5
17	South Carolina	14.3
34	South Dakota	10.4
48	Tennessee	6.0
9	Texas	17.6
3	Utah	20.8
39	Vermont	9.5
26	Virginia	11.8
43	Washington	8.5
17	West Virginia	14.3
47	Wisconsin	6.8
27	Wyoming	11.6

RANK ORDER

RANK	STATE	PERCENT CHANGE
1	Hawaii	25.1
2	Louisiana	21.3
3	Utah	20.8
4	Alaska	20.7
5	New Mexico	20.1
6	Idaho	18.9
7	Nevada	18.6
8	Oklahoma	18.1
9	Texas	17.6
10	Delaware	17.2
11	Ohio	15.7
12	North Carolina	15.3
13	Kentucky	15.2
14	Arkansas	15.0
15	New Hampshire	14.5
16	Maine	14.4
17	Colorado	14.3
17	South Carolina	14.3
17	West Virginia	14.3
20	Iowa	14.0
21	Indiana	13.8
21	Kansas	13.8
23	Missouri	13.6
24	Oregon	13.2
25	Arizona	12.3
26	Virginia	11.8
27	Wyoming	11.6
28	Georgia	11.5
28	Rhode Island	11.5
30	Florida	11.3
31	Alabama	10.8
32	Connecticut	10.7
33	California	10.5
34	Illinois	10.4
34	South Dakota	10.4
36	Nebraska	10.1
37	Pennsylvania	9.9
38	New Jersey	9.6
39	Maryland	9.5
39	Vermont	9.5
41	Mississippi	9.4
42	Minnesota	9.2
43	Massachusetts	8.5
43	Washington	8.5
45	North Dakota	7.8
46	Montana	7.7
47	Wisconsin	6.8
48	Tennessee	6.0
49	New York	4.7
50	Michigan	4.6
	District of Columbia	6.0

Source: U.S. Department of Health and Human Services, Centers for Medicare and Medicaid Services
    "State Health Care Expenditures" (http://www.hcfa.gov/stats/nhe-oact/stateestimates/)
By state of provider. Includes spending for services and products by public and private freestanding home health agencies. Excludes home health care services provided by hospital-based agencies which are included in hospital expenditures.

Per Capita Expenditures for Home Health Care in 1998

National Per Capita = $108*

ALPHA ORDER			RANK ORDER		
RANK	STATE	PER CAPITA	RANK	STATE	PER CAPITA
18	Alabama	$108	1	New York	$236
49	Alaska	15	2	Connecticut	183
36	Arizona	71	3	Massachusetts	163
25	Arkansas	95	4	Maine	151
42	California	60	5	Florida	149
31	Colorado	82	6	Delaware	148
2	Connecticut	183	7	Texas	145
6	Delaware	148	8	Louisiana	144
5	Florida	149	9	Rhode Island	136
19	Georgia	106	10	Kentucky	129
43	Hawaii	50	11	North Carolina	124
45	Idaho	49	12	New Hampshire	122
33	Illinois	81	13	Oklahoma	117
38	Indiana	70	14	New Jersey	116
28	Iowa	87	15	Vermont	115
30	Kansas	83	16	Tennessee	114
10	Kentucky	129	17	Ohio	109
8	Louisiana	144	18	Alabama	108
4	Maine	151	19	Georgia	106
34	Maryland	76	19	Mississippi	106
3	Massachusetts	163	21	Missouri	104
29	Michigan	86	22	Nevada	103
27	Minnesota	89	22	West Virginia	103
19	Mississippi	106	24	South Carolina	102
21	Missouri	104	25	Arkansas	95
40	Montana	64	26	Pennsylvania	92
47	Nebraska	43	27	Minnesota	89
22	Nevada	103	28	Iowa	87
12	New Hampshire	122	29	Michigan	86
14	New Jersey	116	30	Kansas	83
31	New Mexico	82	31	Colorado	82
1	New York	236	31	New Mexico	82
11	North Carolina	124	33	Illinois	81
48	North Dakota	31	34	Maryland	76
17	Ohio	109	35	Wisconsin	75
13	Oklahoma	117	36	Arizona	71
46	Oregon	46	36	Virginia	71
26	Pennsylvania	92	38	Indiana	70
9	Rhode Island	136	39	Utah	65
24	South Carolina	102	40	Montana	64
49	South Dakota	15	40	Washington	64
16	Tennessee	114	42	California	60
7	Texas	145	43	Hawaii	50
39	Utah	65	43	Wyoming	50
15	Vermont	115	45	Idaho	49
36	Virginia	71	46	Oregon	46
40	Washington	64	47	Nebraska	43
22	West Virginia	103	48	North Dakota	31
35	Wisconsin	75	49	Alaska	15
43	Wyoming	50	49	South Dakota	15
				District of Columbia	104

Source: MQ Press using data from U.S. Dept of Health & Human Services, Centers for Medicare and Medicaid Services "State Health Care Expenditures" (http://www.hcfa.gov/stats/nhe-oact/stateestimates/)
*By state of provider. Includes spending for services and products by public and private freestanding home health agencies. Excludes home health care services provided by hospital-based agencies which are included in hospital expenditures.

Expenditures for Drugs and Other Medical Non-Durables in 1998
National Total = $121,906,000,000*

ALPHA ORDER

RANK	STATE	EXPENDITURES	% of USA
21	Alabama	$2,049,000,000	1.7%
49	Alaska	221,000,000	0.2%
20	Arizona	2,066,000,000	1.7%
32	Arkansas	1,177,000,000	1.0%
1	California	11,604,000,000	9.5%
27	Colorado	1,546,000,000	1.3%
26	Connecticut	1,705,000,000	1.4%
44	Delaware	390,000,000	0.3%
4	Florida	8,226,000,000	6.7%
11	Georgia	3,367,000,000	2.8%
41	Hawaii	514,000,000	0.4%
43	Idaho	474,000,000	0.4%
6	Illinois	5,174,000,000	4.2%
15	Indiana	2,649,000,000	2.2%
31	Iowa	1,219,000,000	1.0%
33	Kansas	1,087,000,000	0.9%
24	Kentucky	1,966,000,000	1.6%
23	Louisiana	1,992,000,000	1.6%
39	Maine	559,000,000	0.5%
18	Maryland	2,304,000,000	1.9%
13	Massachusetts	2,882,000,000	2.4%
8	Michigan	4,884,000,000	4.0%
22	Minnesota	2,004,000,000	1.6%
30	Mississippi	1,222,000,000	1.0%
16	Missouri	2,403,000,000	2.0%
45	Montana	349,000,000	0.3%
37	Nebraska	791,000,000	0.6%
36	Nevada	825,000,000	0.7%
40	New Hampshire	539,000,000	0.4%
9	New Jersey	4,564,000,000	3.7%
38	New Mexico	630,000,000	0.5%
2	New York	8,940,000,000	7.3%
10	North Carolina	3,411,000,000	2.8%
47	North Dakota	250,000,000	0.2%
7	Ohio	5,027,000,000	4.1%
28	Oklahoma	1,418,000,000	1.2%
29	Oregon	1,386,000,000	1.1%
5	Pennsylvania	6,162,000,000	5.1%
42	Rhode Island	505,000,000	0.4%
25	South Carolina	1,721,000,000	1.4%
46	South Dakota	268,000,000	0.2%
14	Tennessee	2,751,000,000	2.3%
3	Texas	8,672,000,000	7.1%
35	Utah	828,000,000	0.7%
48	Vermont	237,000,000	0.2%
12	Virginia	2,947,000,000	2.4%
17	Washington	2,365,000,000	1.9%
34	West Virginia	949,000,000	0.8%
19	Wisconsin	2,269,000,000	1.9%
50	Wyoming	178,000,000	0.1%

RANK ORDER

RANK	STATE	EXPENDITURES	% of USA
1	California	$11,604,000,000	9.5%
2	New York	8,940,000,000	7.3%
3	Texas	8,672,000,000	7.1%
4	Florida	8,226,000,000	6.7%
5	Pennsylvania	6,162,000,000	5.1%
6	Illinois	5,174,000,000	4.2%
7	Ohio	5,027,000,000	4.1%
8	Michigan	4,884,000,000	4.0%
9	New Jersey	4,564,000,000	3.7%
10	North Carolina	3,411,000,000	2.8%
11	Georgia	3,367,000,000	2.8%
12	Virginia	2,947,000,000	2.4%
13	Massachusetts	2,882,000,000	2.4%
14	Tennessee	2,751,000,000	2.3%
15	Indiana	2,649,000,000	2.2%
16	Missouri	2,403,000,000	2.0%
17	Washington	2,365,000,000	1.9%
18	Maryland	2,304,000,000	1.9%
19	Wisconsin	2,269,000,000	1.9%
20	Arizona	2,066,000,000	1.7%
21	Alabama	2,049,000,000	1.7%
22	Minnesota	2,004,000,000	1.6%
23	Louisiana	1,992,000,000	1.6%
24	Kentucky	1,966,000,000	1.6%
25	South Carolina	1,721,000,000	1.4%
26	Connecticut	1,705,000,000	1.4%
27	Colorado	1,546,000,000	1.3%
28	Oklahoma	1,418,000,000	1.2%
29	Oregon	1,386,000,000	1.1%
30	Mississippi	1,222,000,000	1.0%
31	Iowa	1,219,000,000	1.0%
32	Arkansas	1,177,000,000	1.0%
33	Kansas	1,087,000,000	0.9%
34	West Virginia	949,000,000	0.8%
35	Utah	828,000,000	0.7%
36	Nevada	825,000,000	0.7%
37	Nebraska	791,000,000	0.6%
38	New Mexico	630,000,000	0.5%
39	Maine	559,000,000	0.5%
40	New Hampshire	539,000,000	0.4%
41	Hawaii	514,000,000	0.4%
42	Rhode Island	505,000,000	0.4%
43	Idaho	474,000,000	0.4%
44	Delaware	390,000,000	0.3%
45	Montana	349,000,000	0.3%
46	South Dakota	268,000,000	0.2%
47	North Dakota	250,000,000	0.2%
48	Vermont	237,000,000	0.2%
49	Alaska	221,000,000	0.2%
50	Wyoming	178,000,000	0.1%
	District of Columbia	239,000,000	0.2%

Source: U.S. Department of Health and Human Services, Centers for Medicare and Medicaid Services
"State Health Care Expenditures" (http://www.hcfa.gov/stats/nhe-oact/stateestimates/)
*Purchases in retail outlets. By state of outlet. Includes prescription drugs, over-the-counter drugs and sundries.

Percent of Total Personal Health Care Expenditures
Spent on Drugs and Other Medical Non-Durables in 1998
National Percent = 12.0%*

ALPHA ORDER

RANK ORDER

RANK	STATE	PERCENT	RANK	STATE	PERCENT
16	Alabama	12.8	1	Nevada	14.7
47	Alaska	9.6	2	Arizona	14.0
2	Arizona	14.0	2	Idaho	14.0
5	Arkansas	13.9	2	New Jersey	14.0
44	California	10.5	5	Arkansas	13.9
40	Colorado	11.3	5	Utah	13.9
41	Connecticut	11.2	7	Florida	13.8
20	Delaware	12.6	7	Mississippi	13.8
7	Florida	13.8	9	Michigan	13.7
24	Georgia	12.4	10	Kentucky	13.6
43	Hawaii	11.0	11	West Virginia	13.5
2	Idaho	14.0	12	Virginia	13.2
32	Illinois	11.7	13	Nebraska	13.0
21	Indiana	12.5	13	South Carolina	13.0
28	Iowa	12.0	15	Oklahoma	12.9
34	Kansas	11.6	16	Alabama	12.8
10	Kentucky	13.6	16	Oregon	12.8
27	Louisiana	12.1	16	Texas	12.8
38	Maine	11.4	19	Wyoming	12.7
32	Maryland	11.7	20	Delaware	12.6
47	Massachusetts	9.6	21	Indiana	12.5
9	Michigan	13.7	21	North Carolina	12.5
46	Minnesota	9.9	21	Tennessee	12.5
7	Mississippi	13.8	24	Georgia	12.4
36	Missouri	11.5	25	Montana	12.3
25	Montana	12.3	25	Washington	12.3
13	Nebraska	13.0	27	Louisiana	12.1
1	Nevada	14.7	28	Iowa	12.0
34	New Hampshire	11.6	28	Pennsylvania	12.0
2	New Jersey	14.0	30	New Mexico	11.8
30	New Mexico	11.8	30	Ohio	11.8
45	New York	10.4	32	Illinois	11.7
21	North Carolina	12.5	32	Maryland	11.7
50	North Dakota	9.3	34	Kansas	11.6
30	Ohio	11.8	34	New Hampshire	11.6
15	Oklahoma	12.9	36	Missouri	11.5
16	Oregon	12.8	36	Vermont	11.5
28	Pennsylvania	12.0	38	Maine	11.4
41	Rhode Island	11.2	38	Wisconsin	11.4
13	South Carolina	13.0	40	Colorado	11.3
49	South Dakota	9.4	41	Connecticut	11.2
21	Tennessee	12.5	41	Rhode Island	11.2
16	Texas	12.8	43	Hawaii	11.0
5	Utah	13.9	44	California	10.5
36	Vermont	11.5	45	New York	10.4
12	Virginia	13.2	46	Minnesota	9.9
25	Washington	12.3	47	Alaska	9.6
11	West Virginia	13.5	47	Massachusetts	9.6
38	Wisconsin	11.4	49	South Dakota	9.4
19	Wyoming	12.7	50	North Dakota	9.3

	District of Columbia	5.6

Source: MQ Press using data from U.S. Dept of Health & Human Services, Centers for Medicare and Medicaid Services
"State Health Care Expenditures" (http://www.hcfa.gov/stats/nhe-oact/stateestimates/)
*Purchases in retail outlets. By state of outlet. Includes prescription drugs, over-the-counter drugs and sundries.

Average Annual Change in Expenditures for Drugs and Other Medical Non-Durables: 1990 to 1998
National Percent Change = 9.3% Average Annual Increase*

ALPHA ORDER

RANK	STATE	PERCENT CHANGE
23	Alabama	9.3
47	Alaska	8.0
3	Arizona	11.4
20	Arkansas	9.5
49	California	7.1
8	Colorado	10.4
29	Connecticut	9.1
3	Delaware	11.4
2	Florida	11.6
12	Georgia	10.2
50	Hawaii	5.6
5	Idaho	10.6
40	Illinois	8.5
31	Indiana	8.9
31	Iowa	8.9
39	Kansas	8.6
17	Kentucky	9.6
44	Louisiana	8.2
8	Maine	10.4
44	Maryland	8.2
37	Massachusetts	8.8
23	Michigan	9.3
14	Minnesota	10.0
23	Mississippi	9.3
37	Missouri	8.8
27	Montana	9.2
13	Nebraska	10.1
1	Nevada	14.3
27	New Hampshire	9.2
16	New Jersey	9.9
31	New Mexico	8.9
22	New York	9.4
8	North Carolina	10.4
48	North Dakota	7.6
40	Ohio	8.5
31	Oklahoma	8.9
5	Oregon	10.6
20	Pennsylvania	9.5
40	Rhode Island	8.5
5	South Carolina	10.6
40	South Dakota	8.5
14	Tennessee	10.0
17	Texas	9.6
11	Utah	10.3
31	Vermont	8.9
31	Virginia	8.9
23	Washington	9.3
30	West Virginia	9.0
17	Wisconsin	9.6
44	Wyoming	8.2

RANK ORDER

RANK	STATE	PERCENT CHANGE
1	Nevada	14.3
2	Florida	11.6
3	Arizona	11.4
3	Delaware	11.4
5	Idaho	10.6
5	Oregon	10.6
5	South Carolina	10.6
8	Colorado	10.4
8	Maine	10.4
8	North Carolina	10.4
11	Utah	10.3
12	Georgia	10.2
13	Nebraska	10.1
14	Minnesota	10.0
14	Tennessee	10.0
16	New Jersey	9.9
17	Kentucky	9.6
17	Texas	9.6
17	Wisconsin	9.6
20	Arkansas	9.5
20	Pennsylvania	9.5
22	New York	9.4
23	Alabama	9.3
23	Michigan	9.3
23	Mississippi	9.3
23	Washington	9.3
27	Montana	9.2
27	New Hampshire	9.2
29	Connecticut	9.1
30	West Virginia	9.0
31	Indiana	8.9
31	Iowa	8.9
31	New Mexico	8.9
31	Oklahoma	8.9
31	Vermont	8.9
31	Virginia	8.9
37	Massachusetts	8.8
37	Missouri	8.8
39	Kansas	8.6
40	Illinois	8.5
40	Ohio	8.5
40	Rhode Island	8.5
40	South Dakota	8.5
44	Louisiana	8.2
44	Maryland	8.2
44	Wyoming	8.2
47	Alaska	8.0
48	North Dakota	7.6
49	California	7.1
50	Hawaii	5.6
	District of Columbia	6.5

Source: U.S. Department of Health and Human Services, Centers for Medicare and Medicaid Services
  "State Health Care Expenditures" (http://www.hcfa.gov/stats/nhe-oact/stateestimates/)
*Purchases in retail outlets. By state of outlet. Includes prescription drugs, over-the-counter drugs and sundries.

Per Capita Expenditures for Drugs and Other Medical Non-Durables in 1998
National Per Capita = $451*

ALPHA ORDER

RANK	STATE	PER CAPITA
14	Alabama	$471
49	Alaska	359
26	Arizona	443
16	Arkansas	464
50	California	355
44	Colorado	390
5	Connecticut	521
3	Delaware	524
2	Florida	552
28	Georgia	441
32	Hawaii	432
45	Idaho	385
33	Illinois	429
21	Indiana	448
34	Iowa	426
39	Kansas	412
9	Kentucky	500
17	Louisiana	457
21	Maine	448
20	Maryland	449
15	Massachusetts	469
10	Michigan	497
36	Minnesota	424
25	Mississippi	444
27	Missouri	442
41	Montana	397
12	Nebraska	476
13	Nevada	473
18	New Hampshire	455
1	New Jersey	564
48	New Mexico	363
11	New York	492
19	North Carolina	452
43	North Dakota	392
24	Ohio	447
35	Oklahoma	425
37	Oregon	422
6	Pennsylvania	513
7	Rhode Island	511
21	South Carolina	448
47	South Dakota	367
8	Tennessee	506
29	Texas	440
42	Utah	394
40	Vermont	401
30	Virginia	434
38	Washington	416
3	West Virginia	524
30	Wisconsin	434
46	Wyoming	371

RANK ORDER

RANK	STATE	PER CAPITA
1	New Jersey	$564
2	Florida	552
3	Delaware	524
3	West Virginia	524
5	Connecticut	521
6	Pennsylvania	513
7	Rhode Island	511
8	Tennessee	506
9	Kentucky	500
10	Michigan	497
11	New York	492
12	Nebraska	476
13	Nevada	473
14	Alabama	471
15	Massachusetts	469
16	Arkansas	464
17	Louisiana	457
18	New Hampshire	455
19	North Carolina	452
20	Maryland	449
21	Indiana	448
21	Maine	448
21	South Carolina	448
24	Ohio	447
25	Mississippi	444
26	Arizona	443
27	Missouri	442
28	Georgia	441
29	Texas	440
30	Virginia	434
30	Wisconsin	434
32	Hawaii	432
33	Illinois	429
34	Iowa	426
35	Oklahoma	425
36	Minnesota	424
37	Oregon	422
38	Washington	416
39	Kansas	412
40	Vermont	401
41	Montana	397
42	Utah	394
43	North Dakota	392
44	Colorado	390
45	Idaho	385
46	Wyoming	371
47	South Dakota	367
48	New Mexico	363
49	Alaska	359
50	California	355
	District of Columbia	458

Source: MQ Press using data from U.S. Dept of Health & Human Services, Centers for Medicare and Medicaid Services
    "State Health Care Expenditures" (http://www.hcfa.gov/stats/nhe-oact/stateestimates/)
*Purchases in retail outlets. By state of outlet. Includes prescription drugs, over-the-counter drugs and sundries.
Per capita calculated using resident population. These figures may be skewed due to residents crossing state
borders to make purchases.

Expenditures for Vision Products and Other Medical Durables in 1998

National Total = $15,499,000,000*

ALPHA ORDER

RANK	STATE	EXPENDITURES	% of USA
25	Alabama	$186,000,000	1.2%
46	Alaska	38,000,000	0.2%
22	Arizona	267,000,000	1.7%
36	Arkansas	87,000,000	0.6%
1	California	1,656,000,000	10.7%
18	Colorado	323,000,000	2.1%
23	Connecticut	231,000,000	1.5%
43	Delaware	49,000,000	0.3%
2	Florida	1,184,000,000	7.6%
10	Georgia	432,000,000	2.8%
38	Hawaii	78,000,000	0.5%
41	Idaho	59,000,000	0.4%
6	Illinois	662,000,000	4.3%
17	Indiana	328,000,000	2.1%
27	Iowa	177,000,000	1.1%
31	Kansas	128,000,000	0.8%
26	Kentucky	185,000,000	1.2%
24	Louisiana	198,000,000	1.3%
42	Maine	58,000,000	0.4%
19	Maryland	322,000,000	2.1%
12	Massachusetts	347,000,000	2.2%
8	Michigan	626,000,000	4.0%
14	Minnesota	343,000,000	2.2%
35	Mississippi	93,000,000	0.6%
20	Missouri	280,000,000	1.8%
44	Montana	41,000,000	0.3%
34	Nebraska	119,000,000	0.8%
32	Nevada	123,000,000	0.8%
40	New Hampshire	68,000,000	0.4%
9	New Jersey	552,000,000	3.6%
39	New Mexico	77,000,000	0.5%
4	New York	1,099,000,000	7.1%
15	North Carolina	338,000,000	2.2%
47	North Dakota	35,000,000	0.2%
7	Ohio	647,000,000	4.2%
30	Oklahoma	142,000,000	0.9%
28	Oregon	169,000,000	1.1%
5	Pennsylvania	688,000,000	4.4%
47	Rhode Island	35,000,000	0.2%
29	South Carolina	168,000,000	1.1%
45	South Dakota	40,000,000	0.3%
21	Tennessee	271,000,000	1.7%
3	Texas	1,176,000,000	7.6%
33	Utah	121,000,000	0.8%
49	Vermont	29,000,000	0.2%
11	Virginia	392,000,000	2.5%
13	Washington	346,000,000	2.2%
36	West Virginia	87,000,000	0.6%
16	Wisconsin	333,000,000	2.1%
50	Wyoming	22,000,000	0.1%

RANK ORDER

RANK	STATE	EXPENDITURES	% of USA
1	California	$1,656,000,000	10.7%
2	Florida	1,184,000,000	7.6%
3	Texas	1,176,000,000	7.6%
4	New York	1,099,000,000	7.1%
5	Pennsylvania	688,000,000	4.4%
6	Illinois	662,000,000	4.3%
7	Ohio	647,000,000	4.2%
8	Michigan	626,000,000	4.0%
9	New Jersey	552,000,000	3.6%
10	Georgia	432,000,000	2.8%
11	Virginia	392,000,000	2.5%
12	Massachusetts	347,000,000	2.2%
13	Washington	346,000,000	2.2%
14	Minnesota	343,000,000	2.2%
15	North Carolina	338,000,000	2.2%
16	Wisconsin	333,000,000	2.1%
17	Indiana	328,000,000	2.1%
18	Colorado	323,000,000	2.1%
19	Maryland	322,000,000	2.1%
20	Missouri	280,000,000	1.8%
21	Tennessee	271,000,000	1.7%
22	Arizona	267,000,000	1.7%
23	Connecticut	231,000,000	1.5%
24	Louisiana	198,000,000	1.3%
25	Alabama	186,000,000	1.2%
26	Kentucky	185,000,000	1.2%
27	Iowa	177,000,000	1.1%
28	Oregon	169,000,000	1.1%
29	South Carolina	168,000,000	1.1%
30	Oklahoma	142,000,000	0.9%
31	Kansas	128,000,000	0.8%
32	Nevada	123,000,000	0.8%
33	Utah	121,000,000	0.8%
34	Nebraska	119,000,000	0.8%
35	Mississippi	93,000,000	0.6%
36	Arkansas	87,000,000	0.6%
36	West Virginia	87,000,000	0.6%
38	Hawaii	78,000,000	0.5%
39	New Mexico	77,000,000	0.5%
40	New Hampshire	68,000,000	0.4%
41	Idaho	59,000,000	0.4%
42	Maine	58,000,000	0.4%
43	Delaware	49,000,000	0.3%
44	Montana	41,000,000	0.3%
45	South Dakota	40,000,000	0.3%
46	Alaska	38,000,000	0.2%
47	North Dakota	35,000,000	0.2%
47	Rhode Island	35,000,000	0.2%
49	Vermont	29,000,000	0.2%
50	Wyoming	22,000,000	0.1%
	District of Columbia	42,000,000	0.3%

Source: U.S. Department of Health and Human Services, Centers for Medicare and Medicaid Services
    "State Health Care Expenditures" (http://www.hcfa.gov/stats/nhe-oact/stateestimates/)
*By state of provider. Includes eyeglasses, hearing aids, surgical appliances and supplies, bulk and cylinder oxygen and medical equipment rentals.

Percent of Total Personal Health Care Expenditures
Spent on Vision Products and Other Medical Durables in 1998
National Percent = 1.5%*

ALPHA ORDER

RANK	STATE	PERCENT
41	Alabama	1.2
10	Alaska	1.7
6	Arizona	1.8
48	Arkansas	1.0
23	California	1.5
1	Colorado	2.4
23	Connecticut	1.5
18	Delaware	1.6
3	Florida	2.0
18	Georgia	1.6
10	Hawaii	1.7
10	Idaho	1.7
23	Illinois	1.5
23	Indiana	1.5
10	Iowa	1.7
29	Kansas	1.4
34	Kentucky	1.3
41	Louisiana	1.2
41	Maine	1.2
18	Maryland	1.6
41	Massachusetts	1.2
6	Michigan	1.8
10	Minnesota	1.7
48	Mississippi	1.0
34	Missouri	1.3
29	Montana	1.4
3	Nebraska	2.0
2	Nevada	2.2
23	New Hampshire	1.5
10	New Jersey	1.7
29	New Mexico	1.4
34	New York	1.3
41	North Carolina	1.2
34	North Dakota	1.3
23	Ohio	1.5
34	Oklahoma	1.3
18	Oregon	1.6
34	Pennsylvania	1.3
50	Rhode Island	0.8
34	South Carolina	1.3
29	South Dakota	1.4
41	Tennessee	1.2
10	Texas	1.7
3	Utah	2.0
29	Vermont	1.4
6	Virginia	1.8
6	Washington	1.8
41	West Virginia	1.2
10	Wisconsin	1.7
18	Wyoming	1.6

RANK ORDER

RANK	STATE	PERCENT
1	Colorado	2.4
2	Nevada	2.2
3	Florida	2.0
3	Nebraska	2.0
3	Utah	2.0
6	Arizona	1.8
6	Michigan	1.8
6	Virginia	1.8
6	Washington	1.8
10	Alaska	1.7
10	Hawaii	1.7
10	Idaho	1.7
10	Iowa	1.7
10	Minnesota	1.7
10	New Jersey	1.7
10	Texas	1.7
10	Wisconsin	1.7
18	Delaware	1.6
18	Georgia	1.6
18	Maryland	1.6
18	Oregon	1.6
18	Wyoming	1.6
23	California	1.5
23	Connecticut	1.5
23	Illinois	1.5
23	Indiana	1.5
23	New Hampshire	1.5
23	Ohio	1.5
29	Kansas	1.4
29	Montana	1.4
29	New Mexico	1.4
29	South Dakota	1.4
29	Vermont	1.4
34	Kentucky	1.3
34	Missouri	1.3
34	New York	1.3
34	North Dakota	1.3
34	Oklahoma	1.3
34	Pennsylvania	1.3
34	South Carolina	1.3
41	Alabama	1.2
41	Louisiana	1.2
41	Maine	1.2
41	Massachusetts	1.2
41	North Carolina	1.2
41	Tennessee	1.2
41	West Virginia	1.2
48	Arkansas	1.0
48	Mississippi	1.0
50	Rhode Island	0.8

| | District of Columbia | 1.0 |

Source: MQ Press using data from U.S. Dept of Health & Human Services, Centers for Medicare and Medicaid Services
"State Health Care Expenditures" (http://www.hcfa.gov/stats/nhe-oact/stateestimates/)
*By state of provider. Includes eyeglasses, hearing aids, surgical appliances and supplies, bulk and cylinder oxygen and medical equipment rentals.

Average Annual Change in Expenditures for Vision Products and Other Medical Durables: 1990 to 1998
National Percent Change = 5.0% Average Annual Increase*

ALPHA ORDER

RANK	STATE	PERCENT CHANGE
22	Alabama	5.2
19	Alaska	5.4
8	Arizona	6.4
16	Arkansas	5.9
45	California	4.0
2	Colorado	7.5
38	Connecticut	4.3
10	Delaware	6.3
10	Florida	6.3
8	Georgia	6.4
41	Hawaii	4.2
2	Idaho	7.5
41	Illinois	4.2
31	Indiana	4.7
38	Iowa	4.3
33	Kansas	4.5
17	Kentucky	5.6
27	Louisiana	4.9
43	Maine	4.1
32	Maryland	4.6
29	Massachusetts	4.8
22	Michigan	5.2
22	Minnesota	5.2
6	Mississippi	6.5
35	Missouri	4.4
45	Montana	4.0
27	Nebraska	4.9
1	Nevada	8.9
13	New Hampshire	6.2
33	New Jersey	4.5
25	New Mexico	5.0
49	New York	3.4
15	North Carolina	6.0
38	North Dakota	4.3
35	Ohio	4.4
35	Oklahoma	4.4
4	Oregon	7.0
47	Pennsylvania	3.9
50	Rhode Island	3.3
13	South Carolina	6.2
25	South Dakota	5.0
21	Tennessee	5.3
10	Texas	6.3
6	Utah	6.5
29	Vermont	4.8
17	Virginia	5.6
5	Washington	6.6
48	West Virginia	3.7
19	Wisconsin	5.4
43	Wyoming	4.1

RANK ORDER

RANK	STATE	PERCENT CHANGE
1	Nevada	8.9
2	Colorado	7.5
2	Idaho	7.5
4	Oregon	7.0
5	Washington	6.6
6	Mississippi	6.5
6	Utah	6.5
8	Arizona	6.4
8	Georgia	6.4
10	Delaware	6.3
10	Florida	6.3
10	Texas	6.3
13	New Hampshire	6.2
13	South Carolina	6.2
15	North Carolina	6.0
16	Arkansas	5.9
17	Kentucky	5.6
17	Virginia	5.6
19	Alaska	5.4
19	Wisconsin	5.4
21	Tennessee	5.3
22	Alabama	5.2
22	Michigan	5.2
22	Minnesota	5.2
25	New Mexico	5.0
25	South Dakota	5.0
27	Louisiana	4.9
27	Nebraska	4.9
29	Massachusetts	4.8
29	Vermont	4.8
31	Indiana	4.7
32	Maryland	4.6
33	Kansas	4.5
33	New Jersey	4.5
35	Missouri	4.4
35	Ohio	4.4
35	Oklahoma	4.4
38	Connecticut	4.3
38	Iowa	4.3
38	North Dakota	4.3
41	Hawaii	4.2
41	Illinois	4.2
43	Maine	4.1
43	Wyoming	4.1
45	California	4.0
45	Montana	4.0
47	Pennsylvania	3.9
48	West Virginia	3.7
49	New York	3.4
50	Rhode Island	3.3
	District of Columbia	3.5

Source: U.S. Department of Health and Human Services, Centers for Medicare and Medicaid Services
"State Health Care Expenditures" (http://www.hcfa.gov/stats/nhe-oact/stateestimates/)
*By state of provider. Includes eyeglasses, hearing aids, surgical appliances and supplies, bulk and cylinder oxygen and medical equipment rentals.

Per Capita Expenditures for Vision Products and Other Medical Durables in 1998

National Per Capita = $57*

ALPHA ORDER

RANK	STATE	PER CAPITA
46	Alabama	$43
13	Alaska	62
21	Arizona	57
49	Arkansas	34
30	California	51
1	Colorado	81
5	Connecticut	71
8	Delaware	66
2	Florida	79
21	Georgia	57
8	Hawaii	66
36	Idaho	48
27	Illinois	55
25	Indiana	56
13	Iowa	62
34	Kansas	49
38	Kentucky	47
42	Louisiana	45
40	Maine	46
12	Maryland	63
25	Massachusetts	56
10	Michigan	64
3	Minnesota	73
49	Mississippi	34
30	Missouri	51
38	Montana	47
4	Nebraska	72
5	Nevada	71
21	New Hampshire	57
7	New Jersey	68
44	New Mexico	44
15	New York	61
42	North Carolina	45
27	North Dakota	55
18	Ohio	58
46	Oklahoma	43
30	Oregon	51
21	Pennsylvania	57
48	Rhode Island	35
44	South Carolina	44
27	South Dakota	55
33	Tennessee	50
17	Texas	60
18	Utah	58
34	Vermont	49
18	Virginia	58
15	Washington	61
36	West Virginia	48
10	Wisconsin	64
40	Wyoming	46

RANK ORDER

RANK	STATE	PER CAPITA
1	Colorado	$81
2	Florida	79
3	Minnesota	73
4	Nebraska	72
5	Connecticut	71
5	Nevada	71
7	New Jersey	68
8	Delaware	66
8	Hawaii	66
10	Michigan	64
10	Wisconsin	64
12	Maryland	63
13	Alaska	62
13	Iowa	62
15	New York	61
15	Washington	61
17	Texas	60
18	Ohio	58
18	Utah	58
18	Virginia	58
21	Arizona	57
21	Georgia	57
21	New Hampshire	57
21	Pennsylvania	57
25	Indiana	56
25	Massachusetts	56
27	Illinois	55
27	North Dakota	55
27	South Dakota	55
30	California	51
30	Missouri	51
30	Oregon	51
33	Tennessee	50
34	Kansas	49
34	Vermont	49
36	Idaho	48
36	West Virginia	48
38	Kentucky	47
38	Montana	47
40	Maine	46
40	Wyoming	46
42	Louisiana	45
42	North Carolina	45
44	New Mexico	44
44	South Carolina	44
46	Alabama	43
46	Oklahoma	43
48	Rhode Island	35
49	Arkansas	34
49	Mississippi	34
	District of Columbia	81

Source: MQ Press using data from U.S. Dept of Health & Human Services, Centers for Medicare and Medicaid Services "State Health Care Expenditures" (http://www.hcfa.gov/stats/nhe-oact/stateestimates/)

*By state of provider. Includes eyeglasses, hearing aids, surgical appliances and supplies, bulk and cylinder oxygen and medical equipment rentals.

Expenditures for Nursing Home Care in 1998

National Total = $87,826,000,000*

ALPHA ORDER

RANK	STATE	EXPENDITURES	% of USA
25	Alabama	$1,064,000,000	1.2%
50	Alaska	42,000,000	0.0%
30	Arizona	839,000,000	1.0%
32	Arkansas	776,000,000	0.9%
3	California	5,626,000,000	6.4%
29	Colorado	904,000,000	1.0%
13	Connecticut	2,264,000,000	2.6%
40	Delaware	290,000,000	0.3%
5	Florida	4,880,000,000	5.6%
20	Georgia	1,545,000,000	1.8%
46	Hawaii	204,000,000	0.2%
43	Idaho	264,000,000	0.3%
7	Illinois	3,924,000,000	4.5%
12	Indiana	2,337,000,000	2.7%
24	Iowa	1,186,000,000	1.4%
27	Kansas	920,000,000	1.0%
22	Kentucky	1,283,000,000	1.5%
23	Louisiana	1,248,000,000	1.4%
36	Maine	476,000,000	0.5%
18	Maryland	1,695,000,000	1.9%
8	Massachusetts	3,568,000,000	4.1%
10	Michigan	2,459,000,000	2.8%
17	Minnesota	1,964,000,000	2.2%
34	Mississippi	687,000,000	0.8%
15	Missouri	2,002,000,000	2.3%
45	Montana	222,000,000	0.3%
33	Nebraska	697,000,000	0.8%
48	Nevada	164,000,000	0.2%
38	New Hampshire	425,000,000	0.5%
9	New Jersey	3,233,000,000	3.7%
44	New Mexico	257,000,000	0.3%
1	New York	10,586,000,000	12.1%
11	North Carolina	2,347,000,000	2.7%
41	North Dakota	287,000,000	0.3%
4	Ohio	4,978,000,000	5.7%
26	Oklahoma	954,000,000	1.1%
31	Oregon	838,000,000	1.0%
2	Pennsylvania	5,883,000,000	6.7%
37	Rhode Island	468,000,000	0.5%
28	South Carolina	907,000,000	1.0%
42	South Dakota	286,000,000	0.3%
16	Tennessee	2,001,000,000	2.3%
6	Texas	4,346,000,000	4.9%
39	Utah	300,000,000	0.3%
47	Vermont	177,000,000	0.2%
19	Virginia	1,546,000,000	1.8%
21	Washington	1,492,000,000	1.7%
35	West Virginia	515,000,000	0.6%
14	Wisconsin	2,110,000,000	2.4%
49	Wyoming	113,000,000	0.1%

RANK ORDER

RANK	STATE	EXPENDITURES	% of USA
1	New York	$10,586,000,000	12.1%
2	Pennsylvania	5,883,000,000	6.7%
3	California	5,626,000,000	6.4%
4	Ohio	4,978,000,000	5.7%
5	Florida	4,880,000,000	5.6%
6	Texas	4,346,000,000	4.9%
7	Illinois	3,924,000,000	4.5%
8	Massachusetts	3,568,000,000	4.1%
9	New Jersey	3,233,000,000	3.7%
10	Michigan	2,459,000,000	2.8%
11	North Carolina	2,347,000,000	2.7%
12	Indiana	2,337,000,000	2.7%
13	Connecticut	2,264,000,000	2.6%
14	Wisconsin	2,110,000,000	2.4%
15	Missouri	2,002,000,000	2.3%
16	Tennessee	2,001,000,000	2.3%
17	Minnesota	1,964,000,000	2.2%
18	Maryland	1,695,000,000	1.9%
19	Virginia	1,546,000,000	1.8%
20	Georgia	1,545,000,000	1.8%
21	Washington	1,492,000,000	1.7%
22	Kentucky	1,283,000,000	1.5%
23	Louisiana	1,248,000,000	1.4%
24	Iowa	1,186,000,000	1.4%
25	Alabama	1,064,000,000	1.2%
26	Oklahoma	954,000,000	1.1%
27	Kansas	920,000,000	1.0%
28	South Carolina	907,000,000	1.0%
29	Colorado	904,000,000	1.0%
30	Arizona	839,000,000	1.0%
31	Oregon	838,000,000	1.0%
32	Arkansas	776,000,000	0.9%
33	Nebraska	697,000,000	0.8%
34	Mississippi	687,000,000	0.8%
35	West Virginia	515,000,000	0.6%
36	Maine	476,000,000	0.5%
37	Rhode Island	468,000,000	0.5%
38	New Hampshire	425,000,000	0.5%
39	Utah	300,000,000	0.3%
40	Delaware	290,000,000	0.3%
41	North Dakota	287,000,000	0.3%
42	South Dakota	286,000,000	0.3%
43	Idaho	264,000,000	0.3%
44	New Mexico	257,000,000	0.3%
45	Montana	222,000,000	0.3%
46	Hawaii	204,000,000	0.2%
47	Vermont	177,000,000	0.2%
48	Nevada	164,000,000	0.2%
49	Wyoming	113,000,000	0.1%
50	Alaska	42,000,000	0.0%
	District of Columbia	245,000,000	0.3%

Source: U.S. Department of Health and Human Services, Centers for Medicare and Medicaid Services
"State Health Care Expenditures" (http://www.hcfa.gov/stats/nhe-oact/stateestimates/)
By state of provider. Includes freestanding nursing and personal-care facilities. Includes Medicare- and Medicaid-certified skilled nursing and intermediate care facilities as well as facilities that are not certified. Excludes hospital-based facilities as they are counted in hospital care expenditures.

Percent of Total Personal Health Care Expenditures
Spent on Nursing Home Care in 1998
National Percent = 8.6%*

ALPHA ORDER

RANK	STATE	PERCENT
40	Alabama	6.6
50	Alaska	1.8
43	Arizona	5.7
19	Arkansas	9.2
45	California	5.1
40	Colorado	6.6
1	Connecticut	14.9
18	Delaware	9.3
28	Florida	8.2
43	Georgia	5.7
48	Hawaii	4.4
30	Idaho	7.8
22	Illinois	8.9
8	Indiana	11.0
5	Iowa	11.6
14	Kansas	9.8
22	Kentucky	8.9
35	Louisiana	7.6
15	Maine	9.7
25	Maryland	8.6
3	Massachusetts	11.9
37	Michigan	6.9
15	Minnesota	9.7
32	Mississippi	7.7
17	Missouri	9.6
30	Montana	7.8
7	Nebraska	11.4
49	Nevada	2.9
20	New Hampshire	9.1
13	New Jersey	9.9
47	New Mexico	4.8
2	New York	12.3
25	North Carolina	8.6
9	North Dakota	10.7
4	Ohio	11.7
24	Oklahoma	8.7
32	Oregon	7.7
6	Pennsylvania	11.5
11	Rhode Island	10.4
37	South Carolina	6.9
12	South Dakota	10.1
20	Tennessee	9.1
42	Texas	6.4
46	Utah	5.0
25	Vermont	8.6
37	Virginia	6.9
32	Washington	7.7
36	West Virginia	7.3
10	Wisconsin	10.6
29	Wyoming	8.0

RANK ORDER

RANK	STATE	PERCENT
1	Connecticut	14.9
2	New York	12.3
3	Massachusetts	11.9
4	Ohio	11.7
5	Iowa	11.6
6	Pennsylvania	11.5
7	Nebraska	11.4
8	Indiana	11.0
9	North Dakota	10.7
10	Wisconsin	10.6
11	Rhode Island	10.4
12	South Dakota	10.1
13	New Jersey	9.9
14	Kansas	9.8
15	Maine	9.7
15	Minnesota	9.7
17	Missouri	9.6
18	Delaware	9.3
19	Arkansas	9.2
20	New Hampshire	9.1
20	Tennessee	9.1
22	Illinois	8.9
22	Kentucky	8.9
24	Oklahoma	8.7
25	Maryland	8.6
25	North Carolina	8.6
25	Vermont	8.6
28	Florida	8.2
29	Wyoming	8.0
30	Idaho	7.8
30	Montana	7.8
32	Mississippi	7.7
32	Oregon	7.7
32	Washington	7.7
35	Louisiana	7.6
36	West Virginia	7.3
37	Michigan	6.9
37	South Carolina	6.9
37	Virginia	6.9
40	Alabama	6.6
40	Colorado	6.6
42	Texas	6.4
43	Arizona	5.7
43	Georgia	5.7
45	California	5.1
46	Utah	5.0
47	New Mexico	4.8
48	Hawaii	4.4
49	Nevada	2.9
50	Alaska	1.8
	District of Columbia	5.8

Source: MQ Press using data from U.S. Dept of Health & Human Services, Centers for Medicare and Medicaid Services
"State Health Care Expenditures" (http://www.hcfa.gov/stats/nhe-oact/stateestimates/)
*By state of provider. Includes freestanding nursing and personal-care facilities. Includes Medicare- and
Medicaid-certified skilled nursing and intermediate care facilities as well as facilities that are not certified.
Excludes hospital-based facilities as they are counted in hospital care expenditures.

Average Annual Change in Expenditures for Nursing Home Care: 1990 to 1998

National Percent Change = 7.1% Average Annual Increase*

ALPHA ORDER

RANK	STATE	PERCENT CHANGE
5	Alabama	10.1
50	Alaska	(0.9)
14	Arizona	8.2
20	Arkansas	7.7
24	California	6.8
22	Colorado	7.3
32	Connecticut	6.1
27	Delaware	6.7
3	Florida	10.2
10	Georgia	9.0
41	Hawaii	4.9
9	Idaho	9.2
24	Illinois	6.8
36	Indiana	5.9
29	Iowa	6.2
32	Kansas	6.1
8	Kentucky	9.5
36	Louisiana	5.9
47	Maine	3.6
16	Maryland	7.9
42	Massachusetts	4.8
28	Michigan	6.4
47	Minnesota	3.6
2	Mississippi	10.5
19	Missouri	7.8
42	Montana	4.8
16	Nebraska	7.9
40	Nevada	5.0
11	New Hampshire	8.8
15	New Jersey	8.1
34	New Mexico	6.0
39	New York	5.3
3	North Carolina	10.2
45	North Dakota	4.6
22	Ohio	7.3
29	Oklahoma	6.2
34	Oregon	6.0
21	Pennsylvania	7.6
49	Rhode Island	2.8
16	South Carolina	7.9
24	South Dakota	6.8
1	Tennessee	12.7
13	Texas	8.4
44	Utah	4.7
46	Vermont	3.9
6	Virginia	9.7
29	Washington	6.2
12	West Virginia	8.7
38	Wisconsin	5.4
6	Wyoming	9.7

RANK ORDER

RANK	STATE	PERCENT CHANGE
1	Tennessee	12.7
2	Mississippi	10.5
3	Florida	10.2
3	North Carolina	10.2
5	Alabama	10.1
6	Virginia	9.7
6	Wyoming	9.7
8	Kentucky	9.5
9	Idaho	9.2
10	Georgia	9.0
11	New Hampshire	8.8
12	West Virginia	8.7
13	Texas	8.4
14	Arizona	8.2
15	New Jersey	8.1
16	Maryland	7.9
16	Nebraska	7.9
16	South Carolina	7.9
19	Missouri	7.8
20	Arkansas	7.7
21	Pennsylvania	7.6
22	Colorado	7.3
22	Ohio	7.3
24	California	6.8
24	Illinois	6.8
24	South Dakota	6.8
27	Delaware	6.7
28	Michigan	6.4
29	Iowa	6.2
29	Oklahoma	6.2
29	Washington	6.2
32	Connecticut	6.1
32	Kansas	6.1
34	New Mexico	6.0
34	Oregon	6.0
36	Indiana	5.9
36	Louisiana	5.9
38	Wisconsin	5.4
39	New York	5.3
40	Nevada	5.0
41	Hawaii	4.9
42	Massachusetts	4.8
42	Montana	4.8
44	Utah	4.7
45	North Dakota	4.6
46	Vermont	3.9
47	Maine	3.6
47	Minnesota	3.6
49	Rhode Island	2.8
50	Alaska	(0.9)

District of Columbia		7.2

Source: U.S. Department of Health and Human Services, Centers for Medicare and Medicaid Services
   "State Health Care Expenditures" (http://www.hcfa.gov/stats/nhe-oact/stateestimates/)

*By state of provider. Includes freestanding nursing and personal-care facilities. Includes Medicare- and Medicaid-certified skilled nursing and intermediate care facilities as well as facilities that are not certified. Excludes hospital-based facilities as they are counted in hospital care expenditures.

Per Capita Expenditures for Nursing Home Care in 1998

National Per Capita = $325*

ALPHA ORDER

RANK ORDER

RANK	STATE	PER CAPITA		RANK	STATE	PER CAPITA
36	Alabama	$245		1	Connecticut	$692
50	Alaska	68		2	New York	583
44	Arizona	180		3	Massachusetts	581
26	Arkansas	306		4	Pennsylvania	490
45	California	172		5	Rhode Island	474
39	Colorado	228		6	North Dakota	450
1	Connecticut	692		7	Ohio	443
15	Delaware	390		8	Nebraska	420
22	Florida	327		9	Minnesota	416
43	Georgia	202		10	Iowa	415
46	Hawaii	171		11	Wisconsin	404
42	Idaho	214		12	New Jersey	399
24	Illinois	325		13	Indiana	396
13	Indiana	396		14	South Dakota	391
10	Iowa	415		15	Delaware	390
20	Kansas	349		16	Maine	382
23	Kentucky	326		17	Missouri	368
28	Louisiana	286		17	Tennessee	368
16	Maine	382		19	New Hampshire	358
21	Maryland	330		20	Kansas	349
3	Massachusetts	581		21	Maryland	330
34	Michigan	250		22	Florida	327
9	Minnesota	416		23	Kentucky	326
34	Mississippi	250		24	Illinois	325
17	Missouri	368		25	North Carolina	311
33	Montana	252		26	Arkansas	306
8	Nebraska	420		27	Vermont	300
49	Nevada	94		28	Louisiana	286
19	New Hampshire	358		28	Oklahoma	286
12	New Jersey	399		30	West Virginia	284
47	New Mexico	148		31	Washington	262
2	New York	583		32	Oregon	255
25	North Carolina	311		33	Montana	252
6	North Dakota	450		34	Michigan	250
7	Ohio	443		34	Mississippi	250
28	Oklahoma	286		36	Alabama	245
32	Oregon	255		37	South Carolina	236
4	Pennsylvania	490		38	Wyoming	235
5	Rhode Island	474		39	Colorado	228
37	South Carolina	236		39	Virginia	228
14	South Dakota	391		41	Texas	220
17	Tennessee	368		42	Idaho	214
41	Texas	220		43	Georgia	202
48	Utah	143		44	Arizona	180
27	Vermont	300		45	California	172
39	Virginia	228		46	Hawaii	171
31	Washington	262		47	New Mexico	148
30	West Virginia	284		48	Utah	143
11	Wisconsin	404		49	Nevada	94
38	Wyoming	235		50	Alaska	68
					District of Columbia	470

Source: MQ Press using data from U.S. Dept of Health & Human Services, Centers for Medicare and Medicaid Services "State Health Care Expenditures" (http://www.hcfa.gov/stats/nhe-oact/stateestimates/)
By state of provider. Includes freestanding nursing and personal-care facilities. Includes Medicare- and Medicaid-certified skilled nursing and intermediate care facilities as well as facilities that are not certified. Excludes hospital-based facilities as they are counted in hospital care expenditures.

Estimated State Funds from the Tobacco Settlement Through 2025

National Total = $195,918,675,920*

ALPHA ORDER

RANK	STATE	FUNDS	% of USA
21	Alabama	$3,166,302,119	1.6%
45	Alaska	668,903,057	0.3%
22	Arizona	2,887,614,909	1.5%
30	Arkansas	1,622,336,126	0.8%
1	California	25,006,972,511	12.8%
23	Colorado	2,685,773,549	1.4%
19	Connecticut	3,637,303,382	1.9%
41	Delaware	774,798,677	0.4%
NA	Florida**	NA	NA
9	Georgia	4,808,740,669	2.5%
35	Hawaii	1,179,165,923	0.6%
43	Idaho	711,700,479	0.4%
5	Illinois	9,118,539,559	4.7%
18	Indiana	3,996,355,551	2.0%
28	Iowa	1,703,839,986	0.9%
29	Kansas	1,633,317,646	0.8%
20	Kentucky	3,450,438,586	1.8%
14	Louisiana	4,418,657,915	2.3%
31	Maine	1,507,301,276	0.8%
13	Maryland	4,428,657,384	2.3%
7	Massachusetts	7,913,114,213	4.0%
6	Michigan	8,526,278,034	4.4%
NA	Minnesota**	NA	NA
NA	Mississippi**	NA	NA
12	Missouri	4,456,368,286	2.3%
39	Montana	832,182,431	0.4%
37	Nebraska	1,165,683,457	0.6%
34	Nevada	1,194,976,855	0.6%
33	New Hampshire	1,304,689,150	0.7%
8	New Jersey	7,576,167,918	3.9%
36	New Mexico	1,168,438,809	0.6%
2	New York	25,003,202,243	12.8%
11	North Carolina	4,569,381,898	2.3%
42	North Dakota	717,089,369	0.4%
4	Ohio	9,869,422,449	5.0%
26	Oklahoma	2,029,985,862	1.0%
25	Oregon	2,248,476,833	1.1%
3	Pennsylvania	11,259,169,603	5.7%
32	Rhode Island	1,408,469,747	0.7%
24	South Carolina	2,304,693,120	1.2%
44	South Dakota	683,650,009	0.3%
10	Tennessee	4,782,168,127	2.4%
NA	Texas**	NA	NA
38	Utah	871,616,513	0.4%
40	Vermont	805,588,329	0.4%
17	Virginia	4,006,037,550	2.0%
16	Washington	4,022,716,267	2.1%
27	West Virginia	1,736,741,427	0.9%
15	Wisconsin	4,059,511,421	2.1%
46	Wyoming	486,553,976	0.2%

RANK ORDER

RANK	STATE	FUNDS	% of USA
1	California	$25,006,972,511	12.8%
2	New York	25,003,202,243	12.8%
3	Pennsylvania	11,259,169,603	5.7%
4	Ohio	9,869,422,449	5.0%
5	Illinois	9,118,539,559	4.7%
6	Michigan	8,526,278,034	4.4%
7	Massachusetts	7,913,114,213	4.0%
8	New Jersey	7,576,167,918	3.9%
9	Georgia	4,808,740,669	2.5%
10	Tennessee	4,782,168,127	2.4%
11	North Carolina	4,569,381,898	2.3%
12	Missouri	4,456,368,286	2.3%
13	Maryland	4,428,657,384	2.3%
14	Louisiana	4,418,657,915	2.3%
15	Wisconsin	4,059,511,421	2.1%
16	Washington	4,022,716,267	2.1%
17	Virginia	4,006,037,550	2.0%
18	Indiana	3,996,355,551	2.0%
19	Connecticut	3,637,303,382	1.9%
20	Kentucky	3,450,438,586	1.8%
21	Alabama	3,166,302,119	1.6%
22	Arizona	2,887,614,909	1.5%
23	Colorado	2,685,773,549	1.4%
24	South Carolina	2,304,693,120	1.2%
25	Oregon	2,248,476,833	1.1%
26	Oklahoma	2,029,985,862	1.0%
27	West Virginia	1,736,741,427	0.9%
28	Iowa	1,703,839,986	0.9%
29	Kansas	1,633,317,646	0.8%
30	Arkansas	1,622,336,126	0.8%
31	Maine	1,507,301,276	0.8%
32	Rhode Island	1,408,469,747	0.7%
33	New Hampshire	1,304,689,150	0.7%
34	Nevada	1,194,976,855	0.6%
35	Hawaii	1,179,165,923	0.6%
36	New Mexico	1,168,438,809	0.6%
37	Nebraska	1,165,683,457	0.6%
38	Utah	871,616,513	0.4%
39	Montana	832,182,431	0.4%
40	Vermont	805,588,329	0.4%
41	Delaware	774,798,677	0.4%
42	North Dakota	717,089,369	0.4%
43	Idaho	711,700,479	0.4%
44	South Dakota	683,650,009	0.3%
45	Alaska	668,903,057	0.3%
46	Wyoming	486,553,976	0.2%
NA	Florida**	NA	NA
NA	Minnesota**	NA	NA
NA	Mississippi**	NA	NA
NA	Texas**	NA	NA
	District of Columbia	1,189,458,106	0.6%

Source: National Association of Attorneys General
"Attorneys General Announce Tobacco Settlement Proposal" (News release, http://www.naag.org/tob2.htm)
*This settlement was reached in November 1998. National total includes $4,640,249,229 for U.S. territories.
**Total does not include $40 billion in previous settlements with Florida, Minnesota, Mississippi and Texas.

State and Local Government Expenditures for Health Programs in 2000

National Total = $51,365,588,000*

ALPHA ORDER

RANK	STATE	EXPENDITURES	% of USA
18	Alabama	$851,603,000	1.7%
42	Alaska	160,201,000	0.3%
17	Arizona	923,391,000	1.8%
34	Arkansas	316,228,000	0.6%
1	California	8,896,217,000	17.3%
27	Colorado	472,937,000	0.9%
28	Connecticut	450,221,000	0.9%
39	Delaware	215,588,000	0.4%
3	Florida	3,137,136,000	6.1%
12	Georgia	1,059,809,000	2.1%
30	Hawaii	408,479,000	0.8%
44	Idaho	139,240,000	0.3%
6	Illinois	2,424,891,000	4.7%
24	Indiana	572,475,000	1.1%
32	Iowa	373,966,000	0.7%
31	Kansas	408,358,000	0.8%
26	Kentucky	544,112,000	1.1%
25	Louisiana	552,240,000	1.1%
37	Maine	293,482,000	0.6%
16	Maryland	933,863,000	1.8%
11	Massachusetts	1,566,025,000	3.0%
5	Michigan	2,502,924,000	4.9%
22	Minnesota	715,323,000	1.4%
35	Mississippi	298,498,000	0.6%
21	Missouri	790,330,000	1.5%
38	Montana	246,150,000	0.5%
46	Nebraska	121,811,000	0.2%
41	Nevada	172,083,000	0.3%
45	New Hampshire	126,450,000	0.2%
14	New Jersey	1,017,852,000	2.0%
33	New Mexico	328,711,000	0.6%
2	New York	3,492,012,000	6.8%
9	North Carolina	1,713,098,000	3.3%
50	North Dakota	48,187,000	0.1%
4	Ohio	2,751,983,000	5.4%
29	Oklahoma	413,461,000	0.8%
23	Oregon	698,276,000	1.4%
7	Pennsylvania	2,392,413,000	4.7%
43	Rhode Island	156,085,000	0.3%
20	South Carolina	831,841,000	1.6%
48	South Dakota	78,428,000	0.2%
19	Tennessee	841,537,000	1.6%
8	Texas	2,317,786,000	4.5%
36	Utah	295,037,000	0.6%
49	Vermont	76,479,000	0.1%
15	Virginia	935,521,000	1.8%
10	Washington	1,702,867,000	3.3%
40	West Virginia	209,259,000	0.4%
13	Wisconsin	1,026,484,000	2.0%
47	Wyoming	90,075,000	0.2%

RANK ORDER

RANK	STATE	EXPENDITURES	% of USA
1	California	$8,896,217,000	17.3%
2	New York	3,492,012,000	6.8%
3	Florida	3,137,136,000	6.1%
4	Ohio	2,751,983,000	5.4%
5	Michigan	2,502,924,000	4.9%
6	Illinois	2,424,891,000	4.7%
7	Pennsylvania	2,392,413,000	4.7%
8	Texas	2,317,786,000	4.5%
9	North Carolina	1,713,098,000	3.3%
10	Washington	1,702,867,000	3.3%
11	Massachusetts	1,566,025,000	3.0%
12	Georgia	1,059,809,000	2.1%
13	Wisconsin	1,026,484,000	2.0%
14	New Jersey	1,017,852,000	2.0%
15	Virginia	935,521,000	1.8%
16	Maryland	933,863,000	1.8%
17	Arizona	923,391,000	1.8%
18	Alabama	851,603,000	1.7%
19	Tennessee	841,537,000	1.6%
20	South Carolina	831,841,000	1.6%
21	Missouri	790,330,000	1.5%
22	Minnesota	715,323,000	1.4%
23	Oregon	698,276,000	1.4%
24	Indiana	572,475,000	1.1%
25	Louisiana	552,240,000	1.1%
26	Kentucky	544,112,000	1.1%
27	Colorado	472,937,000	0.9%
28	Connecticut	450,221,000	0.9%
29	Oklahoma	413,461,000	0.8%
30	Hawaii	408,479,000	0.8%
31	Kansas	408,358,000	0.8%
32	Iowa	373,966,000	0.7%
33	New Mexico	328,711,000	0.6%
34	Arkansas	316,228,000	0.6%
35	Mississippi	298,498,000	0.6%
36	Utah	295,037,000	0.6%
37	Maine	293,482,000	0.6%
38	Montana	246,150,000	0.5%
39	Delaware	215,588,000	0.4%
40	West Virginia	209,259,000	0.4%
41	Nevada	172,083,000	0.3%
42	Alaska	160,201,000	0.3%
43	Rhode Island	156,085,000	0.3%
44	Idaho	139,240,000	0.3%
45	New Hampshire	126,450,000	0.2%
46	Nebraska	121,811,000	0.2%
47	Wyoming	90,075,000	0.2%
48	South Dakota	78,428,000	0.2%
49	Vermont	76,479,000	0.1%
50	North Dakota	48,187,000	0.1%
	District of Columbia	274,165,000	0.5%

Source: U.S. Bureau of the Census, Governments Division
    "State and Local Government Finances: 1999-2000" (http://www.census.gov/govs/www/estimate00.html)
*Includes outpatient health services other than hospital care, research and education, categorical health programs, treatment and immunization clinics, nursing and environmental health activities. Includes capital expenditures.

Per Capita State and Local Government Expenditures for Health Programs in 2000
National Per Capita = $182*

ALPHA ORDER

RANK	STATE	PER CAPITA
17	Alabama	$191
6	Alaska	255
22	Arizona	179
39	Arkansas	118
5	California	262
42	Colorado	109
30	Connecticut	132
3	Delaware	274
14	Florida	195
33	Georgia	129
1	Hawaii	337
43	Idaho	107
14	Illinois	195
47	Indiana	94
34	Iowa	128
24	Kansas	152
29	Kentucky	134
36	Louisiana	124
10	Maine	230
23	Maryland	176
8	Massachusetts	246
7	Michigan	251
27	Minnesota	145
44	Mississippi	105
28	Missouri	141
4	Montana	272
50	Nebraska	71
48	Nevada	85
46	New Hampshire	102
37	New Jersey	121
21	New Mexico	180
19	New York	184
11	North Carolina	212
49	North Dakota	75
9	Ohio	242
38	Oklahoma	120
13	Oregon	204
14	Pennsylvania	195
25	Rhode Island	149
12	South Carolina	207
45	South Dakota	104
26	Tennessee	148
41	Texas	111
30	Utah	132
35	Vermont	125
30	Virginia	132
2	Washington	288
40	West Virginia	116
17	Wisconsin	191
20	Wyoming	182

RANK ORDER

RANK	STATE	PER CAPITA
1	Hawaii	$337
2	Washington	288
3	Delaware	274
4	Montana	272
5	California	262
6	Alaska	255
7	Michigan	251
8	Massachusetts	246
9	Ohio	242
10	Maine	230
11	North Carolina	212
12	South Carolina	207
13	Oregon	204
14	Florida	195
14	Illinois	195
14	Pennsylvania	195
17	Alabama	191
17	Wisconsin	191
19	New York	184
20	Wyoming	182
21	New Mexico	180
22	Arizona	179
23	Maryland	176
24	Kansas	152
25	Rhode Island	149
26	Tennessee	148
27	Minnesota	145
28	Missouri	141
29	Kentucky	134
30	Connecticut	132
30	Utah	132
30	Virginia	132
33	Georgia	129
34	Iowa	128
35	Vermont	125
36	Louisiana	124
37	New Jersey	121
38	Oklahoma	120
39	Arkansas	118
40	West Virginia	116
41	Texas	111
42	Colorado	109
43	Idaho	107
44	Mississippi	105
45	South Dakota	104
46	New Hampshire	102
47	Indiana	94
48	Nevada	85
49	North Dakota	75
50	Nebraska	71

District of Columbia 480

Source: Morgan Quitno Press using data from U.S. Bureau of the Census, Governments Division
"State and Local Government Finances: 1999-2000" (http://www.census.gov/govs/www/estimate00.html)
*Includes outpatient health services other than hospital care, research and education, categorical health programs, treatment and immunization clinics, nursing and environmental health activities. Includes capital expenditures.

State Government Expenditures for Health Programs in 2000

National Total = $42,065,818,000*

ALPHA ORDER

RANK	STATE	EXPENDITURES	% of USA
20	Alabama	$598,894,000	1.4%
43	Alaska	150,313,000	0.4%
12	Arizona	1,028,977,000	2.4%
34	Arkansas	290,306,000	0.7%
1	California	7,546,878,000	17.9%
31	Colorado	308,387,000	0.7%
22	Connecticut	500,735,000	1.2%
39	Delaware	215,020,000	0.5%
4	Florida	2,678,698,000	6.4%
14	Georgia	843,258,000	2.0%
28	Hawaii	398,125,000	0.9%
46	Idaho	98,510,000	0.2%
5	Illinois	2,078,089,000	4.9%
24	Indiana	491,217,000	1.2%
37	Iowa	221,934,000	0.5%
30	Kansas	348,655,000	0.8%
27	Kentucky	419,625,000	1.0%
25	Louisiana	478,003,000	1.1%
35	Maine	279,190,000	0.7%
11	Maryland	1,059,486,000	2.5%
9	Massachusetts	1,486,938,000	3.5%
3	Michigan	2,699,196,000	6.4%
26	Minnesota	455,586,000	1.1%
33	Mississippi	291,496,000	0.7%
21	Missouri	591,534,000	1.4%
38	Montana	215,078,000	0.5%
36	Nebraska	261,953,000	0.6%
45	Nevada	112,244,000	0.3%
44	New Hampshire	132,710,000	0.3%
15	New Jersey	763,044,000	1.8%
32	New Mexico	302,504,000	0.7%
2	New York	3,568,286,000	8.5%
13	North Carolina	886,520,000	2.1%
50	North Dakota	43,080,000	0.1%
6	Ohio	1,615,217,000	3.8%
29	Oklahoma	380,071,000	0.9%
23	Oregon	498,252,000	1.2%
8	Pennsylvania	1,571,394,000	3.7%
42	Rhode Island	152,274,000	0.4%
16	South Carolina	645,473,000	1.5%
49	South Dakota	65,917,000	0.2%
18	Tennessee	633,691,000	1.5%
7	Texas	1,608,023,000	3.8%
40	Utah	208,731,000	0.5%
48	Vermont	72,551,000	0.2%
17	Virginia	642,384,000	1.5%
10	Washington	1,273,277,000	3.0%
41	West Virginia	152,559,000	0.4%
19	Wisconsin	615,676,000	1.5%
47	Wyoming	85,859,000	0.2%

RANK ORDER

RANK	STATE	EXPENDITURES	% of USA
1	California	$7,546,878,000	17.9%
2	New York	3,568,286,000	8.5%
3	Michigan	2,699,196,000	6.4%
4	Florida	2,678,698,000	6.4%
5	Illinois	2,078,089,000	4.9%
6	Ohio	1,615,217,000	3.8%
7	Texas	1,608,023,000	3.8%
8	Pennsylvania	1,571,394,000	3.7%
9	Massachusetts	1,486,938,000	3.5%
10	Washington	1,273,277,000	3.0%
11	Maryland	1,059,486,000	2.5%
12	Arizona	1,028,977,000	2.4%
13	North Carolina	886,520,000	2.1%
14	Georgia	843,258,000	2.0%
15	New Jersey	763,044,000	1.8%
16	South Carolina	645,473,000	1.5%
17	Virginia	642,384,000	1.5%
18	Tennessee	633,691,000	1.5%
19	Wisconsin	615,676,000	1.5%
20	Alabama	598,894,000	1.4%
21	Missouri	591,534,000	1.4%
22	Connecticut	500,735,000	1.2%
23	Oregon	498,252,000	1.2%
24	Indiana	491,217,000	1.2%
25	Louisiana	478,003,000	1.1%
26	Minnesota	455,586,000	1.1%
27	Kentucky	419,625,000	1.0%
28	Hawaii	398,125,000	0.9%
29	Oklahoma	380,071,000	0.9%
30	Kansas	348,655,000	0.8%
31	Colorado	308,387,000	0.7%
32	New Mexico	302,504,000	0.7%
33	Mississippi	291,496,000	0.7%
34	Arkansas	290,306,000	0.7%
35	Maine	279,190,000	0.7%
36	Nebraska	261,953,000	0.6%
37	Iowa	221,934,000	0.5%
38	Montana	215,078,000	0.5%
39	Delaware	215,020,000	0.5%
40	Utah	208,731,000	0.5%
41	West Virginia	152,559,000	0.4%
42	Rhode Island	152,274,000	0.4%
43	Alaska	150,313,000	0.4%
44	New Hampshire	132,710,000	0.3%
45	Nevada	112,244,000	0.3%
46	Idaho	98,510,000	0.2%
47	Wyoming	85,859,000	0.2%
48	Vermont	72,551,000	0.2%
49	South Dakota	65,917,000	0.2%
50	North Dakota	43,080,000	0.1%
	District of Columbia**	NA	NA

Source: U.S. Bureau of the Census, Governments Division
    "2000 State Government Finance Data" (http://www.census.gov/govs/www/state00.html)
*Includes outpatient health services other than hospital care, research and education, categorical health programs, treatment and immunization clinics, nursing and environmental health activities. Includes capital expenditures.
**Not applicable.

Per Capita State Government Expenditures for Health Programs in 2000

National Per Capita = $149*

ALPHA ORDER

RANK	STATE	PER CAPITA
23	Alabama	$135
4	Alaska	239
10	Arizona	199
31	Arkansas	108
7	California	222
48	Colorado	71
19	Connecticut	147
2	Delaware	273
14	Florida	167
36	Georgia	102
1	Hawaii	328
46	Idaho	76
14	Illinois	167
44	Indiana	81
46	Iowa	76
24	Kansas	129
35	Kentucky	104
32	Louisiana	107
8	Maine	219
10	Maryland	199
6	Massachusetts	234
3	Michigan	271
39	Minnesota	92
36	Mississippi	102
34	Missouri	106
5	Montana	238
18	Nebraska	153
50	Nevada	56
32	New Hampshire	107
40	New Jersey	90
16	New Mexico	166
12	New York	188
29	North Carolina	110
49	North Dakota	67
22	Ohio	142
29	Oklahoma	110
20	Oregon	145
25	Pennsylvania	128
20	Rhode Island	145
17	South Carolina	160
42	South Dakota	87
28	Tennessee	111
45	Texas	77
38	Utah	93
26	Vermont	119
40	Virginia	90
9	Washington	215
43	West Virginia	84
27	Wisconsin	115
13	Wyoming	174

RANK ORDER

RANK	STATE	PER CAPITA
1	Hawaii	$328
2	Delaware	273
3	Michigan	271
4	Alaska	239
5	Montana	238
6	Massachusetts	234
7	California	222
8	Maine	219
9	Washington	215
10	Arizona	199
10	Maryland	199
12	New York	188
13	Wyoming	174
14	Florida	167
14	Illinois	167
16	New Mexico	166
17	South Carolina	160
18	Nebraska	153
19	Connecticut	147
20	Oregon	145
20	Rhode Island	145
22	Ohio	142
23	Alabama	135
24	Kansas	129
25	Pennsylvania	128
26	Vermont	119
27	Wisconsin	115
28	Tennessee	111
29	North Carolina	110
29	Oklahoma	110
31	Arkansas	108
32	Louisiana	107
32	New Hampshire	107
34	Missouri	106
35	Kentucky	104
36	Georgia	102
36	Mississippi	102
38	Utah	93
39	Minnesota	92
40	New Jersey	90
40	Virginia	90
42	South Dakota	87
43	West Virginia	84
44	Indiana	81
45	Texas	77
46	Idaho	76
46	Iowa	76
48	Colorado	71
49	North Dakota	67
50	Nevada	56

District of Columbia**   NA

Source: Morgan Quitno Press using data from U.S. Bureau of the Census, Governments Division
    "2000 State Government Finance Data" (http://www.census.gov/govs/www/state00.html)
*Includes outpatient health services other than hospital care, research and education, categorical health programs, treatment and immunization clinics, nursing and environmental health activities. Includes capital expenditures.
**Not applicable.

Local Government Expenditures for Health Programs in 2000

National Total = $23,990,528,000*

ALPHA ORDER

RANK	STATE	EXPENDITURES	% of USA
18	Alabama	$267,601,000	1.1%
35	Alaska	57,733,000	0.2%
25	Arizona	174,735,000	0.7%
42	Arkansas	27,736,000	0.1%
1	California	5,274,867,000	22.0%
24	Colorado	199,740,000	0.8%
29	Connecticut	103,675,000	0.4%
48	Delaware	13,098,000	0.1%
13	Florida	475,794,000	2.0%
9	Georgia	716,591,000	3.0%
41	Hawaii	28,238,000	0.1%
36	Idaho	52,242,000	0.2%
14	Illinois	453,686,000	1.9%
26	Indiana	156,480,000	0.7%
20	Iowa	261,495,000	1.1%
27	Kansas	142,005,000	0.6%
19	Kentucky	266,032,000	1.1%
32	Louisiana	78,728,000	0.3%
47	Maine	14,292,000	0.1%
21	Maryland	239,275,000	1.0%
31	Massachusetts	96,918,000	0.4%
4	Michigan	1,880,940,000	7.8%
15	Minnesota	378,030,000	1.6%
37	Mississippi	48,091,000	0.2%
22	Missouri	228,148,000	1.0%
38	Montana	46,107,000	0.2%
39	Nebraska	33,435,000	0.1%
33	Nevada	68,852,000	0.3%
44	New Hampshire	18,483,000	0.1%
16	New Jersey	283,920,000	1.2%
43	New Mexico	26,207,000	0.1%
2	New York	2,170,552,000	9.0%
7	North Carolina	1,228,614,000	5.1%
45	North Dakota	17,751,000	0.1%
3	Ohio	1,919,239,000	8.0%
30	Oklahoma	99,826,000	0.4%
11	Oregon	510,222,000	2.1%
5	Pennsylvania	1,790,238,000	7.5%
50	Rhode Island	3,811,000	0.0%
17	South Carolina	275,050,000	1.1%
46	South Dakota	14,971,000	0.1%
23	Tennessee	209,186,000	0.9%
6	Texas	1,300,253,000	5.4%
28	Utah	130,670,000	0.5%
49	Vermont	3,928,000	0.0%
12	Virginia	493,712,000	2.1%
10	Washington	587,977,000	2.5%
34	West Virginia	60,453,000	0.3%
8	Wisconsin	755,866,000	3.2%
40	Wyoming	30,870,000	0.1%

RANK ORDER

RANK	STATE	EXPENDITURES	% of USA
1	California	$5,274,867,000	22.0%
2	New York	2,170,552,000	9.0%
3	Ohio	1,919,239,000	8.0%
4	Michigan	1,880,940,000	7.8%
5	Pennsylvania	1,790,238,000	7.5%
6	Texas	1,300,253,000	5.4%
7	North Carolina	1,228,614,000	5.1%
8	Wisconsin	755,866,000	3.2%
9	Georgia	716,591,000	3.0%
10	Washington	587,977,000	2.5%
11	Oregon	510,222,000	2.1%
12	Virginia	493,712,000	2.1%
13	Florida	475,794,000	2.0%
14	Illinois	453,686,000	1.9%
15	Minnesota	378,030,000	1.6%
16	New Jersey	283,920,000	1.2%
17	South Carolina	275,050,000	1.1%
18	Alabama	267,601,000	1.1%
19	Kentucky	266,032,000	1.1%
20	Iowa	261,495,000	1.1%
21	Maryland	239,275,000	1.0%
22	Missouri	228,148,000	1.0%
23	Tennessee	209,186,000	0.9%
24	Colorado	199,740,000	0.8%
25	Arizona	174,735,000	0.7%
26	Indiana	156,480,000	0.7%
27	Kansas	142,005,000	0.6%
28	Utah	130,670,000	0.5%
29	Connecticut	103,675,000	0.4%
30	Oklahoma	99,826,000	0.4%
31	Massachusetts	96,918,000	0.4%
32	Louisiana	78,728,000	0.3%
33	Nevada	68,852,000	0.3%
34	West Virginia	60,453,000	0.3%
35	Alaska	57,733,000	0.2%
36	Idaho	52,242,000	0.2%
37	Mississippi	48,091,000	0.2%
38	Montana	46,107,000	0.2%
39	Nebraska	33,435,000	0.1%
40	Wyoming	30,870,000	0.1%
41	Hawaii	28,238,000	0.1%
42	Arkansas	27,736,000	0.1%
43	New Mexico	26,207,000	0.1%
44	New Hampshire	18,483,000	0.1%
45	North Dakota	17,751,000	0.1%
46	South Dakota	14,971,000	0.1%
47	Maine	14,292,000	0.1%
48	Delaware	13,098,000	0.1%
49	Vermont	3,928,000	0.0%
50	Rhode Island	3,811,000	0.0%
	District of Columbia	274,165,000	1.1%

Source: U.S. Bureau of the Census, Governments Division
"State and Local Government Finances: 1999-2000" (http://www.census.gov/govs/www/estimate00.html)
*Includes outpatient health services other than hospital care, research and education, categorical health programs, treatment and immunization clinics, nursing and environmental health activities. Includes capital expenditures.

Per Capita Local Government Expenditures for Health Programs in 2000

National Per Capita = $85*

ALPHA ORDER

RANK ORDER

RANK	STATE	PER CAPITA	RANK	STATE	PER CAPITA
19	Alabama	$60	1	Michigan	$189
10	Alaska	92	2	Ohio	169
29	Arizona	34	3	California	155
48	Arkansas	10	4	North Carolina	152
3	California	155	5	Oregon	149
23	Colorado	46	6	Pennsylvania	146
33	Connecticut	30	7	Wisconsin	141
42	Delaware	17	8	New York	114
33	Florida	30	9	Washington	99
12	Georgia	87	10	Alaska	92
38	Hawaii	23	11	Iowa	89
26	Idaho	40	12	Georgia	87
28	Illinois	36	13	Minnesota	77
37	Indiana	26	14	Virginia	69
11	Iowa	89	15	South Carolina	68
21	Kansas	53	16	Kentucky	66
16	Kentucky	66	17	Texas	62
41	Louisiana	18	17	Wyoming	62
47	Maine	11	19	Alabama	60
24	Maryland	45	20	Utah	58
44	Massachusetts	15	21	Kansas	53
1	Michigan	189	22	Montana	51
13	Minnesota	77	23	Colorado	46
42	Mississippi	17	24	Maryland	45
25	Missouri	41	25	Missouri	41
22	Montana	51	26	Idaho	40
39	Nebraska	20	27	Tennessee	37
29	Nevada	34	28	Illinois	36
44	New Hampshire	15	29	Arizona	34
29	New Jersey	34	29	Nevada	34
46	New Mexico	14	29	New Jersey	34
8	New York	114	32	West Virginia	33
4	North Carolina	152	33	Connecticut	30
36	North Dakota	28	33	Florida	30
2	Ohio	169	35	Oklahoma	29
35	Oklahoma	29	36	North Dakota	28
5	Oregon	149	37	Indiana	26
6	Pennsylvania	146	38	Hawaii	23
50	Rhode Island	4	39	Nebraska	20
15	South Carolina	68	39	South Dakota	20
39	South Dakota	20	41	Louisiana	18
27	Tennessee	37	42	Delaware	17
17	Texas	62	42	Mississippi	17
20	Utah	58	44	Massachusetts	15
49	Vermont	6	44	New Hampshire	15
14	Virginia	69	46	New Mexico	14
9	Washington	99	47	Maine	11
32	West Virginia	33	48	Arkansas	10
7	Wisconsin	141	49	Vermont	6
17	Wyoming	62	50	Rhode Island	4

District of Columbia 480

Source: Morgan Quitno Press using data from U.S. Bureau of the Census, Governments Division
"State and Local Government Finances: 1999-2000" (http://www.census.gov/govs/www/estimate00.html)
*Includes outpatient health services other than hospital care, research and education, categorical health programs, treatment and immunization clinics, nursing and environmental health activities. Includes capital expenditures.

State and Local Government Expenditures for Hospitals in 2000

National Total = $75,975,990,000*

ALPHA ORDER

RANK	STATE	EXPENDITURES	% of USA
7	Alabama	$2,783,320,000	3.7%
45	Alaska	75,496,000	0.1%
34	Arizona	450,879,000	0.6%
29	Arkansas	654,059,000	0.9%
1	California	9,158,683,000	12.1%
26	Colorado	867,948,000	1.1%
23	Connecticut	1,145,790,000	1.5%
47	Delaware	62,968,000	0.1%
4	Florida	4,170,079,000	5.5%
8	Georgia	2,494,273,000	3.3%
41	Hawaii	192,039,000	0.3%
38	Idaho	373,138,000	0.5%
12	Illinois	1,956,580,000	2.6%
11	Indiana	2,031,205,000	2.7%
21	Iowa	1,304,188,000	1.7%
32	Kansas	525,924,000	0.7%
31	Kentucky	553,180,000	0.7%
6	Louisiana	2,822,725,000	3.7%
43	Maine	103,942,000	0.1%
39	Maryland	360,644,000	0.5%
28	Massachusetts	679,197,000	0.9%
16	Michigan	1,676,070,000	2.2%
24	Minnesota	1,110,804,000	1.5%
14	Mississippi	1,815,109,000	2.4%
19	Missouri	1,376,403,000	1.8%
44	Montana	96,618,000	0.1%
36	Nebraska	399,480,000	0.5%
30	Nevada	564,940,000	0.7%
48	New Hampshire	43,798,000	0.1%
20	New Jersey	1,313,512,000	1.7%
33	New Mexico	483,327,000	0.6%
2	New York	8,075,704,000	10.6%
5	North Carolina	3,823,391,000	5.0%
49	North Dakota	42,548,000	0.1%
9	Ohio	2,210,529,000	2.9%
25	Oklahoma	910,771,000	1.2%
22	Oregon	1,252,602,000	1.6%
18	Pennsylvania	1,553,450,000	2.0%
42	Rhode Island	121,570,000	0.2%
10	South Carolina	2,184,262,000	2.9%
46	South Dakota	71,823,000	0.1%
13	Tennessee	1,897,280,000	2.5%
3	Texas	6,535,751,000	8.6%
35	Utah	445,959,000	0.6%
50	Vermont	2,941,000	0.0%
15	Virginia	1,698,036,000	2.2%
17	Washington	1,614,194,000	2.1%
40	West Virginia	343,014,000	0.5%
27	Wisconsin	812,666,000	1.1%
37	Wyoming	373,784,000	0.5%

RANK ORDER

RANK	STATE	EXPENDITURES	% of USA
1	California	$9,158,683,000	12.1%
2	New York	8,075,704,000	10.6%
3	Texas	6,535,751,000	8.6%
4	Florida	4,170,079,000	5.5%
5	North Carolina	3,823,391,000	5.0%
6	Louisiana	2,822,725,000	3.7%
7	Alabama	2,783,320,000	3.7%
8	Georgia	2,494,273,000	3.3%
9	Ohio	2,210,529,000	2.9%
10	South Carolina	2,184,262,000	2.9%
11	Indiana	2,031,205,000	2.7%
12	Illinois	1,956,580,000	2.6%
13	Tennessee	1,897,280,000	2.5%
14	Mississippi	1,815,109,000	2.4%
15	Virginia	1,698,036,000	2.2%
16	Michigan	1,676,070,000	2.2%
17	Washington	1,614,194,000	2.1%
18	Pennsylvania	1,553,450,000	2.0%
19	Missouri	1,376,403,000	1.8%
20	New Jersey	1,313,512,000	1.7%
21	Iowa	1,304,188,000	1.7%
22	Oregon	1,252,602,000	1.6%
23	Connecticut	1,145,790,000	1.5%
24	Minnesota	1,110,804,000	1.5%
25	Oklahoma	910,771,000	1.2%
26	Colorado	867,948,000	1.1%
27	Wisconsin	812,666,000	1.1%
28	Massachusetts	679,197,000	0.9%
29	Arkansas	654,059,000	0.9%
30	Nevada	564,940,000	0.7%
31	Kentucky	553,180,000	0.7%
32	Kansas	525,924,000	0.7%
33	New Mexico	483,327,000	0.6%
34	Arizona	450,879,000	0.6%
35	Utah	445,959,000	0.6%
36	Nebraska	399,480,000	0.5%
37	Wyoming	373,784,000	0.5%
38	Idaho	373,138,000	0.5%
39	Maryland	360,644,000	0.5%
40	West Virginia	343,014,000	0.5%
41	Hawaii	192,039,000	0.3%
42	Rhode Island	121,570,000	0.2%
43	Maine	103,942,000	0.1%
44	Montana	96,618,000	0.1%
45	Alaska	75,496,000	0.1%
46	South Dakota	71,823,000	0.1%
47	Delaware	62,968,000	0.1%
48	New Hampshire	43,798,000	0.1%
49	North Dakota	42,548,000	0.1%
50	Vermont	2,941,000	0.0%
	District of Columbia	359,397,000	0.5%

Source: U.S. Bureau of the Census, Governments Division
   "State and Local Government Finances: 1999-2000" (http://www.census.gov/govs/www/estimate00.html)
*Financing, construction, acquisition, maintenance or operation of hospital facilities, provision of hospital care and support of public or private hospitals.

Per Capita State and Local Government Expenditures for Hospitals in 2000

National Per Capita = $269*

ALPHA ORDER

RANK	STATE	PER CAPITA
4	Alabama	$625
39	Alaska	120
44	Arizona	87
23	Arkansas	244
18	California	269
27	Colorado	201
10	Connecticut	336
46	Delaware	80
21	Florida	260
14	Georgia	303
33	Hawaii	158
15	Idaho	287
34	Illinois	157
11	Indiana	333
7	Iowa	445
29	Kansas	195
37	Kentucky	137
3	Louisiana	632
45	Maine	81
47	Maryland	68
41	Massachusetts	107
32	Michigan	168
26	Minnesota	225
2	Mississippi	637
22	Missouri	246
41	Montana	107
25	Nebraska	233
16	Nevada	280
49	New Hampshire	35
35	New Jersey	156
19	New Mexico	265
8	New York	425
6	North Carolina	473
48	North Dakota	66
29	Ohio	195
20	Oklahoma	264
9	Oregon	365
38	Pennsylvania	126
40	Rhode Island	116
5	South Carolina	543
43	South Dakota	95
11	Tennessee	333
13	Texas	312
28	Utah	199
50	Vermont	5
24	Virginia	239
17	Washington	273
31	West Virginia	190
36	Wisconsin	151
1	Wyoming	757

RANK ORDER

RANK	STATE	PER CAPITA
1	Wyoming	$757
2	Mississippi	637
3	Louisiana	632
4	Alabama	625
5	South Carolina	543
6	North Carolina	473
7	Iowa	445
8	New York	425
9	Oregon	365
10	Connecticut	336
11	Indiana	333
11	Tennessee	333
13	Texas	312
14	Georgia	303
15	Idaho	287
16	Nevada	280
17	Washington	273
18	California	269
19	New Mexico	265
20	Oklahoma	264
21	Florida	260
22	Missouri	246
23	Arkansas	244
24	Virginia	239
25	Nebraska	233
26	Minnesota	225
27	Colorado	201
28	Utah	199
29	Kansas	195
29	Ohio	195
31	West Virginia	190
32	Michigan	168
33	Hawaii	158
34	Illinois	157
35	New Jersey	156
36	Wisconsin	151
37	Kentucky	137
38	Pennsylvania	126
39	Alaska	120
40	Rhode Island	116
41	Massachusetts	107
41	Montana	107
43	South Dakota	95
44	Arizona	87
45	Maine	81
46	Delaware	80
47	Maryland	68
48	North Dakota	66
49	New Hampshire	35
50	Vermont	5

District of Columbia 629

Source: Morgan Quitno Press using data from U.S. Bureau of the Census, Governments Division
"State and Local Government Finances: 1999-2000" (http://www.census.gov/govs/www/estimate00.html)
*Financing, construction, acquisition, maintenance or operation of hospital facilities, provision of hospital care and support of public or private hospitals.

State Government Expenditures for Hospitals in 2000

National Total = $32,578,358,000*

ALPHA ORDER

RANK	STATE	EXPENDITURES	% of USA
12	Alabama	$1,021,054,000	3.1%
49	Alaska	17,571,000	0.1%
40	Arizona	81,544,000	0.3%
26	Arkansas	383,938,000	1.2%
1	California	3,335,190,000	10.2%
34	Colorado	149,055,000	0.5%
10	Connecticut	1,126,066,000	3.5%
41	Delaware	62,968,000	0.2%
19	Florida	610,607,000	1.9%
17	Georgia	668,219,000	2.1%
32	Hawaii	192,039,000	0.6%
45	Idaho	42,689,000	0.1%
14	Illinois	847,109,000	2.6%
30	Indiana	239,184,000	0.7%
18	Iowa	655,221,000	2.0%
37	Kansas	101,323,000	0.3%
24	Kentucky	451,087,000	1.4%
6	Louisiana	1,376,198,000	4.2%
46	Maine	42,630,000	0.1%
28	Maryland	360,644,000	1.1%
23	Massachusetts	465,869,000	1.4%
11	Michigan	1,112,902,000	3.4%
31	Minnesota	222,650,000	0.7%
20	Mississippi	598,815,000	1.8%
22	Missouri	592,624,000	1.8%
43	Montana	43,787,000	0.1%
33	Nebraska	158,457,000	0.5%
38	Nevada	90,643,000	0.3%
44	New Hampshire	43,492,000	0.1%
9	New Jersey	1,160,401,000	3.6%
29	New Mexico	357,037,000	1.1%
2	New York	3,197,781,000	9.8%
7	North Carolina	1,247,695,000	3.8%
47	North Dakota	42,472,000	0.1%
8	Ohio	1,231,527,000	3.8%
35	Oklahoma	149,035,000	0.5%
13	Oregon	924,106,000	2.8%
4	Pennsylvania	1,681,893,000	5.2%
36	Rhode Island	121,570,000	0.4%
15	South Carolina	772,952,000	2.4%
42	South Dakota	43,836,000	0.1%
27	Tennessee	366,739,000	1.1%
3	Texas	2,947,605,000	9.0%
25	Utah	413,947,000	1.3%
50	Vermont	2,895,000	0.0%
5	Virginia	1,433,577,000	4.4%
16	Washington	681,277,000	2.1%
39	West Virginia	88,518,000	0.3%
21	Wisconsin	594,044,000	1.8%
48	Wyoming	25,876,000	0.1%

RANK ORDER

RANK	STATE	EXPENDITURES	% of USA
1	California	$3,335,190,000	10.2%
2	New York	3,197,781,000	9.8%
3	Texas	2,947,605,000	9.0%
4	Pennsylvania	1,681,893,000	5.2%
5	Virginia	1,433,577,000	4.4%
6	Louisiana	1,376,198,000	4.2%
7	North Carolina	1,247,695,000	3.8%
8	Ohio	1,231,527,000	3.8%
9	New Jersey	1,160,401,000	3.6%
10	Connecticut	1,126,066,000	3.5%
11	Michigan	1,112,902,000	3.4%
12	Alabama	1,021,054,000	3.1%
13	Oregon	924,106,000	2.8%
14	Illinois	847,109,000	2.6%
15	South Carolina	772,952,000	2.4%
16	Washington	681,277,000	2.1%
17	Georgia	668,219,000	2.1%
18	Iowa	655,221,000	2.0%
19	Florida	610,607,000	1.9%
20	Mississippi	598,815,000	1.8%
21	Wisconsin	594,044,000	1.8%
22	Missouri	592,624,000	1.8%
23	Massachusetts	465,869,000	1.4%
24	Kentucky	451,087,000	1.4%
25	Utah	413,947,000	1.3%
26	Arkansas	383,938,000	1.2%
27	Tennessee	366,739,000	1.1%
28	Maryland	360,644,000	1.1%
29	New Mexico	357,037,000	1.1%
30	Indiana	239,184,000	0.7%
31	Minnesota	222,650,000	0.7%
32	Hawaii	192,039,000	0.6%
33	Nebraska	158,457,000	0.5%
34	Colorado	149,055,000	0.5%
35	Oklahoma	149,035,000	0.5%
36	Rhode Island	121,570,000	0.4%
37	Kansas	101,323,000	0.3%
38	Nevada	90,643,000	0.3%
39	West Virginia	88,518,000	0.3%
40	Arizona	81,544,000	0.3%
41	Delaware	62,968,000	0.2%
42	South Dakota	43,836,000	0.1%
43	Montana	43,787,000	0.1%
44	New Hampshire	43,492,000	0.1%
45	Idaho	42,689,000	0.1%
46	Maine	42,630,000	0.1%
47	North Dakota	42,472,000	0.1%
48	Wyoming	25,876,000	0.1%
49	Alaska	17,571,000	0.1%
50	Vermont	2,895,000	0.0%
	District of Columbia**	NA	NA

Source: U.S. Bureau of the Census, Governments Division
"2000 State Government Finance Data" (http://www.census.gov/govs/www/state00.html)
*Financing, construction, acquisition, maintenance or operation of hospital facilities, provision of hospital care and support of public or private hospitals.
**Not applicable.

Per Capita State Government Health Expenditures for Hospitals in 2000

National Per Capita = $116*

ALPHA ORDER

RANK	STATE	PER CAPITA
4	Alabama	$229
48	Alaska	28
49	Arizona	16
14	Arkansas	143
25	California	98
45	Colorado	34
1	Connecticut	330
28	Delaware	80
42	Florida	38
27	Georgia	81
12	Hawaii	158
46	Idaho	33
30	Illinois	68
41	Indiana	39
5	Iowa	224
42	Kansas	38
21	Kentucky	111
2	Louisiana	308
46	Maine	33
30	Maryland	68
29	Massachusetts	73
20	Michigan	112
38	Minnesota	45
6	Mississippi	210
24	Missouri	106
37	Montana	48
26	Nebraska	92
38	Nevada	45
44	New Hampshire	35
16	New Jersey	138
8	New Mexico	196
11	New York	168
13	North Carolina	154
32	North Dakota	66
23	Ohio	108
40	Oklahoma	43
3	Oregon	269
17	Pennsylvania	137
18	Rhode Island	116
9	South Carolina	192
34	South Dakota	58
33	Tennessee	64
15	Texas	141
10	Utah	185
50	Vermont	5
7	Virginia	202
19	Washington	115
36	West Virginia	49
21	Wisconsin	111
35	Wyoming	52

RANK ORDER

RANK	STATE	PER CAPITA
1	Connecticut	$330
2	Louisiana	308
3	Oregon	269
4	Alabama	229
5	Iowa	224
6	Mississippi	210
7	Virginia	202
8	New Mexico	196
9	South Carolina	192
10	Utah	185
11	New York	168
12	Hawaii	158
13	North Carolina	154
14	Arkansas	143
15	Texas	141
16	New Jersey	138
17	Pennsylvania	137
18	Rhode Island	116
19	Washington	115
20	Michigan	112
21	Kentucky	111
21	Wisconsin	111
23	Ohio	108
24	Missouri	106
25	California	98
26	Nebraska	92
27	Georgia	81
28	Delaware	80
29	Massachusetts	73
30	Illinois	68
30	Maryland	68
32	North Dakota	66
33	Tennessee	64
34	South Dakota	58
35	Wyoming	52
36	West Virginia	49
37	Montana	48
38	Minnesota	45
38	Nevada	45
40	Oklahoma	43
41	Indiana	39
42	Florida	38
42	Kansas	38
44	New Hampshire	35
45	Colorado	34
46	Idaho	33
46	Maine	33
48	Alaska	28
49	Arizona	16
50	Vermont	5
	District of Columbia**	NA

Source: Morgan Quitno Press using data from U.S. Bureau of the Census, Governments Division
    "2000 State Government Finance Data" (http://www.census.gov/govs/www/state00.html)
*Financing, construction, acquisition, maintenance or operation of hospital facilities, provision of hospital care and support of public or private hospitals.
**Not applicable.

Local Government Expenditures for Hospitals in 2000

National Total = $43,821,875,000*

ALPHA ORDER

RANK	STATE	EXPENDITURES	% of USA
8	Alabama	$1,762,266,000	4.0%
39	Alaska	57,925,000	0.1%
24	Arizona	369,335,000	0.8%
28	Arkansas	270,121,000	0.6%
1	California	5,823,493,000	13.3%
19	Colorado	720,992,000	1.6%
43	Connecticut	19,724,000	0.0%
47	Delaware	0	0.0%
4	Florida	3,559,622,000	8.1%
6	Georgia	1,826,054,000	4.2%
47	Hawaii	0	0.0%
26	Idaho	330,449,000	0.8%
13	Illinois	1,114,235,000	2.5%
7	Indiana	1,792,021,000	4.1%
20	Iowa	648,967,000	1.5%
23	Kansas	424,601,000	1.0%
36	Kentucky	132,847,000	0.3%
10	Louisiana	1,446,879,000	3.3%
38	Maine	61,312,000	0.1%
47	Maryland	0	0.0%
34	Massachusetts	213,328,000	0.5%
21	Michigan	563,168,000	1.3%
16	Minnesota	888,154,000	2.0%
12	Mississippi	1,216,294,000	2.8%
17	Missouri	784,189,000	1.8%
40	Montana	52,831,000	0.1%
32	Nebraska	241,023,000	0.6%
22	Nevada	474,297,000	1.1%
44	New Hampshire	306,000	0.0%
31	New Jersey	242,526,000	0.6%
37	New Mexico	126,290,000	0.3%
2	New York	4,877,923,000	11.1%
5	North Carolina	2,575,696,000	5.9%
45	North Dakota	76,000	0.0%
14	Ohio	979,002,000	2.2%
18	Oklahoma	762,137,000	1.7%
27	Oregon	328,496,000	0.7%
35	Pennsylvania	154,259,000	0.4%
47	Rhode Island	0	0.0%
11	South Carolina	1,411,310,000	3.2%
42	South Dakota	27,987,000	0.1%
9	Tennessee	1,530,541,000	3.5%
3	Texas	3,597,080,000	8.2%
41	Utah	32,012,000	0.1%
46	Vermont	46,000	0.0%
29	Virginia	268,721,000	0.6%
15	Washington	932,917,000	2.1%
30	West Virginia	254,496,000	0.6%
33	Wisconsin	218,622,000	0.5%
25	Wyoming	347,908,000	0.8%

RANK ORDER

RANK	STATE	EXPENDITURES	% of USA
1	California	$5,823,493,000	13.3%
2	New York	4,877,923,000	11.1%
3	Texas	3,597,080,000	8.2%
4	Florida	3,559,622,000	8.1%
5	North Carolina	2,575,696,000	5.9%
6	Georgia	1,826,054,000	4.2%
7	Indiana	1,792,021,000	4.1%
8	Alabama	1,762,266,000	4.0%
9	Tennessee	1,530,541,000	3.5%
10	Louisiana	1,446,879,000	3.3%
11	South Carolina	1,411,310,000	3.2%
12	Mississippi	1,216,294,000	2.8%
13	Illinois	1,114,235,000	2.5%
14	Ohio	979,002,000	2.2%
15	Washington	932,917,000	2.1%
16	Minnesota	888,154,000	2.0%
17	Missouri	784,189,000	1.8%
18	Oklahoma	762,137,000	1.7%
19	Colorado	720,992,000	1.6%
20	Iowa	648,967,000	1.5%
21	Michigan	563,168,000	1.3%
22	Nevada	474,297,000	1.1%
23	Kansas	424,601,000	1.0%
24	Arizona	369,335,000	0.8%
25	Wyoming	347,908,000	0.8%
26	Idaho	330,449,000	0.8%
27	Oregon	328,496,000	0.7%
28	Arkansas	270,121,000	0.6%
29	Virginia	268,721,000	0.6%
30	West Virginia	254,496,000	0.6%
31	New Jersey	242,526,000	0.6%
32	Nebraska	241,023,000	0.6%
33	Wisconsin	218,622,000	0.5%
34	Massachusetts	213,328,000	0.5%
35	Pennsylvania	154,259,000	0.4%
36	Kentucky	132,847,000	0.3%
37	New Mexico	126,290,000	0.3%
38	Maine	61,312,000	0.1%
39	Alaska	57,925,000	0.1%
40	Montana	52,831,000	0.1%
41	Utah	32,012,000	0.1%
42	South Dakota	27,987,000	0.1%
43	Connecticut	19,724,000	0.0%
44	New Hampshire	306,000	0.0%
45	North Dakota	76,000	0.0%
46	Vermont	46,000	0.0%
47	Delaware	0	0.0%
47	Hawaii	0	0.0%
47	Maryland	0	0.0%
47	Rhode Island	0	0.0%
	District of Columbia	359,397,000	0.8%

Source: U.S. Bureau of the Census, Governments Division
        "State and Local Government Finances: 1999-2000" (http://www.census.gov/govs/www/estimate00.html)
*Financing, construction, acquisition, maintenance or operation of hospital facilities, provision of hospital care and support of public or private hospitals.

Per Capita Local Government Expenditures for Hospitals in 2000

National Per Capita = $155*

ALPHA ORDER

RANK	STATE	PER CAPITA
3	Alabama	$396
27	Alaska	92
30	Arizona	71
25	Arkansas	101
18	California	171
19	Colorado	167
43	Connecticut	6
44	Delaware	0
12	Florida	222
12	Georgia	222
44	Hawaii	0
10	Idaho	254
28	Illinois	90
7	Indiana	294
12	Iowa	222
20	Kansas	158
39	Kentucky	33
5	Louisiana	324
34	Maine	48
44	Maryland	0
38	Massachusetts	34
33	Michigan	57
16	Minnesota	180
2	Mississippi	427
24	Missouri	140
32	Montana	58
22	Nebraska	141
11	Nevada	235
44	New Hampshire	0
40	New Jersey	29
31	New Mexico	69
9	New York	257
6	North Carolina	319
44	North Dakota	0
29	Ohio	86
15	Oklahoma	221
26	Oregon	96
42	Pennsylvania	13
44	Rhode Island	0
4	South Carolina	351
37	South Dakota	37
8	Tennessee	268
17	Texas	172
41	Utah	14
44	Vermont	0
36	Virginia	38
20	Washington	158
22	West Virginia	141
35	Wisconsin	41
1	Wyoming	704

RANK ORDER

RANK	STATE	PER CAPITA
1	Wyoming	$704
2	Mississippi	427
3	Alabama	396
4	South Carolina	351
5	Louisiana	324
6	North Carolina	319
7	Indiana	294
8	Tennessee	268
9	New York	257
10	Idaho	254
11	Nevada	235
12	Florida	222
12	Georgia	222
12	Iowa	222
15	Oklahoma	221
16	Minnesota	180
17	Texas	172
18	California	171
19	Colorado	167
20	Kansas	158
20	Washington	158
22	Nebraska	141
22	West Virginia	141
24	Missouri	140
25	Arkansas	101
26	Oregon	96
27	Alaska	92
28	Illinois	90
29	Ohio	86
30	Arizona	71
31	New Mexico	69
32	Montana	58
33	Michigan	57
34	Maine	48
35	Wisconsin	41
36	Virginia	38
37	South Dakota	37
38	Massachusetts	34
39	Kentucky	33
40	New Jersey	29
41	Utah	14
42	Pennsylvania	13
43	Connecticut	6
44	Delaware	0
44	Hawaii	0
44	Maryland	0
44	New Hampshire	0
44	North Dakota	0
44	Rhode Island	0
44	Vermont	0

| District of Columbia | 629 |

Source: Morgan Quitno Press using data from U.S. Bureau of the Census, Governments Division
"State and Local Government Finances: 1999-2000" (http://www.census.gov/govs/www/estimate00.html)
*Financing, construction, acquisition, maintenance or operation of hospital facilities, provision of hospital care and support of public or private hospitals.

Payroll of Health Care Establishments

National Total = $400,062,158,000*

ALPHA ORDER

RANK	STATE	PAYROLL	% of USA
24	Alabama	$5,671,364,000	1.4%
48	Alaska	1,055,149,000	0.3%
23	Arizona	5,794,326,000	1.4%
33	Arkansas	3,265,294,000	0.8%
1	California	39,988,572,000	10.0%
25	Colorado	5,497,258,000	1.4%
21	Connecticut	6,591,175,000	1.6%
43	Delaware	1,441,629,000	0.4%
4	Florida	21,896,571,000	5.5%
12	Georgia	10,035,050,000	2.5%
42	Hawaii	1,631,635,000	0.4%
44	Idaho	1,360,442,000	0.3%
6	Illinois	18,016,207,000	4.5%
15	Indiana	8,539,554,000	2.1%
28	Iowa	4,627,770,000	1.2%
31	Kansas	3,825,657,000	1.0%
26	Kentucky	5,359,822,000	1.3%
22	Louisiana	5,890,001,000	1.5%
38	Maine	2,104,428,000	0.5%
20	Maryland	7,555,077,000	1.9%
10	Massachusetts	13,111,130,000	3.3%
8	Michigan	14,420,168,000	3.6%
13	Minnesota	8,861,922,000	2.2%
32	Mississippi	3,283,693,000	0.8%
17	Missouri	8,431,668,000	2.1%
46	Montana	1,235,946,000	0.3%
34	Nebraska	2,627,756,000	0.7%
37	Nevada	2,208,338,000	0.6%
40	New Hampshire	1,888,777,000	0.5%
9	New Jersey	13,301,401,000	3.3%
39	New Mexico	1,980,285,000	0.5%
2	New York	35,271,026,000	8.8%
11	North Carolina	11,162,951,000	2.8%
47	North Dakota	1,185,790,000	0.3%
7	Ohio	17,842,592,000	4.5%
30	Oklahoma	4,132,722,000	1.0%
29	Oregon	4,342,549,000	1.1%
5	Pennsylvania	20,409,352,000	5.1%
41	Rhode Island	1,885,438,000	0.5%
27	South Carolina	4,979,067,000	1.2%
45	South Dakota	1,357,558,000	0.3%
16	Tennessee	8,455,136,000	2.1%
3	Texas	25,225,739,000	6.3%
36	Utah	2,298,572,000	0.6%
49	Vermont	936,945,000	0.2%
14	Virginia	8,602,005,000	2.2%
19	Washington	8,085,243,000	2.0%
35	West Virginia	2,501,054,000	0.6%
18	Wisconsin	8,183,073,000	2.0%
50	Wyoming	640,830,000	0.2%

RANK ORDER

RANK	STATE	PAYROLL	% of USA
1	California	$39,988,572,000	10.0%
2	New York	35,271,026,000	8.8%
3	Texas	25,225,739,000	6.3%
4	Florida	21,896,571,000	5.5%
5	Pennsylvania	20,409,352,000	5.1%
6	Illinois	18,016,207,000	4.5%
7	Ohio	17,842,592,000	4.5%
8	Michigan	14,420,168,000	3.6%
9	New Jersey	13,301,401,000	3.3%
10	Massachusetts	13,111,130,000	3.3%
11	North Carolina	11,162,951,000	2.8%
12	Georgia	10,035,050,000	2.5%
13	Minnesota	8,861,922,000	2.2%
14	Virginia	8,602,005,000	2.2%
15	Indiana	8,539,554,000	2.1%
16	Tennessee	8,455,136,000	2.1%
17	Missouri	8,431,668,000	2.1%
18	Wisconsin	8,183,073,000	2.0%
19	Washington	8,085,243,000	2.0%
20	Maryland	7,555,077,000	1.9%
21	Connecticut	6,591,175,000	1.6%
22	Louisiana	5,890,001,000	1.5%
23	Arizona	5,794,326,000	1.4%
24	Alabama	5,671,364,000	1.4%
25	Colorado	5,497,258,000	1.4%
26	Kentucky	5,359,822,000	1.3%
27	South Carolina	4,979,067,000	1.2%
28	Iowa	4,627,770,000	1.2%
29	Oregon	4,342,549,000	1.1%
30	Oklahoma	4,132,722,000	1.0%
31	Kansas	3,825,657,000	1.0%
32	Mississippi	3,283,693,000	0.8%
33	Arkansas	3,265,294,000	0.8%
34	Nebraska	2,627,756,000	0.7%
35	West Virginia	2,501,054,000	0.6%
36	Utah	2,298,572,000	0.6%
37	Nevada	2,208,338,000	0.6%
38	Maine	2,104,428,000	0.5%
39	New Mexico	1,980,285,000	0.5%
40	New Hampshire	1,888,777,000	0.5%
41	Rhode Island	1,885,438,000	0.5%
42	Hawaii	1,631,635,000	0.4%
43	Delaware	1,441,629,000	0.4%
44	Idaho	1,360,442,000	0.3%
45	South Dakota	1,357,558,000	0.3%
46	Montana	1,235,946,000	0.3%
47	North Dakota	1,185,790,000	0.3%
48	Alaska	1,055,149,000	0.3%
49	Vermont	936,945,000	0.2%
50	Wyoming	640,830,000	0.2%
	District of Columbia	1,916,757,000	0.5%

Source: U.S. Bureau of the Census
"County Business Patterns 2000 (NAICS)" (http://censtats.census.gov/cbpnaic/cbpnaic.shtml)
*Includes establishments exempt from as well as subject to the federal income tax. Includes those establishments within the North American Industry Classification System (NAICS) classifications 621 (ambulatory health care services), 622 (hospitals) and 623 (nursing and residential care facilities). See Facilities Chapter for establishments.

Average Pay per Health Care Establishment Employee in 2000

National Average = $32,865 per Employee*

ALPHA ORDER

RANK ORDER

RANK	STATE	AVERAGE PAY	RANK	STATE	AVERAGE PAY
31	Alabama	$31,443	1	Alaska	$45,208
1	Alaska	45,208	2	Delaware	40,634
14	Arizona	33,919	3	Hawaii	38,523
47	Arkansas	28,761	4	Nevada	38,321
8	California	35,286	5	New Jersey	36,639
15	Colorado	33,910	6	Connecticut	36,308
6	Connecticut	36,308	7	Wyoming	35,805
2	Delaware	40,634	8	California	35,286
18	Florida	33,479	9	New York	35,137
13	Georgia	33,969	10	Massachusetts	34,569
3	Hawaii	38,523	11	Maryland	34,268
43	Idaho	29,302	12	Washington	34,019
19	Illinois	33,413	13	Georgia	33,969
36	Indiana	30,575	14	Arizona	33,919
49	Iowa	28,641	15	Colorado	33,910
46	Kansas	28,772	16	New Hampshire	33,623
41	Kentucky	29,809	17	Michigan	33,607
45	Louisiana	28,960	18	Florida	33,479
44	Maine	29,288	19	Illinois	33,413
11	Maryland	34,268	20	Tennessee	33,219
10	Massachusetts	34,569	21	Virginia	33,058
17	Michigan	33,607	22	Oregon	33,039
26	Minnesota	32,382	23	South Carolina	32,902
40	Mississippi	29,901	24	Vermont	32,889
38	Missouri	30,076	25	Rhode Island	32,492
37	Montana	30,298	26	Minnesota	32,382
42	Nebraska	29,658	27	North Carolina	32,349
4	Nevada	38,321	28	Wisconsin	32,004
16	New Hampshire	33,623	29	Pennsylvania	31,686
5	New Jersey	36,639	30	Ohio	31,532
32	New Mexico	31,254	31	Alabama	31,443
9	New York	35,137	32	New Mexico	31,254
27	North Carolina	32,349	33	Texas	31,002
39	North Dakota	29,934	34	South Dakota	30,946
30	Ohio	31,532	35	Utah	30,782
50	Oklahoma	28,457	36	Indiana	30,575
22	Oregon	33,039	37	Montana	30,298
29	Pennsylvania	31,686	38	Missouri	30,076
25	Rhode Island	32,492	39	North Dakota	29,934
23	South Carolina	32,902	40	Mississippi	29,901
34	South Dakota	30,946	41	Kentucky	29,809
20	Tennessee	33,219	42	Nebraska	29,658
33	Texas	31,002	43	Idaho	29,302
35	Utah	30,782	44	Maine	29,288
24	Vermont	32,889	45	Louisiana	28,960
21	Virginia	33,058	46	Kansas	28,772
12	Washington	34,019	47	Arkansas	28,761
48	West Virginia	28,673	48	West Virginia	28,673
28	Wisconsin	32,004	49	Iowa	28,641
7	Wyoming	35,805	50	Oklahoma	28,457
				District of Columbia	40,616

Source: Morgan Quitno Press using data from U.S. Bureau of the Census
"County Business Patterns 2000 (NAICS)" (http://censtats.census.gov/cbpnaic/cbpnaic.shtml)
*Includes establishments exempt from as well as subject to the federal income tax. Includes those establishments within the North American Industry Classification System (NAICS) classifications 621 (ambulatory health care services), 622 (hospitals) and 623 (nursing and residential care facilities). See Facilities Chapter for establishments.

V. INCIDENCE OF DISEASE

V. INCIDENCE OF DISEASE (Continued)

Estimated New Cancer Cases in 2003

National Estimated Total = 1,334,100 New Cases*

ALPHA ORDER

RANK	STATE	CASES	% of USA
20	Alabama	23,600	1.8%
50	Alaska	1,800	0.1%
21	Arizona	23,300	1.7%
32	Arkansas	14,700	1.1%
1	California	125,000	9.4%
30	Colorado	15,200	1.1%
28	Connecticut	16,600	1.2%
45	Delaware	4,100	0.3%
2	Florida	96,100	7.2%
11	Georgia	33,400	2.5%
43	Hawaii	4,900	0.4%
42	Idaho	5,500	0.4%
7	Illinois	59,900	4.5%
14	Indiana	31,200	2.3%
29	Iowa	15,300	1.1%
33	Kansas	12,600	0.9%
23	Kentucky	22,100	1.7%
22	Louisiana	22,600	1.7%
38	Maine	7,300	0.5%
19	Maryland	24,400	1.8%
13	Massachusetts	32,700	2.5%
8	Michigan	47,400	3.6%
24	Minnesota	21,900	1.6%
31	Mississippi	14,900	1.1%
16	Missouri	29,500	2.2%
44	Montana	4,600	0.3%
36	Nebraska	8,100	0.6%
35	Nevada	10,300	0.8%
40	New Hampshire	6,000	0.4%
9	New Jersey	42,300	3.2%
37	New Mexico	7,400	0.6%
3	New York	85,900	6.4%
10	North Carolina	39,600	3.0%
47	North Dakota	3,100	0.2%
6	Ohio	60,300	4.5%
26	Oklahoma	17,700	1.3%
27	Oregon	17,300	1.3%
5	Pennsylvania	70,800	5.3%
41	Rhode Island	5,800	0.4%
25	South Carolina	20,600	1.5%
46	South Dakota	3,900	0.3%
15	Tennessee	30,500	2.3%
4	Texas	83,400	6.3%
39	Utah	6,200	0.5%
47	Vermont	3,100	0.2%
12	Virginia	32,800	2.5%
17	Washington	26,700	2.0%
34	West Virginia	11,300	0.8%
18	Wisconsin	25,800	1.9%
49	Wyoming	2,300	0.2%

RANK ORDER

RANK	STATE	CASES	% of USA
1	California	125,000	9.4%
2	Florida	96,100	7.2%
3	New York	85,900	6.4%
4	Texas	83,400	6.3%
5	Pennsylvania	70,800	5.3%
6	Ohio	60,300	4.5%
7	Illinois	59,900	4.5%
8	Michigan	47,400	3.6%
9	New Jersey	42,300	3.2%
10	North Carolina	39,600	3.0%
11	Georgia	33,400	2.5%
12	Virginia	32,800	2.5%
13	Massachusetts	32,700	2.5%
14	Indiana	31,200	2.3%
15	Tennessee	30,500	2.3%
16	Missouri	29,500	2.2%
17	Washington	26,700	2.0%
18	Wisconsin	25,800	1.9%
19	Maryland	24,400	1.8%
20	Alabama	23,600	1.8%
21	Arizona	23,300	1.7%
22	Louisiana	22,600	1.7%
23	Kentucky	22,100	1.7%
24	Minnesota	21,900	1.6%
25	South Carolina	20,600	1.5%
26	Oklahoma	17,700	1.3%
27	Oregon	17,300	1.3%
28	Connecticut	16,600	1.2%
29	Iowa	15,300	1.1%
30	Colorado	15,200	1.1%
31	Mississippi	14,900	1.1%
32	Arkansas	14,700	1.1%
33	Kansas	12,600	0.9%
34	West Virginia	11,300	0.8%
35	Nevada	10,300	0.8%
36	Nebraska	8,100	0.6%
37	New Mexico	7,400	0.6%
38	Maine	7,300	0.5%
39	Utah	6,200	0.5%
40	New Hampshire	6,000	0.4%
41	Rhode Island	5,800	0.4%
42	Idaho	5,500	0.4%
43	Hawaii	4,900	0.4%
44	Montana	4,600	0.3%
45	Delaware	4,100	0.3%
46	South Dakota	3,900	0.3%
47	North Dakota	3,100	0.2%
47	Vermont	3,100	0.2%
49	Wyoming	2,300	0.2%
50	Alaska	1,800	0.1%
	District of Columbia	2,700	0.2%

Source: American Cancer Society

"Cancer Facts & Figures 2003" (Copyright 2003, Reprinted with permission from the American Cancer Society)
These estimates are offered as a rough guide and should not be regarded as definitive. They are calculated according to the distribution of estimated 2003 cancer deaths by state. Totals do not include basal and squamous cell skin cancers or in situ carcinomas except urinary bladder.

Estimated Rate of New Cancer Cases in 2003

National Estimated Rate = 462.6 New Cases per 100,000 Population*

ALPHA ORDER

RANK	STATE	RATE
10	Alabama	526.0
49	Alaska	279.6
41	Arizona	427.0
5	Arkansas	542.4
47	California	356.0
48	Colorado	337.3
26	Connecticut	479.7
16	Delaware	507.8
2	Florida	575.0
45	Georgia	390.2
44	Hawaii	393.6
42	Idaho	410.1
28	Illinois	475.4
17	Indiana	506.6
11	Iowa	521.0
34	Kansas	463.9
7	Kentucky	540.0
20	Louisiana	504.2
4	Maine	563.9
38	Maryland	447.0
15	Massachusetts	508.7
31	Michigan	471.6
40	Minnesota	436.3
13	Mississippi	518.8
12	Missouri	520.0
19	Montana	505.8
33	Nebraska	468.4
30	Nevada	473.9
32	New Hampshire	470.6
23	New Jersey	492.4
43	New Mexico	398.9
37	New York	448.4
27	North Carolina	476.0
25	North Dakota	488.9
8	Ohio	528.0
17	Oklahoma	506.6
24	Oregon	491.3
3	Pennsylvania	574.0
6	Rhode Island	542.2
22	South Carolina	501.6
14	South Dakota	512.4
9	Tennessee	526.1
46	Texas	382.9
50	Utah	267.7
21	Vermont	502.8
36	Virginia	449.7
39	Washington	439.9
1	West Virginia	627.1
29	Wisconsin	474.2
35	Wyoming	461.2

RANK ORDER

RANK	STATE	RATE
1	West Virginia	627.1
2	Florida	575.0
3	Pennsylvania	574.0
4	Maine	563.9
5	Arkansas	542.4
6	Rhode Island	542.2
7	Kentucky	540.0
8	Ohio	528.0
9	Tennessee	526.1
10	Alabama	526.0
11	Iowa	521.0
12	Missouri	520.0
13	Mississippi	518.8
14	South Dakota	512.4
15	Massachusetts	508.7
16	Delaware	507.8
17	Indiana	506.6
17	Oklahoma	506.6
19	Montana	505.8
20	Louisiana	504.2
21	Vermont	502.8
22	South Carolina	501.6
23	New Jersey	492.4
24	Oregon	491.3
25	North Dakota	488.9
26	Connecticut	479.7
27	North Carolina	476.0
28	Illinois	475.4
29	Wisconsin	474.2
30	Nevada	473.9
31	Michigan	471.6
32	New Hampshire	470.6
33	Nebraska	468.4
34	Kansas	463.9
35	Wyoming	461.2
36	Virginia	449.7
37	New York	448.4
38	Maryland	447.0
39	Washington	439.9
40	Minnesota	436.3
41	Arizona	427.0
42	Idaho	410.1
43	New Mexico	398.9
44	Hawaii	393.6
45	Georgia	390.2
46	Texas	382.9
47	California	356.0
48	Colorado	337.3
49	Alaska	279.6
50	Utah	267.7
	District of Columbia	472.9

Source: Morgan Quitno Press using data from American Cancer Society
"Cancer Facts & Figures 2003" (Copyright 2003, Reprinted with permission from the American Cancer Society)
*These estimates are offered as a rough guide and should not be regarded as definitive. They are calculated according to the distribution of estimated 2003 cancer deaths by state. Totals do not include basal and squamous cell skin cancers or in situ carcinomas except urinary bladder.

Age-Adjusted Rate of New Cancer Cases in Males in 1999

National Rate = 562.6 New Cases per 100,000 Male Population*

ALPHA ORDER

RANK	STATE	RATE
43	Alabama	418.5
29	Alaska	527.2
NA	Arizona**	NA
36	Arkansas	488.8
30	California	526.3
32	Colorado	512.3
8	Connecticut	592.1
5	Delaware	597.4
NA	Florida**	NA
42	Georgia	447.4
37	Hawaii	476.8
33	Idaho	503.6
14	Illinois	566.1
34	Indiana	498.4
18	Iowa	557.5
NA	Kansas**	NA
7	Kentucky	593.7
4	Louisiana	597.9
12	Maine	572.8
3	Maryland	608.9
9	Massachusetts	591.6
6	Michigan	594.4
22	Minnesota	544.1
NA	Mississippi**	NA
15	Missouri	561.6
28	Montana	527.5
21	Nebraska	546.6
40	Nevada	464.0
20	New Hampshire	551.8
2	New Jersey	622.4
38	New Mexico	473.2
18	New York	557.5
31	North Carolina	522.4
23	North Dakota	537.7
25	Ohio	535.8
NA	Oklahoma**	NA
26	Oregon	530.0
10	Pennsylvania	591.1
1	Rhode Island	640.9
11	South Carolina	580.9
NA	South Dakota**	NA
41	Tennessee	461.1
24	Texas	536.7
39	Utah	468.3
NA	Vermont**	NA
35	Virginia	496.4
16	Washington	561.1
13	West Virginia	569.2
17	Wisconsin	557.9
27	Wyoming	527.6

RANK ORDER

RANK	STATE	RATE
1	Rhode Island	640.9
2	New Jersey	622.4
3	Maryland	608.9
4	Louisiana	597.9
5	Delaware	597.4
6	Michigan	594.4
7	Kentucky	593.7
8	Connecticut	592.1
9	Massachusetts	591.6
10	Pennsylvania	591.1
11	South Carolina	580.9
12	Maine	572.8
13	West Virginia	569.2
14	Illinois	566.1
15	Missouri	561.6
16	Washington	561.1
17	Wisconsin	557.9
18	Iowa	557.5
18	New York	557.5
20	New Hampshire	551.8
21	Nebraska	546.6
22	Minnesota	544.1
23	North Dakota	537.7
24	Texas	536.7
25	Ohio	535.8
26	Oregon	530.0
27	Wyoming	527.6
28	Montana	527.5
29	Alaska	527.2
30	California	526.3
31	North Carolina	522.4
32	Colorado	512.3
33	Idaho	503.6
34	Indiana	498.4
35	Virginia	496.4
36	Arkansas	488.8
37	Hawaii	476.8
38	New Mexico	473.2
39	Utah	468.3
40	Nevada	464.0
41	Tennessee	461.1
42	Georgia	447.4
43	Alabama	418.5
NA	Arizona**	NA
NA	Florida**	NA
NA	Kansas**	NA
NA	Mississippi**	NA
NA	Oklahoma**	NA
NA	South Dakota**	NA
NA	Vermont**	NA
	District of Columbia	705.5

Source: American Cancer Society
   "Cancer Facts & Figures 2003" (Copyright 2003, Reprinted with permission from the American Cancer Society)
*For 1995 to 1999. Age-adjusted to the 2000 U.S. standard population.
**Not available.

Age-Adjusted Rate of New Cancer Cases for Females in 1999

National Rate = 424.1 New Cases per 100,000 Female Population*

ALPHA ORDER

RANK	STATE	RATE
43	Alabama	313.7
7	Alaska	443.6
NA	Arizona**	NA
40	Arkansas	347.8
22	California	411.4
26	Colorado	395.0
3	Connecticut	457.1
2	Delaware	458.7
NA	Florida**	NA
42	Georgia	319.3
33	Hawaii	384.2
29	Idaho	391.1
14	Illinois	426.4
28	Indiana	391.4
19	Iowa	420.7
NA	Kansas**	NA
15	Kentucky	425.6
27	Louisiana	391.7
9	Maine	434.0
8	Maryland	442.4
6	Massachusetts	444.5
13	Michigan	427.2
23	Minnesota	409.6
NA	Mississippi**	NA
18	Missouri	422.0
25	Montana	402.0
24	Nebraska	405.2
31	Nevada	387.6
12	New Hampshire	428.4
4	New Jersey	455.9
38	New Mexico	363.3
9	New York	434.0
35	North Carolina	369.7
36	North Dakota	369.6
21	Ohio	415.9
NA	Oklahoma**	NA
16	Oregon	424.9
11	Pennsylvania	430.0
1	Rhode Island	470.3
32	South Carolina	385.7
NA	South Dakota**	NA
39	Tennessee	354.0
34	Texas	380.0
41	Utah	344.6
NA	Vermont**	NA
37	Virginia	365.6
5	Washington	445.7
17	West Virginia	424.0
20	Wisconsin	419.1
30	Wyoming	388.8

RANK ORDER

RANK	STATE	RATE
1	Rhode Island	470.3
2	Delaware	458.7
3	Connecticut	457.1
4	New Jersey	455.9
5	Washington	445.7
6	Massachusetts	444.5
7	Alaska	443.6
8	Maryland	442.4
9	Maine	434.0
9	New York	434.0
11	Pennsylvania	430.0
12	New Hampshire	428.4
13	Michigan	427.2
14	Illinois	426.4
15	Kentucky	425.6
16	Oregon	424.9
17	West Virginia	424.0
18	Missouri	422.0
19	Iowa	420.7
20	Wisconsin	419.1
21	Ohio	415.9
22	California	411.4
23	Minnesota	409.6
24	Nebraska	405.2
25	Montana	402.0
26	Colorado	395.0
27	Louisiana	391.7
28	Indiana	391.4
29	Idaho	391.1
30	Wyoming	388.8
31	Nevada	387.6
32	South Carolina	385.7
33	Hawaii	384.2
34	Texas	380.0
35	North Carolina	369.7
36	North Dakota	369.6
37	Virginia	365.6
38	New Mexico	363.3
39	Tennessee	354.0
40	Arkansas	347.8
41	Utah	344.6
42	Georgia	319.3
43	Alabama	313.7
NA	Arizona**	NA
NA	Florida**	NA
NA	Kansas**	NA
NA	Mississippi**	NA
NA	Oklahoma**	NA
NA	South Dakota**	NA
NA	Vermont**	NA

District of Columbia 438.3

Source: American Cancer Society
   "Cancer Facts & Figures 2003" (Copyright 2003, Reprinted with permission from the American Cancer Society)
*For 1995 to 1999. Age-adjusted to the 2000 U.S. standard population.
**Not available.

Estimated New Cases of Bladder Cancer in 2003

National Estimated Total = 57,400 New Cases*

ALPHA ORDER

RANK	STATE	CASES	% of USA
23	Alabama	800	1.4%
47	Alaska	100	0.2%
18	Arizona	1,000	1.7%
31	Arkansas	500	0.9%
1	California	5,500	9.6%
29	Colorado	600	1.0%
23	Connecticut	800	1.4%
37	Delaware	300	0.5%
2	Florida	4,500	7.8%
13	Georgia	1,200	2.1%
44	Hawaii	200	0.3%
37	Idaho	300	0.5%
7	Illinois	2,600	4.5%
12	Indiana	1,300	2.3%
29	Iowa	600	1.0%
31	Kansas	500	0.9%
21	Kentucky	900	1.6%
23	Louisiana	800	1.4%
35	Maine	400	0.7%
18	Maryland	1,000	1.7%
10	Massachusetts	1,700	3.0%
8	Michigan	2,200	3.8%
21	Minnesota	900	1.6%
31	Mississippi	500	0.9%
17	Missouri	1,100	1.9%
44	Montana	200	0.3%
37	Nebraska	300	0.5%
35	Nevada	400	0.7%
37	New Hampshire	300	0.5%
8	New Jersey	2,200	3.8%
37	New Mexico	300	0.5%
3	New York	4,200	7.3%
11	North Carolina	1,500	2.6%
44	North Dakota	200	0.3%
6	Ohio	2,800	4.9%
27	Oklahoma	700	1.2%
23	Oregon	800	1.4%
4	Pennsylvania	3,400	5.9%
37	Rhode Island	300	0.5%
27	South Carolina	700	1.2%
47	South Dakota	100	0.2%
18	Tennessee	1,000	1.7%
5	Texas	3,000	5.2%
37	Utah	300	0.5%
47	Vermont	100	0.2%
13	Virginia	1,200	2.1%
13	Washington	1,200	2.1%
31	West Virginia	500	0.9%
13	Wisconsin	1,200	2.1%
47	Wyoming	100	0.2%

RANK ORDER

RANK	STATE	CASES	% of USA
1	California	5,500	9.6%
2	Florida	4,500	7.8%
3	New York	4,200	7.3%
4	Pennsylvania	3,400	5.9%
5	Texas	3,000	5.2%
6	Ohio	2,800	4.9%
7	Illinois	2,600	4.5%
8	Michigan	2,200	3.8%
8	New Jersey	2,200	3.8%
10	Massachusetts	1,700	3.0%
11	North Carolina	1,500	2.6%
12	Indiana	1,300	2.3%
13	Georgia	1,200	2.1%
13	Virginia	1,200	2.1%
13	Washington	1,200	2.1%
13	Wisconsin	1,200	2.1%
17	Missouri	1,100	1.9%
18	Arizona	1,000	1.7%
18	Maryland	1,000	1.7%
18	Tennessee	1,000	1.7%
21	Kentucky	900	1.6%
21	Minnesota	900	1.6%
23	Alabama	800	1.4%
23	Connecticut	800	1.4%
23	Louisiana	800	1.4%
23	Oregon	800	1.4%
27	Oklahoma	700	1.2%
27	South Carolina	700	1.2%
29	Colorado	600	1.0%
29	Iowa	600	1.0%
31	Arkansas	500	0.9%
31	Kansas	500	0.9%
31	Mississippi	500	0.9%
31	West Virginia	500	0.9%
35	Maine	400	0.7%
35	Nevada	400	0.7%
37	Delaware	300	0.5%
37	Idaho	300	0.5%
37	Nebraska	300	0.5%
37	New Hampshire	300	0.5%
37	New Mexico	300	0.5%
37	Rhode Island	300	0.5%
37	Utah	300	0.5%
44	Hawaii	200	0.3%
44	Montana	200	0.3%
44	North Dakota	200	0.3%
47	Alaska	100	0.2%
47	South Dakota	100	0.2%
47	Vermont	100	0.2%
47	Wyoming	100	0.2%
	District of Columbia	100	0.2%

Source: American Cancer Society
   "Cancer Facts & Figures 2003" (Copyright 2003, Reprinted with permission from the American Cancer Society)
*These estimates are offered as a rough guide and should be interpreted with caution. They are calculated according to the distribution of estimated 2003 cancer deaths by state.

Estimated Rate of New Bladder Cancer Cases in 2003

National Estimated Rate = 19.9 New Cases per 100,000 Population*

ALPHA ORDER

RANK	STATE	RATE
34	Alabama	17.8
45	Alaska	15.5
30	Arizona	18.3
27	Arkansas	18.4
44	California	15.7
48	Colorado	13.3
12	Connecticut	23.1
1	Delaware	37.2
7	Florida	26.9
46	Georgia	14.0
43	Hawaii	16.1
14	Idaho	22.4
21	Illinois	20.6
20	Indiana	21.1
22	Iowa	20.4
27	Kansas	18.4
16	Kentucky	22.0
34	Louisiana	17.8
3	Maine	30.9
30	Maryland	18.3
8	Massachusetts	26.4
18	Michigan	21.9
33	Minnesota	17.9
36	Mississippi	17.4
26	Missouri	19.4
16	Montana	22.0
37	Nebraska	17.3
27	Nevada	18.4
11	New Hampshire	23.5
9	New Jersey	25.6
41	New Mexico	16.2
18	New York	21.9
32	North Carolina	18.0
2	North Dakota	31.5
10	Ohio	24.5
24	Oklahoma	20.0
13	Oregon	22.7
6	Pennsylvania	27.6
4	Rhode Island	28.0
39	South Carolina	17.0
49	South Dakota	13.1
38	Tennessee	17.2
47	Texas	13.8
50	Utah	13.0
41	Vermont	16.2
40	Virginia	16.5
25	Washington	19.8
5	West Virginia	27.7
15	Wisconsin	22.1
23	Wyoming	20.1

RANK ORDER

RANK	STATE	RATE
1	Delaware	37.2
2	North Dakota	31.5
3	Maine	30.9
4	Rhode Island	28.0
5	West Virginia	27.7
6	Pennsylvania	27.6
7	Florida	26.9
8	Massachusetts	26.4
9	New Jersey	25.6
10	Ohio	24.5
11	New Hampshire	23.5
12	Connecticut	23.1
13	Oregon	22.7
14	Idaho	22.4
15	Wisconsin	22.1
16	Kentucky	22.0
16	Montana	22.0
18	Michigan	21.9
18	New York	21.9
20	Indiana	21.1
21	Illinois	20.6
22	Iowa	20.4
23	Wyoming	20.1
24	Oklahoma	20.0
25	Washington	19.8
26	Missouri	19.4
27	Arkansas	18.4
27	Kansas	18.4
27	Nevada	18.4
30	Arizona	18.3
30	Maryland	18.3
32	North Carolina	18.0
33	Minnesota	17.9
34	Alabama	17.8
34	Louisiana	17.8
36	Mississippi	17.4
37	Nebraska	17.3
38	Tennessee	17.2
39	South Carolina	17.0
40	Virginia	16.5
41	New Mexico	16.2
41	Vermont	16.2
43	Hawaii	16.1
44	California	15.7
45	Alaska	15.5
46	Georgia	14.0
47	Texas	13.8
48	Colorado	13.3
49	South Dakota	13.1
50	Utah	13.0

| | District of Columbia | 17.5 |

Source: Morgan Quitno Press using data from American Cancer Society
    "Cancer Facts & Figures 2003" (Copyright 2003, Reprinted with permission from the American Cancer Society)
*These estimates are offered as a rough guide and should be interpreted with caution. They are calculated
according to the distribution of estimated 2003 cancer deaths by state. Rates calculated using 2002 Census
resident population estimates.

Estimated New Female Breast Cancer Cases in 2003

National Estimated Total = 211,300 New Cases*

ALPHA ORDER

RANK	STATE	CASES	% of USA
22	Alabama	3,400	1.6%
49	Alaska	300	0.1%
18	Arizona	3,900	1.8%
33	Arkansas	2,000	0.9%
1	California	21,100	10.0%
29	Colorado	2,500	1.2%
27	Connecticut	2,600	1.2%
43	Delaware	700	0.3%
4	Florida	13,500	6.4%
11	Georgia	5,400	2.6%
43	Hawaii	700	0.3%
39	Idaho	1,000	0.5%
6	Illinois	10,200	4.8%
13	Indiana	4,700	2.2%
31	Iowa	2,300	1.1%
32	Kansas	2,100	1.0%
25	Kentucky	3,200	1.5%
20	Louisiana	3,800	1.8%
39	Maine	1,000	0.5%
16	Maryland	4,200	2.0%
13	Massachusetts	4,700	2.2%
8	Michigan	7,500	3.5%
22	Minnesota	3,400	1.6%
29	Mississippi	2,500	1.2%
17	Missouri	4,100	1.9%
45	Montana	600	0.3%
37	Nebraska	1,100	0.5%
35	Nevada	1,400	0.7%
41	New Hampshire	800	0.4%
9	New Jersey	7,400	3.5%
36	New Mexico	1,300	0.6%
2	New York	14,800	7.0%
10	North Carolina	6,000	2.8%
47	North Dakota	500	0.2%
7	Ohio	9,900	4.7%
26	Oklahoma	2,700	1.3%
27	Oregon	2,600	1.2%
5	Pennsylvania	11,100	5.3%
41	Rhode Island	800	0.4%
22	South Carolina	3,400	1.6%
45	South Dakota	600	0.3%
15	Tennessee	4,500	2.1%
3	Texas	13,700	6.5%
37	Utah	1,100	0.5%
47	Vermont	500	0.2%
11	Virginia	5,400	2.6%
20	Washington	3,800	1.8%
34	West Virginia	1,600	0.8%
18	Wisconsin	3,900	1.8%
49	Wyoming	300	0.1%

RANK ORDER

RANK	STATE	CASES	% of USA
1	California	21,100	10.0%
2	New York	14,800	7.0%
3	Texas	13,700	6.5%
4	Florida	13,500	6.4%
5	Pennsylvania	11,100	5.3%
6	Illinois	10,200	4.8%
7	Ohio	9,900	4.7%
8	Michigan	7,500	3.5%
9	New Jersey	7,400	3.5%
10	North Carolina	6,000	2.8%
11	Georgia	5,400	2.6%
11	Virginia	5,400	2.6%
13	Indiana	4,700	2.2%
13	Massachusetts	4,700	2.2%
15	Tennessee	4,500	2.1%
16	Maryland	4,200	2.0%
17	Missouri	4,100	1.9%
18	Arizona	3,900	1.8%
18	Wisconsin	3,900	1.8%
20	Louisiana	3,800	1.8%
20	Washington	3,800	1.8%
22	Alabama	3,400	1.6%
22	Minnesota	3,400	1.6%
22	South Carolina	3,400	1.6%
25	Kentucky	3,200	1.5%
26	Oklahoma	2,700	1.3%
27	Connecticut	2,600	1.2%
27	Oregon	2,600	1.2%
29	Colorado	2,500	1.2%
29	Mississippi	2,500	1.2%
31	Iowa	2,300	1.1%
32	Kansas	2,100	1.0%
33	Arkansas	2,000	0.9%
34	West Virginia	1,600	0.8%
35	Nevada	1,400	0.7%
36	New Mexico	1,300	0.6%
37	Nebraska	1,100	0.5%
37	Utah	1,100	0.5%
39	Idaho	1,000	0.5%
39	Maine	1,000	0.5%
41	New Hampshire	800	0.4%
41	Rhode Island	800	0.4%
43	Delaware	700	0.3%
43	Hawaii	700	0.3%
45	Montana	600	0.3%
45	South Dakota	600	0.3%
47	North Dakota	500	0.2%
47	Vermont	500	0.2%
49	Alaska	300	0.1%
49	Wyoming	300	0.1%
	District of Columbia	500	0.2%

Source: American Cancer Society
    "Cancer Facts & Figures 2003" (Copyright 2003, Reprinted with permission from the American Cancer Society)
*These estimates are offered as a rough guide and should be interpreted with caution. They are calculated according to the distribution of estimated 2003 cancer deaths by state.

Age-Adjusted Rate of New Female Breast Cancer Cases in 1999

National Rate = 136.7 New Cases per 100,000 Female Population*

<table>
<tr><td colspan="3">ALPHA ORDER</td><td colspan="3">RANK ORDER</td></tr>
<tr><td>RANK</td><td>STATE</td><td>RATE</td><td>RANK</td><td>STATE</td><td>RATE</td></tr>
<tr><td>42</td><td>Alabama</td><td>105.2</td><td>1</td><td>Connecticut</td><td>145.6</td></tr>
<tr><td>11</td><td>Alaska</td><td>135.9</td><td>2</td><td>Washington</td><td>144.7</td></tr>
<tr><td>NA</td><td>Arizona**</td><td>NA</td><td>3</td><td>Massachusetts</td><td>144.1</td></tr>
<tr><td>40</td><td>Arkansas</td><td>113.2</td><td>4</td><td>Oregon</td><td>142.5</td></tr>
<tr><td>12</td><td>California</td><td>133.2</td><td>5</td><td>Maryland</td><td>141.7</td></tr>
<tr><td>14</td><td>Colorado</td><td>132.6</td><td>6</td><td>Delaware</td><td>140.0</td></tr>
<tr><td>1</td><td>Connecticut</td><td>145.6</td><td>7</td><td>New Jersey</td><td>139.4</td></tr>
<tr><td>6</td><td>Delaware</td><td>140.0</td><td>8</td><td>New Hampshire</td><td>137.7</td></tr>
<tr><td>NA</td><td>Florida**</td><td>NA</td><td>9</td><td>Minnesota</td><td>136.6</td></tr>
<tr><td>43</td><td>Georgia</td><td>104.5</td><td>9</td><td>Rhode Island</td><td>136.6</td></tr>
<tr><td>21</td><td>Hawaii</td><td>130.0</td><td>11</td><td>Alaska</td><td>135.9</td></tr>
<tr><td>25</td><td>Idaho</td><td>127.7</td><td>12</td><td>California</td><td>133.2</td></tr>
<tr><td>13</td><td>Illinois</td><td>133.1</td><td>13</td><td>Illinois</td><td>133.1</td></tr>
<tr><td>28</td><td>Indiana</td><td>124.3</td><td>14</td><td>Colorado</td><td>132.6</td></tr>
<tr><td>19</td><td>Iowa</td><td>130.7</td><td>15</td><td>New York</td><td>132.4</td></tr>
<tr><td>NA</td><td>Kansas**</td><td>NA</td><td>16</td><td>Wisconsin</td><td>131.7</td></tr>
<tr><td>31</td><td>Kentucky</td><td>122.2</td><td>17</td><td>Montana</td><td>131.4</td></tr>
<tr><td>35</td><td>Louisiana</td><td>120.2</td><td>18</td><td>Pennsylvania</td><td>131.3</td></tr>
<tr><td>26</td><td>Maine</td><td>126.9</td><td>19</td><td>Iowa</td><td>130.7</td></tr>
<tr><td>5</td><td>Maryland</td><td>141.7</td><td>20</td><td>Ohio</td><td>130.6</td></tr>
<tr><td>3</td><td>Massachusetts</td><td>144.1</td><td>21</td><td>Hawaii</td><td>130.0</td></tr>
<tr><td>22</td><td>Michigan</td><td>129.8</td><td>22</td><td>Michigan</td><td>129.8</td></tr>
<tr><td>9</td><td>Minnesota</td><td>136.6</td><td>23</td><td>Nebraska</td><td>129.7</td></tr>
<tr><td>NA</td><td>Mississippi**</td><td>NA</td><td>24</td><td>Missouri</td><td>129.0</td></tr>
<tr><td>24</td><td>Missouri</td><td>129.0</td><td>25</td><td>Idaho</td><td>127.7</td></tr>
<tr><td>17</td><td>Montana</td><td>131.4</td><td>26</td><td>Maine</td><td>126.9</td></tr>
<tr><td>23</td><td>Nebraska</td><td>129.7</td><td>27</td><td>South Carolina</td><td>124.4</td></tr>
<tr><td>41</td><td>Nevada</td><td>106.2</td><td>28</td><td>Indiana</td><td>124.3</td></tr>
<tr><td>8</td><td>New Hampshire</td><td>137.7</td><td>29</td><td>North Dakota</td><td>123.8</td></tr>
<tr><td>7</td><td>New Jersey</td><td>139.4</td><td>30</td><td>Virginia</td><td>123.1</td></tr>
<tr><td>34</td><td>New Mexico</td><td>120.3</td><td>31</td><td>Kentucky</td><td>122.2</td></tr>
<tr><td>15</td><td>New York</td><td>132.4</td><td>32</td><td>North Carolina</td><td>122.0</td></tr>
<tr><td>32</td><td>North Carolina</td><td>122.0</td><td>33</td><td>Wyoming</td><td>120.9</td></tr>
<tr><td>29</td><td>North Dakota</td><td>123.8</td><td>34</td><td>New Mexico</td><td>120.3</td></tr>
<tr><td>20</td><td>Ohio</td><td>130.6</td><td>35</td><td>Louisiana</td><td>120.2</td></tr>
<tr><td>NA</td><td>Oklahoma**</td><td>NA</td><td>36</td><td>West Virginia</td><td>118.1</td></tr>
<tr><td>4</td><td>Oregon</td><td>142.5</td><td>37</td><td>Texas</td><td>117.2</td></tr>
<tr><td>18</td><td>Pennsylvania</td><td>131.3</td><td>38</td><td>Utah</td><td>116.9</td></tr>
<tr><td>9</td><td>Rhode Island</td><td>136.6</td><td>39</td><td>Tennessee</td><td>114.4</td></tr>
<tr><td>27</td><td>South Carolina</td><td>124.4</td><td>40</td><td>Arkansas</td><td>113.2</td></tr>
<tr><td>NA</td><td>South Dakota**</td><td>NA</td><td>41</td><td>Nevada</td><td>106.2</td></tr>
<tr><td>39</td><td>Tennessee</td><td>114.4</td><td>42</td><td>Alabama</td><td>105.2</td></tr>
<tr><td>37</td><td>Texas</td><td>117.2</td><td>43</td><td>Georgia</td><td>104.5</td></tr>
<tr><td>38</td><td>Utah</td><td>116.9</td><td>NA</td><td>Arizona**</td><td>NA</td></tr>
<tr><td>NA</td><td>Vermont**</td><td>NA</td><td>NA</td><td>Florida**</td><td>NA</td></tr>
<tr><td>30</td><td>Virginia</td><td>123.1</td><td>NA</td><td>Kansas**</td><td>NA</td></tr>
<tr><td>2</td><td>Washington</td><td>144.7</td><td>NA</td><td>Mississippi**</td><td>NA</td></tr>
<tr><td>36</td><td>West Virginia</td><td>118.1</td><td>NA</td><td>Oklahoma**</td><td>NA</td></tr>
<tr><td>16</td><td>Wisconsin</td><td>131.7</td><td>NA</td><td>South Dakota**</td><td>NA</td></tr>
<tr><td>33</td><td>Wyoming</td><td>120.9</td><td>NA</td><td>Vermont**</td><td>NA</td></tr>
<tr><td></td><td></td><td></td><td></td><td>District of Columbia</td><td>144.1</td></tr>
</table>

Source: American Cancer Society
   "Cancer Facts & Figures 2003" (Copyright 2003, Reprinted with permission from the American Cancer Society)
*For 1995 to 1999. Age-adjusted to the 2000 U.S. standard population.
**Not available.

Percent of Women 40 and Older
Who Have Ever Had a Mammogram: 2000
National Percent = 88.0% of Women 40 and Older

RANK	STATE	PERCENT	RANK	STATE	PERCENT
20	Alabama	88.7	1	Delaware	92.9
41	Alaska	86.2	2	Connecticut	92.7
14	Arizona	89.5	3	Massachusetts	92.1
44	Arkansas	85.3	4	Rhode Island	91.9
NA	California*	NA	5	Michigan	91.2
26	Colorado	87.6	6	New Hampshire	91.0
2	Connecticut	92.7	7	Maryland	90.8
1	Delaware	92.9	8	Maine	90.7
19	Florida	88.9	9	Oregon	90.6
27	Georgia	87.4	10	New York	90.2
14	Hawaii	89.5	11	Pennsylvania	90.0
47	Idaho	84.1	11	South Carolina	90.0
27	Illinois	87.4	13	Ohio	89.6
36	Indiana	86.5	14	Arizona	89.5
35	Iowa	86.9	14	Hawaii	89.5
22	Kansas	88.3	16	Washington	89.3
33	Kentucky	87.1	17	Nevada	89.1
43	Louisiana	85.8	17	North Carolina	89.1
8	Maine	90.7	19	Florida	88.9
7	Maryland	90.8	20	Alabama	88.7
3	Massachusetts	92.1	21	Virginia	88.6
5	Michigan	91.2	22	Kansas	88.3
31	Minnesota	87.3	23	Wisconsin	88.2
48	Mississippi	83.6	24	Tennessee	88.1
44	Missouri	85.3	25	North Dakota	88.0
27	Montana	87.4	26	Colorado	87.6
37	Nebraska	86.4	27	Georgia	87.4
17	Nevada	89.1	27	Illinois	87.4
6	New Hampshire	91.0	27	Montana	87.4
42	New Jersey	86.0	27	Vermont	87.4
31	New Mexico	87.3	31	Minnesota	87.3
10	New York	90.2	31	New Mexico	87.3
17	North Carolina	89.1	33	Kentucky	87.1
25	North Dakota	88.0	34	South Dakota	87.0
13	Ohio	89.6	35	Iowa	86.9
49	Oklahoma	82.3	36	Indiana	86.5
9	Oregon	90.6	37	Nebraska	86.4
11	Pennsylvania	90.0	37	Utah	86.4
4	Rhode Island	91.9	37	West Virginia	86.4
11	South Carolina	90.0	37	Wyoming	86.4
34	South Dakota	87.0	41	Alaska	86.2
24	Tennessee	88.1	42	New Jersey	86.0
46	Texas	84.9	43	Louisiana	85.8
37	Utah	86.4	44	Arkansas	85.3
27	Vermont	87.4	44	Missouri	85.3
21	Virginia	88.6	46	Texas	84.9
16	Washington	89.3	47	Idaho	84.1
37	West Virginia	86.4	48	Mississippi	83.6
23	Wisconsin	88.2	49	Oklahoma	82.3
37	Wyoming	86.4	NA	California*	NA
				District of Columbia	93.0

Source: U.S. Department of Health and Human Services, Centers for Disease Control and Prevention
"2000 Behavioral Risk Factor Surveillance Summary Prevalence Report" (May 3, 2001)
*Not available.

Estimated New Colon and Rectum Cancer Cases in 2003

National Estimated Total = 147,500 New Cases*

ALPHA ORDER

RANK	STATE	CASES	% of USA
25	Alabama	2,200	1.5%
50	Alaska	200	0.1%
21	Arizona	2,500	1.7%
32	Arkansas	1,500	1.0%
1	California	13,000	8.8%
31	Colorado	1,600	1.1%
27	Connecticut	1,900	1.3%
46	Delaware	400	0.3%
3	Florida	10,200	6.9%
14	Georgia	3,300	2.2%
43	Hawaii	500	0.3%
42	Idaho	600	0.4%
7	Illinois	6,800	4.6%
13	Indiana	3,500	2.4%
27	Iowa	1,900	1.3%
33	Kansas	1,300	0.9%
22	Kentucky	2,400	1.6%
20	Louisiana	2,600	1.8%
37	Maine	800	0.5%
17	Maryland	2,900	2.0%
11	Massachusetts	3,700	2.5%
8	Michigan	5,100	3.5%
23	Minnesota	2,300	1.6%
29	Mississippi	1,700	1.2%
14	Missouri	3,300	2.2%
43	Montana	500	0.3%
36	Nebraska	1,100	0.7%
33	Nevada	1,300	0.9%
39	New Hampshire	700	0.5%
9	New Jersey	4,800	3.3%
37	New Mexico	800	0.5%
2	New York	10,300	7.0%
10	North Carolina	4,100	2.8%
48	North Dakota	300	0.2%
6	Ohio	6,900	4.7%
26	Oklahoma	2,000	1.4%
29	Oregon	1,700	1.2%
5	Pennsylvania	8,600	5.8%
39	Rhode Island	700	0.5%
23	South Carolina	2,300	1.6%
43	South Dakota	500	0.3%
16	Tennessee	3,200	2.2%
4	Texas	9,200	6.2%
39	Utah	700	0.5%
46	Vermont	400	0.3%
12	Virginia	3,600	2.4%
19	Washington	2,700	1.8%
35	West Virginia	1,200	0.8%
17	Wisconsin	2,900	2.0%
48	Wyoming	300	0.2%

RANK ORDER

RANK	STATE	CASES	% of USA
1	California	13,000	8.8%
2	New York	10,300	7.0%
3	Florida	10,200	6.9%
4	Texas	9,200	6.2%
5	Pennsylvania	8,600	5.8%
6	Ohio	6,900	4.7%
7	Illinois	6,800	4.6%
8	Michigan	5,100	3.5%
9	New Jersey	4,800	3.3%
10	North Carolina	4,100	2.8%
11	Massachusetts	3,700	2.5%
12	Virginia	3,600	2.4%
13	Indiana	3,500	2.4%
14	Georgia	3,300	2.2%
14	Missouri	3,300	2.2%
16	Tennessee	3,200	2.2%
17	Maryland	2,900	2.0%
17	Wisconsin	2,900	2.0%
19	Washington	2,700	1.8%
20	Louisiana	2,600	1.8%
21	Arizona	2,500	1.7%
22	Kentucky	2,400	1.6%
23	Minnesota	2,300	1.6%
23	South Carolina	2,300	1.6%
25	Alabama	2,200	1.5%
26	Oklahoma	2,000	1.4%
27	Connecticut	1,900	1.3%
27	Iowa	1,900	1.3%
29	Mississippi	1,700	1.2%
29	Oregon	1,700	1.2%
31	Colorado	1,600	1.1%
32	Arkansas	1,500	1.0%
33	Kansas	1,300	0.9%
33	Nevada	1,300	0.9%
35	West Virginia	1,200	0.8%
36	Nebraska	1,100	0.7%
37	Maine	800	0.5%
37	New Mexico	800	0.5%
39	New Hampshire	700	0.5%
39	Rhode Island	700	0.5%
39	Utah	700	0.5%
42	Idaho	600	0.4%
43	Hawaii	500	0.3%
43	Montana	500	0.3%
43	South Dakota	500	0.3%
46	Delaware	400	0.3%
46	Vermont	400	0.3%
48	North Dakota	300	0.2%
48	Wyoming	300	0.2%
50	Alaska	200	0.1%
	District of Columbia	300	0.2%

Source: American Cancer Society

"Cancer Facts & Figures 2003" (Copyright 2003, Reprinted with permission from the American Cancer Society)
These estimates are offered as a rough guide and should be interpreted with caution. They are calculated according to the distribution of estimated 2003 cancer deaths by state.

Estimated Rate of New Colon and Rectum Cancer Cases in 2003

National Estimated Rate = 51.1 New Cases per 100,000 Population*

ALPHA ORDER

RANK	STATE	RATE
35	Alabama	49.0
49	Alaska	31.1
39	Arizona	45.8
22	Arkansas	55.3
47	California	37.0
48	Colorado	35.5
25	Connecticut	54.9
32	Delaware	49.5
9	Florida	61.0
46	Georgia	38.6
45	Hawaii	40.2
41	Idaho	44.7
27	Illinois	54.0
19	Indiana	56.8
6	Iowa	64.7
37	Kansas	47.9
14	Kentucky	58.6
16	Louisiana	58.0
8	Maine	61.8
30	Maryland	53.1
17	Massachusetts	57.6
31	Michigan	50.7
39	Minnesota	45.8
13	Mississippi	59.2
15	Missouri	58.2
24	Montana	55.0
7	Nebraska	63.6
12	Nevada	59.8
25	New Hampshire	54.9
21	New Jersey	55.9
43	New Mexico	43.1
28	New York	53.8
34	North Carolina	49.3
38	North Dakota	47.3
10	Ohio	60.4
18	Oklahoma	57.2
36	Oregon	48.3
1	Pennsylvania	69.7
4	Rhode Island	65.4
20	South Carolina	56.0
3	South Dakota	65.7
23	Tennessee	55.2
44	Texas	42.2
50	Utah	30.2
5	Vermont	64.9
33	Virginia	49.4
42	Washington	44.5
2	West Virginia	66.6
29	Wisconsin	53.3
11	Wyoming	60.2

RANK ORDER

RANK	STATE	RATE
1	Pennsylvania	69.7
2	West Virginia	66.6
3	South Dakota	65.7
4	Rhode Island	65.4
5	Vermont	64.9
6	Iowa	64.7
7	Nebraska	63.6
8	Maine	61.8
9	Florida	61.0
10	Ohio	60.4
11	Wyoming	60.2
12	Nevada	59.8
13	Mississippi	59.2
14	Kentucky	58.6
15	Missouri	58.2
16	Louisiana	58.0
17	Massachusetts	57.6
18	Oklahoma	57.2
19	Indiana	56.8
20	South Carolina	56.0
21	New Jersey	55.9
22	Arkansas	55.3
23	Tennessee	55.2
24	Montana	55.0
25	Connecticut	54.9
25	New Hampshire	54.9
27	Illinois	54.0
28	New York	53.8
29	Wisconsin	53.3
30	Maryland	53.1
31	Michigan	50.7
32	Delaware	49.5
33	Virginia	49.4
34	North Carolina	49.3
35	Alabama	49.0
36	Oregon	48.3
37	Kansas	47.9
38	North Dakota	47.3
39	Arizona	45.8
39	Minnesota	45.8
41	Idaho	44.7
42	Washington	44.5
43	New Mexico	43.1
44	Texas	42.2
45	Hawaii	40.2
46	Georgia	38.6
47	California	37.0
48	Colorado	35.5
49	Alaska	31.1
50	Utah	30.2
	District of Columbia	52.5

Source: Morgan Quitno Press using data from American Cancer Society
   "Cancer Facts & Figures 2003" (Copyright 2003, Reprinted with permission from the American Cancer Society)
These estimates are offered as a rough guide and should be interpreted with caution. They are calculated according to the distribution of estimated 2003 cancer deaths by state. Rates calculated using 2002 Census resident population estimates.

Percent of Adults Receiving Recent Colon and Rectum Cancer Screening: 2001
National Median = 36.6% of Adults*

ALPHA ORDER

RANK	STATE	PERCENT
25	Alabama	37.4
31	Alaska	35.8
25	Arizona	37.4
36	Arkansas	34.5
21	California	39.6
29	Colorado	36.1
4	Connecticut	46.3
1	Delaware	53.6
21	Florida	39.6
12	Georgia	41.6
9	Hawaii	44.3
43	Idaho	33.1
46	Illinois	32.2
40	Indiana	33.5
32	Iowa	35.4
33	Kansas	35.0
42	Kentucky	33.3
45	Louisiana	32.3
18	Maine	39.8
3	Maryland	47.3
8	Massachusetts	45.1
7	Michigan	45.2
2	Minnesota	53.3
46	Mississippi	32.2
34	Missouri	34.9
44	Montana	33.0
48	Nebraska	31.8
38	Nevada	34.0
10	New Hampshire	44.0
28	New Jersey	37.2
30	New Mexico	36.0
15	New York	40.8
13	North Carolina	41.1
14	North Dakota	40.9
24	Ohio	38.0
49	Oklahoma	29.6
18	Oregon	39.8
18	Pennsylvania	39.8
6	Rhode Island	45.3
23	South Carolina	38.8
25	South Dakota	37.4
37	Tennessee	34.1
41	Texas	33.4
39	Utah	33.7
17	Vermont	40.2
11	Virginia	42.8
16	Washington	40.4
50	West Virginia	29.4
5	Wisconsin	45.8
35	Wyoming	34.8

RANK ORDER

RANK	STATE	PERCENT
1	Delaware	53.6
2	Minnesota	53.3
3	Maryland	47.3
4	Connecticut	46.3
5	Wisconsin	45.8
6	Rhode Island	45.3
7	Michigan	45.2
8	Massachusetts	45.1
9	Hawaii	44.3
10	New Hampshire	44.0
11	Virginia	42.8
12	Georgia	41.6
13	North Carolina	41.1
14	North Dakota	40.9
15	New York	40.8
16	Washington	40.4
17	Vermont	40.2
18	Maine	39.8
18	Oregon	39.8
18	Pennsylvania	39.8
21	California	39.6
21	Florida	39.6
23	South Carolina	38.8
24	Ohio	38.0
25	Alabama	37.4
25	Arizona	37.4
25	South Dakota	37.4
28	New Jersey	37.2
29	Colorado	36.1
30	New Mexico	36.0
31	Alaska	35.8
32	Iowa	35.4
33	Kansas	35.0
34	Missouri	34.9
35	Wyoming	34.8
36	Arkansas	34.5
37	Tennessee	34.1
38	Nevada	34.0
39	Utah	33.7
40	Indiana	33.5
41	Texas	33.4
42	Kentucky	33.3
43	Idaho	33.1
44	Montana	33.0
45	Louisiana	32.3
46	Illinois	32.2
46	Mississippi	32.2
48	Nebraska	31.8
49	Oklahoma	29.6
50	West Virginia	29.4
	District of Columbia	48.4

Source: U.S. Department of Health and Human Services, Centers for Disease Control and Prevention
    "2001 Behavioral Risk Factor Surveillance System Public Use Data Tape"
*Persons 50 and older.

Estimated New Leukemia Cases in 2003

National Estimated Total = 30,600 New Cases*

ALPHA ORDER

RANK	STATE	CASES	% of USA
21	Alabama	500	1.6%
NA	Alaska**	NA	NA
21	Arizona	500	1.6%
31	Arkansas	300	1.0%
1	California	3,000	9.8%
24	Colorado	400	1.3%
24	Connecticut	400	1.3%
39	Delaware	100	0.3%
2	Florida	2,200	7.2%
11	Georgia	700	2.3%
39	Hawaii	100	0.3%
39	Idaho	100	0.3%
6	Illinois	1,400	4.6%
11	Indiana	700	2.3%
24	Iowa	400	1.3%
31	Kansas	300	1.0%
24	Kentucky	400	1.3%
21	Louisiana	500	1.6%
39	Maine	100	0.3%
19	Maryland	600	2.0%
11	Massachusetts	700	2.3%
8	Michigan	1,100	3.6%
19	Minnesota	600	2.0%
31	Mississippi	300	1.0%
11	Missouri	700	2.3%
39	Montana	100	0.3%
35	Nebraska	200	0.7%
35	Nevada	200	0.7%
39	New Hampshire	100	0.3%
9	New Jersey	1,000	3.3%
35	New Mexico	200	0.7%
3	New York	2,000	6.5%
10	North Carolina	900	2.9%
39	North Dakota	100	0.3%
6	Ohio	1,400	4.6%
24	Oklahoma	400	1.3%
24	Oregon	400	1.3%
5	Pennsylvania	1,600	5.2%
39	Rhode Island	100	0.3%
24	South Carolina	400	1.3%
39	South Dakota	100	0.3%
11	Tennessee	700	2.3%
4	Texas	1,900	6.2%
35	Utah	200	0.7%
39	Vermont	100	0.3%
11	Virginia	700	2.3%
11	Washington	700	2.3%
31	West Virginia	300	1.0%
11	Wisconsin	700	2.3%
39	Wyoming	100	0.3%

RANK ORDER

RANK	STATE	CASES	% of USA
1	California	3,000	9.8%
2	Florida	2,200	7.2%
3	New York	2,000	6.5%
4	Texas	1,900	6.2%
5	Pennsylvania	1,600	5.2%
6	Illinois	1,400	4.6%
6	Ohio	1,400	4.6%
8	Michigan	1,100	3.6%
9	New Jersey	1,000	3.3%
10	North Carolina	900	2.9%
11	Georgia	700	2.3%
11	Indiana	700	2.3%
11	Massachusetts	700	2.3%
11	Missouri	700	2.3%
11	Tennessee	700	2.3%
11	Virginia	700	2.3%
11	Washington	700	2.3%
11	Wisconsin	700	2.3%
19	Maryland	600	2.0%
19	Minnesota	600	2.0%
21	Alabama	500	1.6%
21	Arizona	500	1.6%
21	Louisiana	500	1.6%
24	Colorado	400	1.3%
24	Connecticut	400	1.3%
24	Iowa	400	1.3%
24	Kentucky	400	1.3%
24	Oklahoma	400	1.3%
24	Oregon	400	1.3%
24	South Carolina	400	1.3%
31	Arkansas	300	1.0%
31	Kansas	300	1.0%
31	Mississippi	300	1.0%
31	West Virginia	300	1.0%
35	Nebraska	200	0.7%
35	Nevada	200	0.7%
35	New Mexico	200	0.7%
35	Utah	200	0.7%
39	Delaware	100	0.3%
39	Hawaii	100	0.3%
39	Idaho	100	0.3%
39	Maine	100	0.3%
39	Montana	100	0.3%
39	New Hampshire	100	0.3%
39	North Dakota	100	0.3%
39	Rhode Island	100	0.3%
39	South Dakota	100	0.3%
39	Vermont	100	0.3%
39	Wyoming	100	0.3%
NA	Alaska**	NA	NA
	District of Columbia**	NA	NA

Source: American Cancer Society
    "Cancer Facts & Figures 2003" (Copyright 2003, Reprinted with permission from the American Cancer Society)
These estimates are offered as a rough guide and should be interpreted with caution. They are calculated according to the distribution of estimated 2003 cancer deaths by state.
**Not available.*

Estimated Rate of New Leukemia Cases in 2003

National Estimated Rate = 10.6 New Cases per 100,000 Population*

ALPHA ORDER

RANK	STATE	RATE		RANK	STATE	RATE
23	Alabama	11.1		1	Wyoming	20.1
NA	Alaska**	NA		2	West Virginia	16.6
39	Arizona	9.2		3	Vermont	16.2
23	Arkansas	11.1		4	North Dakota	15.8
44	California	8.5		5	Iowa	13.6
41	Colorado	8.9		6	Florida	13.2
15	Connecticut	11.6		7	South Dakota	13.1
10	Delaware	12.4		8	Pennsylvania	13.0
6	Florida	13.2		9	Wisconsin	12.9
45	Georgia	8.2		10	Delaware	12.4
46	Hawaii	8.0		11	Missouri	12.3
49	Idaho	7.5		11	Ohio	12.3
23	Illinois	11.1		13	Tennessee	12.1
19	Indiana	11.4		14	Minnesota	12.0
5	Iowa	13.6		15	Connecticut	11.6
26	Kansas	11.0		15	Nebraska	11.6
35	Kentucky	9.8		15	New Jersey	11.6
22	Louisiana	11.2		18	Washington	11.5
48	Maine	7.7		19	Indiana	11.4
26	Maryland	11.0		19	Oklahoma	11.4
29	Massachusetts	10.9		19	Oregon	11.4
29	Michigan	10.9		22	Louisiana	11.2
14	Minnesota	12.0		23	Alabama	11.1
33	Mississippi	10.4		23	Arkansas	11.1
11	Missouri	12.3		23	Illinois	11.1
26	Montana	11.0		26	Kansas	11.0
15	Nebraska	11.6		26	Maryland	11.0
39	Nevada	9.2		26	Montana	11.0
47	New Hampshire	7.8		29	Massachusetts	10.9
15	New Jersey	11.6		29	Michigan	10.9
31	New Mexico	10.8		31	New Mexico	10.8
33	New York	10.4		31	North Carolina	10.8
31	North Carolina	10.8		33	Mississippi	10.4
4	North Dakota	15.8		33	New York	10.4
11	Ohio	12.3		35	Kentucky	9.8
19	Oklahoma	11.4		36	South Carolina	9.7
19	Oregon	11.4		37	Virginia	9.6
8	Pennsylvania	13.0		38	Rhode Island	9.3
38	Rhode Island	9.3		39	Arizona	9.2
36	South Carolina	9.7		39	Nevada	9.2
7	South Dakota	13.1		41	Colorado	8.9
13	Tennessee	12.1		42	Texas	8.7
42	Texas	8.7		43	Utah	8.6
43	Utah	8.6		44	California	8.5
3	Vermont	16.2		45	Georgia	8.2
37	Virginia	9.6		46	Hawaii	8.0
18	Washington	11.5		47	New Hampshire	7.8
2	West Virginia	16.6		48	Maine	7.7
9	Wisconsin	12.9		49	Idaho	7.5
1	Wyoming	20.1		NA	Alaska**	NA
					District of Columbia**	NA

Source: Morgan Quitno Press using data from American Cancer Society
    "Cancer Facts & Figures 2003" (Copyright 2003, Reprinted with permission from the American Cancer Society)
*These estimates are offered as a rough guide and should be interpreted with caution. They are calculated according to the distribution of estimated 2003 cancer deaths by state. Rates calculated using 2002 Census resident population estimates.
**Not available.

Estimated New Lung Cancer Cases in 2003

National Estimated Total = 171,900 New Cases*

ALPHA ORDER

RANK	STATE	CASES	% of USA
19	Alabama	3,300	1.9%
50	Alaska	200	0.1%
21	Arizona	3,000	1.7%
28	Arkansas	2,200	1.3%
1	California	14,400	8.4%
34	Colorado	1,600	0.9%
30	Connecticut	2,000	1.2%
41	Delaware	600	0.3%
2	Florida	13,200	7.7%
11	Georgia	4,600	2.7%
41	Hawaii	600	0.3%
41	Idaho	600	0.3%
7	Illinois	7,400	4.3%
13	Indiana	4,400	2.6%
31	Iowa	1,900	1.1%
32	Kansas	1,700	1.0%
17	Kentucky	3,500	2.0%
21	Louisiana	3,000	1.7%
36	Maine	1,000	0.6%
20	Maryland	3,200	1.9%
16	Massachusetts	4,100	2.4%
8	Michigan	6,100	3.5%
26	Minnesota	2,500	1.5%
28	Mississippi	2,200	1.3%
15	Missouri	4,200	2.4%
41	Montana	600	0.3%
36	Nebraska	1,000	0.6%
35	Nevada	1,500	0.9%
38	New Hampshire	800	0.5%
10	New Jersey	5,000	2.9%
38	New Mexico	800	0.5%
4	New York	10,000	5.8%
9	North Carolina	5,600	3.3%
48	North Dakota	300	0.2%
6	Ohio	8,000	4.7%
25	Oklahoma	2,600	1.5%
27	Oregon	2,300	1.3%
5	Pennsylvania	8,700	5.1%
38	Rhode Island	800	0.5%
24	South Carolina	2,800	1.6%
46	South Dakota	400	0.2%
12	Tennessee	4,500	2.6%
3	Texas	10,900	6.3%
45	Utah	500	0.3%
46	Vermont	400	0.2%
14	Virginia	4,300	2.5%
17	Washington	3,500	2.0%
32	West Virginia	1,700	1.0%
21	Wisconsin	3,000	1.7%
48	Wyoming	300	0.2%

RANK ORDER

RANK	STATE	CASES	% of USA
1	California	14,400	8.4%
2	Florida	13,200	7.7%
3	Texas	10,900	6.3%
4	New York	10,000	5.8%
5	Pennsylvania	8,700	5.1%
6	Ohio	8,000	4.7%
7	Illinois	7,400	4.3%
8	Michigan	6,100	3.5%
9	North Carolina	5,600	3.3%
10	New Jersey	5,000	2.9%
11	Georgia	4,600	2.7%
12	Tennessee	4,500	2.6%
13	Indiana	4,400	2.6%
14	Virginia	4,300	2.5%
15	Missouri	4,200	2.4%
16	Massachusetts	4,100	2.4%
17	Kentucky	3,500	2.0%
17	Washington	3,500	2.0%
19	Alabama	3,300	1.9%
20	Maryland	3,200	1.9%
21	Arizona	3,000	1.7%
21	Louisiana	3,000	1.7%
21	Wisconsin	3,000	1.7%
24	South Carolina	2,800	1.6%
25	Oklahoma	2,600	1.5%
26	Minnesota	2,500	1.5%
27	Oregon	2,300	1.3%
28	Arkansas	2,200	1.3%
28	Mississippi	2,200	1.3%
30	Connecticut	2,000	1.2%
31	Iowa	1,900	1.1%
32	Kansas	1,700	1.0%
32	West Virginia	1,700	1.0%
34	Colorado	1,600	0.9%
35	Nevada	1,500	0.9%
36	Maine	1,000	0.6%
36	Nebraska	1,000	0.6%
38	New Hampshire	800	0.5%
38	New Mexico	800	0.5%
38	Rhode Island	800	0.5%
41	Delaware	600	0.3%
41	Hawaii	600	0.3%
41	Idaho	600	0.3%
41	Montana	600	0.3%
45	Utah	500	0.3%
46	South Dakota	400	0.2%
46	Vermont	400	0.2%
48	North Dakota	300	0.2%
48	Wyoming	300	0.2%
50	Alaska	200	0.1%
	District of Columbia	300	0.2%

Source: American Cancer Society
"Cancer Facts & Figures 2003" (Copyright 2003, Reprinted with permission from the American Cancer Society)
*These estimates are offered as a rough guide and should be interpreted with caution. They are calculated according to the distribution of estimated 2003 cancer deaths by state.

Estimated Rate of New Lung Cancer Cases in 2003

National Estimated Rate = 59.6 New Cases per 100,000 Population*

ALPHA ORDER			RANK ORDER		
RANK	STATE	RATE	RANK	STATE	RATE
12	Alabama	73.6	1	West Virginia	94.3
49	Alaska	31.1	2	Kentucky	85.5
37	Arizona	55.0	3	Arkansas	81.2
3	Arkansas	81.2	4	Florida	79.0
47	California	41.0	5	Tennessee	77.6
48	Colorado	35.5	6	Maine	77.3
33	Connecticut	57.8	7	Mississippi	76.6
10	Delaware	74.3	8	Rhode Island	74.8
4	Florida	79.0	9	Oklahoma	74.4
38	Georgia	53.7	10	Delaware	74.3
43	Hawaii	48.2	11	Missouri	74.0
45	Idaho	44.7	12	Alabama	73.6
30	Illinois	58.7	13	Indiana	71.4
13	Indiana	71.4	14	Pennsylvania	70.5
23	Iowa	64.7	15	Ohio	70.0
26	Kansas	62.6	16	Nevada	69.0
2	Kentucky	85.5	17	South Carolina	68.2
19	Louisiana	66.9	18	North Carolina	67.3
6	Maine	77.3	19	Louisiana	66.9
31	Maryland	58.6	20	Montana	66.0
24	Massachusetts	63.8	21	Oregon	65.3
27	Michigan	60.7	22	Vermont	64.9
42	Minnesota	49.8	23	Iowa	64.7
7	Mississippi	76.6	24	Massachusetts	63.8
11	Missouri	74.0	25	New Hampshire	62.7
20	Montana	66.0	26	Kansas	62.6
33	Nebraska	57.8	27	Michigan	60.7
16	Nevada	69.0	28	Wyoming	60.2
25	New Hampshire	62.7	29	Virginia	59.0
32	New Jersey	58.2	30	Illinois	58.7
46	New Mexico	43.1	31	Maryland	58.6
40	New York	52.2	32	New Jersey	58.2
18	North Carolina	67.3	33	Connecticut	57.8
44	North Dakota	47.3	33	Nebraska	57.8
15	Ohio	70.0	35	Washington	57.7
9	Oklahoma	74.4	36	Wisconsin	55.1
21	Oregon	65.3	37	Arizona	55.0
14	Pennsylvania	70.5	38	Georgia	53.7
8	Rhode Island	74.8	39	South Dakota	52.6
17	South Carolina	68.2	40	New York	52.2
39	South Dakota	52.6	41	Texas	50.0
5	Tennessee	77.6	42	Minnesota	49.8
41	Texas	50.0	43	Hawaii	48.2
50	Utah	21.6	44	North Dakota	47.3
22	Vermont	64.9	45	Idaho	44.7
29	Virginia	59.0	46	New Mexico	43.1
35	Washington	57.7	47	California	41.0
1	West Virginia	94.3	48	Colorado	35.5
36	Wisconsin	55.1	49	Alaska	31.1
28	Wyoming	60.2	50	Utah	21.6
				District of Columbia	52.5

Source: Morgan Quitno Press using data from American Cancer Society
   "Cancer Facts & Figures 2003" (Copyright 2003, Reprinted with permission from the American Cancer Society)
*These estimates are offered as a rough guide and should be interpreted with caution. They are calculated according to the distribution of estimated 2003 cancer deaths by state. Rates calculated using 2002 Census resident population estimates.

Estimated New Non-Hodgkin's Lymphoma Cases in 2003

National Estimated Total = 53,400 New Cases*

<table>
<tr><td colspan="4">ALPHA ORDER</td><td colspan="4">RANK ORDER</td></tr>
<tr><td>RANK</td><td>STATE</td><td>CASES</td><td>% of USA</td><td>RANK</td><td>STATE</td><td>CASES</td><td>% of USA</td></tr>
<tr><td>22</td><td>Alabama</td><td>800</td><td>1.5%</td><td>1</td><td>California</td><td>5,200</td><td>9.7%</td></tr>
<tr><td>47</td><td>Alaska</td><td>100</td><td>0.2%</td><td>2</td><td>Florida</td><td>3,900</td><td>7.3%</td></tr>
<tr><td>20</td><td>Arizona</td><td>1,000</td><td>1.9%</td><td>3</td><td>New York</td><td>3,300</td><td>6.2%</td></tr>
<tr><td>30</td><td>Arkansas</td><td>600</td><td>1.1%</td><td>3</td><td>Texas</td><td>3,300</td><td>6.2%</td></tr>
<tr><td>1</td><td>California</td><td>5,200</td><td>9.7%</td><td>5</td><td>Pennsylvania</td><td>3,000</td><td>5.6%</td></tr>
<tr><td>25</td><td>Colorado</td><td>700</td><td>1.3%</td><td>6</td><td>Ohio</td><td>2,600</td><td>4.9%</td></tr>
<tr><td>25</td><td>Connecticut</td><td>700</td><td>1.3%</td><td>7</td><td>Illinois</td><td>2,400</td><td>4.5%</td></tr>
<tr><td>41</td><td>Delaware</td><td>200</td><td>0.4%</td><td>8</td><td>Michigan</td><td>2,000</td><td>3.7%</td></tr>
<tr><td>2</td><td>Florida</td><td>3,900</td><td>7.3%</td><td>9</td><td>New Jersey</td><td>1,800</td><td>3.4%</td></tr>
<tr><td>16</td><td>Georgia</td><td>1,100</td><td>2.1%</td><td>10</td><td>North Carolina</td><td>1,400</td><td>2.6%</td></tr>
<tr><td>41</td><td>Hawaii</td><td>200</td><td>0.4%</td><td>11</td><td>Indiana</td><td>1,300</td><td>2.4%</td></tr>
<tr><td>41</td><td>Idaho</td><td>200</td><td>0.4%</td><td>11</td><td>Massachusetts</td><td>1,300</td><td>2.4%</td></tr>
<tr><td>7</td><td>Illinois</td><td>2,400</td><td>4.5%</td><td>11</td><td>Virginia</td><td>1,300</td><td>2.4%</td></tr>
<tr><td>11</td><td>Indiana</td><td>1,300</td><td>2.4%</td><td>14</td><td>Tennessee</td><td>1,200</td><td>2.2%</td></tr>
<tr><td>30</td><td>Iowa</td><td>600</td><td>1.1%</td><td>14</td><td>Wisconsin</td><td>1,200</td><td>2.2%</td></tr>
<tr><td>32</td><td>Kansas</td><td>500</td><td>0.9%</td><td>16</td><td>Georgia</td><td>1,100</td><td>2.1%</td></tr>
<tr><td>22</td><td>Kentucky</td><td>800</td><td>1.5%</td><td>16</td><td>Minnesota</td><td>1,100</td><td>2.1%</td></tr>
<tr><td>22</td><td>Louisiana</td><td>800</td><td>1.5%</td><td>16</td><td>Missouri</td><td>1,100</td><td>2.1%</td></tr>
<tr><td>36</td><td>Maine</td><td>300</td><td>0.6%</td><td>16</td><td>Washington</td><td>1,100</td><td>2.1%</td></tr>
<tr><td>21</td><td>Maryland</td><td>900</td><td>1.7%</td><td>20</td><td>Arizona</td><td>1,000</td><td>1.9%</td></tr>
<tr><td>11</td><td>Massachusetts</td><td>1,300</td><td>2.4%</td><td>21</td><td>Maryland</td><td>900</td><td>1.7%</td></tr>
<tr><td>8</td><td>Michigan</td><td>2,000</td><td>3.7%</td><td>22</td><td>Alabama</td><td>800</td><td>1.5%</td></tr>
<tr><td>16</td><td>Minnesota</td><td>1,100</td><td>2.1%</td><td>22</td><td>Kentucky</td><td>800</td><td>1.5%</td></tr>
<tr><td>32</td><td>Mississippi</td><td>500</td><td>0.9%</td><td>22</td><td>Louisiana</td><td>800</td><td>1.5%</td></tr>
<tr><td>16</td><td>Missouri</td><td>1,100</td><td>2.1%</td><td>25</td><td>Colorado</td><td>700</td><td>1.3%</td></tr>
<tr><td>41</td><td>Montana</td><td>200</td><td>0.4%</td><td>25</td><td>Connecticut</td><td>700</td><td>1.3%</td></tr>
<tr><td>34</td><td>Nebraska</td><td>400</td><td>0.7%</td><td>25</td><td>Oklahoma</td><td>700</td><td>1.3%</td></tr>
<tr><td>36</td><td>Nevada</td><td>300</td><td>0.6%</td><td>25</td><td>Oregon</td><td>700</td><td>1.3%</td></tr>
<tr><td>36</td><td>New Hampshire</td><td>300</td><td>0.6%</td><td>25</td><td>South Carolina</td><td>700</td><td>1.3%</td></tr>
<tr><td>9</td><td>New Jersey</td><td>1,800</td><td>3.4%</td><td>30</td><td>Arkansas</td><td>600</td><td>1.1%</td></tr>
<tr><td>36</td><td>New Mexico</td><td>300</td><td>0.6%</td><td>30</td><td>Iowa</td><td>600</td><td>1.1%</td></tr>
<tr><td>3</td><td>New York</td><td>3,300</td><td>6.2%</td><td>32</td><td>Kansas</td><td>500</td><td>0.9%</td></tr>
<tr><td>10</td><td>North Carolina</td><td>1,400</td><td>2.6%</td><td>32</td><td>Mississippi</td><td>500</td><td>0.9%</td></tr>
<tr><td>47</td><td>North Dakota</td><td>100</td><td>0.2%</td><td>34</td><td>Nebraska</td><td>400</td><td>0.7%</td></tr>
<tr><td>6</td><td>Ohio</td><td>2,600</td><td>4.9%</td><td>34</td><td>West Virginia</td><td>400</td><td>0.7%</td></tr>
<tr><td>25</td><td>Oklahoma</td><td>700</td><td>1.3%</td><td>36</td><td>Maine</td><td>300</td><td>0.6%</td></tr>
<tr><td>25</td><td>Oregon</td><td>700</td><td>1.3%</td><td>36</td><td>Nevada</td><td>300</td><td>0.6%</td></tr>
<tr><td>5</td><td>Pennsylvania</td><td>3,000</td><td>5.6%</td><td>36</td><td>New Hampshire</td><td>300</td><td>0.6%</td></tr>
<tr><td>41</td><td>Rhode Island</td><td>200</td><td>0.4%</td><td>36</td><td>New Mexico</td><td>300</td><td>0.6%</td></tr>
<tr><td>25</td><td>South Carolina</td><td>700</td><td>1.3%</td><td>36</td><td>Utah</td><td>300</td><td>0.6%</td></tr>
<tr><td>41</td><td>South Dakota</td><td>200</td><td>0.4%</td><td>41</td><td>Delaware</td><td>200</td><td>0.4%</td></tr>
<tr><td>14</td><td>Tennessee</td><td>1,200</td><td>2.2%</td><td>41</td><td>Hawaii</td><td>200</td><td>0.4%</td></tr>
<tr><td>3</td><td>Texas</td><td>3,300</td><td>6.2%</td><td>41</td><td>Idaho</td><td>200</td><td>0.4%</td></tr>
<tr><td>36</td><td>Utah</td><td>300</td><td>0.6%</td><td>41</td><td>Montana</td><td>200</td><td>0.4%</td></tr>
<tr><td>47</td><td>Vermont</td><td>100</td><td>0.2%</td><td>41</td><td>Rhode Island</td><td>200</td><td>0.4%</td></tr>
<tr><td>11</td><td>Virginia</td><td>1,300</td><td>2.4%</td><td>41</td><td>South Dakota</td><td>200</td><td>0.4%</td></tr>
<tr><td>16</td><td>Washington</td><td>1,100</td><td>2.1%</td><td>47</td><td>Alaska</td><td>100</td><td>0.2%</td></tr>
<tr><td>34</td><td>West Virginia</td><td>400</td><td>0.7%</td><td>47</td><td>North Dakota</td><td>100</td><td>0.2%</td></tr>
<tr><td>14</td><td>Wisconsin</td><td>1,200</td><td>2.2%</td><td>47</td><td>Vermont</td><td>100</td><td>0.2%</td></tr>
<tr><td>47</td><td>Wyoming</td><td>100</td><td>0.2%</td><td>47</td><td>Wyoming</td><td>100</td><td>0.2%</td></tr>
<tr><td></td><td></td><td></td><td></td><td></td><td>District of Columbia**</td><td>NA</td><td>NA</td></tr>
</table>

Source: American Cancer Society
"Cancer Facts & Figures 2003" (Copyright 2003, Reprinted with permission from the American Cancer Society)
*These estimates are offered as a rough guide and should be interpreted with caution. They are calculated according to the distribution of estimated 2003 cancer deaths by state.
**Not available.

Estimated Rate of New Non-Hodgkin's Lymphoma Cases in 2003

National Estimated Rate = 18.5 New Cases per 100,000 Population*

ALPHA ORDER

RANK	STATE	RATE
31	Alabama	17.8
43	Alaska	15.5
29	Arizona	18.3
10	Arkansas	22.1
47	California	14.8
43	Colorado	15.5
18	Connecticut	20.2
2	Delaware	24.8
5	Florida	23.3
50	Georgia	12.9
41	Hawaii	16.1
46	Idaho	14.9
26	Illinois	19.0
14	Indiana	21.1
17	Iowa	20.4
28	Kansas	18.4
24	Kentucky	19.5
31	Louisiana	17.8
6	Maine	23.2
38	Maryland	16.5
18	Massachusetts	20.2
22	Michigan	19.9
13	Minnesota	21.9
34	Mississippi	17.4
25	Missouri	19.4
12	Montana	22.0
7	Nebraska	23.1
48	Nevada	13.8
4	New Hampshire	23.5
15	New Jersey	21.0
39	New Mexico	16.2
35	New York	17.2
37	North Carolina	16.8
42	North Dakota	15.8
8	Ohio	22.8
21	Oklahoma	20.0
22	Oregon	19.9
3	Pennsylvania	24.3
27	Rhode Island	18.7
36	South Carolina	17.0
1	South Dakota	26.3
16	Tennessee	20.7
45	Texas	15.2
49	Utah	13.0
39	Vermont	16.2
31	Virginia	17.8
30	Washington	18.1
9	West Virginia	22.2
10	Wisconsin	22.1
20	Wyoming	20.1

RANK ORDER

RANK	STATE	RATE
1	South Dakota	26.3
2	Delaware	24.8
3	Pennsylvania	24.3
4	New Hampshire	23.5
5	Florida	23.3
6	Maine	23.2
7	Nebraska	23.1
8	Ohio	22.8
9	West Virginia	22.2
10	Arkansas	22.1
10	Wisconsin	22.1
12	Montana	22.0
13	Minnesota	21.9
14	Indiana	21.1
15	New Jersey	21.0
16	Tennessee	20.7
17	Iowa	20.4
18	Connecticut	20.2
18	Massachusetts	20.2
20	Wyoming	20.1
21	Oklahoma	20.0
22	Michigan	19.9
22	Oregon	19.9
24	Kentucky	19.5
25	Missouri	19.4
26	Illinois	19.0
27	Rhode Island	18.7
28	Kansas	18.4
29	Arizona	18.3
30	Washington	18.1
31	Alabama	17.8
31	Louisiana	17.8
31	Virginia	17.8
34	Mississippi	17.4
35	New York	17.2
36	South Carolina	17.0
37	North Carolina	16.8
38	Maryland	16.5
39	New Mexico	16.2
39	Vermont	16.2
41	Hawaii	16.1
42	North Dakota	15.8
43	Alaska	15.5
43	Colorado	15.5
45	Texas	15.2
46	Idaho	14.9
47	California	14.8
48	Nevada	13.8
49	Utah	13.0
50	Georgia	12.9

District of Columbia**   NA

Source: Morgan Quitno Press using data from American Cancer Society
"Cancer Facts & Figures 2003" (Copyright 2003, Reprinted with permission from the American Cancer Society)
These estimates are offered as a rough guide and should be interpreted with caution. They are calculated according to the distribution of estimated 2003 cancer deaths by state. Rates calculated using 2002 Census resident population estimates.
**Not available.*

Estimated New Prostate Cancer Cases in 2003

National Estimated Total = 220,900 New Cases*

ALPHA ORDER

RANK	STATE	CASES	% of USA
15	Alabama	4,700	2.1%
50	Alaska	200	0.1%
19	Arizona	4,300	1.9%
30	Arkansas	2,600	1.2%
1	California	20,500	9.3%
30	Colorado	2,600	1.2%
28	Connecticut	2,800	1.3%
46	Delaware	600	0.3%
2	Florida	15,800	7.2%
11	Georgia	5,700	2.6%
40	Hawaii	900	0.4%
39	Idaho	1,100	0.5%
6	Illinois	10,100	4.6%
14	Indiana	5,000	2.3%
29	Iowa	2,700	1.2%
33	Kansas	2,100	1.0%
25	Kentucky	3,300	1.5%
24	Louisiana	3,600	1.6%
40	Maine	900	0.4%
21	Maryland	3,900	1.8%
12	Massachusetts	5,500	2.5%
8	Michigan	7,800	3.5%
20	Minnesota	4,000	1.8%
27	Mississippi	2,900	1.3%
17	Missouri	4,500	2.0%
44	Montana	800	0.4%
36	Nebraska	1,400	0.6%
35	Nevada	1,600	0.7%
40	New Hampshire	900	0.4%
10	New Jersey	6,600	3.0%
36	New Mexico	1,400	0.6%
3	New York	14,000	6.3%
9	North Carolina	6,800	3.1%
47	North Dakota	500	0.2%
7	Ohio	9,400	4.3%
30	Oklahoma	2,600	1.2%
26	Oregon	3,200	1.4%
5	Pennsylvania	12,000	5.4%
40	Rhode Island	900	0.4%
23	South Carolina	3,800	1.7%
45	South Dakota	700	0.3%
15	Tennessee	4,700	2.1%
4	Texas	13,200	6.0%
36	Utah	1,400	0.6%
49	Vermont	300	0.1%
12	Virginia	5,500	2.5%
21	Washington	3,900	1.8%
34	West Virginia	1,700	0.8%
17	Wisconsin	4,500	2.0%
48	Wyoming	400	0.2%

RANK ORDER

RANK	STATE	CASES	% of USA
1	California	20,500	9.3%
2	Florida	15,800	7.2%
3	New York	14,000	6.3%
4	Texas	13,200	6.0%
5	Pennsylvania	12,000	5.4%
6	Illinois	10,100	4.6%
7	Ohio	9,400	4.3%
8	Michigan	7,800	3.5%
9	North Carolina	6,800	3.1%
10	New Jersey	6,600	3.0%
11	Georgia	5,700	2.6%
12	Massachusetts	5,500	2.5%
12	Virginia	5,500	2.5%
14	Indiana	5,000	2.3%
15	Alabama	4,700	2.1%
15	Tennessee	4,700	2.1%
17	Missouri	4,500	2.0%
17	Wisconsin	4,500	2.0%
19	Arizona	4,300	1.9%
20	Minnesota	4,000	1.8%
21	Maryland	3,900	1.8%
21	Washington	3,900	1.8%
23	South Carolina	3,800	1.7%
24	Louisiana	3,600	1.6%
25	Kentucky	3,300	1.5%
26	Oregon	3,200	1.4%
27	Mississippi	2,900	1.3%
28	Connecticut	2,800	1.3%
29	Iowa	2,700	1.2%
30	Arkansas	2,600	1.2%
30	Colorado	2,600	1.2%
30	Oklahoma	2,600	1.2%
33	Kansas	2,100	1.0%
34	West Virginia	1,700	0.8%
35	Nevada	1,600	0.7%
36	Nebraska	1,400	0.6%
36	New Mexico	1,400	0.6%
36	Utah	1,400	0.6%
39	Idaho	1,100	0.5%
40	Hawaii	900	0.4%
40	Maine	900	0.4%
40	New Hampshire	900	0.4%
40	Rhode Island	900	0.4%
44	Montana	800	0.4%
45	South Dakota	700	0.3%
46	Delaware	600	0.3%
47	North Dakota	500	0.2%
48	Wyoming	400	0.2%
49	Vermont	300	0.1%
50	Alaska	200	0.1%
	District of Columbia	600	0.3%

Source: American Cancer Society
"Cancer Facts & Figures 2003" (Copyright 2003, Reprinted with permission from the American Cancer Society)
*These estimates are offered as a rough guide and should be interpreted with caution. They are calculated according to the distribution of estimated 2003 cancer deaths by state.

Age-Adjusted Rate of New Prostate Cancer Cases in 1999

National Rate = 168.9 New Cases per 100,000 Male Population*

ALPHA ORDER

RANK	STATE	RATE
43	Alabama	93.1
23	Alaska	152.2
NA	Arizona**	NA
37	Arkansas	130.5
21	California	154.3
19	Colorado	156.9
14	Connecticut	165.6
9	Delaware	172.5
NA	Florida**	NA
38	Georgia	130.1
39	Hawaii	124.1
25	Idaho	152.0
22	Illinois	154.2
40	Indiana	120.3
24	Iowa	152.1
NA	Kansas**	NA
33	Kentucky	141.5
11	Louisiana	170.4
29	Maine	147.2
2	Maryland	188.2
6	Massachusetts	174.6
3	Michigan	183.3
7	Minnesota	174.0
NA	Mississippi**	NA
34	Missouri	141.2
16	Montana	164.3
17	Nebraska	161.5
42	Nevada	99.2
26	New Hampshire	150.2
1	New Jersey	188.8
30	New Mexico	147.0
27	New York	150.1
31	North Carolina	146.5
4	North Dakota	179.5
35	Ohio	139.1
NA	Oklahoma**	NA
20	Oregon	154.8
13	Pennsylvania	167.0
10	Rhode Island	172.2
5	South Carolina	177.5
NA	South Dakota**	NA
41	Tennessee	106.6
28	Texas	148.9
8	Utah	172.8
NA	Vermont**	NA
32	Virginia	145.4
15	Washington	165.2
36	West Virginia	138.0
18	Wisconsin	160.3
12	Wyoming	168.0

RANK ORDER

RANK	STATE	RATE
1	New Jersey	188.8
2	Maryland	188.2
3	Michigan	183.3
4	North Dakota	179.5
5	South Carolina	177.5
6	Massachusetts	174.6
7	Minnesota	174.0
8	Utah	172.8
9	Delaware	172.5
10	Rhode Island	172.2
11	Louisiana	170.4
12	Wyoming	168.0
13	Pennsylvania	167.0
14	Connecticut	165.6
15	Washington	165.2
16	Montana	164.3
17	Nebraska	161.5
18	Wisconsin	160.3
19	Colorado	156.9
20	Oregon	154.8
21	California	154.3
22	Illinois	154.2
23	Alaska	152.2
24	Iowa	152.1
25	Idaho	152.0
26	New Hampshire	150.2
27	New York	150.1
28	Texas	148.9
29	Maine	147.2
30	New Mexico	147.0
31	North Carolina	146.5
32	Virginia	145.4
33	Kentucky	141.5
34	Missouri	141.2
35	Ohio	139.1
36	West Virginia	138.0
37	Arkansas	130.5
38	Georgia	130.1
39	Hawaii	124.1
40	Indiana	120.3
41	Tennessee	106.6
42	Nevada	99.2
43	Alabama	93.1
NA	Arizona**	NA
NA	Florida**	NA
NA	Kansas**	NA
NA	Mississippi**	NA
NA	Oklahoma**	NA
NA	South Dakota**	NA
NA	Vermont**	NA

District of Columbia   256.6

Source: American Cancer Society
"Cancer Facts & Figures 2003" (Copyright 2003, Reprinted with permission from the American Cancer Society)
*For 1995 to 1999. Age-adjusted to the 2000 U.S. standard population.
**Not available.

Percent of Males Receiving Recent PSA Test for Prostate Cancer: 2001

National Median = 56.7% of Men 50 and Older*

ALPHA ORDER

RANK	STATE	PERCENT
26	Alabama	55.9
14	Alaska	60.5
11	Arizona	61.4
38	Arkansas	54.2
42	California	53.8
24	Colorado	56.8
17	Connecticut	58.7
4	Delaware	64.1
1	Florida	66.2
12	Georgia	60.9
48	Hawaii	49.5
32	Idaho	54.9
35	Illinois	54.6
33	Indiana	54.8
35	Iowa	54.6
19	Kansas	57.7
40	Kentucky	54.0
28	Louisiana	55.8
48	Maine	49.5
14	Maryland	60.5
6	Massachusetts	63.8
10	Michigan	61.9
44	Minnesota	52.3
30	Mississippi	55.4
7	Missouri	63.4
22	Montana	56.9
50	Nebraska	49.2
26	Nevada	55.9
20	New Hampshire	57.6
3	New Jersey	64.9
45	New Mexico	51.9
16	New York	60.0
37	North Carolina	54.4
22	North Dakota	56.9
9	Ohio	62.8
47	Oklahoma	50.7
33	Oregon	54.8
4	Pennsylvania	64.1
8	Rhode Island	63.2
13	South Carolina	60.6
29	South Dakota	55.6
46	Tennessee	51.8
21	Texas	57.1
42	Utah	53.8
39	Vermont	54.1
25	Virginia	56.7
40	Washington	54.0
18	West Virginia	58.5
31	Wisconsin	55.1
2	Wyoming	65.4

RANK ORDER

RANK	STATE	PERCENT
1	Florida	66.2
2	Wyoming	65.4
3	New Jersey	64.9
4	Delaware	64.1
4	Pennsylvania	64.1
6	Massachusetts	63.8
7	Missouri	63.4
8	Rhode Island	63.2
9	Ohio	62.8
10	Michigan	61.9
11	Arizona	61.4
12	Georgia	60.9
13	South Carolina	60.6
14	Alaska	60.5
14	Maryland	60.5
16	New York	60.0
17	Connecticut	58.7
18	West Virginia	58.5
19	Kansas	57.7
20	New Hampshire	57.6
21	Texas	57.1
22	Montana	56.9
22	North Dakota	56.9
24	Colorado	56.8
25	Virginia	56.7
26	Alabama	55.9
26	Nevada	55.9
28	Louisiana	55.8
29	South Dakota	55.6
30	Mississippi	55.4
31	Wisconsin	55.1
32	Idaho	54.9
33	Indiana	54.8
33	Oregon	54.8
35	Illinois	54.6
35	Iowa	54.6
37	North Carolina	54.4
38	Arkansas	54.2
39	Vermont	54.1
40	Kentucky	54.0
40	Washington	54.0
42	California	53.8
42	Utah	53.8
44	Minnesota	52.3
45	New Mexico	51.9
46	Tennessee	51.8
47	Oklahoma	50.7
48	Hawaii	49.5
48	Maine	49.5
50	Nebraska	49.2
	District of Columbia	63.8

Source: U.S. Department of Health and Human Services, Centers for Disease Control and Prevention
"2001 Behavioral Risk Factor Surveillance System Public Use Data Tape"
*Men 50 and older receiving prostate-specific antigen (PSA) test within the past year.

Estimated New Skin Melanoma Cases in 2003

National Estimated Total = 54,200 New Cases*

ALPHA ORDER

RANK	STATE	CASES	% of USA
22	Alabama	900	1.7%
46	Alaska	100	0.2%
17	Arizona	1,200	2.2%
32	Arkansas	500	0.9%
1	California	5,200	9.6%
24	Colorado	800	1.5%
29	Connecticut	600	1.1%
42	Delaware	200	0.4%
2	Florida	4,100	7.6%
15	Georgia	1,300	2.4%
46	Hawaii	100	0.2%
37	Idaho	300	0.6%
7	Illinois	2,100	3.9%
12	Indiana	1,400	2.6%
29	Iowa	600	1.1%
29	Kansas	600	1.1%
20	Kentucky	1,000	1.8%
27	Louisiana	700	1.3%
37	Maine	300	0.6%
24	Maryland	800	1.5%
11	Massachusetts	1,500	2.8%
8	Michigan	1,800	3.3%
22	Minnesota	900	1.7%
32	Mississippi	500	0.9%
15	Missouri	1,300	2.4%
42	Montana	200	0.4%
37	Nebraska	300	0.6%
34	Nevada	400	0.7%
37	New Hampshire	300	0.6%
9	New Jersey	1,700	3.1%
37	New Mexico	300	0.6%
4	New York	2,900	5.4%
10	North Carolina	1,600	3.0%
46	North Dakota	100	0.2%
6	Ohio	2,300	4.2%
20	Oklahoma	1,000	1.8%
24	Oregon	800	1.5%
5	Pennsylvania	2,700	5.0%
42	Rhode Island	200	0.4%
27	South Carolina	700	1.3%
46	South Dakota	100	0.2%
12	Tennessee	1,400	2.6%
3	Texas	3,500	6.5%
34	Utah	400	0.7%
42	Vermont	200	0.4%
12	Virginia	1,400	2.6%
17	Washington	1,200	2.2%
34	West Virginia	400	0.7%
19	Wisconsin	1,100	2.0%
46	Wyoming	100	0.2%

RANK ORDER

RANK	STATE	CASES	% of USA
1	California	5,200	9.6%
2	Florida	4,100	7.6%
3	Texas	3,500	6.5%
4	New York	2,900	5.4%
5	Pennsylvania	2,700	5.0%
6	Ohio	2,300	4.2%
7	Illinois	2,100	3.9%
8	Michigan	1,800	3.3%
9	New Jersey	1,700	3.1%
10	North Carolina	1,600	3.0%
11	Massachusetts	1,500	2.8%
12	Indiana	1,400	2.6%
12	Tennessee	1,400	2.6%
12	Virginia	1,400	2.6%
15	Georgia	1,300	2.4%
15	Missouri	1,300	2.4%
17	Arizona	1,200	2.2%
17	Washington	1,200	2.2%
19	Wisconsin	1,100	2.0%
20	Kentucky	1,000	1.8%
20	Oklahoma	1,000	1.8%
22	Alabama	900	1.7%
22	Minnesota	900	1.7%
24	Colorado	800	1.5%
24	Maryland	800	1.5%
24	Oregon	800	1.5%
27	Louisiana	700	1.3%
27	South Carolina	700	1.3%
29	Connecticut	600	1.1%
29	Iowa	600	1.1%
29	Kansas	600	1.1%
32	Arkansas	500	0.9%
32	Mississippi	500	0.9%
34	Nevada	400	0.7%
34	Utah	400	0.7%
34	West Virginia	400	0.7%
37	Idaho	300	0.6%
37	Maine	300	0.6%
37	Nebraska	300	0.6%
37	New Hampshire	300	0.6%
37	New Mexico	300	0.6%
42	Delaware	200	0.4%
42	Montana	200	0.4%
42	Rhode Island	200	0.4%
42	Vermont	200	0.4%
46	Alaska	100	0.2%
46	Hawaii	100	0.2%
46	North Dakota	100	0.2%
46	South Dakota	100	0.2%
46	Wyoming	100	0.2%
	District of Columbia**	NA	NA

Source: American Cancer Society
    "Cancer Facts & Figures 2003" (Copyright 2003, Reprinted with permission from the American Cancer Society)
*These estimates are offered as a rough guide and should be interpreted with caution. They are calculated according to the distribution of estimated 2003 cancer deaths by state.
**Not available.

Estimated Rate of New Skin Melanoma Cases in 2003

National Estimated Rate = 18.8 New Cases per 100,000 Population*

ALPHA ORDER

RANK ORDER

RANK	STATE	RATE
21	Alabama	20.1
44	Alaska	15.5
16	Arizona	22.0
29	Arkansas	18.4
47	California	14.8
33	Colorado	17.8
35	Connecticut	17.3
3	Delaware	24.8
4	Florida	24.5
45	Georgia	15.2
50	Hawaii	8.0
13	Idaho	22.4
39	Illinois	16.7
11	Indiana	22.7
19	Iowa	20.4
15	Kansas	22.1
5	Kentucky	24.4
43	Louisiana	15.6
9	Maine	23.2
48	Maryland	14.7
8	Massachusetts	23.3
31	Michigan	17.9
31	Minnesota	17.9
34	Mississippi	17.4
10	Missouri	22.9
16	Montana	22.0
35	Nebraska	17.3
29	Nevada	18.4
7	New Hampshire	23.5
24	New Jersey	19.8
40	New Mexico	16.2
46	New York	15.1
26	North Carolina	19.2
42	North Dakota	15.8
21	Ohio	20.1
2	Oklahoma	28.6
11	Oregon	22.7
18	Pennsylvania	21.9
28	Rhode Island	18.7
38	South Carolina	17.0
49	South Dakota	13.1
6	Tennessee	24.1
41	Texas	16.1
35	Utah	17.3
1	Vermont	32.4
26	Virginia	19.2
24	Washington	19.8
14	West Virginia	22.2
20	Wisconsin	20.2
21	Wyoming	20.1

RANK	STATE	RATE
1	Vermont	32.4
2	Oklahoma	28.6
3	Delaware	24.8
4	Florida	24.5
5	Kentucky	24.4
6	Tennessee	24.1
7	New Hampshire	23.5
8	Massachusetts	23.3
9	Maine	23.2
10	Missouri	22.9
11	Indiana	22.7
11	Oregon	22.7
13	Idaho	22.4
14	West Virginia	22.2
15	Kansas	22.1
16	Arizona	22.0
16	Montana	22.0
18	Pennsylvania	21.9
19	Iowa	20.4
20	Wisconsin	20.2
21	Alabama	20.1
21	Ohio	20.1
21	Wyoming	20.1
24	New Jersey	19.8
24	Washington	19.8
26	North Carolina	19.2
26	Virginia	19.2
28	Rhode Island	18.7
29	Arkansas	18.4
29	Nevada	18.4
31	Michigan	17.9
31	Minnesota	17.9
33	Colorado	17.8
34	Mississippi	17.4
35	Connecticut	17.3
35	Nebraska	17.3
35	Utah	17.3
38	South Carolina	17.0
39	Illinois	16.7
40	New Mexico	16.2
41	Texas	16.1
42	North Dakota	15.8
43	Louisiana	15.6
44	Alaska	15.5
45	Georgia	15.2
46	New York	15.1
47	California	14.8
48	Maryland	14.7
49	South Dakota	13.1
50	Hawaii	8.0

District of Columbia**   NA

Source: Morgan Quitno Press using data from American Cancer Society
    "Cancer Facts & Figures 2003" (Copyright 2003, Reprinted with permission from the American Cancer Society)
*These estimates are offered as a rough guide and should be interpreted with caution. They are calculated according to the distribution of estimated 2003 cancer deaths by state. Rates calculated using 2002 Census resident population estimates.
**Not available.

Estimated New Cervical Cancer Cases in 2003

National Estimated Total = 12,200 New Cases*

ALPHA ORDER

RANK	STATE	CASES	% of USA
15	Alabama	200	1.6%
NA	Alaska**	NA	NA
15	Arizona	200	1.6%
27	Arkansas	100	0.8%
1	California	1,400	11.5%
27	Colorado	100	0.8%
27	Connecticut	100	0.8%
27	Delaware	100	0.8%
3	Florida	900	7.4%
8	Georgia	400	3.3%
NA	Hawaii**	NA	NA
NA	Idaho**	NA	NA
5	Illinois	600	4.9%
11	Indiana	300	2.5%
27	Iowa	100	0.8%
27	Kansas	100	0.8%
15	Kentucky	200	1.6%
15	Louisiana	200	1.6%
NA	Maine**	NA	NA
15	Maryland	200	1.6%
15	Massachusetts	200	1.6%
11	Michigan	300	2.5%
27	Minnesota	100	0.8%
15	Mississippi	200	1.6%
15	Missouri	200	1.6%
NA	Montana**	NA	NA
27	Nebraska	100	0.8%
27	Nevada	100	0.8%
NA	New Hampshire**	NA	NA
8	New Jersey	400	3.3%
27	New Mexico	100	0.8%
3	New York	900	7.4%
8	North Carolina	400	3.3%
NA	North Dakota**	NA	NA
7	Ohio	500	4.1%
15	Oklahoma	200	1.6%
27	Oregon	100	0.8%
5	Pennsylvania	600	4.9%
27	Rhode Island	100	0.8%
15	South Carolina	200	1.6%
NA	South Dakota**	NA	NA
11	Tennessee	300	2.5%
2	Texas	1,000	8.2%
NA	Utah**	NA	NA
NA	Vermont**	NA	NA
11	Virginia	300	2.5%
15	Washington	200	1.6%
27	West Virginia	100	0.8%
15	Wisconsin	200	1.6%
NA	Wyoming**	NA	NA

RANK ORDER

RANK	STATE	CASES	% of USA
1	California	1,400	11.5%
2	Texas	1,000	8.2%
3	Florida	900	7.4%
3	New York	900	7.4%
5	Illinois	600	4.9%
5	Pennsylvania	600	4.9%
7	Ohio	500	4.1%
8	Georgia	400	3.3%
8	New Jersey	400	3.3%
8	North Carolina	400	3.3%
11	Indiana	300	2.5%
11	Michigan	300	2.5%
11	Tennessee	300	2.5%
11	Virginia	300	2.5%
15	Alabama	200	1.6%
15	Arizona	200	1.6%
15	Kentucky	200	1.6%
15	Louisiana	200	1.6%
15	Maryland	200	1.6%
15	Massachusetts	200	1.6%
15	Mississippi	200	1.6%
15	Missouri	200	1.6%
15	Oklahoma	200	1.6%
15	South Carolina	200	1.6%
15	Washington	200	1.6%
15	Wisconsin	200	1.6%
27	Arkansas	100	0.8%
27	Colorado	100	0.8%
27	Connecticut	100	0.8%
27	Delaware	100	0.8%
27	Iowa	100	0.8%
27	Kansas	100	0.8%
27	Minnesota	100	0.8%
27	Nebraska	100	0.8%
27	Nevada	100	0.8%
27	New Mexico	100	0.8%
27	Oregon	100	0.8%
27	Rhode Island	100	0.8%
27	West Virginia	100	0.8%
NA	Alaska**	NA	NA
NA	Hawaii**	NA	NA
NA	Idaho**	NA	NA
NA	Maine**	NA	NA
NA	Montana**	NA	NA
NA	New Hampshire**	NA	NA
NA	North Dakota**	NA	NA
NA	South Dakota**	NA	NA
NA	Utah**	NA	NA
NA	Vermont**	NA	NA
NA	Wyoming**	NA	NA
	District of Columbia**	NA	NA

Source: American Cancer Society
"Cancer Facts & Figures 2003" (Copyright 2003, Reprinted with permission from the American Cancer Society)
*These estimates are offered as a rough guide and should be interpreted with caution. They are calculated according to the distribution of estimated 2003 cancer deaths by state.
**Not available.

Estimated Rate of New Cervical Cancer Cases in 2003

National Estimated Rate = 8.5 New Cases per 100,000 Female Population*

ALPHA ORDER				RANK ORDER		
RANK	STATE	RATE		RANK	STATE	RATE
21	Alabama	8.7		1	Delaware	24.8
NA	Alaska**	NA		2	Rhode Island	18.4
26	Arizona	7.8		3	Mississippi	13.6
29	Arkansas	7.3		4	Nebraska	11.5
25	California	8.2		5	Oklahoma	11.4
38	Colorado	4.7		6	Florida	11.0
37	Connecticut	5.7		7	New Mexico	10.8
1	Delaware	24.8		7	West Virginia	10.8
6	Florida	11.0		9	Tennessee	10.3
15	Georgia	9.6		10	Nevada	10.2
NA	Hawaii**	NA		11	Indiana	9.7
NA	Idaho**	NA		11	Kentucky	9.7
16	Illinois	9.5		11	North Carolina	9.7
11	Indiana	9.7		11	South Carolina	9.7
33	Iowa	6.7		15	Georgia	9.6
27	Kansas	7.4		16	Illinois	9.5
11	Kentucky	9.7		16	Texas	9.5
21	Louisiana	8.7		18	Pennsylvania	9.4
NA	Maine**	NA		19	New Jersey	9.2
29	Maryland	7.3		19	New York	9.2
34	Massachusetts	6.1		21	Alabama	8.7
35	Michigan	5.9		21	Louisiana	8.7
39	Minnesota	4.0		23	Ohio	8.6
3	Mississippi	13.6		24	Virginia	8.3
31	Missouri	7.0		25	California	8.2
NA	Montana**	NA		26	Arizona	7.8
4	Nebraska	11.5		27	Kansas	7.4
10	Nevada	10.2		27	Wisconsin	7.4
NA	New Hampshire**	NA		29	Arkansas	7.3
19	New Jersey	9.2		29	Maryland	7.3
7	New Mexico	10.8		31	Missouri	7.0
19	New York	9.2		32	Washington	6.8
11	North Carolina	9.7		33	Iowa	6.7
NA	North Dakota**	NA		34	Massachusetts	6.1
23	Ohio	8.6		35	Michigan	5.9
5	Oklahoma	11.4		36	Oregon	5.8
36	Oregon	5.8		37	Connecticut	5.7
18	Pennsylvania	9.4		38	Colorado	4.7
2	Rhode Island	18.4		39	Minnesota	4.0
11	South Carolina	9.7		NA	Alaska**	NA
NA	South Dakota**	NA		NA	Hawaii**	NA
9	Tennessee	10.3		NA	Idaho**	NA
16	Texas	9.5		NA	Maine**	NA
NA	Utah**	NA		NA	Montana**	NA
NA	Vermont**	NA		NA	New Hampshire**	NA
24	Virginia	8.3		NA	North Dakota**	NA
32	Washington	6.8		NA	South Dakota**	NA
7	West Virginia	10.8		NA	Utah**	NA
27	Wisconsin	7.4		NA	Vermont**	NA
NA	Wyoming**	NA		NA	Wyoming**	NA
					District of Columbia**	NA

Source: Morgan Quitno Press using data from American Cancer Society
   "Cancer Facts & Figures 2003" (Copyright 2003, Reprinted with permission from the American Cancer Society)
*These estimates are offered as a rough guide and should be interpreted with caution. They are calculated
according to the distribution of estimated 2003 cancer deaths by state. Rates calculated using 2000 Census
female population counts.
**Not available.

Percent of Women 18 Years Old and Older
Who Had a Pap Smear Within the Past Three Years: 2000
National Median = 86.8% of Women 18 Years and Older*

ALPHA ORDER

RANK	STATE	PERCENT
30	Alabama	86.3
3	Alaska	90.1
19	Arizona	87.9
43	Arkansas	83.6
NA	California**	NA
22	Colorado	87.6
16	Connecticut	88.0
1	Delaware	92.0
39	Florida	84.5
8	Georgia	89.1
20	Hawaii	87.8
45	Idaho	83.1
39	Illinois	84.5
37	Indiana	84.7
24	Iowa	86.8
16	Kansas	88.0
29	Kentucky	86.4
21	Louisiana	87.7
9	Maine	89.0
5	Maryland	89.9
6	Massachusetts	89.6
27	Michigan	86.7
31	Minnesota	86.0
13	Mississippi	88.1
37	Missouri	84.7
10	Montana	88.8
31	Nebraska	86.0
42	Nevada	83.8
3	New Hampshire	90.1
48	New Jersey	81.9
36	New Mexico	85.1
33	New York	85.6
7	North Carolina	89.3
41	North Dakota	84.1
28	Ohio	86.5
33	Oklahoma	85.6
16	Oregon	88.0
35	Pennsylvania	85.5
11	Rhode Island	88.5
2	South Carolina	90.8
11	South Dakota	88.5
13	Tennessee	88.1
46	Texas	82.5
44	Utah	83.4
13	Vermont	88.1
24	Virginia	86.8
23	Washington	87.3
47	West Virginia	82.1
24	Wisconsin	86.8
49	Wyoming	81.3

RANK ORDER

RANK	STATE	PERCENT
1	Delaware	92.0
2	South Carolina	90.8
3	Alaska	90.1
3	New Hampshire	90.1
5	Maryland	89.9
6	Massachusetts	89.6
7	North Carolina	89.3
8	Georgia	89.1
9	Maine	89.0
10	Montana	88.8
11	Rhode Island	88.5
11	South Dakota	88.5
13	Mississippi	88.1
13	Tennessee	88.1
13	Vermont	88.1
16	Connecticut	88.0
16	Kansas	88.0
16	Oregon	88.0
19	Arizona	87.9
20	Hawaii	87.8
21	Louisiana	87.7
22	Colorado	87.6
23	Washington	87.3
24	Iowa	86.8
24	Virginia	86.8
24	Wisconsin	86.8
27	Michigan	86.7
28	Ohio	86.5
29	Kentucky	86.4
30	Alabama	86.3
31	Minnesota	86.0
31	Nebraska	86.0
33	New York	85.6
33	Oklahoma	85.6
35	Pennsylvania	85.5
36	New Mexico	85.1
37	Indiana	84.7
37	Missouri	84.7
39	Florida	84.5
39	Illinois	84.5
41	North Dakota	84.1
42	Nevada	83.8
43	Arkansas	83.6
44	Utah	83.4
45	Idaho	83.1
46	Texas	82.5
47	West Virginia	82.1
48	New Jersey	81.9
49	Wyoming	81.3
NA	California**	NA
	District of Columbia	88.7

Source: U.S. Department of Health and Human Services, Centers for Disease Control and Prevention
"2000 Behavioral Risk Factor Surveillance Summary Prevalence Report" (May 3, 2001)
Of women with intact cervix. Pap smear is a test for cancer, especially of the female genital tract. Named after George Papanicolaou (1883-1962), American anatomist.
**Not available.*

AIDS Cases Reported in 2002

National Total = 38,878 New AIDS Cases*

ALPHA ORDER

RANK	STATE	CASES	% of USA
23	Alabama	388	1.0%
43	Alaska	30	0.1%
19	Arizona	559	1.4%
29	Arkansas	223	0.6%
3	California	4,039	10.4%
27	Colorado	286	0.7%
18	Connecticut	562	1.4%
31	Delaware	180	0.5%
2	Florida	4,667	12.0%
7	Georgia	1,536	4.0%
34	Hawaii	108	0.3%
44	Idaho	28	0.1%
5	Illinois	2,094	5.4%
20	Indiana	482	1.2%
36	Iowa	85	0.2%
39	Kansas	68	0.2%
26	Kentucky	288	0.7%
11	Louisiana	905	2.3%
44	Maine	28	0.1%
6	Maryland	1,676	4.3%
16	Massachusetts	754	1.9%
17	Michigan	701	1.8%
33	Minnesota	149	0.4%
22	Mississippi	404	1.0%
24	Missouri	337	0.9%
47	Montana	11	0.0%
40	Nebraska	64	0.2%
28	Nevada	283	0.7%
42	New Hampshire	35	0.1%
9	New Jersey	1,304	3.4%
37	New Mexico	81	0.2%
1	New York	6,236	16.0%
10	North Carolina	971	2.5%
50	North Dakota	3	0.0%
14	Ohio	766	2.0%
30	Oklahoma	181	0.5%
25	Oregon	311	0.8%
8	Pennsylvania	1,458	3.8%
35	Rhode Island	97	0.2%
13	South Carolina	792	2.0%
48	South Dakota	10	0.0%
15	Tennessee	764	2.0%
4	Texas	2,558	6.6%
41	Utah	63	0.2%
46	Vermont	12	0.0%
12	Virginia	816	2.1%
21	Washington	449	1.2%
38	West Virginia	80	0.2%
32	Wisconsin	178	0.5%
49	Wyoming	8	0.0%

RANK ORDER

RANK	STATE	CASES	% of USA
1	New York	6,236	16.0%
2	Florida	4,667	12.0%
3	California	4,039	10.4%
4	Texas	2,558	6.6%
5	Illinois	2,094	5.4%
6	Maryland	1,676	4.3%
7	Georgia	1,536	4.0%
8	Pennsylvania	1,458	3.8%
9	New Jersey	1,304	3.4%
10	North Carolina	971	2.5%
11	Louisiana	905	2.3%
12	Virginia	816	2.1%
13	South Carolina	792	2.0%
14	Ohio	766	2.0%
15	Tennessee	764	2.0%
16	Massachusetts	754	1.9%
17	Michigan	701	1.8%
18	Connecticut	562	1.4%
19	Arizona	559	1.4%
20	Indiana	482	1.2%
21	Washington	449	1.2%
22	Mississippi	404	1.0%
23	Alabama	388	1.0%
24	Missouri	337	0.9%
25	Oregon	311	0.8%
26	Kentucky	288	0.7%
27	Colorado	286	0.7%
28	Nevada	283	0.7%
29	Arkansas	223	0.6%
30	Oklahoma	181	0.5%
31	Delaware	180	0.5%
32	Wisconsin	178	0.5%
33	Minnesota	149	0.4%
34	Hawaii	108	0.3%
35	Rhode Island	97	0.2%
36	Iowa	85	0.2%
37	New Mexico	81	0.2%
38	West Virginia	80	0.2%
39	Kansas	68	0.2%
40	Nebraska	64	0.2%
41	Utah	63	0.2%
42	New Hampshire	35	0.1%
43	Alaska	30	0.1%
44	Idaho	28	0.1%
44	Maine	28	0.1%
46	Vermont	12	0.0%
47	Montana	11	0.0%
48	South Dakota	10	0.0%
49	Wyoming	8	0.0%
50	North Dakota	3	0.0%
	District of Columbia	769	2.0%

Source: U.S. Department of Health and Human Services, National Center for Health Statistics
   "Morbidity and Mortality Weekly Report" (January 3, 2003, Vol. 51, No. 52)
*Provisional data. AIDS is Acquired Immunodeficiency Syndrome. It is a specific group of diseases or conditions which are indicative of severe immunosuppression related to infection with the Human Immunodeficiency Virus (HIV). National total does not include 1,045 new cases in Puerto Rico.

AIDS Rate in 2002

National Rate = 13.5 New AIDS Cases Reported per 100,000 Population*

ALPHA ORDER

RANK	STATE	RATE
24	Alabama	8.6
34	Alaska	4.7
20	Arizona	10.2
25	Arkansas	8.2
18	California	11.5
31	Colorado	6.3
9	Connecticut	16.2
4	Delaware	22.3
3	Florida	27.9
7	Georgia	17.9
23	Hawaii	8.7
45	Idaho	2.1
8	Illinois	16.6
26	Indiana	7.8
40	Iowa	2.9
43	Kansas	2.5
28	Kentucky	7.0
5	Louisiana	20.2
44	Maine	2.2
2	Maryland	30.7
15	Massachusetts	11.7
28	Michigan	7.0
39	Minnesota	3.0
11	Mississippi	14.1
32	Missouri	5.9
49	Montana	1.2
37	Nebraska	3.7
13	Nevada	13.0
41	New Hampshire	2.7
10	New Jersey	15.2
35	New Mexico	4.4
1	New York	32.6
15	North Carolina	11.7
50	North Dakota	0.5
30	Ohio	6.7
33	Oklahoma	5.2
22	Oregon	8.8
14	Pennsylvania	11.8
21	Rhode Island	9.1
6	South Carolina	19.3
48	South Dakota	1.3
12	Tennessee	13.2
15	Texas	11.7
41	Utah	2.7
46	Vermont	1.9
19	Virginia	11.2
27	Washington	7.4
35	West Virginia	4.4
38	Wisconsin	3.3
47	Wyoming	1.6

RANK ORDER

RANK	STATE	RATE
1	New York	32.6
2	Maryland	30.7
3	Florida	27.9
4	Delaware	22.3
5	Louisiana	20.2
6	South Carolina	19.3
7	Georgia	17.9
8	Illinois	16.6
9	Connecticut	16.2
10	New Jersey	15.2
11	Mississippi	14.1
12	Tennessee	13.2
13	Nevada	13.0
14	Pennsylvania	11.8
15	Massachusetts	11.7
15	North Carolina	11.7
15	Texas	11.7
18	California	11.5
19	Virginia	11.2
20	Arizona	10.2
21	Rhode Island	9.1
22	Oregon	8.8
23	Hawaii	8.7
24	Alabama	8.6
25	Arkansas	8.2
26	Indiana	7.8
27	Washington	7.4
28	Kentucky	7.0
28	Michigan	7.0
30	Ohio	6.7
31	Colorado	6.3
32	Missouri	5.9
33	Oklahoma	5.2
34	Alaska	4.7
35	New Mexico	4.4
35	West Virginia	4.4
37	Nebraska	3.7
38	Wisconsin	3.3
39	Minnesota	3.0
40	Iowa	2.9
41	New Hampshire	2.7
41	Utah	2.7
43	Kansas	2.5
44	Maine	2.2
45	Idaho	2.1
46	Vermont	1.9
47	Wyoming	1.6
48	South Dakota	1.3
49	Montana	1.2
50	North Dakota	0.5

| | District of Columbia | 134.7 |

Source: Morgan Quitno Press using data from U.S. Dept. of Health & Human Serv's, National Center for Health Statistics "Morbidity and Mortality Weekly Report" (January 3, 2003, Vol. 51, No. 52)

*Provisional data. AIDS is Acquired Immunodeficiency Syndrome. It is a specific group of diseases or conditions which are indicative of severe immunosuppression related to infection with the Human Immunodeficiency Virus (HIV). National rate does not include cases or population in U.S. territories.

AIDS Cases Reported Through December 2001

National Total = 780,012 Reported AIDS Cases*

ALPHA ORDER

RANK	STATE	CASES	% of USA
23	Alabama	6,632	0.9%
45	Alaska	490	0.1%
21	Arizona	7,925	1.0%
32	Arkansas	3,139	0.4%
2	California	123,200	15.8%
22	Colorado	7,351	0.9%
13	Connecticut	11,972	1.5%
33	Delaware	2,803	0.4%
3	Florida	83,888	10.8%
8	Georgia	24,347	3.1%
34	Hawaii	2,569	0.3%
44	Idaho	514	0.1%
6	Illinois	26,047	3.3%
24	Indiana	6,466	0.8%
39	Iowa	1,392	0.2%
35	Kansas	2,453	0.3%
31	Kentucky	3,648	0.5%
12	Louisiana	13,350	1.7%
42	Maine	995	0.1%
9	Maryland	23,228	3.0%
10	Massachusetts	16,797	2.2%
15	Michigan	11,755	1.5%
29	Minnesota	3,896	0.5%
26	Mississippi	4,821	0.6%
19	Missouri	9,594	1.2%
47	Montana	338	0.0%
41	Nebraska	1,157	0.1%
27	Nevada	4,637	0.6%
43	New Hampshire	910	0.1%
5	New Jersey	43,068	5.5%
36	New Mexico	2,179	0.3%
1	New York	147,065	18.9%
16	North Carolina	11,240	1.4%
50	North Dakota	109	0.0%
14	Ohio	11,834	1.5%
28	Oklahoma	4,004	0.5%
25	Oregon	5,039	0.6%
7	Pennsylvania	26,033	3.3%
37	Rhode Island	2,130	0.3%
17	South Carolina	10,151	1.3%
49	South Dakota	187	0.0%
20	Tennessee	9,114	1.2%
4	Texas	56,344	7.2%
38	Utah	2,076	0.3%
46	Vermont	422	0.1%
11	Virginia	13,842	1.8%
18	Washington	9,971	1.3%
40	West Virginia	1,168	0.1%
30	Wisconsin	3,737	0.5%
48	Wyoming	189	0.0%

RANK ORDER

RANK	STATE	CASES	% of USA
1	New York	147,065	18.9%
2	California	123,200	15.8%
3	Florida	83,888	10.8%
4	Texas	56,344	7.2%
5	New Jersey	43,068	5.5%
6	Illinois	26,047	3.3%
7	Pennsylvania	26,033	3.3%
8	Georgia	24,347	3.1%
9	Maryland	23,228	3.0%
10	Massachusetts	16,797	2.2%
11	Virginia	13,842	1.8%
12	Louisiana	13,350	1.7%
13	Connecticut	11,972	1.5%
14	Ohio	11,834	1.5%
15	Michigan	11,755	1.5%
16	North Carolina	11,240	1.4%
17	South Carolina	10,151	1.3%
18	Washington	9,971	1.3%
19	Missouri	9,594	1.2%
20	Tennessee	9,114	1.2%
21	Arizona	7,925	1.0%
22	Colorado	7,351	0.9%
23	Alabama	6,632	0.9%
24	Indiana	6,466	0.8%
25	Oregon	5,039	0.6%
26	Mississippi	4,821	0.6%
27	Nevada	4,637	0.6%
28	Oklahoma	4,004	0.5%
29	Minnesota	3,896	0.5%
30	Wisconsin	3,737	0.5%
31	Kentucky	3,648	0.5%
32	Arkansas	3,139	0.4%
33	Delaware	2,803	0.4%
34	Hawaii	2,569	0.3%
35	Kansas	2,453	0.3%
36	New Mexico	2,179	0.3%
37	Rhode Island	2,130	0.3%
38	Utah	2,076	0.3%
39	Iowa	1,392	0.2%
40	West Virginia	1,168	0.1%
41	Nebraska	1,157	0.1%
42	Maine	995	0.1%
43	New Hampshire	910	0.1%
44	Idaho	514	0.1%
45	Alaska	490	0.1%
46	Vermont	422	0.1%
47	Montana	338	0.0%
48	Wyoming	189	0.0%
49	South Dakota	187	0.0%
50	North Dakota	109	0.0%
	District of Columbia	13,796	1.8%

Source: U.S. Department of Health and Human Services, Centers for Disease Control and Prevention
      "HIV/AIDS Surveillance Report, 2001" (Year-end Edition, Vol. 13, No. 2)
*Cumulative through December 2001. AIDS is Acquired Immunodeficiency Syndrome. It is a specific group of diseases or conditions which are indicative of severe immunosuppression related to infection with the Human Immunodeficiency Virus (HIV). National total does not include 25,730 cases in Puerto Rico, 501 cases in the Virgin Islands and 63 cases in other U.S. territories.

AIDS Cases in Children 12 Years and Younger Through December 2001

National Total = 8,660 Juvenile AIDS Cases*

ALPHA ORDER

RANK	STATE	CASES	% of USA
18	Alabama	74	0.9%
45	Alaska	5	0.1%
23	Arizona	41	0.5%
24	Arkansas	38	0.4%
4	California	619	7.1%
27	Colorado	30	0.3%
11	Connecticut	176	2.0%
31	Delaware	24	0.3%
2	Florida	1,436	16.6%
9	Georgia	212	2.4%
36	Hawaii	16	0.2%
47	Idaho	3	0.0%
8	Illinois	272	3.1%
22	Indiana	49	0.6%
38	Iowa	10	0.1%
37	Kansas	12	0.1%
29	Kentucky	27	0.3%
13	Louisiana	125	1.4%
41	Maine	9	0.1%
7	Maryland	309	3.6%
10	Massachusetts	211	2.4%
16	Michigan	108	1.2%
32	Minnesota	23	0.3%
20	Mississippi	56	0.6%
19	Missouri	60	0.7%
47	Montana	3	0.0%
38	Nebraska	10	0.1%
28	Nevada	28	0.3%
41	New Hampshire	9	0.1%
3	New Jersey	756	8.7%
43	New Mexico	8	0.1%
1	New York	2,276	26.3%
15	North Carolina	116	1.3%
50	North Dakota	1	0.0%
14	Ohio	124	1.4%
30	Oklahoma	26	0.3%
35	Oregon	17	0.2%
6	Pennsylvania	336	3.9%
32	Rhode Island	23	0.3%
17	South Carolina	86	1.0%
46	South Dakota	4	0.0%
21	Tennessee	52	0.6%
5	Texas	386	4.5%
34	Utah	21	0.2%
44	Vermont	6	0.1%
11	Virginia	176	2.0%
25	Washington	34	0.4%
38	West Virginia	10	0.1%
26	Wisconsin	31	0.4%
47	Wyoming	3	0.0%

RANK ORDER

RANK	STATE	CASES	% of USA
1	New York	2,276	26.3%
2	Florida	1,436	16.6%
3	New Jersey	756	8.7%
4	California	619	7.1%
5	Texas	386	4.5%
6	Pennsylvania	336	3.9%
7	Maryland	309	3.6%
8	Illinois	272	3.1%
9	Georgia	212	2.4%
10	Massachusetts	211	2.4%
11	Connecticut	176	2.0%
11	Virginia	176	2.0%
13	Louisiana	125	1.4%
14	Ohio	124	1.4%
15	North Carolina	116	1.3%
16	Michigan	108	1.2%
17	South Carolina	86	1.0%
18	Alabama	74	0.9%
19	Missouri	60	0.7%
20	Mississippi	56	0.6%
21	Tennessee	52	0.6%
22	Indiana	49	0.6%
23	Arizona	41	0.5%
24	Arkansas	38	0.4%
25	Washington	34	0.4%
26	Wisconsin	31	0.4%
27	Colorado	30	0.3%
28	Nevada	28	0.3%
29	Kentucky	27	0.3%
30	Oklahoma	26	0.3%
31	Delaware	24	0.3%
32	Minnesota	23	0.3%
32	Rhode Island	23	0.3%
34	Utah	21	0.2%
35	Oregon	17	0.2%
36	Hawaii	16	0.2%
37	Kansas	12	0.1%
38	Iowa	10	0.1%
38	Nebraska	10	0.1%
38	West Virginia	10	0.1%
41	Maine	9	0.1%
41	New Hampshire	9	0.1%
43	New Mexico	8	0.1%
44	Vermont	6	0.1%
45	Alaska	5	0.1%
46	South Dakota	4	0.0%
47	Idaho	3	0.0%
47	Montana	3	0.0%
47	Wyoming	3	0.0%
50	North Dakota	1	0.0%
	District of Columbia	173	2.0%

Source: U.S. Department of Health and Human Services, Centers for Disease Control and Prevention
"HIV/AIDS Surveillance Report, 2001" (Year-end Edition, Vol. 13, No. 2)
*Cumulative through December 2001. AIDS is Acquired Immunodeficiency Syndrome. It is a specific group of diseases or conditions which are indicative of severe immunosuppression related to infection with the Human Immunodeficiency Virus (HIV). National total does not include 389 cases in Puerto Rico and 17 cases in the Virgin Islands.

E-Coli Cases Reported in 2002

National Total = 3,784 Cases*

ALPHA ORDER					RANK ORDER			
RANK	STATE		CASES	% of USA	RANK	STATE	CASES	% of USA
37	Alabama		21	0.6%	1	Wisconsin	295	7.8%
47	Alaska		8	0.2%	2	California	282	7.5%
30	Arizona		38	1.0%	3	North Carolina	244	6.4%
43	Arkansas		12	0.3%	4	Oregon	232	6.1%
2	California		282	7.5%	5	Minnesota	201	5.3%
13	Colorado		112	3.0%	6	New York	196	5.2%
20	Connecticut		62	1.6%	7	Ohio	180	4.8%
46	Delaware		9	0.2%	8	Illinois	178	4.7%
14	Florida		92	2.4%	9	Washington	147	3.9%
23	Georgia		51	1.3%	10	Michigan	139	3.7%
27	Hawaii		42	1.1%	11	Massachusetts	125	3.3%
19	Idaho		63	1.7%	12	Iowa	122	3.2%
8	Illinois		178	4.7%	13	Colorado	112	3.0%
16	Indiana		79	2.1%	14	Florida	92	2.4%
12	Iowa		122	3.2%	15	Utah	88	2.3%
29	Kansas		39	1.0%	16	Indiana	79	2.1%
30	Kentucky		38	1.0%	17	Virginia	73	1.9%
49	Louisiana		2	0.1%	18	Missouri	65	1.7%
25	Maine		45	1.2%	19	Idaho	63	1.7%
34	Maryland		29	0.8%	20	Connecticut	62	1.6%
11	Massachusetts		125	3.3%	21	Nebraska	57	1.5%
10	Michigan		139	3.7%	22	New Jersey	55	1.5%
5	Minnesota		201	5.3%	23	Georgia	51	1.3%
44	Mississippi		11	0.3%	24	Tennessee	48	1.3%
18	Missouri		65	1.7%	25	Maine	45	1.2%
33	Montana		31	0.8%	25	Texas	45	1.2%
21	Nebraska		57	1.5%	27	Hawaii	42	1.1%
35	Nevada		28	0.7%	27	South Dakota	42	1.1%
32	New Hampshire		34	0.9%	29	Kansas	39	1.0%
22	New Jersey		55	1.5%	30	Arizona	38	1.0%
40	New Mexico		16	0.4%	30	Kentucky	38	1.0%
6	New York		196	5.2%	32	New Hampshire	34	0.9%
3	North Carolina		244	6.4%	33	Montana	31	0.8%
38	North Dakota		19	0.5%	34	Maryland	29	0.8%
7	Ohio		180	4.8%	35	Nevada	28	0.7%
36	Oklahoma		23	0.6%	36	Oklahoma	23	0.6%
4	Oregon		232	6.1%	37	Alabama	21	0.6%
NA	Pennsylvania**		NA	NA	38	North Dakota	19	0.5%
42	Rhode Island		14	0.4%	39	Wyoming	17	0.4%
48	South Carolina		5	0.1%	40	New Mexico	16	0.4%
27	South Dakota		42	1.1%	40	Vermont	16	0.4%
24	Tennessee		48	1.3%	42	Rhode Island	14	0.4%
25	Texas		45	1.2%	43	Arkansas	12	0.3%
15	Utah		88	2.3%	44	Mississippi	11	0.3%
40	Vermont		16	0.4%	45	West Virginia	10	0.3%
17	Virginia		73	1.9%	46	Delaware	9	0.2%
9	Washington		147	3.9%	47	Alaska	8	0.2%
45	West Virginia		10	0.3%	48	South Carolina	5	0.1%
1	Wisconsin		295	7.8%	49	Louisiana	2	0.1%
39	Wyoming		17	0.4%	NA	Pennsylvania**	NA	NA
						District of Columbia	3	0.1%

Source: U.S. Department of Health and Human Services, National Center for Health Statistics
"Morbidity and Mortality Weekly Report" (January 3, 2003, Vol. 51, No. 52)
*Escherichia Coli is a common bacterium that normally inhabits the intestinal tracts of humans and animals but can cause infection in other parts of the body, especially the urinary tract. One strain, sometimes transmitted in hamburger meat, can cause serious infection resulting in sickness and death. **Not available.

E-Coli Rate in 2002

National Rate = 1.3 Cases per 100,000 Population*

ALPHA ORDER

RANK	STATE	RATE
43	Alabama	0.5
28	Alaska	1.2
37	Arizona	0.7
45	Arkansas	0.4
35	California	0.8
17	Colorado	2.5
20	Connecticut	1.8
29	Delaware	1.1
39	Florida	0.6
39	Georgia	0.6
9	Hawaii	3.4
4	Idaho	4.7
22	Illinois	1.4
25	Indiana	1.3
5	Iowa	4.2
22	Kansas	1.4
33	Kentucky	0.9
49	Louisiana	0.0
8	Maine	3.5
43	Maryland	0.5
19	Massachusetts	1.9
22	Michigan	1.4
6	Minnesota	4.0
45	Mississippi	0.4
29	Missouri	1.1
9	Montana	3.4
12	Nebraska	3.3
25	Nevada	1.3
15	New Hampshire	2.7
39	New Jersey	0.6
33	New Mexico	0.9
31	New York	1.0
14	North Carolina	2.9
13	North Dakota	3.0
21	Ohio	1.6
37	Oklahoma	0.7
1	Oregon	6.6
NA	Pennsylvania**	NA
25	Rhode Island	1.3
48	South Carolina	0.1
2	South Dakota	5.5
35	Tennessee	0.8
47	Texas	0.2
7	Utah	3.8
16	Vermont	2.6
31	Virginia	1.0
18	Washington	2.4
39	West Virginia	0.6
3	Wisconsin	5.4
9	Wyoming	3.4

RANK ORDER

RANK	STATE	RATE
1	Oregon	6.6
2	South Dakota	5.5
3	Wisconsin	5.4
4	Idaho	4.7
5	Iowa	4.2
6	Minnesota	4.0
7	Utah	3.8
8	Maine	3.5
9	Hawaii	3.4
9	Montana	3.4
9	Wyoming	3.4
12	Nebraska	3.3
13	North Dakota	3.0
14	North Carolina	2.9
15	New Hampshire	2.7
16	Vermont	2.6
17	Colorado	2.5
18	Washington	2.4
19	Massachusetts	1.9
20	Connecticut	1.8
21	Ohio	1.6
22	Illinois	1.4
22	Kansas	1.4
22	Michigan	1.4
25	Indiana	1.3
25	Nevada	1.3
25	Rhode Island	1.3
28	Alaska	1.2
29	Delaware	1.1
29	Missouri	1.1
31	New York	1.0
31	Virginia	1.0
33	Kentucky	0.9
33	New Mexico	0.9
35	California	0.8
35	Tennessee	0.8
37	Arizona	0.7
37	Oklahoma	0.7
39	Florida	0.6
39	Georgia	0.6
39	New Jersey	0.6
39	West Virginia	0.6
43	Alabama	0.5
43	Maryland	0.5
45	Arkansas	0.4
45	Mississippi	0.4
47	Texas	0.2
48	South Carolina	0.1
49	Louisiana	0.0
NA	Pennsylvania**	NA

District of Columbia 0.5

Source: Morgan Quitno Press using data from U.S. Dept. of Health & Human Serv's, National Center for Health Statistics
   "Morbidity and Mortality Weekly Report" (January 3, 2003, Vol. 51, No. 52)
*Escherichia Coli is a common bacterium that normally inhabits the intestinal tracts of humans and animals but can cause infection in other parts of the body, especially the urinary tract. One strain, sometimes transmitted in hamburger meat, can cause serious infection resulting in sickness and death. **Not available.

German Measles (Rubella) Cases Reported in 2002

National Total = 17 Cases*

ALPHA ORDER

RANK	STATE	CASES	% of USA
12	Alabama	0	0.0%
12	Alaska	0	0.0%
12	Arizona	0	0.0%
12	Arkansas	0	0.0%
2	California	3	17.6%
12	Colorado	0	0.0%
12	Connecticut	0	0.0%
3	Delaware	1	5.9%
1	Florida	5	29.4%
12	Georgia	0	0.0%
3	Hawaii	1	5.9%
12	Idaho	0	0.0%
3	Illinois	1	5.9%
12	Indiana	0	0.0%
12	Iowa	0	0.0%
12	Kansas	0	0.0%
12	Kentucky	0	0.0%
3	Louisiana	1	5.9%
12	Maine	0	0.0%
12	Maryland	0	0.0%
12	Massachusetts	0	0.0%
3	Michigan	1	5.9%
12	Minnesota	0	0.0%
12	Mississippi	0	0.0%
12	Missouri	0	0.0%
12	Montana	0	0.0%
12	Nebraska	0	0.0%
12	Nevada	0	0.0%
12	New Hampshire	0	0.0%
12	New Jersey	0	0.0%
12	New Mexico	0	0.0%
3	New York	1	5.9%
12	North Carolina	0	0.0%
12	North Dakota	0	0.0%
12	Ohio	0	0.0%
12	Oklahoma	0	0.0%
12	Oregon	0	0.0%
12	Pennsylvania	0	0.0%
12	Rhode Island	0	0.0%
12	South Carolina	0	0.0%
12	South Dakota	0	0.0%
3	Tennessee	1	5.9%
3	Texas	1	5.9%
3	Utah	1	5.9%
12	Vermont	0	0.0%
12	Virginia	0	0.0%
12	Washington	0	0.0%
12	West Virginia	0	0.0%
12	Wisconsin	0	0.0%
12	Wyoming	0	0.0%

RANK ORDER

RANK	STATE	CASES	% of USA
1	Florida	5	29.4%
2	California	3	17.6%
3	Delaware	1	5.9%
3	Hawaii	1	5.9%
3	Illinois	1	5.9%
3	Louisiana	1	5.9%
3	Michigan	1	5.9%
3	New York	1	5.9%
3	Tennessee	1	5.9%
3	Texas	1	5.9%
3	Utah	1	5.9%
12	Alabama	0	0.0%
12	Alaska	0	0.0%
12	Arizona	0	0.0%
12	Arkansas	0	0.0%
12	Colorado	0	0.0%
12	Connecticut	0	0.0%
12	Georgia	0	0.0%
12	Idaho	0	0.0%
12	Indiana	0	0.0%
12	Iowa	0	0.0%
12	Kansas	0	0.0%
12	Kentucky	0	0.0%
12	Maine	0	0.0%
12	Maryland	0	0.0%
12	Massachusetts	0	0.0%
12	Minnesota	0	0.0%
12	Mississippi	0	0.0%
12	Missouri	0	0.0%
12	Montana	0	0.0%
12	Nebraska	0	0.0%
12	Nevada	0	0.0%
12	New Hampshire	0	0.0%
12	New Jersey	0	0.0%
12	New Mexico	0	0.0%
12	North Carolina	0	0.0%
12	North Dakota	0	0.0%
12	Ohio	0	0.0%
12	Oklahoma	0	0.0%
12	Oregon	0	0.0%
12	Pennsylvania	0	0.0%
12	Rhode Island	0	0.0%
12	South Carolina	0	0.0%
12	South Dakota	0	0.0%
12	Vermont	0	0.0%
12	Virginia	0	0.0%
12	Washington	0	0.0%
12	West Virginia	0	0.0%
12	Wisconsin	0	0.0%
12	Wyoming	0	0.0%

District of Columbia	0	0.0%

Source: U.S. Department of Health and Human Services, National Center for Health Statistics
    "Morbidity and Mortality Weekly Report" (January 3, 2003, Vol. 51, No. 52)
*Provisional data. A mild, contagious, eruptive disease caused by a virus and capable of producing congenital defects in infants born to mothers infected during the first three months of pregnancy.

German Measles (Rubella) Rate in 2002

National Rate = 0.01 Cases per 100,000 Population*

ALPHA ORDER

RANK ORDER

RANK	STATE	RATE
11	Alabama	0.00
11	Alaska	0.00
11	Arizona	0.00
11	Arkansas	0.00
7	California	0.01
11	Colorado	0.00
11	Connecticut	0.00
1	Delaware	0.12
4	Florida	0.03
11	Georgia	0.00
2	Hawaii	0.08
11	Idaho	0.00
7	Illinois	0.01
11	Indiana	0.00
11	Iowa	0.00
11	Kansas	0.00
11	Kentucky	0.00
5	Louisiana	0.02
11	Maine	0.00
11	Maryland	0.00
11	Massachusetts	0.00
7	Michigan	0.01
11	Minnesota	0.00
11	Mississippi	0.00
11	Missouri	0.00
11	Montana	0.00
11	Nebraska	0.00
11	Nevada	0.00
11	New Hampshire	0.00
11	New Jersey	0.00
11	New Mexico	0.00
7	New York	0.01
11	North Carolina	0.00
11	North Dakota	0.00
11	Ohio	0.00
11	Oklahoma	0.00
11	Oregon	0.00
11	Pennsylvania	0.00
11	Rhode Island	0.00
11	South Carolina	0.00
11	South Dakota	0.00
5	Tennessee	0.02
11	Texas	0.00
3	Utah	0.04
11	Vermont	0.00
11	Virginia	0.00
11	Washington	0.00
11	West Virginia	0.00
11	Wisconsin	0.00
11	Wyoming	0.00

RANK	STATE	RATE
1	Delaware	0.12
2	Hawaii	0.08
3	Utah	0.04
4	Florida	0.03
5	Louisiana	0.02
5	Tennessee	0.02
7	California	0.01
7	Illinois	0.01
7	Michigan	0.01
7	New York	0.01
11	Alabama	0.00
11	Alaska	0.00
11	Arizona	0.00
11	Arkansas	0.00
11	Colorado	0.00
11	Connecticut	0.00
11	Georgia	0.00
11	Idaho	0.00
11	Indiana	0.00
11	Iowa	0.00
11	Kansas	0.00
11	Kentucky	0.00
11	Maine	0.00
11	Maryland	0.00
11	Massachusetts	0.00
11	Minnesota	0.00
11	Mississippi	0.00
11	Missouri	0.00
11	Montana	0.00
11	Nebraska	0.00
11	Nevada	0.00
11	New Hampshire	0.00
11	New Jersey	0.00
11	New Mexico	0.00
11	North Carolina	0.00
11	North Dakota	0.00
11	Ohio	0.00
11	Oklahoma	0.00
11	Oregon	0.00
11	Pennsylvania	0.00
11	Rhode Island	0.00
11	South Carolina	0.00
11	South Dakota	0.00
11	Texas	0.00
11	Vermont	0.00
11	Virginia	0.00
11	Washington	0.00
11	West Virginia	0.00
11	Wisconsin	0.00
11	Wyoming	0.00

District of Columbia   0.00

Source: Morgan Quitno Press using data from U.S. Dept. of Health & Human Serv's, National Center for Health Statistics "Morbidity and Mortality Weekly Report" (January 3, 2003, Vol. 51, No. 52)
*Provisional data. A mild, contagious, eruptive disease caused by a virus and capable of producing congenital defects in infants born to mothers infected during the first three months of pregnancy.

Hepatitis A and B Cases Reported in 2002

National Total = 14,870 Cases*

ALPHA ORDER

RANK ORDER

RANK	STATE	CASES	% of USA
27	Alabama	145	1.0%
46	Alaska	18	0.1%
6	Arizona	577	3.9%
25	Arkansas	157	1.1%
1	California	1,995	13.4%
26	Colorado	152	1.0%
24	Connecticut	159	1.1%
44	Delaware	20	0.1%
3	Florida	1,616	10.9%
5	Georgia	717	4.8%
47	Hawaii	13	0.1%
40	Idaho	38	0.3%
10	Illinois	441	3.0%
31	Indiana	106	0.7%
32	Iowa	100	0.7%
35	Kansas	92	0.6%
34	Kentucky	94	0.6%
22	Louisiana	173	1.2%
42	Maine	23	0.2%
13	Maryland	421	2.8%
15	Massachusetts	277	1.9%
8	Michigan	549	3.7%
36	Minnesota	86	0.6%
28	Mississippi	137	0.9%
19	Missouri	195	1.3%
42	Montana	23	0.2%
39	Nebraska	39	0.3%
30	Nevada	118	0.8%
41	New Hampshire	33	0.2%
7	New Jersey	555	3.7%
22	New Mexico	173	1.2%
2	New York	1,684	11.3%
12	North Carolina	437	2.9%
48	North Dakota	8	0.1%
9	Ohio	450	3.0%
33	Oklahoma	99	0.7%
20	Oregon	192	1.3%
10	Pennsylvania	441	3.0%
37	Rhode Island	62	0.4%
21	South Carolina	186	1.3%
50	South Dakota	5	0.0%
16	Tennessee	250	1.7%
4	Texas	735	4.9%
29	Utah	129	0.9%
48	Vermont	8	0.1%
14	Virginia	345	2.3%
18	Washington	214	1.4%
38	West Virginia	41	0.3%
17	Wisconsin	221	1.5%
44	Wyoming	20	0.1%

RANK	STATE	CASES	% of USA
1	California	1,995	13.4%
2	New York	1,684	11.3%
3	Florida	1,616	10.9%
4	Texas	735	4.9%
5	Georgia	717	4.8%
6	Arizona	577	3.9%
7	New Jersey	555	3.7%
8	Michigan	549	3.7%
9	Ohio	450	3.0%
10	Illinois	441	3.0%
10	Pennsylvania	441	3.0%
12	North Carolina	437	2.9%
13	Maryland	421	2.8%
14	Virginia	345	2.3%
15	Massachusetts	277	1.9%
16	Tennessee	250	1.7%
17	Wisconsin	221	1.5%
18	Washington	214	1.4%
19	Missouri	195	1.3%
20	Oregon	192	1.3%
21	South Carolina	186	1.3%
22	Louisiana	173	1.2%
22	New Mexico	173	1.2%
24	Connecticut	159	1.1%
25	Arkansas	157	1.1%
26	Colorado	152	1.0%
27	Alabama	145	1.0%
28	Mississippi	137	0.9%
29	Utah	129	0.9%
30	Nevada	118	0.8%
31	Indiana	106	0.7%
32	Iowa	100	0.7%
33	Oklahoma	99	0.7%
34	Kentucky	94	0.6%
35	Kansas	92	0.6%
36	Minnesota	86	0.6%
37	Rhode Island	62	0.4%
38	West Virginia	41	0.3%
39	Nebraska	39	0.3%
40	Idaho	38	0.3%
41	New Hampshire	33	0.2%
42	Maine	23	0.2%
42	Montana	23	0.2%
44	Delaware	20	0.1%
44	Wyoming	20	0.1%
46	Alaska	18	0.1%
47	Hawaii	13	0.1%
48	North Dakota	8	0.1%
48	Vermont	8	0.1%
50	South Dakota	5	0.0%
	District of Columbia	101	0.7%

*Source: U.S. Department of Health and Human Services, National Center for Health Statistics
"Morbidity and Mortality Weekly Report" (January 3, 2003, Vol. 51, No. 52)*
Provisional data. An inflammation of the liver.

Hepatitis A and B Rate in 2002

National Rate = 5.2 Cases per 100,000 Population*

ALPHA ORDER

RANK	STATE	RATE
34	Alabama	3.2
35	Alaska	2.8
1	Arizona	10.6
8	Arkansas	5.8
10	California	5.7
29	Colorado	3.4
18	Connecticut	4.6
39	Delaware	2.5
2	Florida	9.7
5	Georgia	8.4
49	Hawaii	1.0
35	Idaho	2.8
27	Illinois	3.5
45	Indiana	1.7
29	Iowa	3.4
29	Kansas	3.4
41	Kentucky	2.3
24	Louisiana	3.9
44	Maine	1.8
6	Maryland	7.7
20	Massachusetts	4.3
12	Michigan	5.5
45	Minnesota	1.7
16	Mississippi	4.8
29	Missouri	3.4
39	Montana	2.5
41	Nebraska	2.3
14	Nevada	5.4
38	New Hampshire	2.6
7	New Jersey	6.5
3	New Mexico	9.3
4	New York	8.8
15	North Carolina	5.3
47	North Dakota	1.3
24	Ohio	3.9
35	Oklahoma	2.8
12	Oregon	5.5
26	Pennsylvania	3.6
8	Rhode Island	5.8
19	South Carolina	4.5
50	South Dakota	0.7
20	Tennessee	4.3
29	Texas	3.4
11	Utah	5.6
47	Vermont	1.3
17	Virginia	4.7
27	Washington	3.5
41	West Virginia	2.3
22	Wisconsin	4.1
23	Wyoming	4.0

RANK ORDER

RANK	STATE	RATE
1	Arizona	10.6
2	Florida	9.7
3	New Mexico	9.3
4	New York	8.8
5	Georgia	8.4
6	Maryland	7.7
7	New Jersey	6.5
8	Arkansas	5.8
8	Rhode Island	5.8
10	California	5.7
11	Utah	5.6
12	Michigan	5.5
12	Oregon	5.5
14	Nevada	5.4
15	North Carolina	5.3
16	Mississippi	4.8
17	Virginia	4.7
18	Connecticut	4.6
19	South Carolina	4.5
20	Massachusetts	4.3
20	Tennessee	4.3
22	Wisconsin	4.1
23	Wyoming	4.0
24	Louisiana	3.9
24	Ohio	3.9
26	Pennsylvania	3.6
27	Illinois	3.5
27	Washington	3.5
29	Colorado	3.4
29	Iowa	3.4
29	Kansas	3.4
29	Missouri	3.4
29	Texas	3.4
34	Alabama	3.2
35	Alaska	2.8
35	Idaho	2.8
35	Oklahoma	2.8
38	New Hampshire	2.6
39	Delaware	2.5
39	Montana	2.5
41	Kentucky	2.3
41	Nebraska	2.3
41	West Virginia	2.3
44	Maine	1.8
45	Indiana	1.7
45	Minnesota	1.7
47	North Dakota	1.3
47	Vermont	1.3
49	Hawaii	1.0
50	South Dakota	0.7

District of Columbia 17.7

Source: Morgan Quitno Press using data from U.S. Dept. of Health & Human Serv's, National Center for Health Statistics
"Morbidity and Mortality Weekly Report" (January 3, 2003, Vol. 51, No. 52)
*Provisional data. An inflammation of the liver.

Hepatitis C Cases Reported in 2002

National Total = 3,585 Cases*

ALPHA ORDER

RANK	STATE	CASES	% of USA
22	Alabama	11	0.3%
44	Alaska	0	0.0%
26	Arizona	7	0.2%
23	Arkansas	9	0.3%
10	California	64	1.8%
18	Colorado	15	0.4%
44	Connecticut	0	0.0%
27	Delaware	6	0.2%
5	Florida	98	2.7%
8	Georgia	70	2.0%
44	Hawaii	0	0.0%
37	Idaho	1	0.0%
19	Illinois	14	0.4%
44	Indiana	0	0.0%
37	Iowa	1	0.0%
28	Kansas	5	0.1%
31	Kentucky	4	0.1%
7	Louisiana	71	2.0%
44	Maine	0	0.0%
25	Maryland	8	0.2%
23	Massachusetts	9	0.3%
6	Michigan	86	2.4%
37	Minnesota	1	0.0%
3	Mississippi	144	4.0%
2	Missouri	656	18.3%
37	Montana	1	0.0%
20	Nebraska	13	0.4%
13	Nevada	30	0.8%
44	New Hampshire	0	0.0%
1	New Jersey	1,865	52.0%
37	New Mexico	1	0.0%
9	New York	69	1.9%
14	North Carolina	29	0.8%
44	North Dakota	0	0.0%
31	Ohio	4	0.1%
28	Oklahoma	5	0.1%
16	Oregon	17	0.5%
11	Pennsylvania	36	1.0%
37	Rhode Island	1	0.0%
31	South Carolina	4	0.1%
37	South Dakota	1	0.0%
12	Tennessee	34	0.9%
4	Texas	125	3.5%
31	Utah	4	0.1%
20	Vermont	13	0.4%
17	Virginia	16	0.4%
15	Washington	25	0.7%
36	West Virginia	3	0.1%
31	Wisconsin	4	0.1%
28	Wyoming	5	0.1%

RANK ORDER

RANK	STATE	CASES	% of USA
1	New Jersey	1,865	52.0%
2	Missouri	656	18.3%
3	Mississippi	144	4.0%
4	Texas	125	3.5%
5	Florida	98	2.7%
6	Michigan	86	2.4%
7	Louisiana	71	2.0%
8	Georgia	70	2.0%
9	New York	69	1.9%
10	California	64	1.8%
11	Pennsylvania	36	1.0%
12	Tennessee	34	0.9%
13	Nevada	30	0.8%
14	North Carolina	29	0.8%
15	Washington	25	0.7%
16	Oregon	17	0.5%
17	Virginia	16	0.4%
18	Colorado	15	0.4%
19	Illinois	14	0.4%
20	Nebraska	13	0.4%
20	Vermont	13	0.4%
22	Alabama	11	0.3%
23	Arkansas	9	0.3%
23	Massachusetts	9	0.3%
25	Maryland	8	0.2%
26	Arizona	7	0.2%
27	Delaware	6	0.2%
28	Kansas	5	0.1%
28	Oklahoma	5	0.1%
28	Wyoming	5	0.1%
31	Kentucky	4	0.1%
31	Ohio	4	0.1%
31	South Carolina	4	0.1%
31	Utah	4	0.1%
31	Wisconsin	4	0.1%
36	West Virginia	3	0.1%
37	Idaho	1	0.0%
37	Iowa	1	0.0%
37	Minnesota	1	0.0%
37	Montana	1	0.0%
37	New Mexico	1	0.0%
37	Rhode Island	1	0.0%
37	South Dakota	1	0.0%
44	Alaska	0	0.0%
44	Connecticut	0	0.0%
44	Hawaii	0	0.0%
44	Indiana	0	0.0%
44	Maine	0	0.0%
44	New Hampshire	0	0.0%
44	North Dakota	0	0.0%
	District of Columbia	0	0.0%

Source: U.S. Department of Health and Human Services, National Center for Health Statistics
    "Morbidity and Mortality Weekly Report" (January 3, 2003, Vol. 51, No. 52)
*Provisional data. An inflammation of the liver. It is the leading cause for liver transplantation and is transmitted by blood-to-blood contact. Most new cases of C are caused by high-risk drug behaviors.

Hepatitis C Rate in 2002

National Rate = 1.2 Cases per 100,000 Population*

ALPHA ORDER

RANK	STATE	RATE
22	Alabama	0.2
41	Alaska	0.0
28	Arizona	0.1
18	Arkansas	0.3
22	California	0.2
18	Colorado	0.3
41	Connecticut	0.0
11	Delaware	0.7
12	Florida	0.6
9	Georgia	0.8
41	Hawaii	0.0
28	Idaho	0.1
28	Illinois	0.1
41	Indiana	0.0
41	Iowa	0.0
22	Kansas	0.2
28	Kentucky	0.1
5	Louisiana	1.6
41	Maine	0.0
28	Maryland	0.1
28	Massachusetts	0.1
8	Michigan	0.9
41	Minnesota	0.0
3	Mississippi	5.0
2	Missouri	11.6
28	Montana	0.1
9	Nebraska	0.8
6	Nevada	1.4
41	New Hampshire	0.0
1	New Jersey	21.7
28	New Mexico	0.1
16	New York	0.4
18	North Carolina	0.3
41	North Dakota	0.0
41	Ohio	0.0
28	Oklahoma	0.1
15	Oregon	0.5
18	Pennsylvania	0.3
28	Rhode Island	0.1
28	South Carolina	0.1
28	South Dakota	0.1
12	Tennessee	0.6
12	Texas	0.6
22	Utah	0.2
4	Vermont	2.1
22	Virginia	0.2
16	Washington	0.4
22	West Virginia	0.2
28	Wisconsin	0.1
7	Wyoming	1.0

RANK ORDER

RANK	STATE	RATE
1	New Jersey	21.7
2	Missouri	11.6
3	Mississippi	5.0
4	Vermont	2.1
5	Louisiana	1.6
6	Nevada	1.4
7	Wyoming	1.0
8	Michigan	0.9
9	Georgia	0.8
9	Nebraska	0.8
11	Delaware	0.7
12	Florida	0.6
12	Tennessee	0.6
12	Texas	0.6
15	Oregon	0.5
16	New York	0.4
16	Washington	0.4
18	Arkansas	0.3
18	Colorado	0.3
18	North Carolina	0.3
18	Pennsylvania	0.3
22	Alabama	0.2
22	California	0.2
22	Kansas	0.2
22	Utah	0.2
22	Virginia	0.2
22	West Virginia	0.2
28	Arizona	0.1
28	Idaho	0.1
28	Illinois	0.1
28	Kentucky	0.1
28	Maryland	0.1
28	Massachusetts	0.1
28	Montana	0.1
28	New Mexico	0.1
28	Oklahoma	0.1
28	Rhode Island	0.1
28	South Carolina	0.1
28	South Dakota	0.1
28	Wisconsin	0.1
41	Alaska	0.0
41	Connecticut	0.0
41	Hawaii	0.0
41	Indiana	0.0
41	Iowa	0.0
41	Maine	0.0
41	Minnesota	0.0
41	New Hampshire	0.0
41	North Dakota	0.0
41	Ohio	0.0
	District of Columbia	0.0

Source: Morgan Quitno Press using data from U.S. Dept. of Health & Human Serv's, National Center for Health Statistics
"Morbidity and Mortality Weekly Report" (January 3, 2003, Vol. 51, No. 52)
*Provisional data. An inflammation of the liver. It is the leading cause for liver transplantation and is transmitted
by blood-to-blood contact. Most new cases of C are caused by high-risk drug behaviors.

Legionellosis Cases Reported in 2002

National Total = 1,183 Cases*

ALPHA ORDER

RANK	STATE	CASES	% of USA
29	Alabama	8	0.7%
44	Alaska	0	0.0%
22	Arizona	15	1.3%
44	Arkansas	0	0.0%
6	California	63	5.3%
29	Colorado	8	0.7%
16	Connecticut	18	1.5%
25	Delaware	10	0.8%
4	Florida	86	7.3%
17	Georgia	17	1.4%
41	Hawaii	1	0.1%
37	Idaho	3	0.3%
44	Illinois	0	0.0%
13	Indiana	26	2.2%
24	Iowa	12	1.0%
44	Kansas	0	0.0%
14	Kentucky	21	1.8%
35	Louisiana	4	0.3%
33	Maine	6	0.5%
7	Maryland	54	4.6%
10	Massachusetts	30	2.5%
5	Michigan	84	7.1%
17	Minnesota	17	1.4%
44	Mississippi	0	0.0%
17	Missouri	17	1.4%
37	Montana	3	0.3%
25	Nebraska	10	0.8%
34	Nevada	5	0.4%
31	New Hampshire	7	0.6%
12	New Jersey	29	2.5%
40	New Mexico	2	0.2%
1	New York	172	14.5%
23	North Carolina	13	1.1%
41	North Dakota	1	0.1%
3	Ohio	123	10.4%
37	Oklahoma	3	0.3%
NA	Oregon**	NA	NA
2	Pennsylvania	127	10.7%
27	Rhode Island	9	0.8%
27	South Carolina	9	0.8%
35	South Dakota	4	0.3%
15	Tennessee	19	1.6%
17	Texas	17	1.4%
17	Utah	17	1.4%
8	Vermont	35	3.0%
10	Virginia	30	2.5%
31	Washington	7	0.6%
NA	West Virginia**	NA	NA
9	Wisconsin	34	2.9%
41	Wyoming	1	0.1%

RANK ORDER

RANK	STATE	CASES	% of USA
1	New York	172	14.5%
2	Pennsylvania	127	10.7%
3	Ohio	123	10.4%
4	Florida	86	7.3%
5	Michigan	84	7.1%
6	California	63	5.3%
7	Maryland	54	4.6%
8	Vermont	35	3.0%
9	Wisconsin	34	2.9%
10	Massachusetts	30	2.5%
10	Virginia	30	2.5%
12	New Jersey	29	2.5%
13	Indiana	26	2.2%
14	Kentucky	21	1.8%
15	Tennessee	19	1.6%
16	Connecticut	18	1.5%
17	Georgia	17	1.4%
17	Minnesota	17	1.4%
17	Missouri	17	1.4%
17	Texas	17	1.4%
17	Utah	17	1.4%
22	Arizona	15	1.3%
23	North Carolina	13	1.1%
24	Iowa	12	1.0%
25	Delaware	10	0.8%
25	Nebraska	10	0.8%
27	Rhode Island	9	0.8%
27	South Carolina	9	0.8%
29	Alabama	8	0.7%
29	Colorado	8	0.7%
31	New Hampshire	7	0.6%
31	Washington	7	0.6%
33	Maine	6	0.5%
34	Nevada	5	0.4%
35	Louisiana	4	0,3%
35	South Dakota	4	0.3%
37	Idaho	3	0.3%
37	Montana	3	0.3%
37	Oklahoma	3	0.3%
40	New Mexico	2	0.2%
41	Hawaii	1	0.1%
41	North Dakota	1	0.1%
41	Wyoming	1	0.1%
44	Alaska	0	0.0%
44	Arkansas	0	0.0%
44	Illinois	0	0.0%
44	Kansas	0	0.0%
44	Mississippi	0	0.0%
NA	Oregon**	NA	NA
NA	West Virginia**	NA	NA
	District of Columbia	6	0.5%

Source: U.S. Department of Health and Human Services, National Center for Health Statistics "Morbidity and Mortality Weekly Report" (January 3, 2003, Vol. 51, No. 52)
Provisional data. A pneumonia-like disease (Legionnaire's Disease).
**Not notifiable.*

Legionellosis Rate in 2002

National Rate = 0.4 Cases per 100,000 Population*

ALPHA ORDER				RANK ORDER		
RANK	**STATE**	**RATE**		**RANK**	**STATE**	**RATE**
28	Alabama	0.2		1	Vermont	5.7
44	Alaska	0.0		2	Delaware	1.2
22	Arizona	0.3		3	Ohio	1.1
44	Arkansas	0.0		4	Maryland	1.0
28	California	0.2		4	Pennsylvania	1.0
28	Colorado	0.2		6	New York	0.9
12	Connecticut	0.5		7	Michigan	0.8
2	Delaware	1.2		7	Rhode Island	0.8
12	Florida	0.5		9	Utah	0.7
28	Georgia	0.2		10	Nebraska	0.6
38	Hawaii	0.1		10	Wisconsin	0.6
28	Idaho	0.2		12	Connecticut	0.5
44	Illinois	0.0		12	Florida	0.5
19	Indiana	0.4		12	Kentucky	0.5
19	Iowa	0.4		12	Maine	0.5
44	Kansas	0.0		12	Massachusetts	0.5
12	Kentucky	0.5		12	New Hampshire	0.5
38	Louisiana	0.1		12	South Dakota	0.5
12	Maine	0.5		19	Indiana	0.4
4	Maryland	1.0		19	Iowa	0.4
12	Massachusetts	0.5		19	Virginia	0.4
7	Michigan	0.8		22	Arizona	0.3
22	Minnesota	0.3		22	Minnesota	0.3
44	Mississippi	0.0		22	Missouri	0.3
22	Missouri	0.3		22	Montana	0.3
22	Montana	0.3		22	New Jersey	0.3
10	Nebraska	0.6		22	Tennessee	0.3
28	Nevada	0.2		28	Alabama	0.2
12	New Hampshire	0.5		28	California	0.2
22	New Jersey	0.3		28	Colorado	0.2
38	New Mexico	0.1		28	Georgia	0.2
6	New York	0.9		28	Idaho	0.2
28	North Carolina	0.2		28	Nevada	0.2
28	North Dakota	0.2		28	North Carolina	0.2
3	Ohio	1.1		28	North Dakota	0.2
38	Oklahoma	0.1		28	South Carolina	0.2
NA	Oregon**	NA		28	Wyoming	0.2
4	Pennsylvania	1.0		38	Hawaii	0.1
7	Rhode Island	0.8		38	Louisiana	0.1
28	South Carolina	0.2		38	New Mexico	0.1
12	South Dakota	0.5		38	Oklahoma	0.1
22	Tennessee	0.3		38	Texas	0.1
38	Texas	0.1		38	Washington	0.1
9	Utah	0.7		44	Alaska	0.0
1	Vermont	5.7		44	Arkansas	0.0
19	Virginia	0.4		44	Illinois	0.0
38	Washington	0.1		44	Kansas	0.0
NA	West Virginia**	NA		44	Mississippi	0.0
10	Wisconsin	0.6		NA	Oregon**	NA
28	Wyoming	0.2		NA	West Virginia**	NA

	District of Columbia	1.1

Source: Morgan Quitno Press using data from U.S. Dept. of Health & Human Serv's, National Center for Health Statistics
"Morbidity and Mortality Weekly Report" (January 3, 2003, Vol. 51, No. 52)
*Provisional data. A pneumonia-like disease (Legionnaire's Disease).
**Not notifiable.

Lyme Disease Cases in 2002

National Total = 18,181 Cases*

ALPHA ORDER

RANK	STATE	CASES	% of USA
34	Alabama	3	0.0%
34	Alaska	3	0.0%
34	Arizona	3	0.0%
34	Arkansas	3	0.0%
13	California	114	0.6%
40	Colorado	1	0.0%
2	Connecticut	3,978	21.9%
10	Delaware	178	1.0%
16	Florida	81	0.4%
40	Georgia	1	0.0%
NA	Hawaii**	NA	NA
32	Idaho	4	0.0%
45	Illinois	0	0.0%
23	Indiana	20	0.1%
18	Iowa	42	0.2%
29	Kansas	8	0.0%
22	Kentucky	23	0.1%
32	Louisiana	4	0.0%
14	Maine	111	0.6%
6	Maryland	681	3.7%
5	Massachusetts	1,559	8.6%
27	Michigan	13	0.1%
7	Minnesota	404	2.2%
45	Mississippi	0	0.0%
19	Missouri	40	0.2%
45	Montana	0	0.0%
31	Nebraska	6	0.0%
40	Nevada	1	0.0%
9	New Hampshire	246	1.4%
4	New Jersey	1,767	9.7%
40	New Mexico	1	0.0%
1	New York	5,191	28.6%
12	North Carolina	137	0.8%
40	North Dakota	1	0.0%
15	Ohio	82	0.5%
45	Oklahoma	0	0.0%
26	Oregon	15	0.1%
3	Pennsylvania	2,760	15.2%
8	Rhode Island	346	1.9%
23	South Carolina	20	0.1%
38	South Dakota	2	0.0%
21	Tennessee	26	0.1%
17	Texas	61	0.3%
30	Utah	7	0.0%
20	Vermont	37	0.2%
11	Virginia	149	0.8%
28	Washington	11	0.1%
25	West Virginia	17	0.1%
NA	Wisconsin**	NA	NA
38	Wyoming	2	0.0%

RANK ORDER

RANK	STATE	CASES	% of USA
1	New York	5,191	28.6%
2	Connecticut	3,978	21.9%
3	Pennsylvania	2,760	15.2%
4	New Jersey	1,767	9.7%
5	Massachusetts	1,559	8.6%
6	Maryland	681	3.7%
7	Minnesota	404	2.2%
8	Rhode Island	346	1.9%
9	New Hampshire	246	1.4%
10	Delaware	178	1.0%
11	Virginia	149	0.8%
12	North Carolina	137	0.8%
13	California	114	0.6%
14	Maine	111	0.6%
15	Ohio	82	0.5%
16	Florida	81	0.4%
17	Texas	61	0.3%
18	Iowa	42	0.2%
19	Missouri	40	0.2%
20	Vermont	37	0.2%
21	Tennessee	26	0.1%
22	Kentucky	23	0.1%
23	Indiana	20	0.1%
23	South Carolina	20	0.1%
25	West Virginia	17	0.1%
26	Oregon	15	0.1%
27	Michigan	13	0.1%
28	Washington	11	0.1%
29	Kansas	8	0.0%
30	Utah	7	0.0%
31	Nebraska	6	0.0%
32	Idaho	4	0.0%
32	Louisiana	4	0.0%
34	Alabama	3	0.0%
34	Alaska	3	0.0%
34	Arizona	3	0.0%
34	Arkansas	3	0.0%
38	South Dakota	2	0.0%
38	Wyoming	2	0.0%
40	Colorado	1	0.0%
40	Georgia	1	0.0%
40	Nevada	1	0.0%
40	New Mexico	1	0.0%
40	North Dakota	1	0.0%
45	Illinois	0	0.0%
45	Mississippi	0	0.0%
45	Montana	0	0.0%
45	Oklahoma	0	0.0%
NA	Hawaii**	NA	NA
NA	Wisconsin**	NA	NA
	District of Columbia	22	0.1%

Source: U.S. Department of Health and Human Services, National Center for Health Statistics
    "Morbidity and Mortality Weekly Report" (January 3, 2003, Vol. 51, No. 52)
*Provisional data. Caused by ticks-lesions, followed by arthritis of large joints, myalgia, malaise and neurologic and cardiac manifestations. Named after Old Lyme, CT, where the disease was first reported.
**Wisconsin's figure is not available (597 cases in 2001). Lyme disease is not notifiable in Hawaii.

Lyme Disease Rate in 2002

National Rate = 6.3 Cases per 100,000 Population*

ALPHA ORDER				RANK ORDER		
RANK	STATE	RATE		RANK	STATE	RATE
36	Alabama	0.1		1	Connecticut	115.0
20	Alaska	0.5		2	Rhode Island	32.3
36	Arizona	0.1		3	New York	27.1
36	Arkansas	0.1		4	Massachusetts	24.3
26	California	0.3		5	Pennsylvania	22.4
42	Colorado	0.0		6	Delaware	22.0
1	Connecticut	115.0		7	New Jersey	20.6
6	Delaware	22.0		8	New Hampshire	19.3
20	Florida	0.5		9	Maryland	12.5
42	Georgia	0.0		10	Maine	8.6
NA	Hawaii**	NA		11	Minnesota	8.0
26	Idaho	0.3		12	Vermont	6.0
42	Illinois	0.0		13	Virginia	2.0
26	Indiana	0.3		14	North Carolina	1.6
15	Iowa	1.4		15	Iowa	1.4
26	Kansas	0.3		16	West Virginia	0.9
19	Kentucky	0.6		17	Missouri	0.7
36	Louisiana	0.1		17	Ohio	0.7
10	Maine	8.6		19	Kentucky	0.6
9	Maryland	12.5		20	Alaska	0.5
4	Massachusetts	24.3		20	Florida	0.5
36	Michigan	0.1		20	South Carolina	0.5
11	Minnesota	8.0		23	Oregon	0.4
42	Mississippi	0.0		23	Tennessee	0.4
17	Missouri	0.7		23	Wyoming	0.4
42	Montana	0.0		26	California	0.3
26	Nebraska	0.3		26	Idaho	0.3
42	Nevada	0.0		26	Indiana	0.3
8	New Hampshire	19.3		26	Kansas	0.3
7	New Jersey	20.6		26	Nebraska	0.3
36	New Mexico	0.1		26	South Dakota	0.3
3	New York	27.1		26	Texas	0.3
14	North Carolina	1.6		26	Utah	0.3
34	North Dakota	0.2		34	North Dakota	0.2
17	Ohio	0.7		34	Washington	0.2
42	Oklahoma	0.0		36	Alabama	0.1
23	Oregon	0.4		36	Arizona	0.1
5	Pennsylvania	22.4		36	Arkansas	0.1
2	Rhode Island	32.3		36	Louisiana	0.1
20	South Carolina	0.5		36	Michigan	0.1
26	South Dakota	0.3		36	New Mexico	0.1
23	Tennessee	0.4		42	Colorado	0.0
26	Texas	0.3		42	Georgia	0.0
26	Utah	0.3		42	Illinois	0.0
12	Vermont	6.0		42	Mississippi	0.0
13	Virginia	2.0		42	Montana	0.0
34	Washington	0.2		42	Nevada	0.0
16	West Virginia	0.9		42	Oklahoma	0.0
NA	Wisconsin**	NA		NA	Hawaii**	NA
23	Wyoming	0.4		NA	Wisconsin**	NA

District of Columbia   3.9

Source: Morgan Quitno Press using data from U.S. Dept. of Health & Human Serv's, National Center for Health Statistics
    "Morbidity and Mortality Weekly Report" (January 3, 2003, Vol. 51, No. 52)
*Provisional data. Caused by ticks-lesions, followed by arthritis of large joints, myalgia, malaise and neurologic
and cardiac manifestations. Named after Old Lyme, CT, where the disease was first reported.
**Wisconsin's figure is not available. Lyme disease is not notifiable in Hawaii.

Malaria Cases Reported in 2002

National Total = 1,245 Cases

ALPHA ORDER

RANK	STATE	CASES	% of USA
30	Alabama	6	0.5%
44	Alaska	2	0.2%
21	Arizona	13	1.0%
44	Arkansas	2	0.2%
2	California	183	14.7%
13	Colorado	24	1.9%
17	Connecticut	16	1.3%
36	Delaware	4	0.3%
4	Florida	76	6.1%
5	Georgia	49	3.9%
26	Hawaii	8	0.6%
49	Idaho	0	0.0%
7	Illinois	37	3.0%
20	Indiana	14	1.1%
36	Iowa	4	0.3%
21	Kansas	13	1.0%
27	Kentucky	7	0.6%
36	Louisiana	4	0.3%
30	Maine	6	0.5%
3	Maryland	111	8.9%
11	Massachusetts	26	2.1%
6	Michigan	46	3.7%
16	Minnesota	17	1.4%
34	Mississippi	5	0.4%
17	Missouri	16	1.3%
44	Montana	2	0.2%
34	Nebraska	5	0.4%
40	Nevada	3	0.2%
27	New Hampshire	7	0.6%
7	New Jersey	37	3.0%
40	New Mexico	3	0.2%
1	New York	263	21.1%
15	North Carolina	22	1.8%
47	North Dakota	1	0.1%
12	Ohio	25	2.0%
25	Oklahoma	10	0.8%
23	Oregon	12	1.0%
9	Pennsylvania	34	2.7%
24	Rhode Island	11	0.9%
27	South Carolina	7	0.6%
47	South Dakota	1	0.1%
40	Tennessee	3	0.2%
30	Texas	6	0.5%
30	Utah	6	0.5%
36	Vermont	4	0.3%
10	Virginia	32	2.6%
14	Washington	23	1.8%
40	West Virginia	3	0.2%
17	Wisconsin	16	1.3%
49	Wyoming	0	0.0%

RANK ORDER

RANK	STATE	CASES	% of USA
1	New York	263	21.1%
2	California	183	14.7%
3	Maryland	111	8.9%
4	Florida	76	6.1%
5	Georgia	49	3.9%
6	Michigan	46	3.7%
7	Illinois	37	3.0%
7	New Jersey	37	3.0%
9	Pennsylvania	34	2.7%
10	Virginia	32	2.6%
11	Massachusetts	26	2.1%
12	Ohio	25	2.0%
13	Colorado	24	1.9%
14	Washington	23	1.8%
15	North Carolina	22	1.8%
16	Minnesota	17	1.4%
17	Connecticut	16	1.3%
17	Missouri	16	1.3%
17	Wisconsin	16	1.3%
20	Indiana	14	1.1%
21	Arizona	13	1.0%
21	Kansas	13	1.0%
23	Oregon	12	1.0%
24	Rhode Island	11	0.9%
25	Oklahoma	10	0.8%
26	Hawaii	8	0.6%
27	Kentucky	7	0.6%
27	New Hampshire	7	0.6%
27	South Carolina	7	0.6%
30	Alabama	6	0.5%
30	Maine	6	0.5%
30	Texas	6	0.5%
30	Utah	6	0.5%
34	Mississippi	5	0.4%
34	Nebraska	5	0.4%
36	Delaware	4	0.3%
36	Iowa	4	0.3%
36	Louisiana	4	0.3%
36	Vermont	4	0.3%
40	Nevada	3	0.2%
40	New Mexico	3	0.2%
40	Tennessee	3	0.2%
40	West Virginia	3	0.2%
44	Alaska	2	0.2%
44	Arkansas	2	0.2%
44	Montana	2	0.2%
47	North Dakota	1	0.1%
47	South Dakota	1	0.1%
49	Idaho	0	0.0%
49	Wyoming	0	0.0%
	District of Columbia	20	1.6%

Source: U.S. Department of Health and Human Services, National Center for Health Statistics
"Morbidity and Mortality Weekly Report" (January 3, 2003, Vol. 51, No. 52)
*Provisional data. Infectious disease usually transmitted by bites of infected mosquitoes. Symptoms include high fever, shaking chills, sweating and anemia.

Malaria Rate in 2002

National Rate = 0.4 Cases per 100,000 Population*

ALPHA ORDER

RANK	STATE	RATE
41	Alabama	0.1
20	Alaska	0.3
31	Arizona	0.2
41	Arkansas	0.1
7	California	0.5
7	Colorado	0.5
7	Connecticut	0.5
7	Delaware	0.5
7	Florida	0.5
4	Georgia	0.6
4	Hawaii	0.6
48	Idaho	0.0
20	Illinois	0.3
31	Indiana	0.2
41	Iowa	0.1
7	Kansas	0.5
31	Kentucky	0.2
41	Louisiana	0.1
7	Maine	0.5
1	Maryland	2.0
16	Massachusetts	0.4
7	Michigan	0.5
20	Minnesota	0.3
31	Mississippi	0.2
20	Missouri	0.3
31	Montana	0.2
20	Nebraska	0.3
41	Nevada	0.1
7	New Hampshire	0.5
16	New Jersey	0.4
31	New Mexico	0.2
2	New York	1.4
20	North Carolina	0.3
31	North Dakota	0.2
31	Ohio	0.2
20	Oklahoma	0.3
20	Oregon	0.3
20	Pennsylvania	0.3
3	Rhode Island	1.0
31	South Carolina	0.2
41	South Dakota	0.1
41	Tennessee	0.1
48	Texas	0.0
20	Utah	0.3
4	Vermont	0.6
16	Virginia	0.4
16	Washington	0.4
31	West Virginia	0.2
20	Wisconsin	0.3
48	Wyoming	0.0

RANK ORDER

RANK	STATE	RATE
1	Maryland	2.0
2	New York	1.4
3	Rhode Island	1.0
4	Georgia	0.6
4	Hawaii	0.6
4	Vermont	0.6
7	California	0.5
7	Colorado	0.5
7	Connecticut	0.5
7	Delaware	0.5
7	Florida	0.5
7	Kansas	0.5
7	Maine	0.5
7	Michigan	0.5
7	New Hampshire	0.5
16	Massachusetts	0.4
16	New Jersey	0.4
16	Virginia	0.4
16	Washington	0.4
20	Alaska	0.3
20	Illinois	0.3
20	Minnesota	0.3
20	Missouri	0.3
20	Nebraska	0.3
20	North Carolina	0.3
20	Oklahoma	0.3
20	Oregon	0.3
20	Pennsylvania	0.3
20	Utah	0.3
20	Wisconsin	0.3
31	Arizona	0.2
31	Indiana	0.2
31	Kentucky	0.2
31	Mississippi	0.2
31	Montana	0.2
31	New Mexico	0.2
31	North Dakota	0.2
31	Ohio	0.2
31	South Carolina	0.2
31	West Virginia	0.2
41	Alabama	0.1
41	Arkansas	0.1
41	Iowa	0.1
41	Louisiana	0.1
41	Nevada	0.1
41	South Dakota	0.1
41	Tennessee	0.1
48	Idaho	0.0
48	Texas	0.0
48	Wyoming	0.0

District of Columbia   3.5

Source: Morgan Quitno Press using data from U.S. Dept. of Health & Human Serv's, National Center for Health Statistics
"Morbidity and Mortality Weekly Report" (January 3, 2003, Vol. 51, No. 52)
*Provisional data. Infectious disease usually transmitted by bites of infected mosquitoes. Symptoms include high fever, shaking chills, sweating and anemia.

Measles (Rubeloa) Cases Reported in 2002

National Total = 37 Cases*

RANK	STATE	CASES	% of USA
1	Alabama	12	32.4%
14	Alaska	0	0.0%
14	Arizona	0	0.0%
14	Arkansas	0	0.0%
3	California	3	8.1%
14	Colorado	0	0.0%
14	Connecticut	0	0.0%
14	Delaware	0	0.0%
5	Florida	2	5.4%
3	Georgia	3	8.1%
8	Hawaii	1	2.7%
14	Idaho	0	0.0%
14	Illinois	0	0.0%
5	Indiana	2	5.4%
14	Iowa	0	0.0%
14	Kansas	0	0.0%
14	Kentucky	0	0.0%
14	Louisiana	0	0.0%
14	Maine	0	0.0%
14	Maryland	0	0.0%
14	Massachusetts	0	0.0%
14	Michigan	0	0.0%
8	Minnesota	1	2.7%
14	Mississippi	0	0.0%
5	Missouri	2	5.4%
14	Montana	0	0.0%
14	Nebraska	0	0.0%
8	Nevada	1	2.7%
14	New Hampshire	0	0.0%
14	New Jersey	0	0.0%
14	New Mexico	0	0.0%
2	New York	7	18.9%
14	North Carolina	0	0.0%
14	North Dakota	0	0.0%
8	Ohio	1	2.7%
14	Oklahoma	0	0.0%
14	Oregon	0	0.0%
14	Pennsylvania	0	0.0%
14	Rhode Island	0	0.0%
14	South Carolina	0	0.0%
14	South Dakota	0	0.0%
14	Tennessee	0	0.0%
8	Texas	1	2.7%
8	Utah	1	2.7%
14	Vermont	0	0.0%
14	Virginia	0	0.0%
14	Washington	0	0.0%
14	West Virginia	0	0.0%
14	Wisconsin	0	0.0%
14	Wyoming	0	0.0%

RANK	STATE	CASES	% of USA
1	Alabama	12	32.4%
2	New York	7	18.9%
3	California	3	8.1%
3	Georgia	3	8.1%
5	Florida	2	5.4%
5	Indiana	2	5.4%
5	Missouri	2	5.4%
8	Hawaii	1	2.7%
8	Minnesota	1	2.7%
8	Nevada	1	2.7%
8	Ohio	1	2.7%
8	Texas	1	2.7%
8	Utah	1	2.7%
14	Alaska	0	0.0%
14	Arizona	0	0.0%
14	Arkansas	0	0.0%
14	Colorado	0	0.0%
14	Connecticut	0	0.0%
14	Delaware	0	0.0%
14	Idaho	0	0.0%
14	Illinois	0	0.0%
14	Iowa	0	0.0%
14	Kansas	0	0.0%
14	Kentucky	0	0.0%
14	Louisiana	0	0.0%
14	Maine	0	0.0%
14	Maryland	0	0.0%
14	Massachusetts	0	0.0%
14	Michigan	0	0.0%
14	Mississippi	0	0.0%
14	Montana	0	0.0%
14	Nebraska	0	0.0%
14	New Hampshire	0	0.0%
14	New Jersey	0	0.0%
14	New Mexico	0	0.0%
14	North Carolina	0	0.0%
14	North Dakota	0	0.0%
14	Oklahoma	0	0.0%
14	Oregon	0	0.0%
14	Pennsylvania	0	0.0%
14	Rhode Island	0	0.0%
14	South Carolina	0	0.0%
14	South Dakota	0	0.0%
14	Tennessee	0	0.0%
14	Vermont	0	0.0%
14	Virginia	0	0.0%
14	Washington	0	0.0%
14	West Virginia	0	0.0%
14	Wisconsin	0	0.0%
14	Wyoming	0	0.0%
	District of Columbia	0	0.0%

Source: U.S. Department of Health and Human Services, National Center for Health Statistics
    "Morbidity and Mortality Weekly Report" (January 3, 2003, Vol. 51, No. 52)
*Provisional data. Includes indigenous and imported cases.

Measles (Rubeola) Rate in 2002

National Rate = 0.01 Cases per 100,000 Population*

ALPHA ORDER   RANK ORDER

RANK	STATE	RATE	RANK	STATE	RATE
1	Alabama	0.27	1	Alabama	0.27
13	Alaska	0.00	2	Hawaii	0.08
13	Arizona	0.00	3	Nevada	0.05
13	Arkansas	0.00	4	Georgia	0.04
10	California	0.01	4	Missouri	0.04
13	Colorado	0.00	4	New York	0.04
13	Connecticut	0.00	4	Utah	0.04
13	Delaware	0.00	8	Indiana	0.02
10	Florida	0.01	8	Minnesota	0.02
4	Georgia	0.04	10	California	0.01
2	Hawaii	0.08	10	Florida	0.01
13	Idaho	0.00	10	Ohio	0.01
13	Illinois	0.00	13	Alaska	0.00
8	Indiana	0.02	13	Arizona	0.00
13	Iowa	0.00	13	Arkansas	0.00
13	Kansas	0.00	13	Colorado	0.00
13	Kentucky	0.00	13	Connecticut	0.00
13	Louisiana	0.00	13	Delaware	0.00
13	Maine	0.00	13	Idaho	0.00
13	Maryland	0.00	13	Illinois	0.00
13	Massachusetts	0.00	13	Iowa	0.00
13	Michigan	0.00	13	Kansas	0.00
8	Minnesota	0.02	13	Kentucky	0.00
13	Mississippi	0.00	13	Louisiana	0.00
4	Missouri	0.04	13	Maine	0.00
13	Montana	0.00	13	Maryland	0.00
13	Nebraska	0.00	13	Massachusetts	0.00
3	Nevada	0.05	13	Michigan	0.00
13	New Hampshire	0.00	13	Mississippi	0.00
13	New Jersey	0.00	13	Montana	0.00
13	New Mexico	0.00	13	Nebraska	0.00
4	New York	0.04	13	New Hampshire	0.00
13	North Carolina	0.00	13	New Jersey	0.00
13	North Dakota	0.00	13	New Mexico	0.00
10	Ohio	0.01	13	North Carolina	0.00
13	Oklahoma	0.00	13	North Dakota	0.00
13	Oregon	0.00	13	Oklahoma	0.00
13	Pennsylvania	0.00	13	Oregon	0.00
13	Rhode Island	0.00	13	Pennsylvania	0.00
13	South Carolina	0.00	13	Rhode Island	0.00
13	South Dakota	0.00	13	South Carolina	0.00
13	Tennessee	0.00	13	South Dakota	0.00
13	Texas	0.00	13	Tennessee	0.00
4	Utah	0.04	13	Texas	0.00
13	Vermont	0.00	13	Vermont	0.00
13	Virginia	0.00	13	Virginia	0.00
13	Washington	0.00	13	Washington	0.00
13	West Virginia	0.00	13	West Virginia	0.00
13	Wisconsin	0.00	13	Wisconsin	0.00
13	Wyoming	0.00	13	Wyoming	0.00

District of Columbia   0.00

Source: Morgan Quitno Press using data from U.S. Dept. of Health & Human Serv's, National Center for Health Statistics "Morbidity and Mortality Weekly Report" (January 3, 2003, Vol. 51, No. 52)
Provisional data. Includes indigenous and imported cases.

Meningococcal Infections Reported in 2002

National Total = 1,595 Cases*

RANK	STATE	CASES	% of USA
27	Alabama	23	1.4%
43	Alaska	4	0.3%
18	Arizona	32	2.0%
25	Arkansas	24	1.5%
1	California	213	13.4%
25	Colorado	24	1.5%
31	Connecticut	15	0.9%
39	Delaware	7	0.4%
2	Florida	128	8.0%
21	Georgia	30	1.9%
35	Hawaii	10	0.6%
41	Idaho	5	0.3%
15	Illinois	36	2.3%
18	Indiana	32	2.0%
22	Iowa	28	1.8%
38	Kansas	8	0.5%
31	Kentucky	15	0.9%
13	Louisiana	40	2.5%
36	Maine	9	0.6%
36	Maryland	9	0.6%
11	Massachusetts	42	2.6%
10	Michigan	44	2.8%
16	Minnesota	35	2.2%
33	Mississippi	14	0.9%
8	Missouri	51	3.2%
47	Montana	3	0.2%
24	Nebraska	26	1.6%
29	Nevada	20	1.3%
33	New Hampshire	14	0.9%
23	New Jersey	27	1.7%
43	New Mexico	4	0.3%
5	New York	72	4.5%
17	North Carolina	33	2.1%
47	North Dakota	3	0.2%
4	Ohio	74	4.6%
28	Oklahoma	22	1.4%
9	Oregon	45	2.8%
7	Pennsylvania	58	3.6%
41	Rhode Island	5	0.3%
18	South Carolina	32	2.0%
49	South Dakota	2	0.1%
14	Tennessee	38	2.4%
3	Texas	105	6.6%
40	Utah	6	0.4%
43	Vermont	4	0.3%
12	Virginia	41	2.6%
6	Washington	63	3.9%
43	West Virginia	4	0.3%
30	Wisconsin	16	1.0%
50	Wyoming	0	0.0%

RANK	STATE	CASES	% of USA
1	California	213	13.4%
2	Florida	128	8.0%
3	Texas	105	6.6%
4	Ohio	74	4.6%
5	New York	72	4.5%
6	Washington	63	3.9%
7	Pennsylvania	58	3.6%
8	Missouri	51	3.2%
9	Oregon	45	2.8%
10	Michigan	44	2.8%
11	Massachusetts	42	2.6%
12	Virginia	41	2.6%
13	Louisiana	40	2.5%
14	Tennessee	38	2.4%
15	Illinois	36	2.3%
16	Minnesota	35	2.2%
17	North Carolina	33	2.1%
18	Arizona	32	2.0%
18	Indiana	32	2.0%
18	South Carolina	32	2.0%
21	Georgia	30	1.9%
22	Iowa	28	1.8%
23	New Jersey	27	1.7%
24	Nebraska	26	1.6%
25	Arkansas	24	1.5%
25	Colorado	24	1.5%
27	Alabama	23	1.4%
28	Oklahoma	22	1.4%
29	Nevada	20	1.3%
30	Wisconsin	16	1.0%
31	Connecticut	15	0.9%
31	Kentucky	15	0.9%
33	Mississippi	14	0.9%
33	New Hampshire	14	0.9%
35	Hawaii	10	0.6%
36	Maine	9	0.6%
36	Maryland	9	0.6%
38	Kansas	8	0.5%
39	Delaware	7	0.4%
40	Utah	6	0.4%
41	Idaho	5	0.3%
41	Rhode Island	5	0.3%
43	Alaska	4	0.3%
43	New Mexico	4	0.3%
43	Vermont	4	0.3%
43	West Virginia	4	0.3%
47	Montana	3	0.2%
47	North Dakota	3	0.2%
49	South Dakota	2	0.1%
50	Wyoming	0	0.0%
	District of Columbia	0	0.0%

Source: U.S. Department of Health and Human Services, National Center for Health Statistics
   "Morbidity and Mortality Weekly Report" (January 3, 2003, Vol. 51, No. 52)
*Provisional data. A bacterium (Neisseria meningitidis) that causes cerebrospinal meningitis

Meningococcal Infection Rate in 2002

National Rate = 0.6 Cases per 100,000 Population*

ALPHA ORDER

RANK	STATE	RATE
25	Alabama	0.5
18	Alaska	0.6
18	Arizona	0.6
6	Arkansas	0.9
18	California	0.6
25	Colorado	0.5
33	Connecticut	0.4
6	Delaware	0.9
11	Florida	0.8
33	Georgia	0.4
11	Hawaii	0.8
33	Idaho	0.4
40	Illinois	0.3
25	Indiana	0.5
4	Iowa	1.0
40	Kansas	0.3
33	Kentucky	0.4
6	Louisiana	0.9
14	Maine	0.7
47	Maryland	0.2
14	Massachusetts	0.7
33	Michigan	0.4
14	Minnesota	0.7
25	Mississippi	0.5
6	Missouri	0.9
40	Montana	0.3
1	Nebraska	1.5
6	Nevada	0.9
3	New Hampshire	1.1
40	New Jersey	0.3
47	New Mexico	0.2
33	New York	0.4
33	North Carolina	0.4
25	North Dakota	0.5
18	Ohio	0.6
18	Oklahoma	0.6
2	Oregon	1.3
25	Pennsylvania	0.5
25	Rhode Island	0.5
11	South Carolina	0.8
40	South Dakota	0.3
14	Tennessee	0.7
25	Texas	0.5
40	Utah	0.3
18	Vermont	0.6
18	Virginia	0.6
4	Washington	1.0
47	West Virginia	0.2
40	Wisconsin	0.3
50	Wyoming	0.0

RANK ORDER

RANK	STATE	RATE
1	Nebraska	1.5
2	Oregon	1.3
3	New Hampshire	1.1
4	Iowa	1.0
4	Washington	1.0
6	Arkansas	0.9
6	Delaware	0.9
6	Louisiana	0.9
6	Missouri	0.9
6	Nevada	0.9
11	Florida	0.8
11	Hawaii	0.8
11	South Carolina	0.8
14	Maine	0.7
14	Massachusetts	0.7
14	Minnesota	0.7
14	Tennessee	0.7
18	Alaska	0.6
18	Arizona	0.6
18	California	0.6
18	Ohio	0.6
18	Oklahoma	0.6
18	Vermont	0.6
18	Virginia	0.6
25	Alabama	0.5
25	Colorado	0.5
25	Indiana	0.5
25	Mississippi	0.5
25	North Dakota	0.5
25	Pennsylvania	0.5
25	Rhode Island	0.5
25	Texas	0.5
33	Connecticut	0.4
33	Georgia	0.4
33	Idaho	0.4
33	Kentucky	0.4
33	Michigan	0.4
33	New York	0.4
33	North Carolina	0.4
40	Illinois	0.3
40	Kansas	0.3
40	Montana	0.3
40	New Jersey	0.3
40	South Dakota	0.3
40	Utah	0.3
40	Wisconsin	0.3
47	Maryland	0.2
47	New Mexico	0.2
47	West Virginia	0.2
50	Wyoming	0.0
	District of Columbia	0.0

Source: Morgan Quitno Press using data from U.S. Dept. of Health & Human Serv's, National Center for Health Statistics
"Morbidity and Mortality Weekly Report" (January 3, 2003, Vol. 51, No. 52)
*Provisional data. A bacterium (Neisseria meningitidis) that causes cerebrospinal meningitis.

Mumps Cases Reported in 2002

National Total = 238 Cases*

ALPHA ORDER

RANK	STATE	CASES	% of USA
19	Alabama	3	1.3%
36	Alaska	0	0.0%
28	Arizona	1	0.4%
36	Arkansas	0	0.0%
1	California	67	28.2%
19	Colorado	3	1.3%
28	Connecticut	1	0.4%
36	Delaware	0	0.0%
9	Florida	7	2.9%
23	Georgia	2	0.8%
3	Hawaii	16	6.7%
23	Idaho	2	0.8%
4	Illinois	15	6.3%
23	Indiana	2	0.8%
28	Iowa	1	0.4%
11	Kansas	6	2.5%
19	Kentucky	3	1.3%
28	Louisiana	1	0.4%
36	Maine	0	0.0%
13	Maryland	5	2.1%
28	Massachusetts	1	0.4%
9	Michigan	7	2.9%
15	Minnesota	4	1.7%
13	Mississippi	5	2.1%
15	Missouri	4	1.7%
36	Montana	0	0.0%
36	Nebraska	0	0.0%
11	Nevada	6	2.5%
15	New Hampshire	4	1.7%
36	New Jersey	0	0.0%
28	New Mexico	1	0.4%
7	New York	8	3.4%
23	North Carolina	2	0.8%
28	North Dakota	1	0.4%
5	Ohio	14	5.9%
36	Oklahoma	0	0.0%
NA	Oregon**	NA	NA
2	Pennsylvania	17	7.1%
36	Rhode Island	0	0.0%
19	South Carolina	3	1.3%
36	South Dakota	0	0.0%
23	Tennessee	2	0.8%
6	Texas	11	4.6%
7	Utah	8	3.4%
36	Vermont	0	0.0%
15	Virginia	4	1.7%
36	Washington	0	0.0%
36	West Virginia	0	0.0%
28	Wisconsin	1	0.4%
36	Wyoming	0	0.0%

RANK ORDER

RANK	STATE	CASES	% of USA
1	California	67	28.2%
2	Pennsylvania	17	7.1%
3	Hawaii	16	6.7%
4	Illinois	15	6.3%
5	Ohio	14	5.9%
6	Texas	11	4.6%
7	New York	8	3.4%
7	Utah	8	3.4%
9	Florida	7	2.9%
9	Michigan	7	2.9%
11	Kansas	6	2.5%
11	Nevada	6	2.5%
13	Maryland	5	2.1%
13	Mississippi	5	2.1%
15	Minnesota	4	1.7%
15	Missouri	4	1.7%
15	New Hampshire	4	1.7%
15	Virginia	4	1.7%
19	Alabama	3	1.3%
19	Colorado	3	1.3%
19	Kentucky	3	1.3%
19	South Carolina	3	1.3%
23	Georgia	2	0.8%
23	Idaho	2	0.8%
23	Indiana	2	0.8%
23	North Carolina	2	0.8%
23	Tennessee	2	0.8%
28	Arizona	1	0.4%
28	Connecticut	1	0.4%
28	Iowa	1	0.4%
28	Louisiana	1	0.4%
28	Massachusetts	1	0.4%
28	New Mexico	1	0.4%
28	North Dakota	1	0.4%
28	Wisconsin	1	0.4%
36	Alaska	0	0.0%
36	Arkansas	0	0.0%
36	Delaware	0	0.0%
36	Maine	0	0.0%
36	Montana	0	0.0%
36	Nebraska	0	0.0%
36	New Jersey	0	0.0%
36	Oklahoma	0	0.0%
36	Rhode Island	0	0.0%
36	South Dakota	0	0.0%
36	Vermont	0	0.0%
36	Washington	0	0.0%
36	West Virginia	0	0.0%
36	Wyoming	0	0.0%
NA	Oregon**	NA	NA
	District of Columbia	0	0.0%

Source: U.S. Department of Health and Human Services, National Center for Health Statistics
   "Morbidity and Mortality Weekly Report" (January 3, 2003, Vol. 51, No. 52)
*Provisional data. An acute, inflammatory, contagious disease caused by a paramyxovirus and characterized by swelling of the salivary glands, especially the parotids, and sometimes of the pancreas, ovaries, or testes. This disease, mainly affecting children, can be prevented by vaccination.
**Mumps is not a notifiable disease in Oregon.

Mumps Rate in 2002

National Rate = 0.08 Cases per 100,000 Population*

ALPHA ORDER

RANK	STATE	RATE
15	Alabama	0.07
36	Alaska	0.00
30	Arizona	0.02
36	Arkansas	0.00
6	California	0.19
15	Colorado	0.07
26	Connecticut	0.03
36	Delaware	0.00
24	Florida	0.04
30	Georgia	0.02
1	Hawaii	1.29
9	Idaho	0.15
11	Illinois	0.12
26	Indiana	0.03
26	Iowa	0.03
5	Kansas	0.22
15	Kentucky	0.07
30	Louisiana	0.02
36	Maine	0.00
13	Maryland	0.09
30	Massachusetts	0.02
15	Michigan	0.07
14	Minnesota	0.08
7	Mississippi	0.17
15	Missouri	0.07
36	Montana	0.00
36	Nebraska	0.00
4	Nevada	0.28
3	New Hampshire	0.31
36	New Jersey	0.00
21	New Mexico	0.05
24	New York	0.04
30	North Carolina	0.02
8	North Dakota	0.16
11	Ohio	0.12
36	Oklahoma	0.00
NA	Oregon**	NA
10	Pennsylvania	0.14
36	Rhode Island	0.00
15	South Carolina	0.07
36	South Dakota	0.00
26	Tennessee	0.03
21	Texas	0.05
2	Utah	0.35
36	Vermont	0.00
21	Virginia	0.05
36	Washington	0.00
36	West Virginia	0.00
30	Wisconsin	0.02
36	Wyoming	0.00

RANK ORDER

RANK	STATE	RATE
1	Hawaii	1.29
2	Utah	0.35
3	New Hampshire	0.31
4	Nevada	0.28
5	Kansas	0.22
6	California	0.19
7	Mississippi	0.17
8	North Dakota	0.16
9	Idaho	0.15
10	Pennsylvania	0.14
11	Illinois	0.12
11	Ohio	0.12
13	Maryland	0.09
14	Minnesota	0.08
15	Alabama	0.07
15	Colorado	0.07
15	Kentucky	0.07
15	Michigan	0.07
15	Missouri	0.07
15	South Carolina	0.07
21	New Mexico	0.05
21	Texas	0.05
21	Virginia	0.05
24	Florida	0.04
24	New York	0.04
26	Connecticut	0.03
26	Indiana	0.03
26	Iowa	0.03
26	Tennessee	0.03
30	Arizona	0.02
30	Georgia	0.02
30	Louisiana	0.02
30	Massachusetts	0.02
30	North Carolina	0.02
30	Wisconsin	0.02
36	Alaska	0.00
36	Arkansas	0.00
36	Delaware	0.00
36	Maine	0.00
36	Montana	0.00
36	Nebraska	0.00
36	New Jersey	0.00
36	Oklahoma	0.00
36	Rhode Island	0.00
36	South Dakota	0.00
36	Vermont	0.00
36	Washington	0.00
36	West Virginia	0.00
36	Wyoming	0.00
NA	Oregon**	NA

District of Columbia   0.00

Source: Morgan Quitno Press using data from U.S. Dept. of Health & Human Serv's, National Center for Health Statistics
"Morbidity and Mortality Weekly Report" (January 3, 2003, Vol. 51, No. 52)
*Provisional data. An acute, inflammatory, contagious disease caused by a paramyxovirus and characterized by swelling of the salivary glands, especially the parotids, and sometimes of the pancreas, ovaries, or testes. This disease, mainly affecting children, can be prevented by vaccination.
**Mumps is not a notifiable disease in Oregon.

Rabies (Animal) Cases Reported in 2002

National Total = 6,875 Cases*

ALPHA ORDER

RANK	STATE	CASES	% of USA
33	Alabama	34	0.5%
37	Alaska	24	0.3%
16	Arizona	127	1.8%
43	Arkansas	8	0.1%
10	California	235	3.4%
24	Colorado	59	0.9%
7	Connecticut	329	4.8%
25	Delaware	53	0.8%
11	Florida	190	2.8%
5	Georgia	375	5.5%
46	Hawaii	0	0.0%
30	Idaho	38	0.6%
35	Illinois	31	0.5%
34	Indiana	32	0.5%
20	Iowa	79	1.1%
14	Kansas	160	2.3%
36	Kentucky	27	0.4%
46	Louisiana	0	0.0%
23	Maine	61	0.9%
6	Maryland	359	5.2%
8	Massachusetts	297	4.3%
28	Michigan	46	0.7%
31	Minnesota	36	0.5%
45	Mississippi	4	0.1%
26	Missouri	50	0.7%
38	Montana	19	0.3%
46	Nebraska	0	0.0%
42	Nevada	11	0.2%
27	New Hampshire	48	0.7%
12	New Jersey	188	2.7%
44	New Mexico	7	0.1%
2	New York	725	10.5%
3	North Carolina	710	10.3%
31	North Dakota	36	0.5%
29	Ohio	39	0.6%
17	Oklahoma	119	1.7%
40	Oregon	13	0.2%
9	Pennsylvania	245	3.6%
22	Rhode Island	75	1.1%
15	South Carolina	142	2.1%
20	South Dakota	79	1.1%
18	Tennessee	108	1.6%
1	Texas	863	12.6%
40	Utah	13	0.2%
19	Vermont	89	1.3%
4	Virginia	505	7.3%
46	Washington	0	0.0%
13	West Virginia	169	2.5%
46	Wisconsin	0	0.0%
39	Wyoming	18	0.3%

RANK ORDER

RANK	STATE	CASES	% of USA
1	Texas	863	12.6%
2	New York	725	10.5%
3	North Carolina	710	10.3%
4	Virginia	505	7.3%
5	Georgia	375	5.5%
6	Maryland	359	5.2%
7	Connecticut	329	4.8%
8	Massachusetts	297	4.3%
9	Pennsylvania	245	3.6%
10	California	235	3.4%
11	Florida	190	2.8%
12	New Jersey	188	2.7%
13	West Virginia	169	2.5%
14	Kansas	160	2.3%
15	South Carolina	142	2.1%
16	Arizona	127	1.8%
17	Oklahoma	119	1.7%
18	Tennessee	108	1.6%
19	Vermont	89	1.3%
20	Iowa	79	1.1%
20	South Dakota	79	1.1%
22	Rhode Island	75	1.1%
23	Maine	61	0.9%
24	Colorado	59	0.9%
25	Delaware	53	0.8%
26	Missouri	50	0.7%
27	New Hampshire	48	0.7%
28	Michigan	46	0.7%
29	Ohio	39	0.6%
30	Idaho	38	0.6%
31	Minnesota	36	0.5%
31	North Dakota	36	0.5%
33	Alabama	34	0.5%
34	Indiana	32	0.5%
35	Illinois	31	0.5%
36	Kentucky	27	0.4%
37	Alaska	24	0.3%
38	Montana	19	0.3%
39	Wyoming	18	0.3%
40	Oregon	13	0.2%
40	Utah	13	0.2%
42	Nevada	11	0.2%
43	Arkansas	8	0.1%
44	New Mexico	7	0.1%
45	Mississippi	4	0.1%
46	Hawaii	0	0.0%
46	Louisiana	0	0.0%
46	Nebraska	0	0.0%
46	Washington	0	0.0%
46	Wisconsin	0	0.0%
	District of Columbia	0	0.0%

*Source: U.S. Department of Health and Human Services, National Center for Health Statistics
"Morbidity and Mortality Weekly Report" (January 3, 2003, Vol. 51, No. 52)*
Provisional data. An acute, infectious, often fatal viral disease of most warm-blooded animals, especially wolves, cats, and dogs, that attacks the central nervous system and is transmitted by the bite of infected animals.

Rabies (Animal) Rate in 2002

National Rate = 2.4 Cases per 100,000 Human Population*

ALPHA ORDER

RANK	STATE	RATE
32	Alabama	0.8
18	Alaska	3.7
24	Arizona	2.3
42	Arkansas	0.3
33	California	0.7
29	Colorado	1.3
3	Connecticut	9.5
8	Delaware	6.6
30	Florida	1.1
14	Georgia	4.4
46	Hawaii	0.0
22	Idaho	2.8
44	Illinois	0.2
37	Indiana	0.5
23	Iowa	2.7
10	Kansas	5.9
33	Kentucky	0.7
46	Louisiana	0.0
12	Maine	4.7
8	Maryland	6.6
13	Massachusetts	4.6
37	Michigan	0.5
33	Minnesota	0.7
45	Mississippi	0.1
31	Missouri	0.9
26	Montana	2.1
46	Nebraska	0.0
37	Nevada	0.5
16	New Hampshire	3.8
25	New Jersey	2.2
40	New Mexico	0.4
16	New York	3.8
5	North Carolina	8.5
11	North Dakota	5.7
42	Ohio	0.3
21	Oklahoma	3.4
40	Oregon	0.4
27	Pennsylvania	2.0
6	Rhode Island	7.0
20	South Carolina	3.5
2	South Dakota	10.4
28	Tennessee	1.9
15	Texas	4.0
36	Utah	0.6
1	Vermont	14.4
7	Virginia	6.9
46	Washington	0.0
4	West Virginia	9.4
46	Wisconsin	0.0
19	Wyoming	3.6

RANK ORDER

RANK	STATE	RATE
1	Vermont	14.4
2	South Dakota	10.4
3	Connecticut	9.5
4	West Virginia	9.4
5	North Carolina	8.5
6	Rhode Island	7.0
7	Virginia	6.9
8	Delaware	6.6
8	Maryland	6.6
10	Kansas	5.9
11	North Dakota	5.7
12	Maine	4.7
13	Massachusetts	4.6
14	Georgia	4.4
15	Texas	4.0
16	New Hampshire	3.8
16	New York	3.8
18	Alaska	3.7
19	Wyoming	3.6
20	South Carolina	3.5
21	Oklahoma	3.4
22	Idaho	2.8
23	Iowa	2.7
24	Arizona	2.3
25	New Jersey	2.2
26	Montana	2.1
27	Pennsylvania	2.0
28	Tennessee	1.9
29	Colorado	1.3
30	Florida	1.1
31	Missouri	0.9
32	Alabama	0.8
33	California	0.7
33	Kentucky	0.7
33	Minnesota	0.7
36	Utah	0.6
37	Indiana	0.5
37	Michigan	0.5
37	Nevada	0.5
40	New Mexico	0.4
40	Oregon	0.4
42	Arkansas	0.3
42	Ohio	0.3
44	Illinois	0.2
45	Mississippi	0.1
46	Hawaii	0.0
46	Louisiana	0.0
46	Nebraska	0.0
46	Washington	0.0
46	Wisconsin	0.0
	District of Columbia	0.0

Source: Morgan Quitno Press using data from U.S. Dept. of Health & Human Serv's, National Center for Health Statistics
"Morbidity and Mortality Weekly Report" (January 3, 2003, Vol. 51, No. 52)
*Provisional data. An acute, infectious, often fatal viral disease of most warm-blooded animals, especially wolves,
cats, and dogs, that attacks the central nervous system and is transmitted by the bite of infected animals.

Salmonellosis Cases Reported in 2002

National Total = 41,257 Cases*

ALPHA ORDER

RANK	STATE	CASES	% of USA
15	Alabama	877	2.1%
48	Alaska	79	0.2%
22	Arizona	788	1.9%
13	Arkansas	1,047	2.5%
2	California	4,118	10.0%
25	Colorado	602	1.5%
30	Connecticut	445	1.1%
46	Delaware	95	0.2%
1	Florida	4,659	11.3%
4	Georgia	1,712	4.1%
35	Hawaii	278	0.7%
37	Idaho	184	0.4%
5	Illinois	1,658	4.0%
27	Indiana	508	1.2%
26	Iowa	518	1.3%
33	Kansas	336	0.8%
31	Kentucky	398	1.0%
20	Louisiana	813	2.0%
42	Maine	146	0.4%
14	Maryland	954	2.3%
11	Massachusetts	1,168	2.8%
16	Michigan	875	2.1%
24	Minnesota	610	1.5%
12	Mississippi	1,140	2.8%
19	Missouri	820	2.0%
47	Montana	91	0.2%
41	Nebraska	150	0.4%
38	Nevada	183	0.4%
43	New Hampshire	138	0.3%
23	New Jersey	761	1.8%
34	New Mexico	320	0.8%
3	New York	3,012	7.3%
6	North Carolina	1,595	3.9%
50	North Dakota	43	0.1%
7	Ohio	1,447	3.5%
28	Oklahoma	505	1.2%
32	Oregon	354	0.9%
8	Pennsylvania	1,399	3.4%
39	Rhode Island	171	0.4%
20	South Carolina	813	2.0%
44	South Dakota	108	0.3%
18	Tennessee	839	2.0%
9	Texas	1,288	3.1%
36	Utah	202	0.5%
49	Vermont	77	0.2%
10	Virginia	1,244	3.0%
29	Washington	497	1.2%
40	West Virginia	152	0.4%
17	Wisconsin	857	2.1%
45	Wyoming	107	0.3%

RANK ORDER

RANK	STATE	CASES	% of USA
1	Florida	4,659	11.3%
2	California	4,118	10.0%
3	New York	3,012	7.3%
4	Georgia	1,712	4.1%
5	Illinois	1,658	4.0%
6	North Carolina	1,595	3.9%
7	Ohio	1,447	3.5%
8	Pennsylvania	1,399	3.4%
9	Texas	1,288	3.1%
10	Virginia	1,244	3.0%
11	Massachusetts	1,168	2.8%
12	Mississippi	1,140	2.8%
13	Arkansas	1,047	2.5%
14	Maryland	954	2.3%
15	Alabama	877	2.1%
16	Michigan	875	2.1%
17	Wisconsin	857	2.1%
18	Tennessee	839	2.0%
19	Missouri	820	2.0%
20	Louisiana	813	2.0%
20	South Carolina	813	2.0%
22	Arizona	788	1.9%
23	New Jersey	761	1.8%
24	Minnesota	610	1.5%
25	Colorado	602	1.5%
26	Iowa	518	1.3%
27	Indiana	508	1.2%
28	Oklahoma	505	1.2%
29	Washington	497	1.2%
30	Connecticut	445	1.1%
31	Kentucky	398	1.0%
32	Oregon	354	0.9%
33	Kansas	336	0.8%
34	New Mexico	320	0.8%
35	Hawaii	278	0.7%
36	Utah	202	0.5%
37	Idaho	184	0.4%
38	Nevada	183	0.4%
39	Rhode Island	171	0.4%
40	West Virginia	152	0.4%
41	Nebraska	150	0.4%
42	Maine	146	0.4%
43	New Hampshire	138	0.3%
44	South Dakota	108	0.3%
45	Wyoming	107	0.3%
46	Delaware	95	0.2%
47	Montana	91	0.2%
48	Alaska	79	0.2%
49	Vermont	77	0.2%
50	North Dakota	43	0.1%
	District of Columbia	76	0.2%

Source: U.S. Department of Health and Human Services, National Center for Health Statistics
    "Morbidity and Mortality Weekly Report" (January 3, 2003, Vol. 51, No. 52)
*Provisional data. Any disease caused by a salmonella infection, which may be manifested as food poisoning with
acute gastroenteritis, vomiting and diarrhea.

Salmonellosis Rate in 2002

National Rate = 14.3 Cases per 100,000 Population*

ALPHA ORDER

RANK	STATE	RATE
8	Alabama	19.5
31	Alaska	12.3
22	Arizona	14.4
2	Arkansas	38.6
34	California	11.7
25	Colorado	13.4
27	Connecticut	12.9
33	Delaware	11.8
3	Florida	27.9
6	Georgia	20.0
4	Hawaii	22.3
24	Idaho	13.7
26	Illinois	13.2
47	Indiana	8.2
12	Iowa	17.6
30	Kansas	12.4
40	Kentucky	9.7
11	Louisiana	18.1
35	Maine	11.3
13	Maryland	17.5
10	Massachusetts	18.2
42	Michigan	8.7
32	Minnesota	12.2
1	Mississippi	39.7
19	Missouri	14.5
39	Montana	10.0
42	Nebraska	8.7
45	Nevada	8.4
37	New Hampshire	10.8
41	New Jersey	8.9
14	New Mexico	17.3
18	New York	15.7
9	North Carolina	19.2
49	North Dakota	6.8
28	Ohio	12.7
19	Oklahoma	14.5
38	Oregon	10.1
35	Pennsylvania	11.3
16	Rhode Island	16.0
7	South Carolina	19.8
23	South Dakota	14.2
19	Tennessee	14.5
50	Texas	5.9
42	Utah	8.7
29	Vermont	12.5
15	Virginia	17.1
47	Washington	8.2
45	West Virginia	8.4
17	Wisconsin	15.8
5	Wyoming	21.5

RANK ORDER

RANK	STATE	RATE
1	Mississippi	39.7
2	Arkansas	38.6
3	Florida	27.9
4	Hawaii	22.3
5	Wyoming	21.5
6	Georgia	20.0
7	South Carolina	19.8
8	Alabama	19.5
9	North Carolina	19.2
10	Massachusetts	18.2
11	Louisiana	18.1
12	Iowa	17.6
13	Maryland	17.5
14	New Mexico	17.3
15	Virginia	17.1
16	Rhode Island	16.0
17	Wisconsin	15.8
18	New York	15.7
19	Missouri	14.5
19	Oklahoma	14.5
19	Tennessee	14.5
22	Arizona	14.4
23	South Dakota	14.2
24	Idaho	13.7
25	Colorado	13.4
26	Illinois	13.2
27	Connecticut	12.9
28	Ohio	12.7
29	Vermont	12.5
30	Kansas	12.4
31	Alaska	12.3
32	Minnesota	12.2
33	Delaware	11.8
34	California	11.7
35	Maine	11.3
35	Pennsylvania	11.3
37	New Hampshire	10.8
38	Oregon	10.1
39	Montana	10.0
40	Kentucky	9.7
41	New Jersey	8.9
42	Michigan	8.7
42	Nebraska	8.7
42	Utah	8.7
45	Nevada	8.4
45	West Virginia	8.4
47	Indiana	8.2
47	Washington	8.2
49	North Dakota	6.8
50	Texas	5.9
	District of Columbia	13.3

Source: Morgan Quitno Press using data from U.S. Dept. of Health & Human Serv's, National Center for Health Statistics "Morbidity and Mortality Weekly Report" (January 3, 2003, Vol. 51, No. 52)
*Provisional data. Any disease caused by a salmonella infection, which may be manifested as food poisoning with acute gastroenteritis, vomiting and diarrhea.

Shigellosis Cases Reported in 2002

National Total = 19,768 Cases*

ALPHA ORDER

RANK	STATE	CASES	% of USA
6	Alabama	838	4.2%
48	Alaska	6	0.0%
12	Arizona	604	3.1%
25	Arkansas	196	1.0%
1	California	2,675	13.5%
21	Colorado	212	1.1%
36	Connecticut	102	0.5%
16	Delaware	397	2.0%
2	Florida	2,540	12.8%
3	Georgia	1,354	6.8%
38	Hawaii	68	0.3%
41	Idaho	22	0.1%
8	Illinois	819	4.1%
35	Indiana	107	0.5%
33	Iowa	123	0.6%
37	Kansas	91	0.5%
22	Kentucky	201	1.0%
14	Louisiana	445	2.3%
45	Maine	12	0.1%
4	Maryland	1,256	6.4%
26	Massachusetts	187	0.9%
24	Michigan	198	1.0%
20	Minnesota	225	1.1%
17	Mississippi	338	1.7%
22	Missouri	201	1.0%
49	Montana	4	0.0%
27	Nebraska	179	0.9%
39	Nevada	47	0.2%
44	New Hampshire	13	0.1%
15	New Jersey	403	2.0%
19	New Mexico	231	1.2%
7	New York	830	4.2%
10	North Carolina	638	3.2%
43	North Dakota	16	0.1%
9	Ohio	681	3.4%
13	Oklahoma	586	3.0%
34	Oregon	117	0.6%
18	Pennsylvania	254	1.3%
42	Rhode Island	17	0.1%
32	South Carolina	128	0.6%
30	South Dakota	156	0.8%
31	Tennessee	140	0.7%
11	Texas	620	3.1%
40	Utah	42	0.2%
50	Vermont	1	0.0%
5	Virginia	1,015	5.1%
27	Washington	179	0.9%
45	West Virginia	12	0.1%
29	Wisconsin	172	0.9%
47	Wyoming	9	0.0%

RANK ORDER

RANK	STATE	CASES	% of USA
1	California	2,675	13.5%
2	Florida	2,540	12.8%
3	Georgia	1,354	6.8%
4	Maryland	1,256	6.4%
5	Virginia	1,015	5.1%
6	Alabama	838	4.2%
7	New York	830	4.2%
8	Illinois	819	4.1%
9	Ohio	681	3.4%
10	North Carolina	638	3.2%
11	Texas	620	3.1%
12	Arizona	604	3.1%
13	Oklahoma	586	3.0%
14	Louisiana	445	2.3%
15	New Jersey	403	2.0%
16	Delaware	397	2.0%
17	Mississippi	338	1.7%
18	Pennsylvania	254	1.3%
19	New Mexico	231	1.2%
20	Minnesota	225	1.1%
21	Colorado	212	1.1%
22	Kentucky	201	1.0%
22	Missouri	201	1.0%
24	Michigan	198	1.0%
25	Arkansas	196	1.0%
26	Massachusetts	187	0.9%
27	Nebraska	179	0.9%
27	Washington	179	0.9%
29	Wisconsin	172	0.9%
30	South Dakota	156	0.8%
31	Tennessee	140	0.7%
32	South Carolina	128	0.6%
33	Iowa	123	0.6%
34	Oregon	117	0.6%
35	Indiana	107	0.5%
36	Connecticut	102	0.5%
37	Kansas	91	0.5%
38	Hawaii	68	0.3%
39	Nevada	47	0.2%
40	Utah	42	0.2%
41	Idaho	22	0.1%
42	Rhode Island	17	0.1%
43	North Dakota	16	0.1%
44	New Hampshire	13	0.1%
45	Maine	12	0.1%
45	West Virginia	12	0.1%
47	Wyoming	9	0.0%
48	Alaska	6	0.0%
49	Montana	4	0.0%
50	Vermont	1	0.0%
	District of Columbia	61	0.3%

Source: U.S. Department of Health and Human Services, National Center for Health Statistics
    "Morbidity and Mortality Weekly Report" (January 3, 2003, Vol. 51, No. 52)
*Provisional data. Dysentery caused by any of various species of shigellae, occurring most frequently in areas
where poor sanitation and malnutrition are prevalent and commonly affecting children and infants.

Shigellosis Rate in 2002

National Rate = 6.9 Cases per 100,000 Population*

ALPHA ORDER

RANK	STATE	RATE
4	Alabama	18.7
46	Alaska	0.9
11	Arizona	11.1
16	Arkansas	7.2
15	California	7.6
21	Colorado	4.7
31	Connecticut	2.9
1	Delaware	49.2
7	Florida	15.2
6	Georgia	15.8
19	Hawaii	5.5
43	Idaho	1.6
17	Illinois	6.5
42	Indiana	1.7
25	Iowa	4.2
27	Kansas	3.4
20	Kentucky	4.9
13	Louisiana	9.9
46	Maine	0.9
2	Maryland	23.0
31	Massachusetts	2.9
39	Michigan	2.0
23	Minnesota	4.5
10	Mississippi	11.8
26	Missouri	3.5
49	Montana	0.4
12	Nebraska	10.4
37	Nevada	2.2
45	New Hampshire	1.0
21	New Jersey	4.7
9	New Mexico	12.5
24	New York	4.3
14	North Carolina	7.7
35	North Dakota	2.5
18	Ohio	6.0
5	Oklahoma	16.8
28	Oregon	3.3
38	Pennsylvania	2.1
43	Rhode Island	1.6
30	South Carolina	3.1
3	South Dakota	20.5
36	Tennessee	2.4
34	Texas	2.8
40	Utah	1.8
50	Vermont	0.2
8	Virginia	13.9
31	Washington	2.9
48	West Virginia	0.7
29	Wisconsin	3.2
40	Wyoming	1.8

RANK ORDER

RANK	STATE	RATE
1	Delaware	49.2
2	Maryland	23.0
3	South Dakota	20.5
4	Alabama	18.7
5	Oklahoma	16.8
6	Georgia	15.8
7	Florida	15.2
8	Virginia	13.9
9	New Mexico	12.5
10	Mississippi	11.8
11	Arizona	11.1
12	Nebraska	10.4
13	Louisiana	9.9
14	North Carolina	7.7
15	California	7.6
16	Arkansas	7.2
17	Illinois	6.5
18	Ohio	6.0
19	Hawaii	5.5
20	Kentucky	4.9
21	Colorado	4.7
21	New Jersey	4.7
23	Minnesota	4.5
24	New York	4.3
25	Iowa	4.2
26	Missouri	3.5
27	Kansas	3.4
28	Oregon	3.3
29	Wisconsin	3.2
30	South Carolina	3.1
31	Connecticut	2.9
31	Massachusetts	2.9
31	Washington	2.9
34	Texas	2.8
35	North Dakota	2.5
36	Tennessee	2.4
37	Nevada	2.2
38	Pennsylvania	2.1
39	Michigan	2.0
40	Utah	1.8
40	Wyoming	1.8
42	Indiana	1.7
43	Idaho	1.6
43	Rhode Island	1.6
45	New Hampshire	1.0
46	Alaska	0.9
46	Maine	0.9
48	West Virginia	0.7
49	Montana	0.4
50	Vermont	0.2

District of Columbia	10.7

Source: Morgan Quitno Press using data from U.S. Dept. of Health & Human Serv's, National Center for Health Statistics
"Morbidity and Mortality Weekly Report" (January 3, 2003, Vol. 51, No. 52)
*Provisional data. Dysentery caused by any of various species of shigellae, occurring most frequently in areas where poor sanitation and malnutrition are prevalent and commonly affecting children and infants.

Tuberculosis Cases Reported in 2002

National Total = 12,120 Cases*

ALPHA ORDER

RANK	STATE	CASES	% of USA
18	Alabama	207	1.7%
33	Alaska	48	0.4%
15	Arizona	229	1.9%
26	Arkansas	119	1.0%
1	California	2,202	18.2%
32	Colorado	56	0.5%
30	Connecticut	87	0.7%
42	Delaware	15	0.1%
4	Florida	909	7.5%
8	Georgia	400	3.3%
22	Hawaii	139	1.1%
46	Idaho	9	0.1%
5	Illinois	604	5.0%
25	Indiana	120	1.0%
36	Iowa	30	0.2%
29	Kansas	104	0.9%
23	Kentucky	134	1.1%
50	Louisiana	0	0.0%
40	Maine	20	0.2%
11	Maryland	272	2.2%
14	Massachusetts	235	1.9%
13	Michigan	256	2.1%
17	Minnesota	226	1.9%
27	Mississippi	109	0.9%
24	Missouri	126	1.0%
44	Montana	12	0.1%
39	Nebraska	23	0.2%
43	Nevada	14	0.1%
41	New Hampshire	18	0.1%
6	New Jersey	496	4.1%
37	New Mexico	28	0.2%
2	New York	1,334	11.0%
7	North Carolina	417	3.4%
48	North Dakota	4	0.0%
19	Ohio	173	1.4%
21	Oklahoma	142	1.2%
27	Oregon	109	0.9%
12	Pennsylvania	259	2.1%
34	Rhode Island	37	0.3%
20	South Carolina	147	1.2%
44	South Dakota	12	0.1%
9	Tennessee	286	2.4%
3	Texas	1,308	10.8%
35	Utah	31	0.3%
47	Vermont	6	0.0%
10	Virginia	283	2.3%
15	Washington	229	1.9%
37	West Virginia	28	0.2%
31	Wisconsin	65	0.5%
49	Wyoming	3	0.0%

RANK ORDER

RANK	STATE	CASES	% of USA
1	California	2,202	18.2%
2	New York	1,334	11.0%
3	Texas	1,308	10.8%
4	Florida	909	7.5%
5	Illinois	604	5.0%
6	New Jersey	496	4.1%
7	North Carolina	417	3.4%
8	Georgia	400	3.3%
9	Tennessee	286	2.4%
10	Virginia	283	2.3%
11	Maryland	272	2.2%
12	Pennsylvania	259	2.1%
13	Michigan	256	2.1%
14	Massachusetts	235	1.9%
15	Arizona	229	1.9%
15	Washington	229	1.9%
17	Minnesota	226	1.9%
18	Alabama	207	1.7%
19	Ohio	173	1.4%
20	South Carolina	147	1.2%
21	Oklahoma	142	1.2%
22	Hawaii	139	1.1%
23	Kentucky	134	1.1%
24	Missouri	126	1.0%
25	Indiana	120	1.0%
26	Arkansas	119	1.0%
27	Mississippi	109	0.9%
27	Oregon	109	0.9%
29	Kansas	104	0.9%
30	Connecticut	87	0.7%
31	Wisconsin	65	0.5%
32	Colorado	56	0.5%
33	Alaska	48	0.4%
34	Rhode Island	37	0.3%
35	Utah	31	0.3%
36	Iowa	30	0.2%
37	New Mexico	28	0.2%
37	West Virginia	28	0.2%
39	Nebraska	23	0.2%
40	Maine	20	0.2%
41	New Hampshire	18	0.1%
42	Delaware	15	0.1%
43	Nevada	14	0.1%
44	Montana	12	0.1%
44	South Dakota	12	0.1%
46	Idaho	9	0.1%
47	Vermont	6	0.0%
48	North Dakota	4	0.0%
49	Wyoming	3	0.0%
50	Louisiana	0	0.0%
	District of Columbia	0	0.0%

Source: U.S. Department of Health and Human Services, National Center for Health Statistics
"Morbidity and Mortality Weekly Report" (January 3, 2003, Vol. 51, No. 52)
*Provisional data. An infectious disease caused by the tubercle bacillus and causing the formation of tubercles on the lungs and other tissues of the body, often developing long after the initial infection. Characterized by the coughing up of mucus and sputum, fever, weight loss, and chest pain.

Tuberculosis Rate in 2002

National Rate = 4.2 Cases per 100,000 Population*

<u>ALPHA ORDER</u>

RANK	STATE	RATE
13	Alabama	4.6
2	Alaska	7.5
16	Arizona	4.2
15	Arkansas	4.4
4	California	6.3
42	Colorado	1.2
27	Connecticut	2.5
31	Delaware	1.9
7	Florida	5.4
12	Georgia	4.7
1	Hawaii	11.2
46	Idaho	0.7
11	Illinois	4.8
31	Indiana	1.9
44	Iowa	1.0
19	Kansas	3.8
25	Kentucky	3.3
50	Louisiana	0.0
35	Maine	1.5
8	Maryland	5.0
22	Massachusetts	3.7
27	Michigan	2.5
14	Minnesota	4.5
19	Mississippi	3.8
29	Missouri	2.2
39	Montana	1.3
39	Nebraska	1.3
47	Nevada	0.6
38	New Hampshire	1.4
6	New Jersey	5.8
35	New Mexico	1.5
3	New York	7.0
8	North Carolina	5.0
47	North Dakota	0.6
35	Ohio	1.5
17	Oklahoma	4.1
26	Oregon	3.1
30	Pennsylvania	2.1
24	Rhode Island	3.5
23	South Carolina	3.6
33	South Dakota	1.6
10	Tennessee	4.9
5	Texas	6.0
39	Utah	1.3
44	Vermont	1.0
18	Virginia	3.9
19	Washington	3.8
33	West Virginia	1.6
42	Wisconsin	1.2
47	Wyoming	0.6

<u>RANK ORDER</u>

RANK	STATE	RATE
1	Hawaii	11.2
2	Alaska	7.5
3	New York	7.0
4	California	6.3
5	Texas	6.0
6	New Jersey	5.8
7	Florida	5.4
8	Maryland	5.0
8	North Carolina	5.0
10	Tennessee	4.9
11	Illinois	4.8
12	Georgia	4.7
13	Alabama	4.6
14	Minnesota	4.5
15	Arkansas	4.4
16	Arizona	4.2
17	Oklahoma	4.1
18	Virginia	3.9
19	Kansas	3.8
19	Mississippi	3.8
19	Washington	3.8
22	Massachusetts	3.7
23	South Carolina	3.6
24	Rhode Island	3.5
25	Kentucky	3.3
26	Oregon	3.1
27	Connecticut	2.5
27	Michigan	2.5
29	Missouri	2.2
30	Pennsylvania	2.1
31	Delaware	1.9
31	Indiana	1.9
33	South Dakota	1.6
33	West Virginia	1.6
35	Maine	1.5
35	New Mexico	1.5
35	Ohio	1.5
38	New Hampshire	1.4
39	Montana	1.3
39	Nebraska	1.3
39	Utah	1.3
42	Colorado	1.2
42	Wisconsin	1.2
44	Iowa	1.0
44	Vermont	1.0
46	Idaho	0.7
47	Nevada	0.6
47	North Dakota	0.6
47	Wyoming	0.6
50	Louisiana	0.0

| District of Columbia | 0.0 |

Source: Morgan Quitno Press using data from U.S. Dept. of Health & Human Serv's, National Center for Health Statistics "Morbidity and Mortality Weekly Report" (January 3, 2003, Vol. 51, No. 52)

*Provisional data. An infectious disease caused by the tubercle bacillus and causing the formation of tubercles on the lungs and other tissues of the body, often developing long after the initial infection. Characterized by the coughing up of mucus and sputum, fever, weight loss, and chest pain.

Whooping Cough (Pertussis) Cases Reported in 2002

National Total = 8,296 Cases*

ALPHA ORDER

RANK	STATE	CASES	% of USA
34	Alabama	37	0.4%
47	Alaska	5	0.1%
2	Arizona	706	8.5%
5	Arkansas	489	5.9%
3	California	702	8.5%
8	Colorado	432	5.2%
36	Connecticut	27	0.3%
48	Delaware	4	0.0%
30	Florida	53	0.6%
40	Georgia	15	0.2%
37	Hawaii	17	0.2%
16	Idaho	152	1.8%
13	Illinois	166	2.0%
16	Indiana	152	1.8%
19	Iowa	143	1.7%
27	Kansas	64	0.8%
24	Kentucky	93	1.1%
45	Louisiana	7	0.1%
37	Maine	17	0.2%
26	Maryland	65	0.8%
4	Massachusetts	511	6.2%
29	Michigan	60	0.7%
10	Minnesota	379	4.6%
42	Mississippi	9	0.1%
18	Missouri	144	1.7%
42	Montana	9	0.1%
44	Nebraska	8	0.1%
31	Nevada	48	0.6%
28	New Hampshire	61	0.7%
50	New Jersey	1	0.0%
12	New Mexico	188	2.3%
9	New York	389	4.7%
32	North Carolina	45	0.5%
49	North Dakota	3	0.0%
7	Ohio	443	5.3%
25	Oklahoma	66	0.8%
11	Oregon	192	2.3%
21	Pennsylvania	116	1.4%
39	Rhode Island	16	0.2%
33	South Carolina	43	0.5%
46	South Dakota	6	0.1%
22	Tennessee	114	1.4%
1	Texas	1,025	12.4%
23	Utah	107	1.3%
13	Vermont	166	2.0%
15	Virginia	159	1.9%
6	Washington	472	5.7%
35	West Virginia	32	0.4%
20	Wisconsin	125	1.5%
41	Wyoming	11	0.1%

RANK ORDER

RANK	STATE	CASES	% of USA
1	Texas	1,025	12.4%
2	Arizona	706	8.5%
3	California	702	8.5%
4	Massachusetts	511	6.2%
5	Arkansas	489	5.9%
6	Washington	472	5.7%
7	Ohio	443	5.3%
8	Colorado	432	5.2%
9	New York	389	4.7%
10	Minnesota	379	4.6%
11	Oregon	192	2.3%
12	New Mexico	188	2.3%
13	Illinois	166	2.0%
13	Vermont	166	2.0%
15	Virginia	159	1.9%
16	Idaho	152	1.8%
16	Indiana	152	1.8%
18	Missouri	144	1.7%
19	Iowa	143	1.7%
20	Wisconsin	125	1.5%
21	Pennsylvania	116	1.4%
22	Tennessee	114	1.4%
23	Utah	107	1.3%
24	Kentucky	93	1.1%
25	Oklahoma	66	0.8%
26	Maryland	65	0.8%
27	Kansas	64	0.8%
28	New Hampshire	61	0.7%
29	Michigan	60	0.7%
30	Florida	53	0.6%
31	Nevada	48	0.6%
32	North Carolina	45	0.5%
33	South Carolina	43	0.5%
34	Alabama	37	0.4%
35	West Virginia	32	0.4%
36	Connecticut	27	0.3%
37	Hawaii	17	0.2%
37	Maine	17	0.2%
39	Rhode Island	16	0.2%
40	Georgia	15	0.2%
41	Wyoming	11	0.1%
42	Mississippi	9	0.1%
42	Montana	9	0.1%
44	Nebraska	8	0.1%
45	Louisiana	7	0.1%
46	South Dakota	6	0.1%
47	Alaska	5	0.1%
48	Delaware	4	0.0%
49	North Dakota	3	0.0%
50	New Jersey	1	0.0%
	District of Columbia	2	0.0%

Source: U.S. Department of Health and Human Services, National Center for Health Statistics
"Morbidity and Mortality Weekly Report" (January 3, 2003, Vol. 51, No. 52)
*Provisional data. Acute, highly contagious infection of respiratory tract.

Whooping Cough (Pertussis) Rate in 2002

National Rate = 2.9 Cases per 100,000 Population*

ALPHA ORDER

RANK	STATE	RATE
37	Alabama	0.8
37	Alaska	0.8
3	Arizona	12.9
2	Arkansas	18.0
24	California	2.0
6	Colorado	9.6
37	Connecticut	0.8
42	Delaware	0.5
46	Florida	0.3
48	Georgia	0.2
30	Hawaii	1.4
4	Idaho	11.3
31	Illinois	1.3
16	Indiana	2.5
11	Iowa	4.9
18	Kansas	2.4
19	Kentucky	2.3
48	Louisiana	0.2
31	Maine	1.3
33	Maryland	1.2
7	Massachusetts	7.9
41	Michigan	0.6
9	Minnesota	7.6
46	Mississippi	0.3
16	Missouri	2.5
34	Montana	1.0
42	Nebraska	0.5
21	Nevada	2.2
12	New Hampshire	4.8
50	New Jersey	0.0
5	New Mexico	10.1
24	New York	2.0
42	North Carolina	0.5
42	North Dakota	0.5
15	Ohio	3.9
27	Oklahoma	1.9
10	Oregon	5.5
36	Pennsylvania	0.9
29	Rhode Island	1.5
34	South Carolina	1.0
37	South Dakota	0.8
24	Tennessee	2.0
13	Texas	4.7
14	Utah	4.6
1	Vermont	26.9
21	Virginia	2.2
8	Washington	7.8
28	West Virginia	1.8
19	Wisconsin	2.3
21	Wyoming	2.2

RANK ORDER

RANK	STATE	RATE
1	Vermont	26.9
2	Arkansas	18.0
3	Arizona	12.9
4	Idaho	11.3
5	New Mexico	10.1
6	Colorado	9.6
7	Massachusetts	7.9
8	Washington	7.8
9	Minnesota	7.6
10	Oregon	5.5
11	Iowa	4.9
12	New Hampshire	4.8
13	Texas	4.7
14	Utah	4.6
15	Ohio	3.9
16	Indiana	2.5
16	Missouri	2.5
18	Kansas	2.4
19	Kentucky	2.3
19	Wisconsin	2.3
21	Nevada	2.2
21	Virginia	2.2
21	Wyoming	2.2
24	California	2.0
24	New York	2.0
24	Tennessee	2.0
27	Oklahoma	1.9
28	West Virginia	1.8
29	Rhode Island	1.5
30	Hawaii	1.4
31	Illinois	1.3
31	Maine	1.3
33	Maryland	1.2
34	Montana	1.0
34	South Carolina	1.0
36	Pennsylvania	0.9
37	Alabama	0.8
37	Alaska	0.8
37	Connecticut	0.8
37	South Dakota	0.8
41	Michigan	0.6
42	Delaware	0.5
42	Nebraska	0.5
42	North Carolina	0.5
42	North Dakota	0.5
46	Florida	0.3
46	Mississippi	0.3
48	Georgia	0.2
48	Louisiana	0.2
50	New Jersey	0.0

| | District of Columbia | 0.4 |

Source: Morgan Quitno Press using data from U.S. Dept. of Health & Human Serv's, National Center for Health Statistics
"Morbidity and Mortality Weekly Report" (January 3, 2003, Vol. 51, No. 52)
*Provisional data. Acute, highly contagious infection of respiratory tract.

Percent of Children Aged 19 to 35 Months Fully Immunized in 2001

National Percent = 73.7%*

ALPHA ORDER				RANK ORDER		
RANK	STATE	PERCENT		RANK	STATE	PERCENT
7	Alabama	79.1		1	Rhode Island	81.7
35	Alaska	71.2		2	North Carolina	80.4
46	Arizona	68.1		3	Vermont	80.3
44	Arkansas	69.1		4	Mississippi	80.2
33	California	72.6		5	Tennessee	79.7
34	Colorado	71.5		6	Wisconsin	79.5
14	Connecticut	78.4		7	Alabama	79.1
25	Delaware	74.9		8	Nebraska	78.9
30	Florida	73.0		9	Pennsylvania	78.8
13	Georgia	78.5		10	North Dakota	78.7
39	Hawaii	70.8		10	South Carolina	78.7
40	Idaho	70.2		12	Iowa	78.6
32	Illinois	72.7		13	Georgia	78.5
38	Indiana	71.1		14	Connecticut	78.4
12	Iowa	78.6		15	West Virginia	78.1
31	Kansas	72.8		16	Montana	77.9
22	Kentucky	75.9		17	New Hampshire	77.6
49	Louisiana	64.1		18	New York	77.1
24	Maine	75.1		19	Massachusetts	76.6
28	Maryland	73.4		20	South Dakota	76.5
19	Massachusetts	76.6		21	Minnesota	76.3
41	Michigan	70.0		22	Kentucky	75.9
21	Minnesota	76.3		23	Missouri	75.5
4	Mississippi	80.2		24	Maine	75.1
23	Missouri	75.5		25	Delaware	74.9
16	Montana	77.9		25	Virginia	74.9
8	Nebraska	78.9		27	Wyoming	74.3
46	Nevada	68.1		28	Maryland	73.4
17	New Hampshire	77.6		29	New Jersey	73.1
29	New Jersey	73.1		30	Florida	73.0
50	New Mexico	63.2		31	Kansas	72.8
18	New York	77.1		32	Illinois	72.7
2	North Carolina	80.4		33	California	72.6
10	North Dakota	78.7		34	Colorado	71.5
35	Ohio	71.2		35	Alaska	71.2
41	Oklahoma	70.0		35	Ohio	71.2
45	Oregon	68.5		35	Washington	71.2
9	Pennsylvania	78.8		38	Indiana	71.1
1	Rhode Island	81.7		39	Hawaii	70.8
10	South Carolina	78.7		40	Idaho	70.2
20	South Dakota	76.5		41	Michigan	70.0
5	Tennessee	79.7		41	Oklahoma	70.0
43	Texas	69.7		43	Texas	69.7
48	Utah	66.1		44	Arkansas	69.1
3	Vermont	80.3		45	Oregon	68.5
25	Virginia	74.9		46	Arizona	68.1
35	Washington	71.2		46	Nevada	68.1
15	West Virginia	78.1		48	Utah	66.1
6	Wisconsin	79.5		49	Louisiana	64.1
27	Wyoming	74.3		50	New Mexico	63.2
					District of Columbia	68.9

Source: U.S. Department of Health and Human Services, Centers for Disease Control and Prevention
"State Vaccination Coverage Levels" (Morbidity and Mortality Weekly Report, Vol. 51, No. 30, August 2, 2002)
*Fully immunized children received four doses of DTP/DT/DTaP (Diphtheria, Tetanus, Pertussis (Whooping Cough), Acellular Pertussis), three doses of OPV (Oral Poliovirus Vaccine), one dose of MCV (Measles-Containing Vaccine) and three doses of Hib (Haemophilus influenzae type b).

Reported Rate of Adverse Events After Immunization: 1991-2001

National Average = 44.1 Events per 1,000,000 Population*

ALPHA ORDER

RANK	STATE	RATE
50	Alabama	27.7
1	Alaska	113.2
44	Arizona	32.6
21	Arkansas	48.1
48	California	28.4
11	Colorado	52.7
33	Connecticut	41.4
5	Delaware	66.5
46	Florida	30.3
18	Georgia	49.0
29	Hawaii	43.6
2	Idaho	81.4
42	Illinois	33.8
43	Indiana	33.5
26	Iowa	44.8
23	Kansas	46.9
47	Kentucky	29.9
48	Louisiana	28.4
9	Maine	59.7
15	Maryland	50.0
13	Massachusetts	51.7
25	Michigan	45.5
17	Minnesota	49.7
39	Mississippi	35.5
27	Missouri	43.9
8	Montana	59.8
24	Nebraska	46.6
40	Nevada	35.2
4	New Hampshire	74.6
28	New Jersey	43.7
31	New Mexico	42.5
38	New York	35.8
36	North Carolina	40.4
6	North Dakota	66.0
37	Ohio	39.4
40	Oklahoma	35.2
19	Oregon	48.4
10	Pennsylvania	54.3
35	Rhode Island	40.7
14	South Carolina	50.6
7	South Dakota	60.2
34	Tennessee	41.1
45	Texas	32.0
32	Utah	41.5
22	Vermont	47.0
30	Virginia	42.8
12	Washington	52.3
20	West Virginia	48.2
15	Wisconsin	50.0
3	Wyoming	75.2

RANK ORDER

RANK	STATE	RATE
1	Alaska	113.2
2	Idaho	81.4
3	Wyoming	75.2
4	New Hampshire	74.6
5	Delaware	66.5
6	North Dakota	66.0
7	South Dakota	60.2
8	Montana	59.8
9	Maine	59.7
10	Pennsylvania	54.3
11	Colorado	52.7
12	Washington	52.3
13	Massachusetts	51.7
14	South Carolina	50.6
15	Maryland	50.0
15	Wisconsin	50.0
17	Minnesota	49.7
18	Georgia	49.0
19	Oregon	48.4
20	West Virginia	48.2
21	Arkansas	48.1
22	Vermont	47.0
23	Kansas	46.9
24	Nebraska	46.6
25	Michigan	45.5
26	Iowa	44.8
27	Missouri	43.9
28	New Jersey	43.7
29	Hawaii	43.6
30	Virginia	42.8
31	New Mexico	42.5
32	Utah	41.5
33	Connecticut	41.4
34	Tennessee	41.1
35	Rhode Island	40.7
36	North Carolina	40.4
37	Ohio	39.4
38	New York	35.8
39	Mississippi	35.5
40	Nevada	35.2
40	Oklahoma	35.2
42	Illinois	33.8
43	Indiana	33.5
44	Arizona	32.6
45	Texas	32.0
46	Florida	30.3
47	Kentucky	29.9
48	California	28.4
48	Louisiana	28.4
50	Alabama	27.7
	District of Columbia	61.7

Source: U.S. Department of Health and Human Services, National Center for Health Statistics
   "Morbidity and Mortality Weekly Report" (January 24, 2003, Vol. 52, No. SS-1)
*These population-based reported rates were calculated by using the 11-year (1991-2001) average number of reports in each state as numerator and the average of 1990 and 2000 Bureau of the Census data for each state as denominator.

Sexually Transmitted Diseases in 2001

National Total = 1,151,088 Cases*

ALPHA ORDER				RANK ORDER			
RANK	STATE	CASES	% of USA	RANK	STATE	CASES	% of USA
15	Alabama	25,848	2.2%	1	California	125,787	10.9%
41	Alaska	3,201	0.3%	2	Texas	100,260	8.7%
22	Arizona	18,446	1.6%	3	New York	68,999	6.0%
28	Arkansas	11,933	1.0%	4	Illinois	68,150	5.9%
1	California	125,787	10.9%	5	Florida	59,642	5.2%
24	Colorado	16,452	1.4%	6	Ohio	58,897	5.1%
30	Connecticut	10,276	0.9%	7	Georgia	53,174	4.6%
37	Delaware	4,540	0.4%	8	Michigan	48,638	4.2%
5	Florida	59,642	5.2%	9	Pennsylvania	42,715	3.7%
7	Georgia	53,174	4.6%	10	North Carolina	39,132	3.4%
36	Hawaii	4,647	0.4%	11	Louisiana	30,266	2.6%
44	Idaho	2,100	0.2%	12	Virginia	29,534	2.6%
4	Illinois	68,150	5.9%	13	South Carolina	26,384	2.3%
19	Indiana	22,381	1.9%	14	Tennessee	26,036	2.3%
34	Iowa	7,122	0.6%	15	Alabama	25,848	2.2%
31	Kansas	8,744	0.8%	16	New Jersey	25,374	2.2%
27	Kentucky	12,517	1.1%	17	Maryland	25,333	2.2%
11	Louisiana	30,266	2.6%	18	Missouri	22,698	2.0%
47	Maine	1,480	0.1%	19	Indiana	22,381	1.9%
17	Maryland	25,333	2.2%	20	Wisconsin	22,317	1.9%
26	Massachusetts	13,664	1.2%	21	Mississippi	19,692	1.7%
8	Michigan	48,638	4.2%	22	Arizona	18,446	1.6%
29	Minnesota	11,057	1.0%	23	Washington	16,679	1.4%
21	Mississippi	19,692	1.7%	24	Colorado	16,452	1.4%
18	Missouri	22,698	2.0%	25	Oklahoma	15,322	1.3%
45	Montana	2,023	0.2%	26	Massachusetts	13,664	1.2%
38	Nebraska	4,405	0.4%	27	Kentucky	12,517	1.1%
35	Nevada	6,595	0.6%	28	Arkansas	11,933	1.0%
46	New Hampshire	1,560	0.1%	29	Minnesota	11,057	1.0%
16	New Jersey	25,374	2.2%	30	Connecticut	10,276	0.9%
33	New Mexico	7,313	0.6%	31	Kansas	8,744	0.8%
3	New York	68,999	6.0%	32	Oregon	8,611	0.7%
10	North Carolina	39,132	3.4%	33	New Mexico	7,313	0.6%
48	North Dakota	1,118	0.1%	34	Iowa	7,122	0.6%
6	Ohio	58,897	5.1%	35	Nevada	6,595	0.6%
25	Oklahoma	15,322	1.3%	36	Hawaii	4,647	0.4%
32	Oregon	8,611	0.7%	37	Delaware	4,540	0.4%
9	Pennsylvania	42,715	3.7%	38	Nebraska	4,405	0.4%
39	Rhode Island	3,751	0.3%	39	Rhode Island	3,751	0.3%
13	South Carolina	26,384	2.3%	40	Utah	3,235	0.3%
43	South Dakota	2,111	0.2%	41	Alaska	3,201	0.3%
14	Tennessee	26,036	2.3%	42	West Virginia	3,083	0.3%
2	Texas	100,260	8.7%	43	South Dakota	2,111	0.2%
40	Utah	3,235	0.3%	44	Idaho	2,100	0.2%
50	Vermont	717	0.1%	45	Montana	2,023	0.2%
12	Virginia	29,534	2.6%	46	New Hampshire	1,560	0.1%
23	Washington	16,679	1.4%	47	Maine	1,480	0.1%
42	West Virginia	3,083	0.3%	48	North Dakota	1,118	0.1%
20	Wisconsin	22,317	1.9%	49	Wyoming	917	0.1%
49	Wyoming	917	0.1%	50	Vermont	717	0.1%
					District of Columbia	6,212	0.5%

Source: Morgan Quitno Press using data from U.S. Dept. of Health and Human Services, Nat'l Center for Health Statistics
"Sexually Transmitted Disease Surveillance 2001" (http://www.cdc.gov/std/stats/TOC2001.htm)
*Includes chancroid, chlamydia, gonorrhea and primary and secondary syphilis.

Sexually Transmitted Disease Rate in 2001

National Rate = 409.0 Cases per 100,000 Population*

ALPHA ORDER

RANK	STATE	RATE
5	Alabama	581.2
9	Alaska	510.6
27	Arizona	359.5
15	Arkansas	446.3
24	California	371.4
22	Colorado	382.5
33	Connecticut	301.8
6	Delaware	579.4
23	Florida	373.1
4	Georgia	649.6
21	Hawaii	383.6
46	Idaho	162.3
7	Illinois	548.7
25	Indiana	368.1
39	Iowa	243.4
31	Kansas	325.2
32	Kentucky	309.7
2	Louisiana	677.3
50	Maine	116.1
13	Maryland	478.3
42	Massachusetts	215.1
10	Michigan	489.4
40	Minnesota	224.8
1	Mississippi	692.3
19	Missouri	405.7
41	Montana	224.2
37	Nebraska	257.4
30	Nevada	330.1
48	New Hampshire	126.2
34	New Jersey	301.5
20	New Mexico	402.0
26	New York	363.6
11	North Carolina	486.1
44	North Dakota	174.1
8	Ohio	518.8
16	Oklahoma	444.0
38	Oregon	251.7
29	Pennsylvania	347.8
28	Rhode Island	357.9
3	South Carolina	657.7
36	South Dakota	279.6
14	Tennessee	457.6
12	Texas	480.8
47	Utah	144.8
49	Vermont	117.8
17	Virginia	417.2
35	Washington	283.0
45	West Virginia	170.5
18	Wisconsin	416.1
43	Wyoming	185.7

RANK ORDER

RANK	STATE	RATE
1	Mississippi	692.3
2	Louisiana	677.3
3	South Carolina	657.7
4	Georgia	649.6
5	Alabama	581.2
6	Delaware	579.4
7	Illinois	548.7
8	Ohio	518.8
9	Alaska	510.6
10	Michigan	489.4
11	North Carolina	486.1
12	Texas	480.8
13	Maryland	478.3
14	Tennessee	457.6
15	Arkansas	446.3
16	Oklahoma	444.0
17	Virginia	417.2
18	Wisconsin	416.1
19	Missouri	405.7
20	New Mexico	402.0
21	Hawaii	383.6
22	Colorado	382.5
23	Florida	373.1
24	California	371.4
25	Indiana	368.1
26	New York	363.6
27	Arizona	359.5
28	Rhode Island	357.9
29	Pennsylvania	347.8
30	Nevada	330.1
31	Kansas	325.2
32	Kentucky	309.7
33	Connecticut	301.8
34	New Jersey	301.5
35	Washington	283.0
36	South Dakota	279.6
37	Nebraska	257.4
38	Oregon	251.7
39	Iowa	243.4
40	Minnesota	224.8
41	Montana	224.2
42	Massachusetts	215.1
43	Wyoming	185.7
44	North Dakota	174.1
45	West Virginia	170.5
46	Idaho	162.3
47	Utah	144.8
48	New Hampshire	126.2
49	Vermont	117.8
50	Maine	116.1

District of Columbia 1,086.4

Source: Morgan Quitno Press using data from U.S. Dept. of Health and Human Services, Nat'l Center for Health Statistics
"Sexually Transmitted Disease Surveillance 2001" (http://www.cdc.gov/std/stats/TOC2001.htm)
*Includes chancroid, chlamydia, gonorrhea and primary and secondary syphilis.

Chlamydia Cases Reported in 2001

National Total = 783,242 Cases*

ALPHA ORDER

RANK	STATE	CASES	% of USA
19	Alabama	14,524	1.9%
41	Alaska	2,744	0.4%
20	Arizona	14,346	1.8%
31	Arkansas	7,280	0.9%
1	California	101,944	13.0%
23	Colorado	13,239	1.7%
29	Connecticut	7,718	1.0%
40	Delaware	2,793	0.4%
6	Florida	37,625	4.8%
7	Georgia	33,840	4.3%
36	Hawaii	4,031	0.5%
43	Idaho	2,023	0.3%
4	Illinois	43,716	5.6%
18	Indiana	15,258	1.9%
34	Iowa	5,699	0.7%
33	Kansas	6,050	0.8%
27	Kentucky	8,881	1.1%
12	Louisiana	17,840	2.3%
47	Maine	1,338	0.2%
15	Maryland	15,640	2.0%
26	Massachusetts	10,402	1.3%
8	Michigan	31,090	4.0%
28	Minnesota	8,323	1.1%
24	Mississippi	11,793	1.5%
21	Missouri	13,949	1.8%
44	Montana	1,919	0.2%
37	Nebraska	3,206	0.4%
35	Nevada	4,831	0.6%
46	New Hampshire	1,383	0.2%
13	New Jersey	16,312	2.1%
32	New Mexico	6,254	0.8%
3	New York	46,393	5.9%
10	North Carolina	22,101	2.8%
48	North Dakota	1,062	0.1%
5	Ohio	37,653	4.8%
25	Oklahoma	10,478	1.3%
30	Oregon	7,454	1.0%
9	Pennsylvania	28,371	3.6%
39	Rhode Island	2,912	0.4%
17	South Carolina	15,329	2.0%
45	South Dakota	1,821	0.2%
16	Tennessee	15,560	2.0%
2	Texas	69,752	8.9%
38	Utah	3,004	0.4%
50	Vermont	638	0.1%
11	Virginia	18,337	2.3%
22	Washington	13,631	1.7%
42	West Virginia	2,346	0.3%
14	Wisconsin	16,284	2.1%
49	Wyoming	839	0.1%

RANK ORDER

RANK	STATE	CASES	% of USA
1	California	101,944	13.0%
2	Texas	69,752	8.9%
3	New York	46,393	5.9%
4	Illinois	43,716	5.6%
5	Ohio	37,653	4.8%
6	Florida	37,625	4.8%
7	Georgia	33,840	4.3%
8	Michigan	31,090	4.0%
9	Pennsylvania	28,371	3.6%
10	North Carolina	22,101	2.8%
11	Virginia	18,337	2.3%
12	Louisiana	17,840	2.3%
13	New Jersey	16,312	2.1%
14	Wisconsin	16,284	2.1%
15	Maryland	15,640	2.0%
16	Tennessee	15,560	2.0%
17	South Carolina	15,329	2.0%
18	Indiana	15,258	1.9%
19	Alabama	14,524	1.9%
20	Arizona	14,346	1.8%
21	Missouri	13,949	1.8%
22	Washington	13,631	1.7%
23	Colorado	13,239	1.7%
24	Mississippi	11,793	1.5%
25	Oklahoma	10,478	1.3%
26	Massachusetts	10,402	1.3%
27	Kentucky	8,881	1.1%
28	Minnesota	8,323	1.1%
29	Connecticut	7,718	1.0%
30	Oregon	7,454	1.0%
31	Arkansas	7,280	0.9%
32	New Mexico	6,254	0.8%
33	Kansas	6,050	0.8%
34	Iowa	5,699	0.7%
35	Nevada	4,831	0.6%
36	Hawaii	4,031	0.5%
37	Nebraska	3,206	0.4%
38	Utah	3,004	0.4%
39	Rhode Island	2,912	0.4%
40	Delaware	2,793	0.4%
41	Alaska	2,744	0.4%
42	West Virginia	2,346	0.3%
43	Idaho	2,023	0.3%
44	Montana	1,919	0.2%
45	South Dakota	1,821	0.2%
46	New Hampshire	1,383	0.2%
47	Maine	1,338	0.2%
48	North Dakota	1,062	0.1%
49	Wyoming	839	0.1%
50	Vermont	638	0.1%
	District of Columbia	3,286	0.4%

Source: U.S. Department of Health and Human Services, National Center for Health Statistics
   "Sexually Transmitted Disease Surveillance 2001" (http://www.cdc.gov/std/stats/TOC2001.htm)
*Any of several common, often asymptomatic, sexually transmitted diseases caused by the microorganism Chlamydia trachomatis, including nonspecific urethritis in men.

Chlamydia Rate in 2001

National Rate = 278.3 Cases per 100,000 Population*

ALPHA ORDER

ALPHA ORDER

RANK	STATE	RATE
12	Alabama	326.6
1	Alaska	437.7
19	Arizona	279.6
23	Arkansas	272.3
17	California	301.0
14	Colorado	307.8
33	Connecticut	226.6
6	Delaware	356.4
30	Florida	235.4
3	Georgia	413.4
10	Hawaii	332.7
45	Idaho	156.3
7	Illinois	352.0
25	Indiana	250.9
38	Iowa	194.7
34	Kansas	225.0
35	Kentucky	219.7
4	Louisiana	399.2
49	Maine	104.9
18	Maryland	295.3
44	Massachusetts	163.8
13	Michigan	312.8
42	Minnesota	169.2
2	Mississippi	414.6
26	Missouri	249.3
37	Montana	212.7
40	Nebraska	187.3
28	Nevada	241.8
48	New Hampshire	111.9
39	New Jersey	193.9
8	New Mexico	343.8
27	New York	244.5
21	North Carolina	274.6
43	North Dakota	165.4
11	Ohio	331.7
15	Oklahoma	303.7
36	Oregon	217.9
32	Pennsylvania	231.0
20	Rhode Island	277.8
5	South Carolina	382.1
29	South Dakota	241.2
22	Tennessee	273.5
9	Texas	334.5
46	Utah	134.5
50	Vermont	104.8
24	Virginia	259.1
31	Washington	231.3
47	West Virginia	129.7
16	Wisconsin	303.6
41	Wyoming	169.9

RANK ORDER

RANK	STATE	RATE
1	Alaska	437.7
2	Mississippi	414.6
3	Georgia	413.4
4	Louisiana	399.2
5	South Carolina	382.1
6	Delaware	356.4
7	Illinois	352.0
8	New Mexico	343.8
9	Texas	334.5
10	Hawaii	332.7
11	Ohio	331.7
12	Alabama	326.6
13	Michigan	312.8
14	Colorado	307.8
15	Oklahoma	303.7
16	Wisconsin	303.6
17	California	301.0
18	Maryland	295.3
19	Arizona	279.6
20	Rhode Island	277.8
21	North Carolina	274.6
22	Tennessee	273.5
23	Arkansas	272.3
24	Virginia	259.1
25	Indiana	250.9
26	Missouri	249.3
27	New York	244.5
28	Nevada	241.8
29	South Dakota	241.2
30	Florida	235.4
31	Washington	231.3
32	Pennsylvania	231.0
33	Connecticut	226.6
34	Kansas	225.0
35	Kentucky	219.7
36	Oregon	217.9
37	Montana	212.7
38	Iowa	194.7
39	New Jersey	193.9
40	Nebraska	187.3
41	Wyoming	169.9
42	Minnesota	169.2
43	North Dakota	165.4
44	Massachusetts	163.8
45	Idaho	156.3
46	Utah	134.5
47	West Virginia	129.7
48	New Hampshire	111.9
49	Maine	104.9
50	Vermont	104.8
	District of Columbia	574.7

Source: U.S. Department of Health and Human Services, National Center for Health Statistics
"Sexually Transmitted Disease Surveillance 2001" (http://www.cdc.gov/std/stats/TOC2001.htm)
*Any of several common, often asymptomatic, sexually transmitted diseases caused by the microorganism Chlamydia trachomatis, including nonspecific urethritis in men.

Gonorrhea Cases Reported in 2001

National Total = 361,705 Cases*

ALPHA ORDER

RANK	STATE	CASES	% of USA
12	Alabama	11,182	3.1%
41	Alaska	457	0.1%
24	Arizona	3,920	1.1%
23	Arkansas	4,604	1.3%
3	California	23,296	6.4%
27	Colorado	3,190	0.9%
31	Connecticut	2,546	0.7%
33	Delaware	1,733	0.5%
5	Florida	21,531	6.0%
7	Georgia	18,920	5.2%
40	Hawaii	604	0.2%
48	Idaho	76	0.0%
2	Illinois	24,025	6.6%
20	Indiana	6,972	1.9%
34	Iowa	1,418	0.4%
30	Kansas	2,669	0.7%
25	Kentucky	3,588	1.0%
11	Louisiana	12,253	3.4%
45	Maine	141	0.0%
16	Maryland	9,427	2.6%
26	Massachusetts	3,214	0.9%
8	Michigan	17,120	4.7%
29	Minnesota	2,701	0.7%
19	Mississippi	7,759	2.1%
18	Missouri	8,723	2.4%
46	Montana	104	0.0%
35	Nebraska	1,189	0.3%
32	Nevada	1,756	0.5%
44	New Hampshire	176	0.0%
17	New Jersey	8,921	2.5%
37	New Mexico	1,040	0.3%
4	New York	22,299	6.2%
9	North Carolina	16,583	4.6%
50	North Dakota	56	0.0%
6	Ohio	21,163	5.9%
22	Oklahoma	4,784	1.3%
36	Oregon	1,144	0.3%
10	Pennsylvania	14,244	3.9%
38	Rhode Island	830	0.2%
14	South Carolina	10,805	3.0%
42	South Dakota	289	0.1%
15	Tennessee	10,145	2.8%
1	Texas	30,024	8.3%
43	Utah	219	0.1%
48	Vermont	76	0.0%
13	Virginia	11,095	3.1%
28	Washington	2,991	0.8%
39	West Virginia	732	0.2%
21	Wisconsin	6,011	1.7%
47	Wyoming	77	0.0%

RANK ORDER

RANK	STATE	CASES	% of USA
1	Texas	30,024	8.3%
2	Illinois	24,025	6.6%
3	California	23,296	6.4%
4	New York	22,299	6.2%
5	Florida	21,531	6.0%
6	Ohio	21,163	5.9%
7	Georgia	18,920	5.2%
8	Michigan	17,120	4.7%
9	North Carolina	16,583	4.6%
10	Pennsylvania	14,244	3.9%
11	Louisiana	12,253	3.4%
12	Alabama	11,182	3.1%
13	Virginia	11,095	3.1%
14	South Carolina	10,805	3.0%
15	Tennessee	10,145	2.8%
16	Maryland	9,427	2.6%
17	New Jersey	8,921	2.5%
18	Missouri	8,723	2.4%
19	Mississippi	7,759	2.1%
20	Indiana	6,972	1.9%
21	Wisconsin	6,011	1.7%
22	Oklahoma	4,784	1.3%
23	Arkansas	4,604	1.3%
24	Arizona	3,920	1.1%
25	Kentucky	3,588	1.0%
26	Massachusetts	3,214	0.9%
27	Colorado	3,190	0.9%
28	Washington	2,991	0.8%
29	Minnesota	2,701	0.7%
30	Kansas	2,669	0.7%
31	Connecticut	2,546	0.7%
32	Nevada	1,756	0.5%
33	Delaware	1,733	0.5%
34	Iowa	1,418	0.4%
35	Nebraska	1,189	0.3%
36	Oregon	1,144	0.3%
37	New Mexico	1,040	0.3%
38	Rhode Island	830	0.2%
39	West Virginia	732	0.2%
40	Hawaii	604	0.2%
41	Alaska	457	0.1%
42	South Dakota	289	0.1%
43	Utah	219	0.1%
44	New Hampshire	176	0.0%
45	Maine	141	0.0%
46	Montana	104	0.0%
47	Wyoming	77	0.0%
48	Idaho	76	0.0%
48	Vermont	76	0.0%
50	North Dakota	56	0.0%
	District of Columbia	2,883	0.8%

Source: U.S. Department of Health and Human Services, National Center for Health Statistics
    "Sexually Transmitted Disease Surveillance 2001" (http://www.cdc.gov/std/stats/TOC2001.htm)
*Gonorrhea is a sexually transmitted disease caused by gonococcal bacteria that affects the mucous membrane chiefly of the genital and urinary tracts and is characterized by an acute purulent discharge and painful or difficult urination, though women often have no symptoms.

Gonorrhea Rate in 2001

National Rate = 128.5 Cases per 100,000 Population*

RANK	STATE	RATE
4	Alabama	251.4
31	Alaska	72.9
28	Arizona	76.4
13	Arkansas	172.2
33	California	68.8
30	Colorado	74.2
29	Connecticut	74.8
6	Delaware	221.2
18	Florida	134.7
5	Georgia	231.1
38	Hawaii	49.9
50	Idaho	5.9
8	Illinois	193.4
21	Indiana	114.7
39	Iowa	48.5
24	Kansas	99.3
25	Kentucky	88.8
1	Louisiana	274.2
47	Maine	11.1
11	Maryland	178.0
37	Massachusetts	50.6
12	Michigan	172.3
35	Minnesota	54.9
2	Mississippi	272.8
15	Missouri	155.9
46	Montana	11.5
32	Nebraska	69.5
26	Nevada	87.9
44	New Hampshire	14.2
23	New Jersey	106.0
34	New Mexico	57.2
19	New York	117.5
7	North Carolina	206.0
49	North Dakota	8.7
9	Ohio	186.4
17	Oklahoma	138.6
42	Oregon	33.4
20	Pennsylvania	116.0
27	Rhode Island	79.2
3	South Carolina	269.3
41	South Dakota	38.3
10	Tennessee	178.3
16	Texas	144.0
48	Utah	9.8
45	Vermont	12.5
14	Virginia	156.7
36	Washington	50.7
40	West Virginia	40.5
22	Wisconsin	112.1
43	Wyoming	15.6

RANK	STATE	RATE
1	Louisiana	274.2
2	Mississippi	272.8
3	South Carolina	269.3
4	Alabama	251.4
5	Georgia	231.1
6	Delaware	221.2
7	North Carolina	206.0
8	Illinois	193.4
9	Ohio	186.4
10	Tennessee	178.3
11	Maryland	178.0
12	Michigan	172.3
13	Arkansas	172.2
14	Virginia	156.7
15	Missouri	155.9
16	Texas	144.0
17	Oklahoma	138.6
18	Florida	134.7
19	New York	117.5
20	Pennsylvania	116.0
21	Indiana	114.7
22	Wisconsin	112.1
23	New Jersey	106.0
24	Kansas	99.3
25	Kentucky	88.8
26	Nevada	87.9
27	Rhode Island	79.2
28	Arizona	76.4
29	Connecticut	74.8
30	Colorado	74.2
31	Alaska	72.9
32	Nebraska	69.5
33	California	68.8
34	New Mexico	57.2
35	Minnesota	54.9
36	Washington	50.7
37	Massachusetts	50.6
38	Hawaii	49.9
39	Iowa	48.5
40	West Virginia	40.5
41	South Dakota	38.3
42	Oregon	33.4
43	Wyoming	15.6
44	New Hampshire	14.2
45	Vermont	12.5
46	Montana	11.5
47	Maine	11.1
48	Utah	9.8
49	North Dakota	8.7
50	Idaho	5.9

| | District of Columbia | 504.2 |

Source: U.S. Department of Health and Human Services, National Center for Health Statistics
"Sexually Transmitted Disease Surveillance 2001" (http://www.cdc.gov/std/stats/TOC2001.htm)
*Gonorrhea is a sexually transmitted disease caused by gonococcal bacteria that affects the mucous membrane chiefly of the genital and urinary tracts and is characterized by an acute purulent discharge and painful or difficult urination, though women often have no symptoms.

Syphilis Cases Reported in 2001

National Total = 6,103 Cases*

ALPHA ORDER

RANK	STATE	CASES	% of USA
15	Alabama	142	2.3%
48	Alaska	0	0.0%
12	Arizona	180	2.9%
23	Arkansas	49	0.8%
1	California	545	8.9%
29	Colorado	23	0.4%
34	Connecticut	12	0.2%
32	Delaware	14	0.2%
2	Florida	484	7.9%
6	Georgia	414	6.8%
34	Hawaii	12	0.2%
43	Idaho	1	0.0%
7	Illinois	409	6.7%
14	Indiana	151	2.5%
40	Iowa	5	0.1%
28	Kansas	25	0.4%
24	Kentucky	48	0.8%
13	Louisiana	173	2.8%
43	Maine	1	0.0%
10	Maryland	266	4.4%
25	Massachusetts	46	0.8%
5	Michigan	428	7.0%
26	Minnesota	33	0.5%
16	Mississippi	140	2.3%
27	Missouri	26	0.4%
48	Montana	0	0.0%
37	Nebraska	10	0.2%
39	Nevada	8	0.1%
43	New Hampshire	1	0.0%
17	New Jersey	137	2.2%
31	New Mexico	19	0.3%
9	New York	304	5.0%
4	North Carolina	445	7.3%
48	North Dakota	0	0.0%
20	Ohio	81	1.3%
21	Oklahoma	60	1.0%
33	Oregon	13	0.2%
19	Pennsylvania	100	1.6%
38	Rhode Island	9	0.1%
11	South Carolina	235	3.9%
43	South Dakota	1	0.0%
8	Tennessee	331	5.4%
3	Texas	478	7.8%
36	Utah	11	0.2%
42	Vermont	3	0.0%
18	Virginia	102	1.7%
22	Washington	57	0.9%
40	West Virginia	5	0.1%
30	Wisconsin	22	0.4%
43	Wyoming	1	0.0%

RANK ORDER

RANK	STATE	CASES	% of USA
1	California	545	8.9%
2	Florida	484	7.9%
3	Texas	478	7.8%
4	North Carolina	445	7.3%
5	Michigan	428	7.0%
6	Georgia	414	6.8%
7	Illinois	409	6.7%
8	Tennessee	331	5.4%
9	New York	304	5.0%
10	Maryland	266	4.4%
11	South Carolina	235	3.9%
12	Arizona	180	2.9%
13	Louisiana	173	2.8%
14	Indiana	151	2.5%
15	Alabama	142	2.3%
16	Mississippi	140	2.3%
17	New Jersey	137	2.2%
18	Virginia	102	1.7%
19	Pennsylvania	100	1.6%
20	Ohio	81	1.3%
21	Oklahoma	60	1.0%
22	Washington	57	0.9%
23	Arkansas	49	0.8%
24	Kentucky	48	0.8%
25	Massachusetts	46	0.8%
26	Minnesota	33	0.5%
27	Missouri	26	0.4%
28	Kansas	25	0.4%
29	Colorado	23	0.4%
30	Wisconsin	22	0.4%
31	New Mexico	19	0.3%
32	Delaware	14	0.2%
33	Oregon	13	0.2%
34	Connecticut	12	0.2%
34	Hawaii	12	0.2%
36	Utah	11	0.2%
37	Nebraska	10	0.2%
38	Rhode Island	9	0.1%
39	Nevada	8	0.1%
40	Iowa	5	0.1%
40	West Virginia	5	0.1%
42	Vermont	3	0.0%
43	Idaho	1	0.0%
43	Maine	1	0.0%
43	New Hampshire	1	0.0%
43	South Dakota	1	0.0%
43	Wyoming	1	0.0%
48	Alaska	0	0.0%
48	Montana	0	0.0%
48	North Dakota	0	0.0%
	District of Columbia	43	0.7%

*Source: U.S. Department of Health and Human Services, National Center for Health Statistics
"Sexually Transmitted Disease Surveillance 2001" (http://www.cdc.gov/std/stats/TOC2001.htm)*
Includes only primary and secondary cases. Does not include 26,118 cases in other stages. A chronic infectious disease caused by a spirochete (Treponema pallidum), either transmitted by direct contact, usually in sexual intercourse, or passed from mother to child in utero, and progressing through three stages characterized respectively by local formation of chancres, ulcerous skin eruptions, and systemic infection leading to general paresis.

Syphilis Rate in 2001

National Rate = 2.2 Cases per 100,000 Population*

ALPHA ORDER

RANK	STATE	RATE
11	Alabama	3.2
48	Alaska	0.0
9	Arizona	3.5
15	Arkansas	1.8
18	California	1.6
33	Colorado	0.5
37	Connecticut	0.4
15	Delaware	1.8
12	Florida	3.0
4	Georgia	5.1
23	Hawaii	1.0
44	Idaho	0.1
10	Illinois	3.3
13	Indiana	2.5
42	Iowa	0.2
26	Kansas	0.9
22	Kentucky	1.2
8	Louisiana	3.9
44	Maine	0.1
5	Maryland	5.0
29	Massachusetts	0.7
7	Michigan	4.3
29	Minnesota	0.7
6	Mississippi	4.9
33	Missouri	0.5
48	Montana	0.0
32	Nebraska	0.6
37	Nevada	0.4
44	New Hampshire	0.1
18	New Jersey	1.6
23	New Mexico	1.0
18	New York	1.6
3	North Carolina	5.5
48	North Dakota	0.0
29	Ohio	0.7
17	Oklahoma	1.7
37	Oregon	0.4
28	Pennsylvania	0.8
26	Rhode Island	0.9
1	South Carolina	5.9
44	South Dakota	0.1
2	Tennessee	5.8
14	Texas	2.3
33	Utah	0.5
33	Vermont	0.5
21	Virginia	1.4
23	Washington	1.0
41	West Virginia	0.3
37	Wisconsin	0.4
42	Wyoming	0.2

RANK ORDER

RANK	STATE	RATE
1	South Carolina	5.9
2	Tennessee	5.8
3	North Carolina	5.5
4	Georgia	5.1
5	Maryland	5.0
6	Mississippi	4.9
7	Michigan	4.3
8	Louisiana	3.9
9	Arizona	3.5
10	Illinois	3.3
11	Alabama	3.2
12	Florida	3.0
13	Indiana	2.5
14	Texas	2.3
15	Arkansas	1.8
15	Delaware	1.8
17	Oklahoma	1.7
18	California	1.6
18	New Jersey	1.6
18	New York	1.6
21	Virginia	1.4
22	Kentucky	1.2
23	Hawaii	1.0
23	New Mexico	1.0
23	Washington	1.0
26	Kansas	0.9
26	Rhode Island	0.9
28	Pennsylvania	0.8
29	Massachusetts	0.7
29	Minnesota	0.7
29	Ohio	0.7
32	Nebraska	0.6
33	Colorado	0.5
33	Missouri	0.5
33	Utah	0.5
33	Vermont	0.5
37	Connecticut	0.4
37	Nevada	0.4
37	Oregon	0.4
37	Wisconsin	0.4
41	West Virginia	0.3
42	Iowa	0.2
42	Wyoming	0.2
44	Idaho	0.1
44	Maine	0.1
44	New Hampshire	0.1
44	South Dakota	0.1
48	Alaska	0.0
48	Montana	0.0
48	North Dakota	0.0
	District of Columbia	7.5

*Source: U.S. Department of Health and Human Services, National Center for Health Statistics
    "Sexually Transmitted Disease Surveillance 2001" (http://www.cdc.gov/std/stats/TOC2001.htm)*
*Includes only primary and secondary cases. Does not include 26,118 cases in other stages. A chronic infectious disease caused by a spirochete (Treponema pallidum), either transmitted by direct contact, usually in sexual intercourse, or passed from mother to child in utero, and progressing through three stages characterized respectively by local formation of chancres, ulcerous skin eruptions, and systemic infection leading to general paresis.

VI. PROVIDERS

VI. PROVIDERS (continued)

Physicians in 2001

National Total = 820,924 Physicians*

ALPHA ORDER

RANK	STATE	PHYSICIANS	% of USA
25	Alabama	10,009	1.2%
49	Alaska	1,414	0.2%
22	Arizona	12,660	1.5%
32	Arkansas	5,857	0.7%
1	California	99,567	12.1%
24	Colorado	12,095	1.5%
21	Connecticut	13,657	1.7%
46	Delaware	2,153	0.3%
4	Florida	47,305	5.8%
14	Georgia	19,839	2.4%
39	Hawaii	4,044	0.5%
43	Idaho	2,448	0.3%
6	Illinois	36,361	4.4%
20	Indiana	13,895	1.7%
31	Iowa	6,041	0.7%
30	Kansas	6,534	0.8%
28	Kentucky	9,678	1.2%
23	Louisiana	12,439	1.5%
41	Maine	3,708	0.5%
11	Maryland	23,858	2.9%
8	Massachusetts	29,338	3.6%
10	Michigan	25,710	3.1%
17	Minnesota	14,752	1.8%
33	Mississippi	5,544	0.7%
19	Missouri	14,350	1.7%
45	Montana	2,292	0.3%
37	Nebraska	4,399	0.5%
38	Nevada	4,281	0.5%
42	New Hampshire	3,609	0.4%
9	New Jersey	28,179	3.4%
35	New Mexico	4,678	0.6%
2	New York	79,541	9.7%
12	North Carolina	21,900	2.7%
48	North Dakota	1,602	0.2%
7	Ohio	30,880	3.8%
29	Oklahoma	6,572	0.8%
27	Oregon	9,749	1.2%
5	Pennsylvania	40,065	4.9%
40	Rhode Island	3,942	0.5%
26	South Carolina	9,940	1.2%
47	South Dakota	1,755	0.2%
16	Tennessee	15,695	1.9%
3	Texas	48,343	5.9%
34	Utah	5,165	0.6%
44	Vermont	2,403	0.3%
13	Virginia	20,881	2.5%
15	Washington	17,404	2.1%
36	West Virginia	4,499	0.5%
18	Wisconsin	14,375	1.8%
50	Wyoming	1,029	0.1%

RANK ORDER

RANK	STATE	PHYSICIANS	% of USA
1	California	99,567	12.1%
2	New York	79,541	9.7%
3	Texas	48,343	5.9%
4	Florida	47,305	5.8%
5	Pennsylvania	40,065	4.9%
6	Illinois	36,361	4.4%
7	Ohio	30,880	3.8%
8	Massachusetts	29,338	3.6%
9	New Jersey	28,179	3.4%
10	Michigan	25,710	3.1%
11	Maryland	23,858	2.9%
12	North Carolina	21,900	2.7%
13	Virginia	20,881	2.5%
14	Georgia	19,839	2.4%
15	Washington	17,404	2.1%
16	Tennessee	15,695	1.9%
17	Minnesota	14,752	1.8%
18	Wisconsin	14,375	1.8%
19	Missouri	14,350	1.7%
20	Indiana	13,895	1.7%
21	Connecticut	13,657	1.7%
22	Arizona	12,660	1.5%
23	Louisiana	12,439	1.5%
24	Colorado	12,095	1.5%
25	Alabama	10,009	1.2%
26	South Carolina	9,940	1.2%
27	Oregon	9,749	1.2%
28	Kentucky	9,678	1.2%
29	Oklahoma	6,572	0.8%
30	Kansas	6,534	0.8%
31	Iowa	6,041	0.7%
32	Arkansas	5,857	0.7%
33	Mississippi	5,544	0.7%
34	Utah	5,165	0.6%
35	New Mexico	4,678	0.6%
36	West Virginia	4,499	0.5%
37	Nebraska	4,399	0.5%
38	Nevada	4,281	0.5%
39	Hawaii	4,044	0.5%
40	Rhode Island	3,942	0.5%
41	Maine	3,708	0.5%
42	New Hampshire	3,609	0.4%
43	Idaho	2,448	0.3%
44	Vermont	2,403	0.3%
45	Montana	2,292	0.3%
46	Delaware	2,153	0.3%
47	South Dakota	1,755	0.2%
48	North Dakota	1,602	0.2%
49	Alaska	1,414	0.2%
50	Wyoming	1,029	0.1%
	District of Columbia	4,490	0.5%

Source: American Medical Association (Chicago, Illinois)
"Physician Characteristics and Distribution in the U.S." (2003-2004 Edition)
As of December 31, 2001. Comprised of federal and nonfederal physicians. Total does not include 15,232
physicians in the U.S. territories and possessions, at APO's and FPO's and whose addresses are unknown.

Male Physicians in 2001

National Total = 619,126 Physicians*

<table>
<tr><td colspan="4">ALPHA ORDER</td><td colspan="4">RANK ORDER</td></tr>
<tr><td>RANK</td><td>STATE</td><td>PHYSICIANS</td><td>% of USA</td><td>RANK</td><td>STATE</td><td>PHYSICIANS</td><td>% of USA</td></tr>
<tr><td>25</td><td>Alabama</td><td>8,113</td><td>1.3%</td><td>1</td><td>California</td><td>74,937</td><td>12.1%</td></tr>
<tr><td>49</td><td>Alaska</td><td>1,022</td><td>0.2%</td><td>2</td><td>New York</td><td>56,663</td><td>9.2%</td></tr>
<tr><td>22</td><td>Arizona</td><td>9,879</td><td>1.6%</td><td>3</td><td>Florida</td><td>38,604</td><td>6.2%</td></tr>
<tr><td>32</td><td>Arkansas</td><td>4,778</td><td>0.8%</td><td>4</td><td>Texas</td><td>37,061</td><td>6.0%</td></tr>
<tr><td>1</td><td>California</td><td>74,937</td><td>12.1%</td><td>5</td><td>Pennsylvania</td><td>29,911</td><td>4.8%</td></tr>
<tr><td>24</td><td>Colorado</td><td>9,016</td><td>1.5%</td><td>6</td><td>Illinois</td><td>26,012</td><td>4.2%</td></tr>
<tr><td>21</td><td>Connecticut</td><td>10,114</td><td>1.6%</td><td>7</td><td>Ohio</td><td>23,169</td><td>3.7%</td></tr>
<tr><td>46</td><td>Delaware</td><td>1,596</td><td>0.3%</td><td>8</td><td>Massachusetts</td><td>20,456</td><td>3.3%</td></tr>
<tr><td>3</td><td>Florida</td><td>38,604</td><td>6.2%</td><td>9</td><td>New Jersey</td><td>20,219</td><td>3.3%</td></tr>
<tr><td>14</td><td>Georgia</td><td>15,319</td><td>2.5%</td><td>10</td><td>Michigan</td><td>19,017</td><td>3.1%</td></tr>
<tr><td>39</td><td>Hawaii</td><td>3,089</td><td>0.5%</td><td>11</td><td>Maryland</td><td>16,920</td><td>2.7%</td></tr>
<tr><td>43</td><td>Idaho</td><td>2,074</td><td>0.3%</td><td>12</td><td>North Carolina</td><td>16,826</td><td>2.7%</td></tr>
<tr><td>6</td><td>Illinois</td><td>26,012</td><td>4.2%</td><td>13</td><td>Virginia</td><td>15,552</td><td>2.5%</td></tr>
<tr><td>20</td><td>Indiana</td><td>10,869</td><td>1.8%</td><td>14</td><td>Georgia</td><td>15,319</td><td>2.5%</td></tr>
<tr><td>31</td><td>Iowa</td><td>4,830</td><td>0.8%</td><td>15</td><td>Washington</td><td>13,128</td><td>2.1%</td></tr>
<tr><td>30</td><td>Kansas</td><td>5,103</td><td>0.8%</td><td>16</td><td>Tennessee</td><td>12,500</td><td>2.0%</td></tr>
<tr><td>27</td><td>Kentucky</td><td>7,579</td><td>1.2%</td><td>17</td><td>Minnesota</td><td>11,051</td><td>1.8%</td></tr>
<tr><td>23</td><td>Louisiana</td><td>9,677</td><td>1.6%</td><td>18</td><td>Wisconsin</td><td>11,024</td><td>1.8%</td></tr>
<tr><td>40</td><td>Maine</td><td>2,834</td><td>0.5%</td><td>19</td><td>Missouri</td><td>10,927</td><td>1.8%</td></tr>
<tr><td>11</td><td>Maryland</td><td>16,920</td><td>2.7%</td><td>20</td><td>Indiana</td><td>10,869</td><td>1.8%</td></tr>
<tr><td>8</td><td>Massachusetts</td><td>20,456</td><td>3.3%</td><td>21</td><td>Connecticut</td><td>10,114</td><td>1.6%</td></tr>
<tr><td>10</td><td>Michigan</td><td>19,017</td><td>3.1%</td><td>22</td><td>Arizona</td><td>9,879</td><td>1.6%</td></tr>
<tr><td>17</td><td>Minnesota</td><td>11,051</td><td>1.8%</td><td>23</td><td>Louisiana</td><td>9,677</td><td>1.6%</td></tr>
<tr><td>33</td><td>Mississippi</td><td>4,541</td><td>0.7%</td><td>24</td><td>Colorado</td><td>9,016</td><td>1.5%</td></tr>
<tr><td>19</td><td>Missouri</td><td>10,927</td><td>1.8%</td><td>25</td><td>Alabama</td><td>8,113</td><td>1.3%</td></tr>
<tr><td>44</td><td>Montana</td><td>1,893</td><td>0.3%</td><td>26</td><td>South Carolina</td><td>7,952</td><td>1.3%</td></tr>
<tr><td>36</td><td>Nebraska</td><td>3,490</td><td>0.6%</td><td>27</td><td>Kentucky</td><td>7,579</td><td>1.2%</td></tr>
<tr><td>37</td><td>Nevada</td><td>3,458</td><td>0.6%</td><td>28</td><td>Oregon</td><td>7,417</td><td>1.2%</td></tr>
<tr><td>42</td><td>New Hampshire</td><td>2,790</td><td>0.5%</td><td>29</td><td>Oklahoma</td><td>5,291</td><td>0.9%</td></tr>
<tr><td>9</td><td>New Jersey</td><td>20,219</td><td>3.3%</td><td>30</td><td>Kansas</td><td>5,103</td><td>0.8%</td></tr>
<tr><td>38</td><td>New Mexico</td><td>3,354</td><td>0.5%</td><td>31</td><td>Iowa</td><td>4,830</td><td>0.8%</td></tr>
<tr><td>2</td><td>New York</td><td>56,663</td><td>9.2%</td><td>32</td><td>Arkansas</td><td>4,778</td><td>0.8%</td></tr>
<tr><td>12</td><td>North Carolina</td><td>16,826</td><td>2.7%</td><td>33</td><td>Mississippi</td><td>4,541</td><td>0.7%</td></tr>
<tr><td>48</td><td>North Dakota</td><td>1,312</td><td>0.2%</td><td>34</td><td>Utah</td><td>4,261</td><td>0.7%</td></tr>
<tr><td>7</td><td>Ohio</td><td>23,169</td><td>3.7%</td><td>35</td><td>West Virginia</td><td>3,569</td><td>0.6%</td></tr>
<tr><td>29</td><td>Oklahoma</td><td>5,291</td><td>0.9%</td><td>36</td><td>Nebraska</td><td>3,490</td><td>0.6%</td></tr>
<tr><td>28</td><td>Oregon</td><td>7,417</td><td>1.2%</td><td>37</td><td>Nevada</td><td>3,458</td><td>0.6%</td></tr>
<tr><td>5</td><td>Pennsylvania</td><td>29,911</td><td>4.8%</td><td>38</td><td>New Mexico</td><td>3,354</td><td>0.5%</td></tr>
<tr><td>41</td><td>Rhode Island</td><td>2,813</td><td>0.5%</td><td>39</td><td>Hawaii</td><td>3,089</td><td>0.5%</td></tr>
<tr><td>26</td><td>South Carolina</td><td>7,952</td><td>1.3%</td><td>40</td><td>Maine</td><td>2,834</td><td>0.5%</td></tr>
<tr><td>47</td><td>South Dakota</td><td>1,440</td><td>0.2%</td><td>41</td><td>Rhode Island</td><td>2,813</td><td>0.5%</td></tr>
<tr><td>16</td><td>Tennessee</td><td>12,500</td><td>2.0%</td><td>42</td><td>New Hampshire</td><td>2,790</td><td>0.5%</td></tr>
<tr><td>4</td><td>Texas</td><td>37,061</td><td>6.0%</td><td>43</td><td>Idaho</td><td>2,074</td><td>0.3%</td></tr>
<tr><td>34</td><td>Utah</td><td>4,261</td><td>0.7%</td><td>44</td><td>Montana</td><td>1,893</td><td>0.3%</td></tr>
<tr><td>45</td><td>Vermont</td><td>1,754</td><td>0.3%</td><td>45</td><td>Vermont</td><td>1,754</td><td>0.3%</td></tr>
<tr><td>13</td><td>Virginia</td><td>15,552</td><td>2.5%</td><td>46</td><td>Delaware</td><td>1,596</td><td>0.3%</td></tr>
<tr><td>15</td><td>Washington</td><td>13,128</td><td>2.1%</td><td>47</td><td>South Dakota</td><td>1,440</td><td>0.2%</td></tr>
<tr><td>35</td><td>West Virginia</td><td>3,569</td><td>0.6%</td><td>48</td><td>North Dakota</td><td>1,312</td><td>0.2%</td></tr>
<tr><td>18</td><td>Wisconsin</td><td>11,024</td><td>1.8%</td><td>49</td><td>Alaska</td><td>1,022</td><td>0.2%</td></tr>
<tr><td>50</td><td>Wyoming</td><td>857</td><td>0.1%</td><td>50</td><td>Wyoming</td><td>857</td><td>0.1%</td></tr>
<tr><td></td><td></td><td></td><td></td><td colspan="2">District of Columbia</td><td>3,065</td><td>0.5%</td></tr>
</table>

Source: American Medical Association (Chicago, Illinois)
   "Physician Characteristics and Distribution in the U.S." (2003-2004 Edition)
*As of December 31, 2001. Comprised of federal and nonfederal physicians. Total does not include 11,127 male physicians in the U.S. territories and possessions, at APO's and FPO's and whose addresses are unknown.

Female Physicians in 2001

National Total = 201,798 Physicians*

ALPHA ORDER

RANK	STATE	PHYSICIANS	% of USA
28	Alabama	1,896	0.9%
46	Alaska	392	0.2%
23	Arizona	2,781	1.4%
34	Arkansas	1,079	0.5%
1	California	24,630	12.2%
21	Colorado	3,079	1.5%
17	Connecticut	3,543	1.8%
44	Delaware	557	0.3%
7	Florida	8,701	4.3%
14	Georgia	4,520	2.2%
36	Hawaii	955	0.5%
47	Idaho	374	0.2%
4	Illinois	10,349	5.1%
22	Indiana	3,026	1.5%
32	Iowa	1,211	0.6%
29	Kansas	1,431	0.7%
26	Kentucky	2,099	1.0%
24	Louisiana	2,762	1.4%
40	Maine	874	0.4%
10	Maryland	6,938	3.4%
6	Massachusetts	8,882	4.4%
11	Michigan	6,693	3.3%
16	Minnesota	3,701	1.8%
35	Mississippi	1,003	0.5%
18	Missouri	3,423	1.7%
45	Montana	399	0.2%
38	Nebraska	909	0.5%
41	Nevada	823	0.4%
42	New Hampshire	819	0.4%
8	New Jersey	7,960	3.9%
30	New Mexico	1,324	0.7%
2	New York	22,878	11.3%
13	North Carolina	5,074	2.5%
49	North Dakota	290	0.1%
9	Ohio	7,711	3.8%
31	Oklahoma	1,281	0.6%
25	Oregon	2,332	1.2%
5	Pennsylvania	10,154	5.0%
33	Rhode Island	1,129	0.6%
27	South Carolina	1,988	1.0%
48	South Dakota	315	0.2%
20	Tennessee	3,195	1.6%
3	Texas	11,282	5.6%
39	Utah	904	0.4%
43	Vermont	649	0.3%
12	Virginia	5,329	2.6%
15	Washington	4,276	2.1%
37	West Virginia	930	0.5%
19	Wisconsin	3,351	1.7%
50	Wyoming	172	0.1%

RANK ORDER

RANK	STATE	PHYSICIANS	% of USA
1	California	24,630	12.2%
2	New York	22,878	11.3%
3	Texas	11,282	5.6%
4	Illinois	10,349	5.1%
5	Pennsylvania	10,154	5.0%
6	Massachusetts	8,882	4.4%
7	Florida	8,701	4.3%
8	New Jersey	7,960	3.9%
9	Ohio	7,711	3.8%
10	Maryland	6,938	3.4%
11	Michigan	6,693	3.3%
12	Virginia	5,329	2.6%
13	North Carolina	5,074	2.5%
14	Georgia	4,520	2.2%
15	Washington	4,276	2.1%
16	Minnesota	3,701	1.8%
17	Connecticut	3,543	1.8%
18	Missouri	3,423	1.7%
19	Wisconsin	3,351	1.7%
20	Tennessee	3,195	1.6%
21	Colorado	3,079	1.5%
22	Indiana	3,026	1.5%
23	Arizona	2,781	1.4%
24	Louisiana	2,762	1.4%
25	Oregon	2,332	1.2%
26	Kentucky	2,099	1.0%
27	South Carolina	1,988	1.0%
28	Alabama	1,896	0.9%
29	Kansas	1,431	0.7%
30	New Mexico	1,324	0.7%
31	Oklahoma	1,281	0.6%
32	Iowa	1,211	0.6%
33	Rhode Island	1,129	0.6%
34	Arkansas	1,079	0.5%
35	Mississippi	1,003	0.5%
36	Hawaii	955	0.5%
37	West Virginia	930	0.5%
38	Nebraska	909	0.5%
39	Utah	904	0.4%
40	Maine	874	0.4%
41	Nevada	823	0.4%
42	New Hampshire	819	0.4%
43	Vermont	649	0.3%
44	Delaware	557	0.3%
45	Montana	399	0.2%
46	Alaska	392	0.2%
47	Idaho	374	0.2%
48	South Dakota	315	0.2%
49	North Dakota	290	0.1%
50	Wyoming	172	0.1%
	District of Columbia	1,425	0.7%

Source: American Medical Association (Chicago, Illinois)
  "Physician Characteristics and Distribution in the U.S." (2003-2004 Edition)
*As of December 31, 2001. Comprised of federal and nonfederal physicians. Total does not include 4,105 female physicians in the U.S. territories and possessions, at APO's and FPO's and whose addresses are unknown.

Percent of Physicians Who Are Female: 2001

National Percent = 24.6% of Physicians*

ALPHA ORDER

ALPHA ORDER

RANK	STATE	PERCENT
41	Alabama	18.9
8	Alaska	27.7
30	Arizona	22.0
42	Arkansas	18.4
18	California	24.7
13	Colorado	25.5
11	Connecticut	25.9
11	Delaware	25.9
42	Florida	18.4
27	Georgia	22.8
22	Hawaii	23.6
50	Idaho	15.3
5	Illinois	28.5
32	Indiana	21.8
37	Iowa	20.0
31	Kansas	21.9
33	Kentucky	21.7
29	Louisiana	22.2
22	Maine	23.6
2	Maryland	29.1
1	Massachusetts	30.3
10	Michigan	26.0
16	Minnesota	25.1
44	Mississippi	18.1
20	Missouri	23.9
48	Montana	17.4
34	Nebraska	20.7
40	Nevada	19.2
28	New Hampshire	22.7
7	New Jersey	28.2
6	New Mexico	28.3
3	New York	28.8
26	North Carolina	23.2
44	North Dakota	18.1
17	Ohio	25.0
39	Oklahoma	19.5
20	Oregon	23.9
15	Pennsylvania	25.3
4	Rhode Island	28.6
37	South Carolina	20.0
46	South Dakota	17.9
36	Tennessee	20.4
24	Texas	23.3
47	Utah	17.5
9	Vermont	27.0
13	Virginia	25.5
19	Washington	24.6
34	West Virginia	20.7
24	Wisconsin	23.3
49	Wyoming	16.7

RANK ORDER

RANK	STATE	PERCENT
1	Massachusetts	30.3
2	Maryland	29.1
3	New York	28.8
4	Rhode Island	28.6
5	Illinois	28.5
6	New Mexico	28.3
7	New Jersey	28.2
8	Alaska	27.7
9	Vermont	27.0
10	Michigan	26.0
11	Connecticut	25.9
11	Delaware	25.9
13	Colorado	25.5
13	Virginia	25.5
15	Pennsylvania	25.3
16	Minnesota	25.1
17	Ohio	25.0
18	California	24.7
19	Washington	24.6
20	Missouri	23.9
20	Oregon	23.9
22	Hawaii	23.6
22	Maine	23.6
24	Texas	23.3
24	Wisconsin	23.3
26	North Carolina	23.2
27	Georgia	22.8
28	New Hampshire	22.7
29	Louisiana	22.2
30	Arizona	22.0
31	Kansas	21.9
32	Indiana	21.8
33	Kentucky	21.7
34	Nebraska	20.7
34	West Virginia	20.7
36	Tennessee	20.4
37	Iowa	20.0
37	South Carolina	20.0
39	Oklahoma	19.5
40	Nevada	19.2
41	Alabama	18.9
42	Arkansas	18.4
42	Florida	18.4
44	Mississippi	18.1
44	North Dakota	18.1
46	South Dakota	17.9
47	Utah	17.5
48	Montana	17.4
49	Wyoming	16.7
50	Idaho	15.3

| | District of Columbia | 31.7 |

Source: Morgan Quitno Press using data from American Medical Association (Chicago, Illinois)
    "Physician Characteristics and Distribution in the U.S." (2003-2004 Edition)
As of December 31, 2001. Comprised of federal and nonfederal physicians. National percent does not include physicians in the U.S. territories and possessions, at APO's and FPO's and whose addresses are unknown.

Physicians Under 35 Years Old in 2001

National Total = 136,691 Physicians*

ALPHA ORDER

RANK	STATE	PHYSICIANS	% of USA
26	Alabama	1,614	1.2%
49	Alaska	150	0.1%
24	Arizona	1,693	1.2%
31	Arkansas	956	0.7%
2	California	14,051	10.3%
23	Colorado	1,713	1.3%
19	Connecticut	2,317	1.7%
43	Delaware	369	0.3%
9	Florida	4,697	3.4%
14	Georgia	3,188	2.3%
39	Hawaii	526	0.4%
46	Idaho	197	0.1%
4	Illinois	7,660	5.6%
22	Indiana	2,200	1.6%
30	Iowa	1,004	0.7%
29	Kansas	1,020	0.7%
27	Kentucky	1,554	1.1%
18	Louisiana	2,512	1.8%
42	Maine	377	0.3%
12	Maryland	4,022	2.9%
7	Massachusetts	5,835	4.3%
8	Michigan	5,233	3.8%
16	Minnesota	2,657	1.9%
35	Mississippi	820	0.6%
15	Missouri	2,865	2.1%
48	Montana	163	0.1%
36	Nebraska	806	0.6%
41	Nevada	468	0.3%
40	New Hampshire	469	0.3%
10	New Jersey	4,225	3.1%
38	New Mexico	625	0.5%
1	New York	15,794	11.6%
11	North Carolina	4,027	2.9%
45	North Dakota	200	0.1%
6	Ohio	6,147	4.5%
32	Oklahoma	934	0.7%
28	Oregon	1,133	0.8%
5	Pennsylvania	7,316	5.4%
33	Rhode Island	850	0.6%
25	South Carolina	1,688	1.2%
47	South Dakota	179	0.1%
17	Tennessee	2,624	1.9%
3	Texas	8,819	6.5%
34	Utah	822	0.6%
44	Vermont	341	0.2%
13	Virginia	3,533	2.6%
20	Washington	2,251	1.6%
37	West Virginia	749	0.5%
21	Wisconsin	2,208	1.6%
50	Wyoming	95	0.1%

RANK ORDER

RANK	STATE	PHYSICIANS	% of USA
1	New York	15,794	11.6%
2	California	14,051	10.3%
3	Texas	8,819	6.5%
4	Illinois	7,660	5.6%
5	Pennsylvania	7,316	5.4%
6	Ohio	6,147	4.5%
7	Massachusetts	5,835	4.3%
8	Michigan	5,233	3.8%
9	Florida	4,697	3.4%
10	New Jersey	4,225	3.1%
11	North Carolina	4,027	2.9%
12	Maryland	4,022	2.9%
13	Virginia	3,533	2.6%
14	Georgia	3,188	2.3%
15	Missouri	2,865	2.1%
16	Minnesota	2,657	1.9%
17	Tennessee	2,624	1.9%
18	Louisiana	2,512	1.8%
19	Connecticut	2,317	1.7%
20	Washington	2,251	1.6%
21	Wisconsin	2,208	1.6%
22	Indiana	2,200	1.6%
23	Colorado	1,713	1.3%
24	Arizona	1,693	1.2%
25	South Carolina	1,688	1.2%
26	Alabama	1,614	1.2%
27	Kentucky	1,554	1.1%
28	Oregon	1,133	0.8%
29	Kansas	1,020	0.7%
30	Iowa	1,004	0.7%
31	Arkansas	956	0.7%
32	Oklahoma	934	0.7%
33	Rhode Island	850	0.6%
34	Utah	822	0.6%
35	Mississippi	820	0.6%
36	Nebraska	806	0.6%
37	West Virginia	749	0.5%
38	New Mexico	625	0.5%
39	Hawaii	526	0.4%
40	New Hampshire	469	0.3%
41	Nevada	468	0.3%
42	Maine	377	0.3%
43	Delaware	369	0.3%
44	Vermont	341	0.2%
45	North Dakota	200	0.1%
46	Idaho	197	0.1%
47	South Dakota	179	0.1%
48	Montana	163	0.1%
49	Alaska	150	0.1%
50	Wyoming	95	0.1%
	District of Columbia	995	0.7%

Source: American Medical Association (Chicago, Illinois)
    "Physician Characteristics and Distribution in the U.S." (2003-2004 Edition)
*As of December 31, 2001. Comprised of federal and nonfederal physicians. Total does not include 2,216
physicians in the U.S. territories and possessions, at APO's and FPO's and whose addresses are unknown.

Percent of Physicians Under 35 Years Old in 2001

National Percent = 16.7% of Physicians*

ALPHA ORDER

RANK	STATE	PERCENT
23	Alabama	16.1
44	Alaska	10.6
36	Arizona	13.4
22	Arkansas	16.3
35	California	14.1
32	Colorado	14.2
15	Connecticut	17.0
14	Delaware	17.1
47	Florida	9.9
23	Georgia	16.1
38	Hawaii	13.0
49	Idaho	8.0
2	Illinois	21.1
27	Indiana	15.8
20	Iowa	16.6
28	Kansas	15.6
23	Kentucky	16.1
4	Louisiana	20.2
45	Maine	10.2
17	Maryland	16.9
6	Massachusetts	19.9
3	Michigan	20.4
13	Minnesota	18.0
31	Mississippi	14.8
5	Missouri	20.0
50	Montana	7.1
10	Nebraska	18.3
43	Nevada	10.9
38	New Hampshire	13.0
30	New Jersey	15.0
36	New Mexico	13.4
6	New York	19.9
9	North Carolina	18.4
41	North Dakota	12.5
6	Ohio	19.9
32	Oklahoma	14.2
42	Oregon	11.6
10	Pennsylvania	18.3
1	Rhode Island	21.6
15	South Carolina	17.0
45	South Dakota	10.2
19	Tennessee	16.7
12	Texas	18.2
26	Utah	15.9
32	Vermont	14.2
17	Virginia	16.9
40	Washington	12.9
20	West Virginia	16.6
29	Wisconsin	15.4
48	Wyoming	9.2

RANK ORDER

RANK	STATE	PERCENT
1	Rhode Island	21.6
2	Illinois	21.1
3	Michigan	20.4
4	Louisiana	20.2
5	Missouri	20.0
6	Massachusetts	19.9
6	New York	19.9
6	Ohio	19.9
9	North Carolina	18.4
10	Nebraska	18.3
10	Pennsylvania	18.3
12	Texas	18.2
13	Minnesota	18.0
14	Delaware	17.1
15	Connecticut	17.0
15	South Carolina	17.0
17	Maryland	16.9
17	Virginia	16.9
19	Tennessee	16.7
20	Iowa	16.6
20	West Virginia	16.6
22	Arkansas	16.3
23	Alabama	16.1
23	Georgia	16.1
23	Kentucky	16.1
26	Utah	15.9
27	Indiana	15.8
28	Kansas	15.6
29	Wisconsin	15.4
30	New Jersey	15.0
31	Mississippi	14.8
32	Colorado	14.2
32	Oklahoma	14.2
32	Vermont	14.2
35	California	14.1
36	Arizona	13.4
36	New Mexico	13.4
38	Hawaii	13.0
38	New Hampshire	13.0
40	Washington	12.9
41	North Dakota	12.5
42	Oregon	11.6
43	Nevada	10.9
44	Alaska	10.6
45	Maine	10.2
45	South Dakota	10.2
47	Florida	9.9
48	Wyoming	9.2
49	Idaho	8.0
50	Montana	7.1

District of Columbia   22.2

Source: Morgan Quitno Press using data from American Medical Association (Chicago, Illinois)
"Physician Characteristics and Distribution in the U.S." (2003-2004 Edition)
*As of December 31, 2001. Comprised of federal and nonfederal physicians. National percent does not include physicians in the U.S. territories and possessions, at APO's and FPO's and whose addresses are unknown.

Physicians 35 to 44 Years Old in 2001

National Total = 207,272 Physicians*

ALPHA ORDER

RANK	STATE	PHYSICIANS	% of USA
26	Alabama	2,737	1.3%
49	Alaska	422	0.2%
24	Arizona	3,107	1.5%
33	Arkansas	1,452	0.7%
1	California	21,588	10.4%
23	Colorado	3,116	1.5%
21	Connecticut	3,295	1.6%
46	Delaware	564	0.3%
4	Florida	11,240	5.4%
13	Georgia	5,539	2.7%
40	Hawaii	976	0.5%
43	Idaho	649	0.3%
6	Illinois	9,267	4.5%
20	Indiana	3,776	1.8%
31	Iowa	1,535	0.7%
29	Kansas	1,629	0.8%
27	Kentucky	2,657	1.3%
22	Louisiana	3,152	1.5%
41	Maine	892	0.4%
12	Maryland	6,122	3.0%
8	Massachusetts	7,875	3.8%
10	Michigan	6,576	3.2%
18	Minnesota	4,030	1.9%
32	Mississippi	1,526	0.7%
19	Missouri	3,826	1.8%
45	Montana	570	0.3%
36	Nebraska	1,202	0.6%
35	Nevada	1,262	0.6%
42	New Hampshire	881	0.4%
9	New Jersey	7,112	3.4%
37	New Mexico	1,099	0.5%
2	New York	19,610	9.5%
11	North Carolina	6,208	3.0%
48	North Dakota	445	0.2%
7	Ohio	8,050	3.9%
30	Oklahoma	1,584	0.8%
28	Oregon	2,351	1.1%
5	Pennsylvania	9,897	4.8%
39	Rhode Island	1,014	0.5%
25	South Carolina	2,800	1.4%
47	South Dakota	505	0.2%
15	Tennessee	4,196	2.0%
3	Texas	13,150	6.3%
34	Utah	1,428	0.7%
44	Vermont	603	0.3%
14	Virginia	5,261	2.5%
16	Washington	4,194	2.0%
38	West Virginia	1,048	0.5%
17	Wisconsin	4,056	2.0%
50	Wyoming	244	0.1%

RANK ORDER

RANK	STATE	PHYSICIANS	% of USA
1	California	21,588	10.4%
2	New York	19,610	9.5%
3	Texas	13,150	6.3%
4	Florida	11,240	5.4%
5	Pennsylvania	9,897	4.8%
6	Illinois	9,267	4.5%
7	Ohio	8,050	3.9%
8	Massachusetts	7,875	3.8%
9	New Jersey	7,112	3.4%
10	Michigan	6,576	3.2%
11	North Carolina	6,208	3.0%
12	Maryland	6,122	3.0%
13	Georgia	5,539	2.7%
14	Virginia	5,261	2.5%
15	Tennessee	4,196	2.0%
16	Washington	4,194	2.0%
17	Wisconsin	4,056	2.0%
18	Minnesota	4,030	1.9%
19	Missouri	3,826	1.8%
20	Indiana	3,776	1.8%
21	Connecticut	3,295	1.6%
22	Louisiana	3,152	1.5%
23	Colorado	3,116	1.5%
24	Arizona	3,107	1.5%
25	South Carolina	2,800	1.4%
26	Alabama	2,737	1.3%
27	Kentucky	2,657	1.3%
28	Oregon	2,351	1.1%
29	Kansas	1,629	0.8%
30	Oklahoma	1,584	0.8%
31	Iowa	1,535	0.7%
32	Mississippi	1,526	0.7%
33	Arkansas	1,452	0.7%
34	Utah	1,428	0.7%
35	Nevada	1,262	0.6%
36	Nebraska	1,202	0.6%
37	New Mexico	1,099	0.5%
38	West Virginia	1,048	0.5%
39	Rhode Island	1,014	0.5%
40	Hawaii	976	0.5%
41	Maine	892	0.4%
42	New Hampshire	881	0.4%
43	Idaho	649	0.3%
44	Vermont	603	0.3%
45	Montana	570	0.3%
46	Delaware	564	0.3%
47	South Dakota	505	0.2%
48	North Dakota	445	0.2%
49	Alaska	422	0.2%
50	Wyoming	244	0.1%
	District of Columbia	954	0.5%

Source: American Medical Association (Chicago, Illinois)
    "Physician Characteristics and Distribution in the U.S." (2003-2004 Edition)
*As of December 31, 2001. Comprised of federal and nonfederal physicians. Total does not include 4,078 physicians in the U.S. territories and possessions, at APO's and FPO's and whose addresses are unknown.

Physicians 45 to 54 Years Old in 2001

National Total = 204,781 Physicians*

ALPHA ORDER

ALPHA ORDER

RANK	STATE	PHYSICIANS	% of USA
26	Alabama	2,655	1.3%
49	Alaska	404	0.2%
24	Arizona	3,058	1.5%
31	Arkansas	1,605	0.8%
1	California	24,863	12.1%
22	Colorado	3,232	1.6%
21	Connecticut	3,505	1.7%
47	Delaware	463	0.2%
4	Florida	11,671	5.7%
13	Georgia	5,269	2.6%
38	Hawaii	1,073	0.5%
43	Idaho	677	0.3%
6	Illinois	8,457	4.1%
19	Indiana	3,646	1.8%
32	Iowa	1,603	0.8%
30	Kansas	1,634	0.8%
27	Kentucky	2,586	1.3%
23	Louisiana	3,087	1.5%
39	Maine	1,039	0.5%
11	Maryland	5,931	2.9%
9	Massachusetts	6,972	3.4%
10	Michigan	6,016	2.9%
17	Minnesota	3,854	1.9%
33	Mississippi	1,361	0.7%
20	Missouri	3,535	1.7%
44	Montana	647	0.3%
36	Nebraska	1,133	0.6%
40	Nevada	1,016	0.5%
41	New Hampshire	1,002	0.5%
7	New Jersey	7,369	3.6%
34	New Mexico	1,325	0.6%
2	New York	18,385	9.0%
12	North Carolina	5,416	2.6%
48	North Dakota	462	0.2%
8	Ohio	7,262	3.5%
29	Oklahoma	1,792	0.9%
25	Oregon	2,684	1.3%
5	Pennsylvania	10,048	4.9%
42	Rhode Island	852	0.4%
28	South Carolina	2,442	1.2%
46	South Dakota	543	0.3%
16	Tennessee	4,317	2.1%
3	Texas	11,879	5.8%
34	Utah	1,325	0.6%
45	Vermont	621	0.3%
14	Virginia	5,161	2.5%
15	Washington	4,895	2.4%
37	West Virginia	1,092	0.5%
18	Wisconsin	3,716	1.8%
50	Wyoming	285	0.1%

RANK ORDER

RANK	STATE	PHYSICIANS	% of USA
1	California	24,863	12.1%
2	New York	18,385	9.0%
3	Texas	11,879	5.8%
4	Florida	11,671	5.7%
5	Pennsylvania	10,048	4.9%
6	Illinois	8,457	4.1%
7	New Jersey	7,369	3.6%
8	Ohio	7,262	3.5%
9	Massachusetts	6,972	3.4%
10	Michigan	6,016	2.9%
11	Maryland	5,931	2.9%
12	North Carolina	5,416	2.6%
13	Georgia	5,269	2.6%
14	Virginia	5,161	2.5%
15	Washington	4,895	2.4%
16	Tennessee	4,317	2.1%
17	Minnesota	3,854	1.9%
18	Wisconsin	3,716	1.8%
19	Indiana	3,646	1.8%
20	Missouri	3,535	1.7%
21	Connecticut	3,505	1.7%
22	Colorado	3,232	1.6%
23	Louisiana	3,087	1.5%
24	Arizona	3,058	1.5%
25	Oregon	2,684	1.3%
26	Alabama	2,655	1.3%
27	Kentucky	2,586	1.3%
28	South Carolina	2,442	1.2%
29	Oklahoma	1,792	0.9%
30	Kansas	1,634	0.8%
31	Arkansas	1,605	0.8%
32	Iowa	1,603	0.8%
33	Mississippi	1,361	0.7%
34	New Mexico	1,325	0.6%
34	Utah	1,325	0.6%
36	Nebraska	1,133	0.6%
37	West Virginia	1,092	0.5%
38	Hawaii	1,073	0.5%
39	Maine	1,039	0.5%
40	Nevada	1,016	0.5%
41	New Hampshire	1,002	0.5%
42	Rhode Island	852	0.4%
43	Idaho	677	0.3%
44	Montana	647	0.3%
45	Vermont	621	0.3%
46	South Dakota	543	0.3%
47	Delaware	463	0.2%
48	North Dakota	462	0.2%
49	Alaska	404	0.2%
50	Wyoming	285	0.1%
	District of Columbia	916	0.4%

Source: American Medical Association (Chicago, Illinois)
   "Physician Characteristics and Distribution in the U.S." (2003-2004 Edition)
*As of December 31, 2001. Comprised of federal and nonfederal physicians. Total does not include 3,674 physicians in the U.S. territories and possessions, at APO's and FPO's and whose addresses are unknown.

Physicians 55 to 64 Years Old in 2001

National Total = 124,182 Physicians*

ALPHA ORDER

RANK	STATE	PHYSICIANS	% of USA
26	Alabama	1,492	1.2%
47	Alaska	274	0.2%
20	Arizona	1,953	1.6%
33	Arkansas	836	0.7%
1	California	17,470	14.1%
22	Colorado	1,918	1.5%
18	Connecticut	2,010	1.6%
45	Delaware	356	0.3%
3	Florida	7,371	5.9%
13	Georgia	2,846	2.3%
38	Hawaii	668	0.5%
43	Idaho	432	0.3%
6	Illinois	5,621	4.5%
21	Indiana	1,932	1.6%
32	Iowa	848	0.7%
30	Kansas	995	0.8%
27	Kentucky	1,425	1.1%
24	Louisiana	1,770	1.4%
39	Maine	600	0.5%
10	Maryland	3,800	3.1%
9	Massachusetts	4,064	3.3%
11	Michigan	3,717	3.0%
23	Minnesota	1,909	1.5%
34	Mississippi	829	0.7%
17	Missouri	2,050	1.7%
44	Montana	427	0.3%
40	Nebraska	553	0.4%
37	Nevada	671	0.5%
42	New Hampshire	499	0.4%
7	New Jersey	4,626	3.7%
35	New Mexico	826	0.7%
2	New York	11,483	9.2%
15	North Carolina	2,753	2.2%
48	North Dakota	247	0.2%
8	Ohio	4,299	3.5%
29	Oklahoma	1,042	0.8%
25	Oregon	1,671	1.3%
5	Pennsylvania	5,628	4.5%
41	Rhode Island	515	0.4%
28	South Carolina	1,359	1.1%
49	South Dakota	246	0.2%
16	Tennessee	2,147	1.7%
4	Texas	7,029	5.7%
36	Utah	782	0.6%
46	Vermont	339	0.3%
12	Virginia	3,197	2.6%
14	Washington	2,808	2.3%
31	West Virginia	852	0.7%
19	Wisconsin	1,989	1.6%
50	Wyoming	200	0.2%

RANK ORDER

RANK	STATE	PHYSICIANS	% of USA
1	California	17,470	14.1%
2	New York	11,483	9.2%
3	Florida	7,371	5.9%
4	Texas	7,029	5.7%
5	Pennsylvania	5,628	4.5%
6	Illinois	5,621	4.5%
7	New Jersey	4,626	3.7%
8	Ohio	4,299	3.5%
9	Massachusetts	4,064	3.3%
10	Maryland	3,800	3.1%
11	Michigan	3,717	3.0%
12	Virginia	3,197	2.6%
13	Georgia	2,846	2.3%
14	Washington	2,808	2.3%
15	North Carolina	2,753	2.2%
16	Tennessee	2,147	1.7%
17	Missouri	2,050	1.7%
18	Connecticut	2,010	1.6%
19	Wisconsin	1,989	1.6%
20	Arizona	1,953	1.6%
21	Indiana	1,932	1.6%
22	Colorado	1,918	1.5%
23	Minnesota	1,909	1.5%
24	Louisiana	1,770	1.4%
25	Oregon	1,671	1.3%
26	Alabama	1,492	1.2%
27	Kentucky	1,425	1.1%
28	South Carolina	1,359	1.1%
29	Oklahoma	1,042	0.8%
30	Kansas	995	0.8%
31	West Virginia	852	0.7%
32	Iowa	848	0.7%
33	Arkansas	836	0.7%
34	Mississippi	829	0.7%
35	New Mexico	826	0.7%
36	Utah	782	0.6%
37	Nevada	671	0.5%
38	Hawaii	668	0.5%
39	Maine	600	0.5%
40	Nebraska	553	0.4%
41	Rhode Island	515	0.4%
42	New Hampshire	499	0.4%
43	Idaho	432	0.3%
44	Montana	427	0.3%
45	Delaware	356	0.3%
46	Vermont	339	0.3%
47	Alaska	274	0.2%
48	North Dakota	247	0.2%
49	South Dakota	246	0.2%
50	Wyoming	200	0.2%
	District of Columbia	808	0.7%

Source: American Medical Association (Chicago, Illinois)
 "Physician Characteristics and Distribution in the U.S." (2003-2004 Edition)
*As of December 31, 2001. Comprised of federal and nonfederal physicians. Total does not include 2,036 physicians in the U.S. territories and possessions, at APO's and FPO's and whose addresses are unknown.

427

Physicians 65 Years Old and Older in 2001

National Total = 147,998 Physicians*

ALPHA ORDER

RANK	STATE	PHYSICIANS	% of USA
27	Alabama	1,511	1.0%
50	Alaska	164	0.1%
16	Arizona	2,849	1.9%
32	Arkansas	1,008	0.7%
1	California	21,595	14.6%
22	Colorado	2,116	1.4%
17	Connecticut	2,530	1.7%
46	Delaware	401	0.3%
3	Florida	12,326	8.3%
15	Georgia	2,997	2.0%
37	Hawaii	801	0.5%
44	Idaho	493	0.3%
6	Illinois	5,356	3.6%
20	Indiana	2,341	1.6%
31	Iowa	1,051	0.7%
29	Kansas	1,256	0.8%
28	Kentucky	1,456	1.0%
24	Louisiana	1,918	1.3%
38	Maine	800	0.5%
11	Maryland	3,983	2.7%
9	Massachusetts	4,592	3.1%
10	Michigan	4,168	2.8%
21	Minnesota	2,302	1.6%
32	Mississippi	1,008	0.7%
23	Missouri	2,074	1.4%
45	Montana	485	0.3%
42	Nebraska	705	0.5%
34	Nevada	864	0.6%
39	New Hampshire	758	0.5%
8	New Jersey	4,847	3.3%
36	New Mexico	803	0.5%
2	New York	14,269	9.6%
13	North Carolina	3,496	2.4%
48	North Dakota	248	0.2%
7	Ohio	5,122	3.5%
30	Oklahoma	1,220	0.8%
25	Oregon	1,910	1.3%
5	Pennsylvania	7,176	4.8%
41	Rhode Island	711	0.5%
26	South Carolina	1,651	1.1%
47	South Dakota	282	0.2%
18	Tennessee	2,411	1.6%
4	Texas	7,466	5.0%
35	Utah	808	0.5%
43	Vermont	499	0.3%
12	Virginia	3,729	2.5%
14	Washington	3,256	2.2%
39	West Virginia	758	0.5%
19	Wisconsin	2,406	1.6%
49	Wyoming	205	0.1%

RANK ORDER

RANK	STATE	PHYSICIANS	% of USA
1	California	21,595	14.6%
2	New York	14,269	9.6%
3	Florida	12,326	8.3%
4	Texas	7,466	5.0%
5	Pennsylvania	7,176	4.8%
6	Illinois	5,356	3.6%
7	Ohio	5,122	3.5%
8	New Jersey	4,847	3.3%
9	Massachusetts	4,592	3.1%
10	Michigan	4,168	2.8%
11	Maryland	3,983	2.7%
12	Virginia	3,729	2.5%
13	North Carolina	3,496	2.4%
14	Washington	3,256	2.2%
15	Georgia	2,997	2.0%
16	Arizona	2,849	1.9%
17	Connecticut	2,530	1.7%
18	Tennessee	2,411	1.6%
19	Wisconsin	2,406	1.6%
20	Indiana	2,341	1.6%
21	Minnesota	2,302	1.6%
22	Colorado	2,116	1.4%
23	Missouri	2,074	1.4%
24	Louisiana	1,918	1.3%
25	Oregon	1,910	1.3%
26	South Carolina	1,651	1.1%
27	Alabama	1,511	1.0%
28	Kentucky	1,456	1.0%
29	Kansas	1,256	0.8%
30	Oklahoma	1,220	0.8%
31	Iowa	1,051	0.7%
32	Arkansas	1,008	0.7%
32	Mississippi	1,008	0.7%
34	Nevada	864	0.6%
35	Utah	808	0.5%
36	New Mexico	803	0.5%
37	Hawaii	801	0.5%
38	Maine	800	0.5%
39	New Hampshire	758	0.5%
39	West Virginia	758	0.5%
41	Rhode Island	711	0.5%
42	Nebraska	705	0.5%
43	Vermont	499	0.3%
44	Idaho	493	0.3%
45	Montana	485	0.3%
46	Delaware	401	0.3%
47	South Dakota	282	0.2%
48	North Dakota	248	0.2%
49	Wyoming	205	0.1%
50	Alaska	164	0.1%
	District of Columbia	817	0.6%

Source: American Medical Association (Chicago, Illinois)
    "Physician Characteristics and Distribution in the U.S." (2003-2004 Edition)
*As of December 31, 2001. Comprised of federal and nonfederal physicians. Total does not include 3,228 physicians in the U.S. territories and possessions, at APO's and FPO's and whose addresses are unknown.

Percent of Physicians 65 Years Old and Older in 2001

National Percent = 18.0% of Physicians*

ALPHA ORDER

RANK	STATE	PERCENT
45	Alabama	15.1
50	Alaska	11.6
2	Arizona	22.5
25	Arkansas	17.2
3	California	21.7
23	Colorado	17.5
17	Connecticut	18.5
15	Delaware	18.6
1	Florida	26.1
45	Georgia	15.1
11	Hawaii	19.8
9	Idaho	20.1
48	Illinois	14.7
28	Indiana	16.8
24	Iowa	17.4
13	Kansas	19.2
47	Kentucky	15.0
42	Louisiana	15.4
4	Maine	21.6
30	Maryland	16.7
38	Massachusetts	15.7
34	Michigan	16.2
39	Minnesota	15.6
18	Mississippi	18.2
49	Missouri	14.5
5	Montana	21.2
36	Nebraska	16.0
8	Nevada	20.2
6	New Hampshire	21.0
25	New Jersey	17.2
25	New Mexico	17.2
20	New York	17.9
36	North Carolina	16.0
41	North Dakota	15.5
32	Ohio	16.6
15	Oklahoma	18.6
12	Oregon	19.6
20	Pennsylvania	17.9
19	Rhode Island	18.0
32	South Carolina	16.6
35	South Dakota	16.1
42	Tennessee	15.4
42	Texas	15.4
39	Utah	15.6
7	Vermont	20.8
20	Virginia	17.9
14	Washington	18.7
28	West Virginia	16.8
30	Wisconsin	16.7
10	Wyoming	19.9

RANK ORDER

RANK	STATE	PERCENT
1	Florida	26.1
2	Arizona	22.5
3	California	21.7
4	Maine	21.6
5	Montana	21.2
6	New Hampshire	21.0
7	Vermont	20.8
8	Nevada	20.2
9	Idaho	20.1
10	Wyoming	19.9
11	Hawaii	19.8
12	Oregon	19.6
13	Kansas	19.2
14	Washington	18.7
15	Delaware	18.6
15	Oklahoma	18.6
17	Connecticut	18.5
18	Mississippi	18.2
19	Rhode Island	18.0
20	New York	17.9
20	Pennsylvania	17.9
20	Virginia	17.9
23	Colorado	17.5
24	Iowa	17.4
25	Arkansas	17.2
25	New Jersey	17.2
25	New Mexico	17.2
28	Indiana	16.8
28	West Virginia	16.8
30	Maryland	16.7
30	Wisconsin	16.7
32	Ohio	16.6
32	South Carolina	16.6
34	Michigan	16.2
35	South Dakota	16.1
36	Nebraska	16.0
36	North Carolina	16.0
38	Massachusetts	15.7
39	Minnesota	15.6
39	Utah	15.6
41	North Dakota	15.5
42	Louisiana	15.4
42	Tennessee	15.4
42	Texas	15.4
45	Alabama	15.1
45	Georgia	15.1
47	Kentucky	15.0
48	Illinois	14.7
49	Missouri	14.5
50	Alaska	11.6

| | District of Columbia | 18.2 |

Source: Morgan Quitno Press using data from American Medical Association (Chicago, Illinois)
    "Physician Characteristics and Distribution in the U.S." (2003-2004 Edition)
*As of December 31, 2001. Comprised of federal and nonfederal physicians. National percent does not include physicians in the U.S. territories and possessions, at APO's and FPO's and whose addresses are unknown.

Federal Physicians in 2001

National Total = 20,359 Physicians*

ALPHA ORDER

RANK	STATE	PHYSICIANS	% of USA
27	Alabama	212	1.0%
35	Alaska	147	0.7%
13	Arizona	454	2.2%
34	Arkansas	158	0.8%
1	California	2,218	10.9%
16	Colorado	368	1.8%
32	Connecticut	184	0.9%
47	Delaware	52	0.3%
4	Florida	1,247	6.1%
7	Georgia	868	4.3%
23	Hawaii	259	1.3%
42	Idaho	86	0.4%
11	Illinois	560	2.8%
29	Indiana	192	0.9%
39	Iowa	106	0.5%
32	Kansas	184	0.9%
30	Kentucky	186	0.9%
26	Louisiana	230	1.1%
44	Maine	74	0.4%
2	Maryland	1,866	9.2%
14	Massachusetts	433	2.1%
17	Michigan	319	1.6%
20	Minnesota	287	1.4%
24	Mississippi	251	1.2%
19	Missouri	298	1.5%
46	Montana	68	0.3%
41	Nebraska	87	0.4%
37	Nevada	131	0.6%
45	New Hampshire	72	0.4%
18	New Jersey	315	1.5%
25	New Mexico	248	1.2%
6	New York	966	4.7%
8	North Carolina	598	2.9%
49	North Dakota	44	0.2%
12	Ohio	515	2.5%
31	Oklahoma	185	0.9%
22	Oregon	263	1.3%
10	Pennsylvania	578	2.8%
43	Rhode Island	79	0.4%
21	South Carolina	271	1.3%
40	South Dakota	91	0.4%
15	Tennessee	417	2.0%
3	Texas	1,624	8.0%
38	Utah	119	0.6%
50	Vermont	42	0.2%
5	Virginia	1,067	5.2%
9	Washington	596	2.9%
35	West Virginia	147	0.7%
28	Wisconsin	194	1.0%
48	Wyoming	46	0.2%

RANK ORDER

RANK	STATE	PHYSICIANS	% of USA
1	California	2,218	10.9%
2	Maryland	1,866	9.2%
3	Texas	1,624	8.0%
4	Florida	1,247	6.1%
5	Virginia	1,067	5.2%
6	New York	966	4.7%
7	Georgia	868	4.3%
8	North Carolina	598	2.9%
9	Washington	596	2.9%
10	Pennsylvania	578	2.8%
11	Illinois	560	2.8%
12	Ohio	515	2.5%
13	Arizona	454	2.2%
14	Massachusetts	433	2.1%
15	Tennessee	417	2.0%
16	Colorado	368	1.8%
17	Michigan	319	1.6%
18	New Jersey	315	1.5%
19	Missouri	298	1.5%
20	Minnesota	287	1.4%
21	South Carolina	271	1.3%
22	Oregon	263	1.3%
23	Hawaii	259	1.3%
24	Mississippi	251	1.2%
25	New Mexico	248	1.2%
26	Louisiana	230	1.1%
27	Alabama	212	1.0%
28	Wisconsin	194	1.0%
29	Indiana	192	0.9%
30	Kentucky	186	0.9%
31	Oklahoma	185	0.9%
32	Connecticut	184	0.9%
32	Kansas	184	0.9%
34	Arkansas	158	0.8%
35	Alaska	147	0.7%
35	West Virginia	147	0.7%
37	Nevada	131	0.6%
38	Utah	119	0.6%
39	Iowa	106	0.5%
40	South Dakota	91	0.4%
41	Nebraska	87	0.4%
42	Idaho	86	0.4%
43	Rhode Island	79	0.4%
44	Maine	74	0.4%
45	New Hampshire	72	0.4%
46	Montana	68	0.3%
47	Delaware	52	0.3%
48	Wyoming	46	0.2%
49	North Dakota	44	0.2%
50	Vermont	42	0.2%
	District of Columbia	357	1.8%

Source: American Medical Association (Chicago, Illinois)
    "Physician Characteristics and Distribution in the U.S." (2003-2004 Edition)
*As of December 31, 2001. Total does not include 1,021 physicians in U.S. territories and possessions, at APO's and FPO's and whose addresses are unknown.

Rate of Federal Physicians in 2001

National Rate = 7.1 Physicians per 100,000 Population*

ALPHA ORDER			RANK ORDER		
RANK	STATE	RATE	RANK	STATE	RATE
41	Alabama	4.7	1	Maryland	34.6
2	Alaska	23.2	2	Alaska	23.2
11	Arizona	8.6	3	Hawaii	21.1
30	Arkansas	5.9	4	Virginia	14.8
28	California	6.4	5	New Mexico	13.5
12	Colorado	8.3	6	South Dakota	12.0
34	Connecticut	5.4	7	Georgia	10.3
26	Delaware	6.5	8	Washington	9.9
14	Florida	7.6	9	Wyoming	9.3
7	Georgia	10.3	10	Mississippi	8.8
3	Hawaii	21.1	11	Arizona	8.6
26	Idaho	6.5	12	Colorado	8.3
44	Illinois	4.5	13	West Virginia	8.2
50	Indiana	3.1	14	Florida	7.6
47	Iowa	3.6	14	Oregon	7.6
23	Kansas	6.8	14	Texas	7.6
43	Kentucky	4.6	17	Montana	7.5
38	Louisiana	5.1	17	Rhode Island	7.5
31	Maine	5.8	19	North Carolina	7.3
1	Maryland	34.6	19	Tennessee	7.3
23	Massachusetts	6.8	21	North Dakota	6.9
49	Michigan	3.2	21	Vermont	6.9
31	Minnesota	5.8	23	Kansas	6.8
10	Mississippi	8.8	23	Massachusetts	6.8
35	Missouri	5.3	25	South Carolina	6.7
17	Montana	7.5	26	Delaware	6.5
38	Nebraska	5.1	26	Idaho	6.5
29	Nevada	6.2	28	California	6.4
33	New Hampshire	5.7	29	Nevada	6.2
46	New Jersey	3.7	30	Arkansas	5.9
5	New Mexico	13.5	31	Maine	5.8
38	New York	5.1	31	Minnesota	5.8
19	North Carolina	7.3	33	New Hampshire	5.7
21	North Dakota	6.9	34	Connecticut	5.4
44	Ohio	4.5	35	Missouri	5.3
35	Oklahoma	5.3	35	Oklahoma	5.3
14	Oregon	7.6	37	Utah	5.2
41	Pennsylvania	4.7	38	Louisiana	5.1
17	Rhode Island	7.5	38	Nebraska	5.1
25	South Carolina	6.7	38	New York	5.1
6	South Dakota	12.0	41	Alabama	4.7
19	Tennessee	7.3	41	Pennsylvania	4.7
14	Texas	7.6	43	Kentucky	4.6
37	Utah	5.2	44	Illinois	4.5
21	Vermont	6.9	44	Ohio	4.5
4	Virginia	14.8	46	New Jersey	3.7
8	Washington	9.9	47	Iowa	3.6
13	West Virginia	8.2	47	Wisconsin	3.6
47	Wisconsin	3.6	49	Michigan	3.2
9	Wyoming	9.3	50	Indiana	3.1
				District of Columbia	62.2

Source: Morgan Quitno Press using data from American Medical Association (Chicago, Illinois)
    "Physician Characteristics and Distribution in the U.S." (2003-2004 Edition)
*As of December 31, 2001. National rate does not include physicians in U.S. territories and possessions, at APO's and FPO's and whose addresses are unknown.

Nonfederal Physicians in 2001

National Total = 800,565 Physicians*

ALPHA ORDER

RANK	STATE	PHYSICIANS	% of USA
25	Alabama	9,797	1.2%
49	Alaska	1,267	0.2%
23	Arizona	12,206	1.5%
32	Arkansas	5,699	0.7%
1	California	97,349	12.2%
24	Colorado	11,727	1.5%
21	Connecticut	13,473	1.7%
46	Delaware	2,101	0.3%
4	Florida	46,058	5.8%
14	Georgia	18,971	2.4%
40	Hawaii	3,785	0.5%
43	Idaho	2,362	0.3%
6	Illinois	35,801	4.5%
20	Indiana	13,703	1.7%
31	Iowa	5,935	0.7%
30	Kansas	6,350	0.8%
27	Kentucky	9,492	1.2%
22	Louisiana	12,209	1.5%
41	Maine	3,634	0.5%
11	Maryland	21,992	2.7%
8	Massachusetts	28,905	3.6%
10	Michigan	25,391	3.2%
17	Minnesota	14,465	1.8%
33	Mississippi	5,293	0.7%
19	Missouri	14,052	1.8%
45	Montana	2,224	0.3%
37	Nebraska	4,312	0.5%
38	Nevada	4,150	0.5%
42	New Hampshire	3,537	0.4%
9	New Jersey	27,864	3.5%
35	New Mexico	4,430	0.6%
2	New York	78,575	9.8%
12	North Carolina	21,302	2.7%
48	North Dakota	1,558	0.2%
7	Ohio	30,365	3.8%
29	Oklahoma	6,387	0.8%
28	Oregon	9,486	1.2%
5	Pennsylvania	39,487	4.9%
39	Rhode Island	3,863	0.5%
26	South Carolina	9,669	1.2%
47	South Dakota	1,664	0.2%
16	Tennessee	15,278	1.9%
3	Texas	46,719	5.8%
34	Utah	5,046	0.6%
44	Vermont	2,361	0.3%
13	Virginia	19,814	2.5%
15	Washington	16,808	2.1%
36	West Virginia	4,352	0.5%
18	Wisconsin	14,181	1.8%
50	Wyoming	983	0.1%

RANK ORDER

RANK	STATE	PHYSICIANS	% of USA
1	California	97,349	12.2%
2	New York	78,575	9.8%
3	Texas	46,719	5.8%
4	Florida	46,058	5.8%
5	Pennsylvania	39,487	4.9%
6	Illinois	35,801	4.5%
7	Ohio	30,365	3.8%
8	Massachusetts	28,905	3.6%
9	New Jersey	27,864	3.5%
10	Michigan	25,391	3.2%
11	Maryland	21,992	2.7%
12	North Carolina	21,302	2.7%
13	Virginia	19,814	2.5%
14	Georgia	18,971	2.4%
15	Washington	16,808	2.1%
16	Tennessee	15,278	1.9%
17	Minnesota	14,465	1.8%
18	Wisconsin	14,181	1.8%
19	Missouri	14,052	1.8%
20	Indiana	13,703	1.7%
21	Connecticut	13,473	1.7%
22	Louisiana	12,209	1.5%
23	Arizona	12,206	1.5%
24	Colorado	11,727	1.5%
25	Alabama	9,797	1.2%
26	South Carolina	9,669	1.2%
27	Kentucky	9,492	1.2%
28	Oregon	9,486	1.2%
29	Oklahoma	6,387	0.8%
30	Kansas	6,350	0.8%
31	Iowa	5,935	0.7%
32	Arkansas	5,699	0.7%
33	Mississippi	5,293	0.7%
34	Utah	5,046	0.6%
35	New Mexico	4,430	0.6%
36	West Virginia	4,352	0.5%
37	Nebraska	4,312	0.5%
38	Nevada	4,150	0.5%
39	Rhode Island	3,863	0.5%
40	Hawaii	3,785	0.5%
41	Maine	3,634	0.5%
42	New Hampshire	3,537	0.4%
43	Idaho	2,362	0.3%
44	Vermont	2,361	0.3%
45	Montana	2,224	0.3%
46	Delaware	2,101	0.3%
47	South Dakota	1,664	0.2%
48	North Dakota	1,558	0.2%
49	Alaska	1,267	0.2%
50	Wyoming	983	0.1%
	District of Columbia	4,133	0.5%

Source: American Medical Association (Chicago, Illinois)
   "Physician Characteristics and Distribution in the U.S." (2003-2004 Edition)
*As of December 31, 2001. Total does not include 14,211 physicians in U.S. territories and possessions, at APO's and FPO's and whose addresses are unknown.

Rate of Nonfederal Physicians in 2001

National Rate = 281 Physicians per 100,000 Population*

ALPHA ORDER

RANK	STATE	RATE
40	Alabama	219
45	Alaska	200
36	Arizona	230
43	Arkansas	211
13	California	281
22	Colorado	265
4	Connecticut	392
23	Delaware	264
13	Florida	281
37	Georgia	226
9	Hawaii	308
50	Idaho	179
11	Illinois	286
38	Indiana	224
44	Iowa	202
34	Kansas	235
35	Kentucky	233
18	Louisiana	273
12	Maine	283
3	Maryland	408
1	Massachusetts	452
26	Michigan	254
10	Minnesota	290
48	Mississippi	185
28	Missouri	249
29	Montana	246
27	Nebraska	251
47	Nevada	198
13	New Hampshire	281
7	New Jersey	327
31	New Mexico	242
2	New York	412
25	North Carolina	260
30	North Dakota	245
20	Ohio	267
49	Oklahoma	184
18	Oregon	273
8	Pennsylvania	321
6	Rhode Island	365
33	South Carolina	238
40	South Dakota	219
21	Tennessee	266
40	Texas	219
39	Utah	221
5	Vermont	385
17	Virginia	275
16	Washington	280
31	West Virginia	242
24	Wisconsin	262
46	Wyoming	199

RANK ORDER

RANK	STATE	RATE
1	Massachusetts	452
2	New York	412
3	Maryland	408
4	Connecticut	392
5	Vermont	385
6	Rhode Island	365
7	New Jersey	327
8	Pennsylvania	321
9	Hawaii	308
10	Minnesota	290
11	Illinois	286
12	Maine	283
13	California	281
13	Florida	281
13	New Hampshire	281
16	Washington	280
17	Virginia	275
18	Louisiana	273
18	Oregon	273
20	Ohio	267
21	Tennessee	266
22	Colorado	265
23	Delaware	264
24	Wisconsin	262
25	North Carolina	260
26	Michigan	254
27	Nebraska	251
28	Missouri	249
29	Montana	246
30	North Dakota	245
31	New Mexico	242
31	West Virginia	242
33	South Carolina	238
34	Kansas	235
35	Kentucky	233
36	Arizona	230
37	Georgia	226
38	Indiana	224
39	Utah	221
40	Alabama	219
40	South Dakota	219
40	Texas	219
43	Arkansas	211
44	Iowa	202
45	Alaska	200
46	Wyoming	199
47	Nevada	198
48	Mississippi	185
49	Oklahoma	184
50	Idaho	179
	District of Columbia	720

Source: Morgan Quitno Press using data from American Medical Association (Chicago, Illinois)
      "Physician Characteristics and Distribution in the U.S." (2003-2004 Edition)
*As of December 31, 2001. National rate does not include physicians in U.S. territories and possessions, at APO's and FPO's and whose addresses are unknown.

Nonfederal Physicians in Patient Care in 2001

National Total = 643,223 Physicians*

ALPHA ORDER

RANK	STATE	PHYSICIANS	% of USA
25	Alabama	8,229	1.3%
49	Alaska	1,083	0.2%
23	Arizona	9,405	1.5%
31	Arkansas	4,759	0.7%
1	California	75,598	11.8%
24	Colorado	9,385	1.5%
21	Connecticut	10,634	1.7%
46	Delaware	1,731	0.3%
4	Florida	34,960	5.4%
14	Georgia	15,741	2.4%
40	Hawaii	3,063	0.5%
43	Idaho	1,957	0.3%
6	Illinois	29,116	4.5%
20	Indiana	11,418	1.8%
32	Iowa	4,631	0.7%
30	Kansas	5,128	0.8%
27	Kentucky	7,983	1.2%
22	Louisiana	10,298	1.6%
41	Maine	2,880	0.4%
12	Maryland	17,057	2.7%
9	Massachusetts	22,443	3.5%
10	Michigan	20,623	3.2%
17	Minnesota	11,807	1.8%
33	Mississippi	4,474	0.7%
18	Missouri	11,698	1.8%
45	Montana	1,796	0.3%
36	Nebraska	3,566	0.6%
38	Nevada	3,389	0.5%
42	New Hampshire	2,849	0.4%
8	New Jersey	22,842	3.6%
37	New Mexico	3,481	0.5%
2	New York	62,553	9.7%
11	North Carolina	17,341	2.7%
48	North Dakota	1,296	0.2%
7	Ohio	24,903	3.9%
29	Oklahoma	5,187	0.8%
28	Oregon	7,428	1.2%
5	Pennsylvania	31,706	4.9%
39	Rhode Island	3,160	0.5%
26	South Carolina	8,106	1.3%
47	South Dakota	1,383	0.2%
16	Tennessee	12,784	2.0%
3	Texas	38,910	6.0%
34	Utah	4,097	0.6%
44	Vermont	1,847	0.3%
13	Virginia	16,154	2.5%
15	Washington	13,175	2.0%
35	West Virginia	3,597	0.6%
19	Wisconsin	11,632	1.8%
50	Wyoming	813	0.1%

RANK ORDER

RANK	STATE	PHYSICIANS	% of USA
1	California	75,598	11.8%
2	New York	62,553	9.7%
3	Texas	38,910	6.0%
4	Florida	34,960	5.4%
5	Pennsylvania	31,706	4.9%
6	Illinois	29,116	4.5%
7	Ohio	24,903	3.9%
8	New Jersey	22,842	3.6%
9	Massachusetts	22,443	3.5%
10	Michigan	20,623	3.2%
11	North Carolina	17,341	2.7%
12	Maryland	17,057	2.7%
13	Virginia	16,154	2.5%
14	Georgia	15,741	2.4%
15	Washington	13,175	2.0%
16	Tennessee	12,784	2.0%
17	Minnesota	11,807	1.8%
18	Missouri	11,698	1.8%
19	Wisconsin	11,632	1.8%
20	Indiana	11,418	1.8%
21	Connecticut	10,634	1.7%
22	Louisiana	10,298	1.6%
23	Arizona	9,405	1.5%
24	Colorado	9,385	1.5%
25	Alabama	8,229	1.3%
26	South Carolina	8,106	1.3%
27	Kentucky	7,983	1.2%
28	Oregon	7,428	1.2%
29	Oklahoma	5,187	0.8%
30	Kansas	5,128	0.8%
31	Arkansas	4,759	0.7%
32	Iowa	4,631	0.7%
33	Mississippi	4,474	0.7%
34	Utah	4,097	0.6%
35	West Virginia	3,597	0.6%
36	Nebraska	3,566	0.6%
37	New Mexico	3,481	0.5%
38	Nevada	3,389	0.5%
39	Rhode Island	3,160	0.5%
40	Hawaii	3,063	0.5%
41	Maine	2,880	0.4%
42	New Hampshire	2,849	0.4%
43	Idaho	1,957	0.3%
44	Vermont	1,847	0.3%
45	Montana	1,796	0.3%
46	Delaware	1,731	0.3%
47	South Dakota	1,383	0.2%
48	North Dakota	1,296	0.2%
49	Alaska	1,083	0.2%
50	Wyoming	813	0.1%
	District of Columbia	3,127	0.5%

Source: American Medical Association (Chicago, Illinois)
    "Physician Characteristics and Distribution in the U.S." (2003-2004 Edition)
*As of December 31, 2001. Total does not include 9,105 physicians in U.S. territories and possessions.

Rate of Nonfederal Physicians in Patient Care in 2001

National Rate = 225 Physicians per 100,000 Population*

ALPHA ORDER

RANK	STATE	RATE
38	Alabama	184
44	Alaska	171
42	Arizona	177
42	Arkansas	177
19	California	218
24	Colorado	212
4	Connecticut	310
20	Delaware	217
22	Florida	214
36	Georgia	187
9	Hawaii	250
50	Idaho	148
11	Illinois	233
37	Indiana	186
47	Iowa	158
34	Kansas	190
33	Kentucky	196
12	Louisiana	230
14	Maine	224
3	Maryland	317
1	Massachusetts	351
28	Michigan	206
10	Minnesota	237
48	Mississippi	156
26	Missouri	208
32	Montana	198
27	Nebraska	207
46	Nevada	162
13	New Hampshire	226
7	New Jersey	268
34	New Mexico	190
2	New York	328
25	North Carolina	211
29	North Dakota	204
18	Ohio	219
49	Oklahoma	149
22	Oregon	214
8	Pennsylvania	258
6	Rhode Island	298
30	South Carolina	200
39	South Dakota	182
16	Tennessee	222
39	Texas	182
41	Utah	180
5	Vermont	301
14	Virginia	224
17	Washington	220
30	West Virginia	200
21	Wisconsin	215
45	Wyoming	165

RANK ORDER

RANK	STATE	RATE
1	Massachusetts	351
2	New York	328
3	Maryland	317
4	Connecticut	310
5	Vermont	301
6	Rhode Island	298
7	New Jersey	268
8	Pennsylvania	258
9	Hawaii	250
10	Minnesota	237
11	Illinois	233
12	Louisiana	230
13	New Hampshire	226
14	Maine	224
14	Virginia	224
16	Tennessee	222
17	Washington	220
18	Ohio	219
19	California	218
20	Delaware	217
21	Wisconsin	215
22	Florida	214
22	Oregon	214
24	Colorado	212
25	North Carolina	211
26	Missouri	208
27	Nebraska	207
28	Michigan	206
29	North Dakota	204
30	South Carolina	200
30	West Virginia	200
32	Montana	198
33	Kentucky	196
34	Kansas	190
34	New Mexico	190
36	Georgia	187
37	Indiana	186
38	Alabama	184
39	South Dakota	182
39	Texas	182
41	Utah	180
42	Arizona	177
42	Arkansas	177
44	Alaska	171
45	Wyoming	165
46	Nevada	162
47	Iowa	158
48	Mississippi	156
49	Oklahoma	149
50	Idaho	148
	District of Columbia	545

Source: Morgan Quitno Press using data from American Medical Association (Chicago, Illinois)
"Physician Characteristics and Distribution in the U.S." (2003-2004 Edition)
*As of December 31, 2001. National rate does not include physicians in U.S. territories and possessions.

Physicians in Primary Care in 2001

National Total = 278,149 Physicians*

ALPHA ORDER

RANK	STATE	PHYSICIANS	% of USA
25	Alabama	3,689	1.3%
49	Alaska	628	0.2%
24	Arizona	4,068	1.5%
31	Arkansas	2,187	0.8%
1	California	33,204	11.9%
23	Colorado	4,091	1.5%
21	Connecticut	4,413	1.6%
46	Delaware	730	0.3%
4	Florida	14,146	5.1%
14	Georgia	7,144	2.6%
39	Hawaii	1,466	0.5%
43	Idaho	870	0.3%
5	Illinois	13,228	4.8%
19	Indiana	4,970	1.8%
32	Iowa	2,056	0.7%
30	Kansas	2,305	0.8%
27	Kentucky	3,450	1.2%
22	Louisiana	4,169	1.5%
41	Maine	1,305	0.5%
12	Maryland	7,460	2.7%
10	Massachusetts	8,832	3.2%
9	Michigan	8,913	3.2%
16	Minnesota	5,476	2.0%
33	Mississippi	1,980	0.7%
20	Missouri	4,838	1.7%
45	Montana	801	0.3%
36	Nebraska	1,680	0.6%
38	Nevada	1,475	0.5%
42	New Hampshire	1,239	0.4%
8	New Jersey	9,896	3.6%
35	New Mexico	1,687	0.6%
2	New York	26,217	9.4%
11	North Carolina	7,581	2.7%
48	North Dakota	635	0.2%
7	Ohio	10,762	3.9%
29	Oklahoma	2,308	0.8%
28	Oregon	3,355	1.2%
6	Pennsylvania	12,755	4.6%
40	Rhode Island	1,358	0.5%
26	South Carolina	3,597	1.3%
47	South Dakota	685	0.2%
17	Tennessee	5,466	2.0%
3	Texas	16,472	5.9%
34	Utah	1,736	0.6%
44	Vermont	869	0.3%
13	Virginia	7,416	2.7%
15	Washington	5,988	2.2%
37	West Virginia	1,638	0.6%
18	Wisconsin	5,187	1.9%
50	Wyoming	421	0.2%

RANK ORDER

RANK	STATE	PHYSICIANS	% of USA
1	California	33,204	11.9%
2	New York	26,217	9.4%
3	Texas	16,472	5.9%
4	Florida	14,146	5.1%
5	Illinois	13,228	4.8%
6	Pennsylvania	12,755	4.6%
7	Ohio	10,762	3.9%
8	New Jersey	9,896	3.6%
9	Michigan	8,913	3.2%
10	Massachusetts	8,832	3.2%
11	North Carolina	7,581	2.7%
12	Maryland	7,460	2.7%
13	Virginia	7,416	2.7%
14	Georgia	7,144	2.6%
15	Washington	5,988	2.2%
16	Minnesota	5,476	2.0%
17	Tennessee	5,466	2.0%
18	Wisconsin	5,187	1.9%
19	Indiana	4,970	1.8%
20	Missouri	4,838	1.7%
21	Connecticut	4,413	1.6%
22	Louisiana	4,169	1.5%
23	Colorado	4,091	1.5%
24	Arizona	4,068	1.5%
25	Alabama	3,689	1.3%
26	South Carolina	3,597	1.3%
27	Kentucky	3,450	1.2%
28	Oregon	3,355	1.2%
29	Oklahoma	2,308	0.8%
30	Kansas	2,305	0.8%
31	Arkansas	2,187	0.8%
32	Iowa	2,056	0.7%
33	Mississippi	1,980	0.7%
34	Utah	1,736	0.6%
35	New Mexico	1,687	0.6%
36	Nebraska	1,680	0.6%
37	West Virginia	1,638	0.6%
38	Nevada	1,475	0.5%
39	Hawaii	1,466	0.5%
40	Rhode Island	1,358	0.5%
41	Maine	1,305	0.5%
42	New Hampshire	1,239	0.4%
43	Idaho	870	0.3%
44	Vermont	869	0.3%
45	Montana	801	0.3%
46	Delaware	730	0.3%
47	South Dakota	685	0.2%
48	North Dakota	635	0.2%
49	Alaska	628	0.2%
50	Wyoming	421	0.2%
	District of Columbia	1,307	0.5%

Source: American Medical Association (Chicago, Illinois)
   "Physician Characteristics and Distribution in the U.S." (2003-2004 Edition)
*Federal and nonfederal physicians as of December 31, 2001. National total does not include 5,434 physicians in U.S. territories and possessions. Primary Care Specialties include Family Practice, General Practice, Internal Medicine, Obstetrics/Gynecology and Pediatrics excluding subspecialties within each category.

Rate of Physicians in Primary Care in 2001

National Rate = 97 Physicians per 100,000 Population*

ALPHA ORDER

RANK	STATE	RATE
40	Alabama	83
16	Alaska	99
43	Arizona	77
41	Arkansas	81
20	California	96
25	Colorado	92
5	Connecticut	128
25	Delaware	92
34	Florida	86
36	Georgia	85
7	Hawaii	119
50	Idaho	66
10	Illinois	106
41	Indiana	81
46	Iowa	70
36	Kansas	85
36	Kentucky	85
24	Louisiana	93
13	Maine	102
2	Maryland	139
3	Massachusetts	138
31	Michigan	89
9	Minnesota	110
48	Mississippi	69
34	Missouri	86
33	Montana	88
17	Nebraska	98
46	Nevada	70
17	New Hampshire	98
8	New Jersey	116
25	New Mexico	92
4	New York	137
25	North Carolina	92
14	North Dakota	100
23	Ohio	94
49	Oklahoma	67
19	Oregon	97
11	Pennsylvania	104
5	Rhode Island	128
31	South Carolina	89
30	South Dakota	90
22	Tennessee	95
43	Texas	77
45	Utah	76
1	Vermont	142
12	Virginia	103
14	Washington	100
29	West Virginia	91
20	Wisconsin	96
36	Wyoming	85

RANK ORDER

RANK	STATE	RATE
1	Vermont	142
2	Maryland	139
3	Massachusetts	138
4	New York	137
5	Connecticut	128
5	Rhode Island	128
7	Hawaii	119
8	New Jersey	116
9	Minnesota	110
10	Illinois	106
11	Pennsylvania	104
12	Virginia	103
13	Maine	102
14	North Dakota	100
14	Washington	100
16	Alaska	99
17	Nebraska	98
17	New Hampshire	98
19	Oregon	97
20	California	96
20	Wisconsin	96
22	Tennessee	95
23	Ohio	94
24	Louisiana	93
25	Colorado	92
25	Delaware	92
25	New Mexico	92
25	North Carolina	92
29	West Virginia	91
30	South Dakota	90
31	Michigan	89
31	South Carolina	89
33	Montana	88
34	Florida	86
34	Missouri	86
36	Georgia	85
36	Kansas	85
36	Kentucky	85
36	Wyoming	85
40	Alabama	83
41	Arkansas	81
41	Indiana	81
43	Arizona	77
43	Texas	77
45	Utah	76
46	Iowa	70
46	Nevada	70
48	Mississippi	69
49	Oklahoma	67
50	Idaho	66

	District of Columbia	228

Source: Morgan Quitno Press using data from American Medical Association (Chicago, Illinois)
"Physician Characteristics and Distribution in the U.S." (2003-2004 Edition)
*Federal and nonfederal physicians as of December 31, 2001. National rate does not include physicians in U.S. territories and possessions. Primary Care Specialties include Family Practice, General Practice, Internal Medicine, Obstetrics/Gynecology and Pediatrics excluding subspecialties within each category.

Percent of Physicians in Primary Care in 2001

National Percent = 33.9% of Physicians*

<table>
<tr><td colspan="3">ALPHA ORDER</td><td colspan="3">RANK ORDER</td></tr>
<tr><td>RANK</td><td>STATE</td><td>PERCENT</td><td>RANK</td><td>STATE</td><td>PERCENT</td></tr>
<tr><td>8</td><td>Alabama</td><td>36.9</td><td>1</td><td>Alaska</td><td>44.4</td></tr>
<tr><td>1</td><td>Alaska</td><td>44.4</td><td>2</td><td>Wyoming</td><td>40.9</td></tr>
<tr><td>46</td><td>Arizona</td><td>32.1</td><td>3</td><td>North Dakota</td><td>39.6</td></tr>
<tr><td>6</td><td>Arkansas</td><td>37.3</td><td>4</td><td>South Dakota</td><td>39.0</td></tr>
<tr><td>43</td><td>California</td><td>33.3</td><td>5</td><td>Nebraska</td><td>38.2</td></tr>
<tr><td>39</td><td>Colorado</td><td>33.8</td><td>6</td><td>Arkansas</td><td>37.3</td></tr>
<tr><td>45</td><td>Connecticut</td><td>32.3</td><td>7</td><td>Minnesota</td><td>37.1</td></tr>
<tr><td>38</td><td>Delaware</td><td>33.9</td><td>8</td><td>Alabama</td><td>36.9</td></tr>
<tr><td>50</td><td>Florida</td><td>29.9</td><td>9</td><td>Illinois</td><td>36.4</td></tr>
<tr><td>16</td><td>Georgia</td><td>36.0</td><td>9</td><td>West Virginia</td><td>36.4</td></tr>
<tr><td>11</td><td>Hawaii</td><td>36.3</td><td>11</td><td>Hawaii</td><td>36.3</td></tr>
<tr><td>20</td><td>Idaho</td><td>35.5</td><td>12</td><td>South Carolina</td><td>36.2</td></tr>
<tr><td>9</td><td>Illinois</td><td>36.4</td><td>12</td><td>Vermont</td><td>36.2</td></tr>
<tr><td>17</td><td>Indiana</td><td>35.8</td><td>14</td><td>New Mexico</td><td>36.1</td></tr>
<tr><td>37</td><td>Iowa</td><td>34.0</td><td>14</td><td>Wisconsin</td><td>36.1</td></tr>
<tr><td>22</td><td>Kansas</td><td>35.3</td><td>16</td><td>Georgia</td><td>36.0</td></tr>
<tr><td>19</td><td>Kentucky</td><td>35.6</td><td>17</td><td>Indiana</td><td>35.8</td></tr>
<tr><td>42</td><td>Louisiana</td><td>33.5</td><td>18</td><td>Mississippi</td><td>35.7</td></tr>
<tr><td>23</td><td>Maine</td><td>35.2</td><td>19</td><td>Kentucky</td><td>35.6</td></tr>
<tr><td>48</td><td>Maryland</td><td>31.3</td><td>20</td><td>Idaho</td><td>35.5</td></tr>
<tr><td>49</td><td>Massachusetts</td><td>30.1</td><td>20</td><td>Virginia</td><td>35.5</td></tr>
<tr><td>29</td><td>Michigan</td><td>34.7</td><td>22</td><td>Kansas</td><td>35.3</td></tr>
<tr><td>7</td><td>Minnesota</td><td>37.1</td><td>23</td><td>Maine</td><td>35.2</td></tr>
<tr><td>18</td><td>Mississippi</td><td>35.7</td><td>24</td><td>New Jersey</td><td>35.1</td></tr>
<tr><td>40</td><td>Missouri</td><td>33.7</td><td>24</td><td>Oklahoma</td><td>35.1</td></tr>
<tr><td>26</td><td>Montana</td><td>34.9</td><td>26</td><td>Montana</td><td>34.9</td></tr>
<tr><td>5</td><td>Nebraska</td><td>38.2</td><td>26</td><td>Ohio</td><td>34.9</td></tr>
<tr><td>31</td><td>Nevada</td><td>34.5</td><td>28</td><td>Tennessee</td><td>34.8</td></tr>
<tr><td>35</td><td>New Hampshire</td><td>34.3</td><td>29</td><td>Michigan</td><td>34.7</td></tr>
<tr><td>24</td><td>New Jersey</td><td>35.1</td><td>30</td><td>North Carolina</td><td>34.6</td></tr>
<tr><td>14</td><td>New Mexico</td><td>36.1</td><td>31</td><td>Nevada</td><td>34.5</td></tr>
<tr><td>44</td><td>New York</td><td>33.0</td><td>32</td><td>Oregon</td><td>34.4</td></tr>
<tr><td>30</td><td>North Carolina</td><td>34.6</td><td>32</td><td>Rhode Island</td><td>34.4</td></tr>
<tr><td>3</td><td>North Dakota</td><td>39.6</td><td>32</td><td>Washington</td><td>34.4</td></tr>
<tr><td>26</td><td>Ohio</td><td>34.9</td><td>35</td><td>New Hampshire</td><td>34.3</td></tr>
<tr><td>24</td><td>Oklahoma</td><td>35.1</td><td>36</td><td>Texas</td><td>34.1</td></tr>
<tr><td>32</td><td>Oregon</td><td>34.4</td><td>37</td><td>Iowa</td><td>34.0</td></tr>
<tr><td>47</td><td>Pennsylvania</td><td>31.8</td><td>38</td><td>Delaware</td><td>33.9</td></tr>
<tr><td>32</td><td>Rhode Island</td><td>34.4</td><td>39</td><td>Colorado</td><td>33.8</td></tr>
<tr><td>12</td><td>South Carolina</td><td>36.2</td><td>40</td><td>Missouri</td><td>33.7</td></tr>
<tr><td>4</td><td>South Dakota</td><td>39.0</td><td>41</td><td>Utah</td><td>33.6</td></tr>
<tr><td>28</td><td>Tennessee</td><td>34.8</td><td>42</td><td>Louisiana</td><td>33.5</td></tr>
<tr><td>36</td><td>Texas</td><td>34.1</td><td>43</td><td>California</td><td>33.3</td></tr>
<tr><td>41</td><td>Utah</td><td>33.6</td><td>44</td><td>New York</td><td>33.0</td></tr>
<tr><td>12</td><td>Vermont</td><td>36.2</td><td>45</td><td>Connecticut</td><td>32.3</td></tr>
<tr><td>20</td><td>Virginia</td><td>35.5</td><td>46</td><td>Arizona</td><td>32.1</td></tr>
<tr><td>32</td><td>Washington</td><td>34.4</td><td>47</td><td>Pennsylvania</td><td>31.8</td></tr>
<tr><td>9</td><td>West Virginia</td><td>36.4</td><td>48</td><td>Maryland</td><td>31.3</td></tr>
<tr><td>14</td><td>Wisconsin</td><td>36.1</td><td>49</td><td>Massachusetts</td><td>30.1</td></tr>
<tr><td>2</td><td>Wyoming</td><td>40.9</td><td>50</td><td>Florida</td><td>29.9</td></tr>
<tr><td></td><td></td><td></td><td></td><td>District of Columbia</td><td>29.1</td></tr>
</table>

Source: Morgan Quitno Press using data from American Medical Association (Chicago, Illinois)
"Physician Characteristics and Distribution in the U.S." (2003-2004 Edition)
*Federal and nonfederal physicians as of December 31, 2001. National percent does not include physicians in U.S. territories and possessions. Primary Care Specialties include Family Practice, General Practice, Internal Medicine, Obstetrics/Gynecology and Pediatrics excluding subspecialties within each category.

Percent of Population Lacking Access to Primary Care in 2002

National Percent = 11.3% of Population*

ALPHA ORDER

RANK	STATE	PERCENT
2	Alabama	26.1
19	Alaska	12.6
20	Arizona	12.1
29	Arkansas	9.8
33	California	8.8
30	Colorado	9.4
43	Connecticut	6.5
37	Delaware	8.1
14	Florida	15.3
12	Georgia	16.2
48	Hawaii	4.1
4	Idaho	20.3
20	Illinois	12.1
38	Indiana	7.8
35	Iowa	8.4
17	Kansas	14.9
16	Kentucky	15.0
8	Louisiana	18.1
36	Maine	8.3
39	Maryland	7.7
47	Massachusetts	4.9
25	Michigan	10.9
22	Minnesota	11.3
1	Mississippi	27.0
3	Missouri	25.1
10	Montana	17.6
45	Nebraska	5.5
22	Nevada	11.3
46	New Hampshire	5.1
49	New Jersey	3.3
5	New Mexico	19.5
28	New York	10.1
32	North Carolina	9.0
7	North Dakota	18.7
42	Ohio	7.2
33	Oklahoma	8.8
39	Oregon	7.7
44	Pennsylvania	6.3
31	Rhode Island	9.2
11	South Carolina	16.9
6	South Dakota	19.1
26	Tennessee	10.8
15	Texas	15.1
13	Utah	15.7
49	Vermont	3.3
41	Virginia	7.5
22	Washington	11.3
18	West Virginia	13.4
27	Wisconsin	10.4
9	Wyoming	17.9

RANK ORDER

RANK	STATE	PERCENT
1	Mississippi	27.0
2	Alabama	26.1
3	Missouri	25.1
4	Idaho	20.3
5	New Mexico	19.5
6	South Dakota	19.1
7	North Dakota	18.7
8	Louisiana	18.1
9	Wyoming	17.9
10	Montana	17.6
11	South Carolina	16.9
12	Georgia	16.2
13	Utah	15.7
14	Florida	15.3
15	Texas	15.1
16	Kentucky	15.0
17	Kansas	14.9
18	West Virginia	13.4
19	Alaska	12.6
20	Arizona	12.1
20	Illinois	12.1
22	Minnesota	11.3
22	Nevada	11.3
22	Washington	11.3
25	Michigan	10.9
26	Tennessee	10.8
27	Wisconsin	10.4
28	New York	10.1
29	Arkansas	9.8
30	Colorado	9.4
31	Rhode Island	9.2
32	North Carolina	9.0
33	California	8.8
33	Oklahoma	8.8
35	Iowa	8.4
36	Maine	8.3
37	Delaware	8.1
38	Indiana	7.8
39	Maryland	7.7
39	Oregon	7.7
41	Virginia	7.5
42	Ohio	7.2
43	Connecticut	6.5
44	Pennsylvania	6.3
45	Nebraska	5.5
46	New Hampshire	5.1
47	Massachusetts	4.9
48	Hawaii	4.1
49	New Jersey	3.3
49	Vermont	3.3
	District of Columbia	15.3

Source: Morgan Quitno Press using data from U.S. Dept. of Health and Human Services, Div. of Shortage Designation
    "Selected Statistics on Health Professional Shortage Areas, As of December 31, 2002"
*Percent of population considered under-served by primary medical practitioners (Family & General Practice doctors, Internists, Ob/Gyns and Pediatricians). An under-served population does not have primary medical care within reasonable economic and geographic bounds.

Nonfederal Physicians in General/Family Practice in 2001

National Total = 84,792 Physicians*

ALPHA ORDER

RANK	STATE	PHYSICIANS	% of USA
25	Alabama	1,255	1.5%
46	Alaska	295	0.3%
20	Arizona	1,349	1.6%
29	Arkansas	1,139	1.3%
1	California	10,179	12.0%
18	Colorado	1,573	1.9%
37	Connecticut	604	0.7%
49	Delaware	226	0.3%
3	Florida	4,531	5.3%
15	Georgia	2,023	2.4%
43	Hawaii	355	0.4%
39	Idaho	488	0.6%
6	Illinois	3,722	4.4%
13	Indiana	2,333	2.8%
27	Iowa	1,146	1.4%
30	Kansas	1,064	1.3%
21	Kentucky	1,316	1.6%
23	Louisiana	1,285	1.5%
38	Maine	554	0.7%
24	Maryland	1,279	1.5%
26	Massachusetts	1,214	1.4%
9	Michigan	2,639	3.1%
10	Minnesota	2,606	3.1%
33	Mississippi	763	0.9%
22	Missouri	1,300	1.5%
42	Montana	384	0.5%
32	Nebraska	871	1.0%
40	Nevada	466	0.5%
41	New Hampshire	426	0.5%
17	New Jersey	1,645	1.9%
34	New Mexico	673	0.8%
5	New York	3,799	4.5%
11	North Carolina	2,591	3.1%
45	North Dakota	344	0.4%
7	Ohio	3,383	4.0%
31	Oklahoma	982	1.2%
27	Oregon	1,146	1.4%
4	Pennsylvania	3,891	4.6%
49	Rhode Island	226	0.3%
19	South Carolina	1,464	1.7%
44	South Dakota	353	0.4%
16	Tennessee	1,792	2.1%
2	Texas	5,873	6.9%
36	Utah	634	0.7%
47	Vermont	294	0.3%
12	Virginia	2,371	2.8%
8	Washington	2,643	3.1%
35	West Virginia	666	0.8%
14	Wisconsin	2,238	2.6%
48	Wyoming	237	0.3%

RANK ORDER

RANK	STATE	PHYSICIANS	% of USA
1	California	10,179	12.0%
2	Texas	5,873	6.9%
3	Florida	4,531	5.3%
4	Pennsylvania	3,891	4.6%
5	New York	3,799	4.5%
6	Illinois	3,722	4.4%
7	Ohio	3,383	4.0%
8	Washington	2,643	3.1%
9	Michigan	2,639	3.1%
10	Minnesota	2,606	3.1%
11	North Carolina	2,591	3.1%
12	Virginia	2,371	2.8%
13	Indiana	2,333	2.8%
14	Wisconsin	2,238	2.6%
15	Georgia	2,023	2.4%
16	Tennessee	1,792	2.1%
17	New Jersey	1,645	1.9%
18	Colorado	1,573	1.9%
19	South Carolina	1,464	1.7%
20	Arizona	1,349	1.6%
21	Kentucky	1,316	1.6%
22	Missouri	1,300	1.5%
23	Louisiana	1,285	1.5%
24	Maryland	1,279	1.5%
25	Alabama	1,255	1.5%
26	Massachusetts	1,214	1.4%
27	Iowa	1,146	1.4%
27	Oregon	1,146	1.4%
29	Arkansas	1,139	1.3%
30	Kansas	1,064	1.3%
31	Oklahoma	982	1.2%
32	Nebraska	871	1.0%
33	Mississippi	763	0.9%
34	New Mexico	673	0.8%
35	West Virginia	666	0.8%
36	Utah	634	0.7%
37	Connecticut	604	0.7%
38	Maine	554	0.7%
39	Idaho	488	0.6%
40	Nevada	466	0.5%
41	New Hampshire	426	0.5%
42	Montana	384	0.5%
43	Hawaii	355	0.4%
44	South Dakota	353	0.4%
45	North Dakota	344	0.4%
46	Alaska	295	0.3%
47	Vermont	294	0.3%
48	Wyoming	237	0.3%
49	Delaware	226	0.3%
49	Rhode Island	226	0.3%
	District of Columbia	162	0.2%

Source: American Medical Association (Chicago, Illinois)
"Physician Characteristics and Distribution in the U.S." (2003-2004 Edition)
*As of December 31, 2001. Total does not include 2,297 physicians in U.S. territories and possessions.

Rate of Nonfederal Physicians in General/Family Practice in 2001

National Rate = 30 Physicians per 100,000 Population*

ALPHA ORDER

RANK ORDER

RANK	STATE	RATE	RANK	STATE	RATE
33	Alabama	28	1	North Dakota	54
6	Alaska	47	2	Minnesota	52
41	Arizona	25	3	Nebraska	51
10	Arkansas	42	4	Vermont	48
30	California	29	4	Wyoming	48
20	Colorado	35	6	Alaska	47
50	Connecticut	18	6	South Dakota	47
33	Delaware	28	8	Washington	44
33	Florida	28	9	Maine	43
42	Georgia	24	10	Arkansas	42
30	Hawaii	29	10	Montana	42
16	Idaho	37	12	Wisconsin	41
28	Illinois	30	13	Iowa	39
15	Indiana	38	13	Kansas	39
13	Iowa	39	15	Indiana	38
13	Kansas	39	16	Idaho	37
24	Kentucky	32	16	New Mexico	37
30	Louisiana	29	16	West Virginia	37
9	Maine	43	19	South Carolina	36
42	Maryland	24	20	Colorado	35
48	Massachusetts	19	21	New Hampshire	34
40	Michigan	26	22	Oregon	33
2	Minnesota	52	22	Virginia	33
38	Mississippi	27	24	Kentucky	32
44	Missouri	23	24	North Carolina	32
10	Montana	42	24	Pennsylvania	32
3	Nebraska	51	27	Tennessee	31
45	Nevada	22	28	Illinois	30
21	New Hampshire	34	28	Ohio	30
48	New Jersey	19	30	California	29
16	New Mexico	37	30	Hawaii	29
47	New York	20	30	Louisiana	29
24	North Carolina	32	33	Alabama	28
1	North Dakota	54	33	Delaware	28
28	Ohio	30	33	Florida	28
33	Oklahoma	28	33	Oklahoma	28
22	Oregon	33	33	Utah	28
24	Pennsylvania	32	38	Mississippi	27
46	Rhode Island	21	38	Texas	27
19	South Carolina	36	40	Michigan	26
6	South Dakota	47	41	Arizona	25
27	Tennessee	31	42	Georgia	24
38	Texas	27	42	Maryland	24
33	Utah	28	44	Missouri	23
4	Vermont	48	45	Nevada	22
22	Virginia	33	46	Rhode Island	21
8	Washington	44	47	New York	20
16	West Virginia	37	48	Massachusetts	19
12	Wisconsin	41	48	New Jersey	19
4	Wyoming	48	50	Connecticut	18
				District of Columbia	28

Source: Morgan Quitno Press using data from American Medical Association (Chicago, Illinois)
  "Physician Characteristics and Distribution in the U.S." (2003-2004 Edition)
*As of December 31, 2001. National rate does not include physicians in U.S. territories and possessions.

Percent of Nonfederal Physicians Who Are Specialists in 2001

National Percent = 74.8% of Physicians*

ALPHA ORDER

RANK ORDER

RANK	STATE	PERCENT	RANK	STATE	PERCENT
16	Alabama	75.6	1	Connecticut	81.4
44	Alaska	66.3	1	Rhode Island	81.4
34	Arizona	70.2	3	New Jersey	81.2
42	Arkansas	67.0	4	Massachusetts	81.1
27	California	72.3	5	New York	80.7
28	Colorado	71.9	6	Maryland	79.9
1	Connecticut	81.4	7	Missouri	79.3
12	Delaware	75.9	8	Louisiana	77.9
36	Florida	69.7	9	Georgia	76.6
9	Georgia	76.6	10	Pennsylvania	76.5
12	Hawaii	75.9	11	Tennessee	76.3
48	Idaho	64.2	12	Delaware	75.9
14	Illinois	75.8	12	Hawaii	75.9
32	Indiana	70.6	14	Illinois	75.8
49	Iowa	63.8	15	Michigan	75.7
41	Kansas	68.0	16	Alabama	75.6
22	Kentucky	73.9	17	Ohio	75.2
8	Louisiana	77.9	17	Texas	75.2
38	Maine	68.7	19	North Carolina	74.5
6	Maryland	79.9	20	Utah	74.1
4	Massachusetts	81.1	21	Virginia	74.0
15	Michigan	75.7	22	Kentucky	73.9
39	Minnesota	68.6	23	Mississippi	73.4
23	Mississippi	73.4	23	Nevada	73.4
7	Missouri	79.3	25	South Carolina	72.8
45	Montana	66.2	26	New Hampshire	72.6
43	Nebraska	66.8	27	California	72.3
23	Nevada	73.4	28	Colorado	71.9
26	New Hampshire	72.6	29	Vermont	71.7
3	New Jersey	81.2	30	West Virginia	71.5
37	New Mexico	68.9	31	Wisconsin	70.8
5	New York	80.7	32	Indiana	70.6
19	North Carolina	74.5	33	Oregon	70.5
47	North Dakota	64.5	34	Arizona	70.2
17	Ohio	75.2	35	Oklahoma	69.9
35	Oklahoma	69.9	36	Florida	69.7
33	Oregon	70.5	37	New Mexico	68.9
10	Pennsylvania	76.5	38	Maine	68.7
1	Rhode Island	81.4	39	Minnesota	68.6
25	South Carolina	72.8	40	Washington	68.1
46	South Dakota	64.8	41	Kansas	68.0
11	Tennessee	76.3	42	Arkansas	67.0
17	Texas	75.2	43	Nebraska	66.8
20	Utah	74.1	44	Alaska	66.3
29	Vermont	71.7	45	Montana	66.2
21	Virginia	74.0	46	South Dakota	64.8
40	Washington	68.1	47	North Dakota	64.5
30	West Virginia	71.5	48	Idaho	64.2
31	Wisconsin	70.8	49	Iowa	63.8
50	Wyoming	62.0	50	Wyoming	62.0
				District of Columbia	81.9

Source: Morgan Quitno Press using data from American Medical Association (Chicago, Illinois)
"Physician Characteristics and Distribution in the U.S." (2003-2004 Edition)
*As of December 31, 2001. National percent does not include physicians in U.S. territories and possessions.
Includes physicians in medical, surgical and other specialties.

Nonfederal Physicians in Medical Specialties in 2001

National Total = 252,841 Physicians*

<u>ALPHA ORDER</u>

RANK	STATE	PHYSICIANS	% of USA
25	Alabama	3,089	1.2%
49	Alaska	278	0.1%
23	Arizona	3,362	1.3%
32	Arkansas	1,457	0.6%
2	California	29,279	11.6%
24	Colorado	3,252	1.3%
15	Connecticut	5,004	2.0%
44	Delaware	679	0.3%
4	Florida	13,570	5.4%
14	Georgia	5,895	2.3%
39	Hawaii	1,182	0.5%
46	Idaho	476	0.2%
6	Illinois	12,175	4.8%
22	Indiana	3,709	1.5%
35	Iowa	1,388	0.5%
30	Kansas	1,616	0.6%
26	Kentucky	2,791	1.1%
21	Louisiana	3,812	1.5%
42	Maine	957	0.4%
11	Maryland	7,890	3.1%
7	Massachusetts	10,914	4.3%
10	Michigan	8,152	3.2%
19	Minnesota	4,196	1.7%
33	Mississippi	1,441	0.6%
17	Missouri	4,822	1.9%
45	Montana	490	0.2%
40	Nebraska	1,085	0.4%
36	Nevada	1,233	0.5%
41	New Hampshire	999	0.4%
8	New Jersey	10,822	4.3%
37	New Mexico	1,214	0.5%
1	New York	29,657	11.7%
12	North Carolina	6,496	2.6%
48	North Dakota	378	0.1%
9	Ohio	9,713	3.8%
29	Oklahoma	1,700	0.7%
27	Oregon	2,607	1.0%
5	Pennsylvania	12,608	5.0%
31	Rhode Island	1,511	0.6%
28	South Carolina	2,606	1.0%
47	South Dakota	387	0.2%
16	Tennessee	4,907	1.9%
3	Texas	13,824	5.5%
34	Utah	1,417	0.6%
43	Vermont	685	0.3%
13	Virginia	5,964	2.4%
18	Washington	4,352	1.7%
38	West Virginia	1,202	0.5%
20	Wisconsin	3,961	1.6%
50	Wyoming	173	0.1%

<u>RANK ORDER</u>

RANK	STATE	PHYSICIANS	% of USA
1	New York	29,657	11.7%
2	California	29,279	11.6%
3	Texas	13,824	5.5%
4	Florida	13,570	5.4%
5	Pennsylvania	12,608	5.0%
6	Illinois	12,175	4.8%
7	Massachusetts	10,914	4.3%
8	New Jersey	10,822	4.3%
9	Ohio	9,713	3.8%
10	Michigan	8,152	3.2%
11	Maryland	7,890	3.1%
12	North Carolina	6,496	2.6%
13	Virginia	5,964	2.4%
14	Georgia	5,895	2.3%
15	Connecticut	5,004	2.0%
16	Tennessee	4,907	1.9%
17	Missouri	4,822	1.9%
18	Washington	4,352	1.7%
19	Minnesota	4,196	1.7%
20	Wisconsin	3,961	1.6%
21	Louisiana	3,812	1.5%
22	Indiana	3,709	1.5%
23	Arizona	3,362	1.3%
24	Colorado	3,252	1.3%
25	Alabama	3,089	1.2%
26	Kentucky	2,791	1.1%
27	Oregon	2,607	1.0%
28	South Carolina	2,606	1.0%
29	Oklahoma	1,700	0.7%
30	Kansas	1,616	0.6%
31	Rhode Island	1,511	0.6%
32	Arkansas	1,457	0.6%
33	Mississippi	1,441	0.6%
34	Utah	1,417	0.6%
35	Iowa	1,388	0.5%
36	Nevada	1,233	0.5%
37	New Mexico	1,214	0.5%
38	West Virginia	1,202	0.5%
39	Hawaii	1,182	0.5%
40	Nebraska	1,085	0.4%
41	New Hampshire	999	0.4%
42	Maine	957	0.4%
43	Vermont	685	0.3%
44	Delaware	679	0.3%
45	Montana	490	0.2%
46	Idaho	476	0.2%
47	South Dakota	387	0.2%
48	North Dakota	378	0.1%
49	Alaska	278	0.1%
50	Wyoming	173	0.1%
	District of Columbia	1,464	0.6%

Source: American Medical Association (Chicago, Illinois)
    "Physician Characteristics and Distribution in the U.S." (2003-2004 Edition)
*As of December 31, 2001. Total does not include 3,113 physicians in U.S. territories and possessions. Medical Specialties are Allergy/Immunology, Cardiovascular Diseases, Dermatology, Gastroenterology, Internal Medicine, Pediatrics, Pediatric Cardiology and Pulmonary Diseases.

Rate of Nonfederal Physicians in Medical Specialties in 2001

National Rate = 89 Physicians per 100,000 Population*

ALPHA ORDER

RANK	STATE	RATE
29	Alabama	69
48	Alaska	44
35	Arizona	63
42	Arkansas	54
12	California	85
25	Colorado	73
3	Connecticut	146
12	Delaware	85
18	Florida	83
28	Georgia	70
10	Hawaii	96
49	Idaho	36
9	Illinois	97
38	Indiana	61
47	Iowa	47
39	Kansas	60
29	Kentucky	69
12	Louisiana	85
23	Maine	75
3	Maryland	146
1	Massachusetts	171
20	Michigan	81
17	Minnesota	84
45	Mississippi	50
11	Missouri	86
42	Montana	54
35	Nebraska	63
40	Nevada	59
21	New Hampshire	79
6	New Jersey	127
32	New Mexico	66
2	New York	155
21	North Carolina	79
40	North Dakota	59
12	Ohio	85
46	Oklahoma	49
23	Oregon	75
8	Pennsylvania	102
5	Rhode Island	143
34	South Carolina	64
44	South Dakota	51
12	Tennessee	85
33	Texas	65
37	Utah	62
7	Vermont	112
18	Virginia	83
25	Washington	73
31	West Virginia	67
25	Wisconsin	73
50	Wyoming	35

RANK ORDER

RANK	STATE	RATE
1	Massachusetts	171
2	New York	155
3	Connecticut	146
3	Maryland	146
5	Rhode Island	143
6	New Jersey	127
7	Vermont	112
8	Pennsylvania	102
9	Illinois	97
10	Hawaii	96
11	Missouri	86
12	California	85
12	Delaware	85
12	Louisiana	85
12	Ohio	85
12	Tennessee	85
17	Minnesota	84
18	Florida	83
18	Virginia	83
20	Michigan	81
21	New Hampshire	79
21	North Carolina	79
23	Maine	75
23	Oregon	75
25	Colorado	73
25	Washington	73
25	Wisconsin	73
28	Georgia	70
29	Alabama	69
29	Kentucky	69
31	West Virginia	67
32	New Mexico	66
33	Texas	65
34	South Carolina	64
35	Arizona	63
35	Nebraska	63
37	Utah	62
38	Indiana	61
39	Kansas	60
40	Nevada	59
40	North Dakota	59
42	Arkansas	54
42	Montana	54
44	South Dakota	51
45	Mississippi	50
46	Oklahoma	49
47	Iowa	47
48	Alaska	44
49	Idaho	36
50	Wyoming	35

District of Columbia 255

Source: Morgan Quitno Press using data from American Medical Association (Chicago, Illinois)
    "Physician Characteristics and Distribution in the U.S." (2003-2004 Edition)

*As of December 31, 2001. National rate does not include physicians in U.S. territories and possessions. Medical Specialties are Allergy/Immunology, Cardiovascular Diseases, Dermatology, Gastroenterology, Internal Medicine, Pediatrics, Pediatric Cardiology and Pulmonary Diseases.

Nonfederal Physicians in Internal Medicine in 2001

National Total = 134,500 Physicians*

ALPHA ORDER

RANK	STATE	PHYSICIANS	% of USA
25	Alabama	1,657	1.2%
49	Alaska	137	0.1%
24	Arizona	1,662	1.2%
37	Arkansas	643	0.5%
2	California	15,359	11.4%
23	Colorado	1,663	1.2%
15	Connecticut	2,912	2.2%
44	Delaware	336	0.2%
6	Florida	6,637	4.9%
14	Georgia	3,098	2.3%
34	Hawaii	664	0.5%
47	Idaho	232	0.2%
4	Illinois	6,894	5.1%
22	Indiana	1,841	1.4%
38	Iowa	632	0.5%
31	Kansas	828	0.6%
27	Kentucky	1,373	1.0%
21	Louisiana	1,884	1.4%
40	Maine	531	0.4%
11	Maryland	4,383	3.3%
7	Massachusetts	6,331	4.7%
10	Michigan	4,501	3.3%
19	Minnesota	2,271	1.7%
32	Mississippi	713	0.5%
16	Missouri	2,545	1.9%
45	Montana	263	0.2%
42	Nebraska	521	0.4%
33	Nevada	677	0.5%
41	New Hampshire	528	0.4%
8	New Jersey	5,783	4.3%
35	New Mexico	648	0.5%
1	New York	16,908	12.6%
12	North Carolina	3,258	2.4%
46	North Dakota	236	0.2%
9	Ohio	4,993	3.7%
29	Oklahoma	873	0.6%
26	Oregon	1,538	1.1%
3	Pennsylvania	6,946	5.2%
30	Rhode Island	847	0.6%
28	South Carolina	1,286	1.0%
48	South Dakota	220	0.2%
17	Tennessee	2,484	1.8%
5	Texas	6,661	5.0%
39	Utah	609	0.5%
43	Vermont	400	0.3%
13	Virginia	3,114	2.3%
18	Washington	2,324	1.7%
35	West Virginia	648	0.5%
20	Wisconsin	2,136	1.6%
50	Wyoming	90	0.1%

RANK ORDER

RANK	STATE	PHYSICIANS	% of USA
1	New York	16,908	12.6%
2	California	15,359	11.4%
3	Pennsylvania	6,946	5.2%
4	Illinois	6,894	5.1%
5	Texas	6,661	5.0%
6	Florida	6,637	4.9%
7	Massachusetts	6,331	4.7%
8	New Jersey	5,783	4.3%
9	Ohio	4,993	3.7%
10	Michigan	4,501	3.3%
11	Maryland	4,383	3.3%
12	North Carolina	3,258	2.4%
13	Virginia	3,114	2.3%
14	Georgia	3,098	2.3%
15	Connecticut	2,912	2.2%
16	Missouri	2,545	1.9%
17	Tennessee	2,484	1.8%
18	Washington	2,324	1.7%
19	Minnesota	2,271	1.7%
20	Wisconsin	2,136	1.6%
21	Louisiana	1,884	1.4%
22	Indiana	1,841	1.4%
23	Colorado	1,663	1.2%
24	Arizona	1,662	1.2%
25	Alabama	1,657	1.2%
26	Oregon	1,538	1.1%
27	Kentucky	1,373	1.0%
28	South Carolina	1,286	1.0%
29	Oklahoma	873	0.6%
30	Rhode Island	847	0.6%
31	Kansas	828	0.6%
32	Mississippi	713	0.5%
33	Nevada	677	0.5%
34	Hawaii	664	0.5%
35	New Mexico	648	0.5%
35	West Virginia	648	0.5%
37	Arkansas	643	0.5%
38	Iowa	632	0.5%
39	Utah	609	0.5%
40	Maine	531	0.4%
41	New Hampshire	528	0.4%
42	Nebraska	521	0.4%
43	Vermont	400	0.3%
44	Delaware	336	0.2%
45	Montana	263	0.2%
46	North Dakota	236	0.2%
47	Idaho	232	0.2%
48	South Dakota	220	0.2%
49	Alaska	137	0.1%
50	Wyoming	90	0.1%
	District of Columbia	782	0.6%

Source: American Medical Association (Chicago, Illinois)
"Physician Characteristics and Distribution in the U.S." (2003-2004 Edition)
*As of December 31, 2001. Total does not include 1,434 physicians in U.S. territories and possessions. Internal Medicine includes Diabetes, Endocrinology, Geriatrics, Hematology, Infectious Diseases, Nephrology, Nutrition, Medical Oncology and Rheumatology.

Rate of Nonfederal Physicians in Internal Medicine in 2001

National Rate = 47 Physicians per 100,000 Population*

ALPHA ORDER

RANK	STATE	RATE
28	Alabama	37
47	Alaska	22
36	Arizona	31
46	Arkansas	24
14	California	44
27	Colorado	38
3	Connecticut	85
19	Delaware	42
22	Florida	41
28	Georgia	37
10	Hawaii	54
49	Idaho	18
9	Illinois	55
39	Indiana	30
47	Iowa	22
36	Kansas	31
33	Kentucky	34
19	Louisiana	42
22	Maine	41
4	Maryland	81
1	Massachusetts	99
12	Michigan	45
11	Minnesota	46
44	Mississippi	25
12	Missouri	45
41	Montana	29
39	Nebraska	30
34	Nevada	32
19	New Hampshire	42
6	New Jersey	68
32	New Mexico	35
2	New York	89
24	North Carolina	40
28	North Dakota	37
14	Ohio	44
44	Oklahoma	25
14	Oregon	44
8	Pennsylvania	56
5	Rhode Island	80
34	South Carolina	32
41	South Dakota	29
17	Tennessee	43
36	Texas	31
43	Utah	27
7	Vermont	65
17	Virginia	43
26	Washington	39
31	West Virginia	36
24	Wisconsin	40
49	Wyoming	18

RANK ORDER

RANK	STATE	RATE
1	Massachusetts	99
2	New York	89
3	Connecticut	85
4	Maryland	81
5	Rhode Island	80
6	New Jersey	68
7	Vermont	65
8	Pennsylvania	56
9	Illinois	55
10	Hawaii	54
11	Minnesota	46
12	Michigan	45
12	Missouri	45
14	California	44
14	Ohio	44
14	Oregon	44
17	Tennessee	43
17	Virginia	43
19	Delaware	42
19	Louisiana	42
19	New Hampshire	42
22	Florida	41
22	Maine	41
24	North Carolina	40
24	Wisconsin	40
26	Washington	39
27	Colorado	38
28	Alabama	37
28	Georgia	37
28	North Dakota	37
31	West Virginia	36
32	New Mexico	35
33	Kentucky	34
34	Nevada	32
34	South Carolina	32
36	Arizona	31
36	Kansas	31
36	Texas	31
39	Indiana	30
39	Nebraska	30
41	Montana	29
41	South Dakota	29
43	Utah	27
44	Mississippi	25
44	Oklahoma	25
46	Arkansas	24
47	Alaska	22
47	Iowa	22
49	Idaho	18
49	Wyoming	18

District of Columbia 136

Source: Morgan Quitno Press using data from American Medical Association (Chicago, Illinois)
    "Physician Characteristics and Distribution in the U.S." (2003-2004 Edition)
*As of December 31, 2001. National rate does not include physicians in U.S. territories and possessions. Internal Medicine includes Diabetes, Endocrinology, Geriatrics, Hematology, Infectious Diseases, Nephrology, Nutrition, Medical Oncology and Rheumatology.

Nonfederal Physicians in Pediatrics in 2001

National Total = 62,878 Physicians*

RANK	STATE	PHYSICIANS	% of USA
26	Alabama	750	1.2%
47	Alaska	97	0.2%
23	Arizona	871	1.4%
30	Arkansas	432	0.7%
1	California	7,578	12.1%
24	Colorado	834	1.3%
18	Connecticut	1,066	1.7%
43	Delaware	211	0.3%
4	Florida	3,197	5.1%
14	Georgia	1,533	2.4%
36	Hawaii	332	0.5%
46	Idaho	103	0.2%
5	Illinois	2,869	4.6%
21	Indiana	943	1.5%
35	Iowa	342	0.5%
31	Kansas	406	0.6%
25	Kentucky	762	1.2%
19	Louisiana	1,025	1.6%
42	Maine	220	0.3%
11	Maryland	1,941	3.1%
9	Massachusetts	2,392	3.8%
10	Michigan	2,009	3.2%
22	Minnesota	928	1.5%
33	Mississippi	375	0.6%
16	Missouri	1,181	1.9%
45	Montana	104	0.2%
39	Nebraska	299	0.5%
40	Nevada	257	0.4%
41	New Hampshire	246	0.4%
6	New Jersey	2,746	4.4%
37	New Mexico	316	0.5%
2	New York	7,067	11.2%
12	North Carolina	1,724	2.7%
48	North Dakota	72	0.1%
8	Ohio	2,665	4.2%
32	Oklahoma	402	0.6%
28	Oregon	551	0.9%
7	Pennsylvania	2,679	4.3%
34	Rhode Island	367	0.6%
27	South Carolina	679	1.1%
49	South Dakota	69	0.1%
15	Tennessee	1,337	2.1%
3	Texas	3,867	6.2%
29	Utah	462	0.7%
44	Vermont	176	0.3%
13	Virginia	1,582	2.5%
17	Washington	1,083	1.7%
38	West Virginia	306	0.5%
20	Wisconsin	983	1.6%
50	Wyoming	44	0.1%

RANK	STATE	PHYSICIANS	% of USA
1	California	7,578	12.1%
2	New York	7,067	11.2%
3	Texas	3,867	6.2%
4	Florida	3,197	5.1%
5	Illinois	2,869	4.6%
6	New Jersey	2,746	4.4%
7	Pennsylvania	2,679	4.3%
8	Ohio	2,665	4.2%
9	Massachusetts	2,392	3.8%
10	Michigan	2,009	3.2%
11	Maryland	1,941	3.1%
12	North Carolina	1,724	2.7%
13	Virginia	1,582	2.5%
14	Georgia	1,533	2.4%
15	Tennessee	1,337	2.1%
16	Missouri	1,181	1.9%
17	Washington	1,083	1.7%
18	Connecticut	1,066	1.7%
19	Louisiana	1,025	1.6%
20	Wisconsin	983	1.6%
21	Indiana	943	1.5%
22	Minnesota	928	1.5%
23	Arizona	871	1.4%
24	Colorado	834	1.3%
25	Kentucky	762	1.2%
26	Alabama	750	1.2%
27	South Carolina	679	1.1%
28	Oregon	551	0.9%
29	Utah	462	0.7%
30	Arkansas	432	0.7%
31	Kansas	406	0.6%
32	Oklahoma	402	0.6%
33	Mississippi	375	0.6%
34	Rhode Island	367	0.6%
35	Iowa	342	0.5%
36	Hawaii	332	0.5%
37	New Mexico	316	0.5%
38	West Virginia	306	0.5%
39	Nebraska	299	0.5%
40	Nevada	257	0.4%
41	New Hampshire	246	0.4%
42	Maine	220	0.3%
43	Delaware	211	0.3%
44	Vermont	176	0.3%
45	Montana	104	0.2%
46	Idaho	103	0.2%
47	Alaska	97	0.2%
48	North Dakota	72	0.1%
49	South Dakota	69	0.1%
50	Wyoming	44	0.1%
	District of Columbia	398	0.6%

Source: American Medical Association (Chicago, Illinois)
"Physician Characteristics and Distribution in the U.S." (2003-2004 Edition)
As of December 31, 2001. Total does not include 1,132 physicians in U.S. territories and possessions. Pediatrics includes Adolescent Medicine, Neonatal-Perinatal, Pediatric Allergy, Pediatric Endocrinology, Pediatric Pulmonology, Pediatric Hematology-Oncology and Pediatric Nephrology.

Rate of Nonfederal Physicians in Pediatrics in 2001

National Rate = 87 Physicians per 100,000 Population 17 Years and Younger*

<table>
<tr><td colspan="3">ALPHA ORDER</td><td colspan="3">RANK ORDER</td></tr>
<tr><td>RANK</td><td>STATE</td><td>RATE</td><td>RANK</td><td>STATE</td><td>RATE</td></tr>
<tr><td>30</td><td>Alabama</td><td>67</td><td>1</td><td>Massachusetts</td><td>159</td></tr>
<tr><td>41</td><td>Alaska</td><td>51</td><td>2</td><td>New York</td><td>151</td></tr>
<tr><td>35</td><td>Arizona</td><td>64</td><td>3</td><td>Rhode Island</td><td>148</td></tr>
<tr><td>37</td><td>Arkansas</td><td>63</td><td>4</td><td>Maryland</td><td>143</td></tr>
<tr><td>19</td><td>California</td><td>82</td><td>5</td><td>New Jersey</td><td>132</td></tr>
<tr><td>23</td><td>Colorado</td><td>76</td><td>6</td><td>Connecticut</td><td>127</td></tr>
<tr><td>6</td><td>Connecticut</td><td>127</td><td>7</td><td>Vermont</td><td>119</td></tr>
<tr><td>9</td><td>Delaware</td><td>108</td><td>8</td><td>Hawaii</td><td>112</td></tr>
<tr><td>14</td><td>Florida</td><td>88</td><td>9</td><td>Delaware</td><td>108</td></tr>
<tr><td>29</td><td>Georgia</td><td>71</td><td>10</td><td>Tennessee</td><td>96</td></tr>
<tr><td>8</td><td>Hawaii</td><td>112</td><td>11</td><td>Ohio</td><td>92</td></tr>
<tr><td>50</td><td>Idaho</td><td>28</td><td>11</td><td>Pennsylvania</td><td>92</td></tr>
<tr><td>14</td><td>Illinois</td><td>88</td><td>13</td><td>Virginia</td><td>91</td></tr>
<tr><td>39</td><td>Indiana</td><td>60</td><td>14</td><td>Florida</td><td>88</td></tr>
<tr><td>44</td><td>Iowa</td><td>47</td><td>14</td><td>Illinois</td><td>88</td></tr>
<tr><td>40</td><td>Kansas</td><td>57</td><td>14</td><td>North Carolina</td><td>88</td></tr>
<tr><td>21</td><td>Kentucky</td><td>77</td><td>17</td><td>Louisiana</td><td>84</td></tr>
<tr><td>17</td><td>Louisiana</td><td>84</td><td>18</td><td>Missouri</td><td>83</td></tr>
<tr><td>25</td><td>Maine</td><td>73</td><td>19</td><td>California</td><td>82</td></tr>
<tr><td>4</td><td>Maryland</td><td>143</td><td>20</td><td>New Hampshire</td><td>79</td></tr>
<tr><td>1</td><td>Massachusetts</td><td>159</td><td>21</td><td>Kentucky</td><td>77</td></tr>
<tr><td>21</td><td>Michigan</td><td>77</td><td>21</td><td>Michigan</td><td>77</td></tr>
<tr><td>26</td><td>Minnesota</td><td>72</td><td>23</td><td>Colorado</td><td>76</td></tr>
<tr><td>43</td><td>Mississippi</td><td>48</td><td>23</td><td>West Virginia</td><td>76</td></tr>
<tr><td>18</td><td>Missouri</td><td>83</td><td>25</td><td>Maine</td><td>73</td></tr>
<tr><td>45</td><td>Montana</td><td>45</td><td>26</td><td>Minnesota</td><td>72</td></tr>
<tr><td>32</td><td>Nebraska</td><td>66</td><td>26</td><td>Washington</td><td>72</td></tr>
<tr><td>42</td><td>Nevada</td><td>50</td><td>26</td><td>Wisconsin</td><td>72</td></tr>
<tr><td>20</td><td>New Hampshire</td><td>79</td><td>29</td><td>Georgia</td><td>71</td></tr>
<tr><td>5</td><td>New Jersey</td><td>132</td><td>30</td><td>Alabama</td><td>67</td></tr>
<tr><td>38</td><td>New Mexico</td><td>62</td><td>30</td><td>South Carolina</td><td>67</td></tr>
<tr><td>2</td><td>New York</td><td>151</td><td>32</td><td>Nebraska</td><td>66</td></tr>
<tr><td>14</td><td>North Carolina</td><td>88</td><td>32</td><td>Texas</td><td>66</td></tr>
<tr><td>45</td><td>North Dakota</td><td>45</td><td>34</td><td>Oregon</td><td>65</td></tr>
<tr><td>11</td><td>Ohio</td><td>92</td><td>35</td><td>Arizona</td><td>64</td></tr>
<tr><td>45</td><td>Oklahoma</td><td>45</td><td>35</td><td>Utah</td><td>64</td></tr>
<tr><td>34</td><td>Oregon</td><td>65</td><td>37</td><td>Arkansas</td><td>63</td></tr>
<tr><td>11</td><td>Pennsylvania</td><td>92</td><td>38</td><td>New Mexico</td><td>62</td></tr>
<tr><td>3</td><td>Rhode Island</td><td>148</td><td>39</td><td>Indiana</td><td>60</td></tr>
<tr><td>30</td><td>South Carolina</td><td>67</td><td>40</td><td>Kansas</td><td>57</td></tr>
<tr><td>48</td><td>South Dakota</td><td>34</td><td>41</td><td>Alaska</td><td>51</td></tr>
<tr><td>10</td><td>Tennessee</td><td>96</td><td>42</td><td>Nevada</td><td>50</td></tr>
<tr><td>32</td><td>Texas</td><td>66</td><td>43</td><td>Mississippi</td><td>48</td></tr>
<tr><td>35</td><td>Utah</td><td>64</td><td>44</td><td>Iowa</td><td>47</td></tr>
<tr><td>7</td><td>Vermont</td><td>119</td><td>45</td><td>Montana</td><td>45</td></tr>
<tr><td>13</td><td>Virginia</td><td>91</td><td>45</td><td>North Dakota</td><td>45</td></tr>
<tr><td>26</td><td>Washington</td><td>72</td><td>45</td><td>Oklahoma</td><td>45</td></tr>
<tr><td>23</td><td>West Virginia</td><td>76</td><td>48</td><td>South Dakota</td><td>34</td></tr>
<tr><td>26</td><td>Wisconsin</td><td>72</td><td>48</td><td>Wyoming</td><td>34</td></tr>
<tr><td>48</td><td>Wyoming</td><td>34</td><td>50</td><td>Idaho</td><td>28</td></tr>
<tr><td colspan="3"></td><td></td><td>District of Columbia</td><td>346</td></tr>
</table>

Source: Morgan Quitno Press using data from American Medical Association (Chicago, Illinois)
   "Physician Characteristics and Distribution in the U.S." (2003-2004 Edition)
*As of December 31, 2001. National rate does not include physicians in U.S. territories and possessions. Pediatrics includes Adolescent Medicine, Neonatal-Perinatal, Pediatric Allergy, Pediatric Endocrinology, Pediatric Pulmonology, Pediatric Hematology-Oncology and Pediatric Nephrology.

Nonfederal Physicians in Surgical Specialties in 2001

National Total = 152,803 Physicians*

ALPHA ORDER

RANK	STATE	PHYSICIANS	% of USA
25	Alabama	2,188	1.4%
49	Alaska	258	0.2%
23	Arizona	2,276	1.5%
33	Arkansas	1,104	0.7%
1	California	17,493	11.4%
24	Colorado	2,211	1.4%
21	Connecticut	2,531	1.7%
46	Delaware	412	0.3%
4	Florida	8,628	5.6%
12	Georgia	4,126	2.7%
38	Hawaii	768	0.5%
43	Idaho	538	0.4%
6	Illinois	6,398	4.2%
20	Indiana	2,577	1.7%
32	Iowa	1,118	0.7%
31	Kansas	1,209	0.8%
27	Kentucky	1,951	1.3%
18	Louisiana	2,838	1.9%
42	Maine	650	0.4%
14	Maryland	3,990	2.6%
10	Massachusetts	4,592	3.0%
9	Michigan	4,893	3.2%
22	Minnesota	2,495	1.6%
30	Mississippi	1,257	0.8%
16	Missouri	2,944	1.9%
44	Montana	465	0.3%
36	Nebraska	849	0.6%
37	Nevada	824	0.5%
41	New Hampshire	686	0.4%
8	New Jersey	5,348	3.5%
39	New Mexico	746	0.5%
2	New York	14,043	9.2%
11	North Carolina	4,373	2.9%
48	North Dakota	279	0.2%
7	Ohio	5,976	3.9%
29	Oklahoma	1,271	0.8%
28	Oregon	1,784	1.2%
5	Pennsylvania	7,545	4.9%
40	Rhode Island	732	0.5%
26	South Carolina	2,121	1.4%
47	South Dakota	340	0.2%
15	Tennessee	3,305	2.2%
3	Texas	9,783	6.4%
34	Utah	1,051	0.7%
45	Vermont	418	0.3%
13	Virginia	3,992	2.6%
17	Washington	2,936	1.9%
35	West Virginia	898	0.6%
19	Wisconsin	2,586	1.7%
50	Wyoming	212	0.1%

RANK ORDER

RANK	STATE	PHYSICIANS	% of USA
1	California	17,493	11.4%
2	New York	14,043	9.2%
3	Texas	9,783	6.4%
4	Florida	8,628	5.6%
5	Pennsylvania	7,545	4.9%
6	Illinois	6,398	4.2%
7	Ohio	5,976	3.9%
8	New Jersey	5,348	3.5%
9	Michigan	4,893	3.2%
10	Massachusetts	4,592	3.0%
11	North Carolina	4,373	2.9%
12	Georgia	4,126	2.7%
13	Virginia	3,992	2.6%
14	Maryland	3,990	2.6%
15	Tennessee	3,305	2.2%
16	Missouri	2,944	1.9%
17	Washington	2,936	1.9%
18	Louisiana	2,838	1.9%
19	Wisconsin	2,586	1.7%
20	Indiana	2,577	1.7%
21	Connecticut	2,531	1.7%
22	Minnesota	2,495	1.6%
23	Arizona	2,276	1.5%
24	Colorado	2,211	1.4%
25	Alabama	2,188	1.4%
26	South Carolina	2,121	1.4%
27	Kentucky	1,951	1.3%
28	Oregon	1,784	1.2%
29	Oklahoma	1,271	0.8%
30	Mississippi	1,257	0.8%
31	Kansas	1,209	0.8%
32	Iowa	1,118	0.7%
33	Arkansas	1,104	0.7%
34	Utah	1,051	0.7%
35	West Virginia	898	0.6%
36	Nebraska	849	0.6%
37	Nevada	824	0.5%
38	Hawaii	768	0.5%
39	New Mexico	746	0.5%
40	Rhode Island	732	0.5%
41	New Hampshire	686	0.4%
42	Maine	650	0.4%
43	Idaho	538	0.4%
44	Montana	465	0.3%
45	Vermont	418	0.3%
46	Delaware	412	0.3%
47	South Dakota	340	0.2%
48	North Dakota	279	0.2%
49	Alaska	258	0.2%
50	Wyoming	212	0.1%
	District of Columbia	795	0.5%

Source: American Medical Association (Chicago, Illinois)
"Physician Characteristics and Distribution in the U.S." (2003-2004 Edition)
*As of December 31, 2001. Total does not include 1,763 physicians in U.S. territories and possessions. Surgical Specialties include Colon and Rectal, General, Neurological, Obstetrics & Gynecology, Ophthalmology, Orthopedic, Otolaryngology, Plastic, Thoracic and Urological Surgeries.

Rate of Nonfederal Physicians in Surgical Specialties in 2001

National Rate = 54 Physicians per 100,000 Population*

ALPHA ORDER

RANK	STATE	RATE
28	Alabama	49
44	Alaska	41
41	Arizona	43
44	Arkansas	41
20	California	51
25	Colorado	50
1	Connecticut	74
16	Delaware	52
14	Florida	53
28	Georgia	49
7	Hawaii	63
44	Idaho	41
20	Illinois	51
43	Indiana	42
49	Iowa	38
37	Kansas	45
33	Kentucky	48
7	Louisiana	63
20	Maine	51
1	Maryland	74
4	Massachusetts	72
28	Michigan	49
25	Minnesota	50
39	Mississippi	44
16	Missouri	52
20	Montana	51
28	Nebraska	49
48	Nevada	39
13	New Hampshire	54
7	New Jersey	63
44	New Mexico	41
1	New York	74
14	North Carolina	53
39	North Dakota	44
16	Ohio	52
50	Oklahoma	37
20	Oregon	51
10	Pennsylvania	61
5	Rhode Island	69
16	South Carolina	52
37	South Dakota	45
11	Tennessee	57
35	Texas	46
35	Utah	46
6	Vermont	68
12	Virginia	55
28	Washington	49
25	West Virginia	50
33	Wisconsin	48
41	Wyoming	43

RANK ORDER

RANK	STATE	RATE
1	Connecticut	74
1	Maryland	74
1	New York	74
4	Massachusetts	72
5	Rhode Island	69
6	Vermont	68
7	Hawaii	63
7	Louisiana	63
7	New Jersey	63
10	Pennsylvania	61
11	Tennessee	57
12	Virginia	55
13	New Hampshire	54
14	Florida	53
14	North Carolina	53
16	Delaware	52
16	Missouri	52
16	Ohio	52
16	South Carolina	52
20	California	51
20	Illinois	51
20	Maine	51
20	Montana	51
20	Oregon	51
25	Colorado	50
25	Minnesota	50
25	West Virginia	50
28	Alabama	49
28	Georgia	49
28	Michigan	49
28	Nebraska	49
28	Washington	49
33	Kentucky	48
33	Wisconsin	48
35	Texas	46
35	Utah	46
37	Kansas	45
37	South Dakota	45
39	Mississippi	44
39	North Dakota	44
41	Arizona	43
41	Wyoming	43
43	Indiana	42
44	Alaska	41
44	Arkansas	41
44	Idaho	41
44	New Mexico	41
48	Nevada	39
49	Iowa	38
50	Oklahoma	37

| | District of Columbia | 139 |

Source: Morgan Quitno Press using data from American Medical Association (Chicago, Illinois)
   "Physician Characteristics and Distribution in the U.S." (2003-2004 Edition)
As of December 31, 2001. National rate does not include physicians in U.S. territories and possessions. Surgical Specialties include Colon and Rectal, General, Neurological, Obstetrics & Gynecology, Ophthalmology, Orthopedic, Otolaryngology, Plastic, Thoracic and Urological Surgeries.

Nonfederal Physicians in General Surgery in 2001

National Total = 36,034 Physicians*

ALPHA ORDER

RANK	STATE	PHYSICIANS	% of USA
23	Alabama	528	1.5%
49	Alaska	53	0.1%
24	Arizona	523	1.5%
33	Arkansas	265	0.7%
1	California	3,733	10.4%
27	Colorado	490	1.4%
20	Connecticut	596	1.7%
45	Delaware	107	0.3%
5	Florida	1,735	4.8%
12	Georgia	973	2.7%
42	Hawaii	169	0.5%
43	Idaho	121	0.3%
6	Illinois	1,558	4.3%
22	Indiana	565	1.6%
31	Iowa	286	0.8%
29	Kansas	301	0.8%
26	Kentucky	507	1.4%
17	Louisiana	650	1.8%
41	Maine	170	0.5%
13	Maryland	928	2.6%
10	Massachusetts	1,202	3.3%
9	Michigan	1,250	3.5%
21	Minnesota	568	1.6%
30	Mississippi	292	0.8%
16	Missouri	703	2.0%
46	Montana	101	0.3%
35	Nebraska	226	0.6%
39	Nevada	183	0.5%
40	New Hampshire	171	0.5%
8	New Jersey	1,281	3.6%
37	New Mexico	193	0.5%
2	New York	3,583	9.9%
11	North Carolina	1,024	2.8%
48	North Dakota	75	0.2%
7	Ohio	1,532	4.3%
32	Oklahoma	282	0.8%
28	Oregon	408	1.1%
4	Pennsylvania	1,963	5.4%
38	Rhode Island	186	0.5%
25	South Carolina	514	1.4%
47	South Dakota	88	0.2%
15	Tennessee	814	2.3%
3	Texas	2,137	5.9%
36	Utah	196	0.5%
44	Vermont	120	0.3%
14	Virginia	912	2.5%
18	Washington	640	1.8%
34	West Virginia	251	0.7%
19	Wisconsin	619	1.7%
50	Wyoming	48	0.1%

RANK ORDER

RANK	STATE	PHYSICIANS	% of USA
1	California	3,733	10.4%
2	New York	3,583	9.9%
3	Texas	2,137	5.9%
4	Pennsylvania	1,963	5.4%
5	Florida	1,735	4.8%
6	Illinois	1,558	4.3%
7	Ohio	1,532	4.3%
8	New Jersey	1,281	3.6%
9	Michigan	1,250	3.5%
10	Massachusetts	1,202	3.3%
11	North Carolina	1,024	2.8%
12	Georgia	973	2.7%
13	Maryland	928	2.6%
14	Virginia	912	2.5%
15	Tennessee	814	2.3%
16	Missouri	703	2.0%
17	Louisiana	650	1.8%
18	Washington	640	1.8%
19	Wisconsin	619	1.7%
20	Connecticut	596	1.7%
21	Minnesota	568	1.6%
22	Indiana	565	1.6%
23	Alabama	528	1.5%
24	Arizona	523	1.5%
25	South Carolina	514	1.4%
26	Kentucky	507	1.4%
27	Colorado	490	1.4%
28	Oregon	408	1.1%
29	Kansas	301	0.8%
30	Mississippi	292	0.8%
31	Iowa	286	0.8%
32	Oklahoma	282	0.8%
33	Arkansas	265	0.7%
34	West Virginia	251	0.7%
35	Nebraska	226	0.6%
36	Utah	196	0.5%
37	New Mexico	193	0.5%
38	Rhode Island	186	0.5%
39	Nevada	183	0.5%
40	New Hampshire	171	0.5%
41	Maine	170	0.5%
42	Hawaii	169	0.5%
43	Idaho	121	0.3%
44	Vermont	120	0.3%
45	Delaware	107	0.3%
46	Montana	101	0.3%
47	South Dakota	88	0.2%
48	North Dakota	75	0.2%
49	Alaska	53	0.1%
50	Wyoming	48	0.1%
	District of Columbia	214	0.6%

Source: American Medical Association (Chicago, Illinois)
"Physician Characteristics and Distribution in the U.S." (2003-2004 Edition)
*As of December 31, 2001. Total does not include 478 physicians in U.S. territories and possessions. General Surgery includes Abdominal, Cardiovascular, Hand, Head and Neck, Pediatric, Traumatic and Vascular Surgeries.

Rate of Nonfederal Physicians in General Surgery in 2001

National Rate = 12.6 Physicians per 100,000 Population*

ALPHA ORDER

RANK	STATE	RATE
25	Alabama	11.8
49	Alaska	8.4
41	Arizona	9.9
42	Arkansas	9.8
35	California	10.8
33	Colorado	11.1
5	Connecticut	17.4
15	Delaware	13.4
37	Florida	10.6
28	Georgia	11.6
12	Hawaii	13.8
45	Idaho	9.2
24	Illinois	12.4
45	Indiana	9.2
42	Iowa	9.8
33	Kansas	11.1
20	Kentucky	12.5
9	Louisiana	14.5
16	Maine	13.2
6	Maryland	17.2
2	Massachusetts	18.8
20	Michigan	12.5
31	Minnesota	11.4
39	Mississippi	10.2
20	Missouri	12.5
32	Montana	11.2
17	Nebraska	13.1
47	Nevada	8.7
13	New Hampshire	13.6
8	New Jersey	15.1
38	New Mexico	10.5
2	New York	18.8
20	North Carolina	12.5
25	North Dakota	11.8
14	Ohio	13.5
50	Oklahoma	8.1
27	Oregon	11.7
7	Pennsylvania	16.0
4	Rhode Island	17.6
18	South Carolina	12.7
28	South Dakota	11.6
10	Tennessee	14.2
40	Texas	10.0
48	Utah	8.6
1	Vermont	19.6
18	Virginia	12.7
36	Washington	10.7
11	West Virginia	13.9
30	Wisconsin	11.5
44	Wyoming	9.7

RANK ORDER

RANK	STATE	RATE
1	Vermont	19.6
2	Massachusetts	18.8
2	New York	18.8
4	Rhode Island	17.6
5	Connecticut	17.4
6	Maryland	17.2
7	Pennsylvania	16.0
8	New Jersey	15.1
9	Louisiana	14.5
10	Tennessee	14.2
11	West Virginia	13.9
12	Hawaii	13.8
13	New Hampshire	13.6
14	Ohio	13.5
15	Delaware	13.4
16	Maine	13.2
17	Nebraska	13.1
18	South Carolina	12.7
18	Virginia	12.7
20	Kentucky	12.5
20	Michigan	12.5
20	Missouri	12.5
20	North Carolina	12.5
24	Illinois	12.4
25	Alabama	11.8
25	North Dakota	11.8
27	Oregon	11.7
28	Georgia	11.6
28	South Dakota	11.6
30	Wisconsin	11.5
31	Minnesota	11.4
32	Montana	11.2
33	Colorado	11.1
33	Kansas	11.1
35	California	10.8
36	Washington	10.7
37	Florida	10.6
38	New Mexico	10.5
39	Mississippi	10.2
40	Texas	10.0
41	Arizona	9.9
42	Arkansas	9.8
42	Iowa	9.8
44	Wyoming	9.7
45	Idaho	9.2
45	Indiana	9.2
47	Nevada	8.7
48	Utah	8.6
49	Alaska	8.4
50	Oklahoma	8.1

	District of Columbia	37.3

Source: Morgan Quitno Press using data from American Medical Association (Chicago, Illinois)
"Physician Characteristics and Distribution in the U.S." (2003-2004 Edition)
*As of December 31, 2001. National rate does not include physicians in U.S. territories and possessions. General Surgery includes Abdominal, Cardiovascular, Hand, Head and Neck, Pediatric, Traumatic and Vascular Surgeries.

Nonfederal Physicians in Obstetrics and Gynecology in 2001

National Total = 39,906 Physicians*

ALPHA ORDER

RANK	STATE	PHYSICIANS	% of USA
21	Alabama	624	1.6%
47	Alaska	70	0.2%
22	Arizona	616	1.5%
33	Arkansas	250	0.6%
1	California	4,655	11.7%
23	Colorado	577	1.4%
19	Connecticut	695	1.7%
44	Delaware	106	0.3%
4	Florida	2,071	5.2%
10	Georgia	1,283	3.2%
35	Hawaii	236	0.6%
43	Idaho	115	0.3%
5	Illinois	1,826	4.6%
20	Indiana	650	1.6%
36	Iowa	213	0.5%
31	Kansas	272	0.7%
27	Kentucky	480	1.2%
16	Louisiana	730	1.8%
42	Maine	154	0.4%
14	Maryland	1,118	2.8%
12	Massachusetts	1,141	2.9%
9	Michigan	1,353	3.4%
26	Minnesota	550	1.4%
29	Mississippi	328	0.8%
16	Missouri	730	1.8%
46	Montana	99	0.2%
41	Nebraska	176	0.4%
34	Nevada	243	0.6%
39	New Hampshire	185	0.5%
7	New Jersey	1,560	3.9%
39	New Mexico	185	0.5%
2	New York	3,714	9.3%
11	North Carolina	1,197	3.0%
50	North Dakota	50	0.1%
8	Ohio	1,540	3.9%
30	Oklahoma	298	0.7%
28	Oregon	446	1.1%
6	Pennsylvania	1,770	4.4%
38	Rhode Island	198	0.5%
24	South Carolina	574	1.4%
48	South Dakota	67	0.2%
15	Tennessee	825	2.1%
3	Texas	2,691	6.7%
32	Utah	265	0.7%
45	Vermont	101	0.3%
13	Virginia	1,131	2.8%
18	Washington	704	1.8%
37	West Virginia	211	0.5%
25	Wisconsin	561	1.4%
49	Wyoming	52	0.1%

RANK ORDER

RANK	STATE	PHYSICIANS	% of USA
1	California	4,655	11.7%
2	New York	3,714	9.3%
3	Texas	2,691	6.7%
4	Florida	2,071	5.2%
5	Illinois	1,826	4.6%
6	Pennsylvania	1,770	4.4%
7	New Jersey	1,560	3.9%
8	Ohio	1,540	3.9%
9	Michigan	1,353	3.4%
10	Georgia	1,283	3.2%
11	North Carolina	1,197	3.0%
12	Massachusetts	1,141	2.9%
13	Virginia	1,131	2.8%
14	Maryland	1,118	2.8%
15	Tennessee	825	2.1%
16	Louisiana	730	1.8%
16	Missouri	730	1.8%
18	Washington	704	1.8%
19	Connecticut	695	1.7%
20	Indiana	650	1.6%
21	Alabama	624	1.6%
22	Arizona	616	1.5%
23	Colorado	577	1.4%
24	South Carolina	574	1.4%
25	Wisconsin	561	1.4%
26	Minnesota	550	1.4%
27	Kentucky	480	1.2%
28	Oregon	446	1.1%
29	Mississippi	328	0.8%
30	Oklahoma	298	0.7%
31	Kansas	272	0.7%
32	Utah	265	0.7%
33	Arkansas	250	0.6%
34	Nevada	243	0.6%
35	Hawaii	236	0.6%
36	Iowa	213	0.5%
37	West Virginia	211	0.5%
38	Rhode Island	198	0.5%
39	New Hampshire	185	0.5%
39	New Mexico	185	0.5%
41	Nebraska	176	0.4%
42	Maine	154	0.4%
43	Idaho	115	0.3%
44	Delaware	106	0.3%
45	Vermont	101	0.3%
46	Montana	99	0.2%
47	Alaska	70	0.2%
48	South Dakota	67	0.2%
49	Wyoming	52	0.1%
50	North Dakota	50	0.1%
	District of Columbia	220	0.6%

Source: American Medical Association (Chicago, Illinois)
  "Physician Characteristics and Distribution in the U.S." (2003-2004 Edition)
*As of December 31, 2001. Total does not include 548 physicians in U.S. territories and possessions. Obstetrics and Gynecology includes Gynecology and Oncology, Maternal and Fetal Medicine and Reproductive Endocrinology.

Rate of Nonfederal Physicians in Obstetrics and Gynecology in 2001

National Rate = 28 Physicians per 100,000 Female Population*

ALPHA ORDER

RANK	STATE	RATE
18	Alabama	27
33	Alaska	23
29	Arizona	24
45	Arkansas	18
18	California	27
18	Colorado	27
2	Connecticut	40
22	Delaware	26
26	Florida	25
10	Georgia	31
3	Hawaii	39
45	Idaho	18
12	Illinois	29
39	Indiana	21
50	Iowa	14
42	Kansas	20
33	Kentucky	23
9	Louisiana	32
29	Maine	24
1	Maryland	41
7	Massachusetts	35
18	Michigan	27
36	Minnesota	22
36	Mississippi	22
26	Missouri	25
36	Montana	22
42	Nebraska	20
26	Nevada	25
12	New Hampshire	29
5	New Jersey	36
42	New Mexico	20
4	New York	38
12	North Carolina	29
49	North Dakota	16
22	Ohio	26
48	Oklahoma	17
22	Oregon	26
15	Pennsylvania	28
5	Rhode Island	36
15	South Carolina	28
45	South Dakota	18
15	Tennessee	28
22	Texas	26
29	Utah	24
8	Vermont	33
10	Virginia	31
29	Washington	24
33	West Virginia	23
39	Wisconsin	21
39	Wyoming	21

RANK ORDER

RANK	STATE	RATE
1	Maryland	41
2	Connecticut	40
3	Hawaii	39
4	New York	38
5	New Jersey	36
5	Rhode Island	36
7	Massachusetts	35
8	Vermont	33
9	Louisiana	32
10	Georgia	31
10	Virginia	31
12	Illinois	29
12	New Hampshire	29
12	North Carolina	29
15	Pennsylvania	28
15	South Carolina	28
15	Tennessee	28
18	Alabama	27
18	California	27
18	Colorado	27
18	Michigan	27
22	Delaware	26
22	Ohio	26
22	Oregon	26
22	Texas	26
26	Florida	25
26	Missouri	25
26	Nevada	25
29	Arizona	24
29	Maine	24
29	Utah	24
29	Washington	24
33	Alaska	23
33	Kentucky	23
33	West Virginia	23
36	Minnesota	22
36	Mississippi	22
36	Montana	22
39	Indiana	21
39	Wisconsin	21
39	Wyoming	21
42	Kansas	20
42	Nebraska	20
42	New Mexico	20
45	Arkansas	18
45	Idaho	18
45	South Dakota	18
48	Oklahoma	17
49	North Dakota	16
50	Iowa	14

District of Columbia	73

Source: Morgan Quitno Press using data from American Medical Association (Chicago, Illinois)
"Physician Characteristics and Distribution in the U.S." (2003-2004 Edition)
*As of December 31, 2001. National rate does not include physicians in U.S. territories and possessions. Obstetrics and Gynecology includes Gynecology and Oncology, Maternal and Fetal Medicine and Reproductive Endocrinology.

Nonfederal Physicians in Ophthalmology in 2001

National Total = 18,008 Physicians*

ALPHA ORDER

RANK	STATE	PHYSICIANS	% of USA
27	Alabama	212	1.2%
49	Alaska	26	0.1%
23	Arizona	268	1.5%
33	Arkansas	138	0.8%
1	California	2,194	12.2%
24	Colorado	258	1.4%
21	Connecticut	313	1.7%
46	Delaware	42	0.2%
3	Florida	1,133	6.3%
14	Georgia	407	2.3%
37	Hawaii	94	0.5%
43	Idaho	59	0.3%
6	Illinois	712	4.0%
22	Indiana	292	1.6%
29	Iowa	164	0.9%
30	Kansas	154	0.9%
28	Kentucky	194	1.1%
18	Louisiana	336	1.9%
41	Maine	77	0.4%
11	Maryland	523	2.9%
10	Massachusetts	542	3.0%
9	Michigan	585	3.2%
20	Minnesota	317	1.8%
32	Mississippi	139	0.8%
16	Missouri	341	1.9%
44	Montana	53	0.3%
36	Nebraska	96	0.5%
38	Nevada	83	0.5%
42	New Hampshire	71	0.4%
7	New Jersey	648	3.6%
40	New Mexico	79	0.4%
2	New York	1,779	9.9%
12	North Carolina	432	2.4%
48	North Dakota	37	0.2%
8	Ohio	636	3.5%
31	Oklahoma	147	0.8%
26	Oregon	222	1.2%
5	Pennsylvania	931	5.2%
39	Rhode Island	80	0.4%
25	South Carolina	250	1.4%
47	South Dakota	39	0.2%
17	Tennessee	340	1.9%
4	Texas	1,068	5.9%
34	Utah	119	0.7%
45	Vermont	47	0.3%
13	Virginia	430	2.4%
15	Washington	348	1.9%
35	West Virginia	100	0.6%
19	Wisconsin	331	1.8%
50	Wyoming	18	0.1%

RANK ORDER

RANK	STATE	PHYSICIANS	% of USA
1	California	2,194	12.2%
2	New York	1,779	9.9%
3	Florida	1,133	6.3%
4	Texas	1,068	5.9%
5	Pennsylvania	931	5.2%
6	Illinois	712	4.0%
7	New Jersey	648	3.6%
8	Ohio	636	3.5%
9	Michigan	585	3.2%
10	Massachusetts	542	3.0%
11	Maryland	523	2.9%
12	North Carolina	432	2.4%
13	Virginia	430	2.4%
14	Georgia	407	2.3%
15	Washington	348	1.9%
16	Missouri	341	1.9%
17	Tennessee	340	1.9%
18	Louisiana	336	1.9%
19	Wisconsin	331	1.8%
20	Minnesota	317	1.8%
21	Connecticut	313	1.7%
22	Indiana	292	1.6%
23	Arizona	268	1.5%
24	Colorado	258	1.4%
25	South Carolina	250	1.4%
26	Oregon	222	1.2%
27	Alabama	212	1.2%
28	Kentucky	194	1.1%
29	Iowa	164	0.9%
30	Kansas	154	0.9%
31	Oklahoma	147	0.8%
32	Mississippi	139	0.8%
33	Arkansas	138	0.8%
34	Utah	119	0.7%
35	West Virginia	100	0.6%
36	Nebraska	96	0.5%
37	Hawaii	94	0.5%
38	Nevada	83	0.5%
39	Rhode Island	80	0.4%
40	New Mexico	79	0.4%
41	Maine	77	0.4%
42	New Hampshire	71	0.4%
43	Idaho	59	0.3%
44	Montana	53	0.3%
45	Vermont	47	0.3%
46	Delaware	42	0.2%
47	South Dakota	39	0.2%
48	North Dakota	37	0.2%
49	Alaska	26	0.1%
50	Wyoming	18	0.1%
	District of Columbia	104	0.6%

Source: American Medical Association (Chicago, Illinois)
"Physician Characteristics and Distribution in the U.S." (2003-2004 Edition)
*As of December 31, 2001. Total does not include 186 physicians in U.S. territories and possessions.
Ophthalmology is the branch of medicine dealing with the anatomy, functions and diseases of the eye.

Rate of Nonfederal Physicians in Ophthalmology in 2001

National Rate = 6.3 Physicians per 100,000 Population*

ALPHA ORDER

RANK ORDER

RANK	STATE	RATE		RANK	STATE	RATE
44	Alabama	4.7		1	Maryland	9.7
48	Alaska	4.1		2	New York	9.3
38	Arizona	5.0		3	Connecticut	9.1
36	Arkansas	5.1		4	Massachusetts	8.5
14	California	6.3		5	Hawaii	7.7
22	Colorado	5.8		5	Vermont	7.7
3	Connecticut	9.1		7	New Jersey	7.6
33	Delaware	5.3		7	Pennsylvania	7.6
11	Florida	6.9		9	Louisiana	7.5
41	Georgia	4.8		9	Rhode Island	7.5
5	Hawaii	7.7		11	Florida	6.9
45	Idaho	4.5		12	Minnesota	6.4
26	Illinois	5.7		12	Oregon	6.4
41	Indiana	4.8		14	California	6.3
28	Iowa	5.6		15	South Carolina	6.2
26	Kansas	5.7		16	Wisconsin	6.1
41	Kentucky	4.8		17	Maine	6.0
9	Louisiana	7.5		17	Missouri	6.0
17	Maine	6.0		17	Virginia	6.0
1	Maryland	9.7		20	Montana	5.9
4	Massachusetts	8.5		20	Tennessee	5.9
22	Michigan	5.8		22	Colorado	5.8
12	Minnesota	6.4		22	Michigan	5.8
40	Mississippi	4.9		22	North Dakota	5.8
17	Missouri	6.0		22	Washington	5.8
20	Montana	5.9		26	Illinois	5.7
28	Nebraska	5.6		26	Kansas	5.7
49	Nevada	4.0		28	Iowa	5.6
28	New Hampshire	5.6		28	Nebraska	5.6
7	New Jersey	7.6		28	New Hampshire	5.6
46	New Mexico	4.3		28	Ohio	5.6
2	New York	9.3		28	West Virginia	5.6
33	North Carolina	5.3		33	Delaware	5.3
22	North Dakota	5.8		33	North Carolina	5.3
28	Ohio	5.6		35	Utah	5.2
47	Oklahoma	4.2		36	Arkansas	5.1
12	Oregon	6.4		36	South Dakota	5.1
7	Pennsylvania	7.6		38	Arizona	5.0
9	Rhode Island	7.5		38	Texas	5.0
15	South Carolina	6.2		40	Mississippi	4.9
36	South Dakota	5.1		41	Georgia	4.8
20	Tennessee	5.9		41	Indiana	4.8
38	Texas	5.0		41	Kentucky	4.8
35	Utah	5.2		44	Alabama	4.7
5	Vermont	7.7		45	Idaho	4.5
17	Virginia	6.0		46	New Mexico	4.3
22	Washington	5.8		47	Oklahoma	4.2
28	West Virginia	5.6		48	Alaska	4.1
16	Wisconsin	6.1		49	Nevada	4.0
50	Wyoming	3.6		50	Wyoming	3.6
					District of Columbia	18.1

Source: Morgan Quitno Press using data from American Medical Association (Chicago, Illinois)
    "Physician Characteristics and Distribution in the U.S." (2003-2004 Edition)
*As of December 31, 2001. National rate does not include physicians in U.S. territories and possessions.
Ophthalmology is the branch of medicine dealing with the anatomy, functions and diseases of the eye.

Nonfederal Physicians in Orthopedic Surgery in 2001

National Total = 22,253 Physicians*

ALPHA ORDER

RANK	STATE	PHYSICIANS	% of USA
25	Alabama	328	1.5%
48	Alaska	53	0.2%
24	Arizona	330	1.5%
33	Arkansas	173	0.8%
1	California	2,679	12.0%
22	Colorado	384	1.7%
23	Connecticut	377	1.7%
46	Delaware	62	0.3%
4	Florida	1,244	5.6%
13	Georgia	542	2.4%
41	Hawaii	112	0.5%
43	Idaho	102	0.5%
7	Illinois	847	3.8%
19	Indiana	418	1.9%
33	Iowa	173	0.8%
30	Kansas	194	0.9%
28	Kentucky	273	1.2%
21	Louisiana	408	1.8%
39	Maine	114	0.5%
14	Maryland	534	2.4%
8	Massachusetts	686	3.1%
11	Michigan	619	2.8%
18	Minnesota	429	1.9%
32	Mississippi	177	0.8%
20	Missouri	409	1.8%
44	Montana	100	0.4%
35	Nebraska	147	0.7%
39	Nevada	114	0.5%
37	New Hampshire	118	0.5%
9	New Jersey	681	3.1%
36	New Mexico	137	0.6%
2	New York	1,753	7.9%
10	North Carolina	637	2.9%
50	North Dakota	41	0.2%
6	Ohio	868	3.9%
29	Oklahoma	211	0.9%
27	Oregon	286	1.3%
5	Pennsylvania	1,076	4.8%
38	Rhode Island	117	0.5%
26	South Carolina	312	1.4%
47	South Dakota	58	0.3%
16	Tennessee	497	2.2%
3	Texas	1,413	6.3%
31	Utah	184	0.8%
45	Vermont	76	0.3%
12	Virginia	563	2.5%
15	Washington	515	2.3%
42	West Virginia	110	0.5%
17	Wisconsin	438	2.0%
49	Wyoming	49	0.2%

RANK ORDER

RANK	STATE	PHYSICIANS	% of USA
1	California	2,679	12.0%
2	New York	1,753	7.9%
3	Texas	1,413	6.3%
4	Florida	1,244	5.6%
5	Pennsylvania	1,076	4.8%
6	Ohio	868	3.9%
7	Illinois	847	3.8%
8	Massachusetts	686	3.1%
9	New Jersey	681	3.1%
10	North Carolina	637	2.9%
11	Michigan	619	2.8%
12	Virginia	563	2.5%
13	Georgia	542	2.4%
14	Maryland	534	2.4%
15	Washington	515	2.3%
16	Tennessee	497	2.2%
17	Wisconsin	438	2.0%
18	Minnesota	429	1.9%
19	Indiana	418	1.9%
20	Missouri	409	1.8%
21	Louisiana	408	1.8%
22	Colorado	384	1.7%
23	Connecticut	377	1.7%
24	Arizona	330	1.5%
25	Alabama	328	1.5%
26	South Carolina	312	1.4%
27	Oregon	286	1.3%
28	Kentucky	273	1.2%
29	Oklahoma	211	0.9%
30	Kansas	194	0.9%
31	Utah	184	0.8%
32	Mississippi	177	0.8%
33	Arkansas	173	0.8%
33	Iowa	173	0.8%
35	Nebraska	147	0.7%
36	New Mexico	137	0.6%
37	New Hampshire	118	0.5%
38	Rhode Island	117	0.5%
39	Maine	114	0.5%
39	Nevada	114	0.5%
41	Hawaii	112	0.5%
42	West Virginia	110	0.5%
43	Idaho	102	0.5%
44	Montana	100	0.4%
45	Vermont	76	0.3%
46	Delaware	62	0.3%
47	South Dakota	58	0.3%
48	Alaska	53	0.2%
49	Wyoming	49	0.2%
50	North Dakota	41	0.2%
	District of Columbia	85	0.4%

Source: American Medical Association (Chicago, Illinois)
  "Physician Characteristics and Distribution in the U.S." (2003-2004 Edition)
As of December 31, 2001. Total does not include 172 physicians in U.S. territories and possessions.
Orthopedics is the branch of medicine dealing with the skeletal system.

Rate of Nonfederal Physicians in Orthopedic Surgery in 2001

National Rate = 7.8 Physicians per 100,000 Population*

ALPHA ORDER

RANK	STATE	RATE
34	Alabama	7.3
19	Alaska	8.4
44	Arizona	6.2
41	Arkansas	6.4
27	California	7.7
13	Colorado	8.7
2	Connecticut	11.0
24	Delaware	7.8
30	Florida	7.6
41	Georgia	6.4
10	Hawaii	9.1
27	Idaho	7.7
37	Illinois	6.8
37	Indiana	6.8
49	Iowa	5.9
36	Kansas	7.2
39	Kentucky	6.7
10	Louisiana	9.1
12	Maine	8.9
6	Maryland	9.9
5	Massachusetts	10.7
44	Michigan	6.2
15	Minnesota	8.6
44	Mississippi	6.2
34	Missouri	7.3
2	Montana	11.0
18	Nebraska	8.5
50	Nevada	5.4
8	New Hampshire	9.4
23	New Jersey	8.0
33	New Mexico	7.5
9	New York	9.2
24	North Carolina	7.8
41	North Dakota	6.4
30	Ohio	7.6
47	Oklahoma	6.1
20	Oregon	8.2
13	Pennsylvania	8.7
2	Rhode Island	11.0
27	South Carolina	7.7
30	South Dakota	7.6
15	Tennessee	8.6
40	Texas	6.6
21	Utah	8.1
1	Vermont	12.4
24	Virginia	7.8
15	Washington	8.6
47	West Virginia	6.1
21	Wisconsin	8.1
6	Wyoming	9.9

RANK ORDER

RANK	STATE	RATE
1	Vermont	12.4
2	Connecticut	11.0
2	Montana	11.0
2	Rhode Island	11.0
5	Massachusetts	10.7
6	Maryland	9.9
6	Wyoming	9.9
8	New Hampshire	9.4
9	New York	9.2
10	Hawaii	9.1
10	Louisiana	9.1
12	Maine	8.9
13	Colorado	8.7
13	Pennsylvania	8.7
15	Minnesota	8.6
15	Tennessee	8.6
15	Washington	8.6
18	Nebraska	8.5
19	Alaska	8.4
20	Oregon	8.2
21	Utah	8.1
21	Wisconsin	8.1
23	New Jersey	8.0
24	Delaware	7.8
24	North Carolina	7.8
24	Virginia	7.8
27	California	7.7
27	Idaho	7.7
27	South Carolina	7.7
30	Florida	7.6
30	Ohio	7.6
30	South Dakota	7.6
33	New Mexico	7.5
34	Alabama	7.3
34	Missouri	7.3
36	Kansas	7.2
37	Illinois	6.8
37	Indiana	6.8
39	Kentucky	6.7
40	Texas	6.6
41	Arkansas	6.4
41	Georgia	6.4
41	North Dakota	6.4
44	Arizona	6.2
44	Michigan	6.2
44	Mississippi	6.2
47	Oklahoma	6.1
47	West Virginia	6.1
49	Iowa	5.9
50	Nevada	5.4

| | District of Columbia | 14.8 |

Source: Morgan Quitno Press using data from American Medical Association (Chicago, Illinois)
    "Physician Characteristics and Distribution in the U.S." (2003-2004 Edition)
*As of December 31, 2001. National rate does not include physicians in U.S. territories and possessions.
Orthopedics is the branch of medicine dealing with the skeletal system.

Nonfederal Physicians in Plastic Surgery in 2001

National Total = 6,323 Physicians*

ALPHA ORDER

RANK	STATE	PHYSICIANS	% of USA
24	Alabama	84	1.3%
49	Alaska	6	0.1%
17	Arizona	122	1.9%
35	Arkansas	31	0.5%
1	California	927	14.7%
20	Colorado	94	1.5%
19	Connecticut	96	1.5%
42	Delaware	18	0.3%
3	Florida	501	7.9%
13	Georgia	157	2.5%
34	Hawaii	33	0.5%
40	Idaho	23	0.4%
6	Illinois	230	3.6%
22	Indiana	88	1.4%
38	Iowa	25	0.4%
30	Kansas	53	0.8%
21	Kentucky	89	1.4%
23	Louisiana	86	1.4%
45	Maine	14	0.2%
14	Maryland	150	2.4%
10	Massachusetts	174	2.8%
9	Michigan	190	3.0%
25	Minnesota	82	1.3%
33	Mississippi	39	0.6%
16	Missouri	128	2.0%
44	Montana	17	0.3%
37	Nebraska	27	0.4%
31	Nevada	42	0.7%
42	New Hampshire	18	0.3%
7	New Jersey	205	3.2%
41	New Mexico	22	0.3%
2	New York	621	9.8%
12	North Carolina	159	2.5%
46	North Dakota	10	0.2%
8	Ohio	196	3.1%
31	Oklahoma	42	0.7%
29	Oregon	59	0.9%
5	Pennsylvania	247	3.9%
39	Rhode Island	24	0.4%
28	South Carolina	64	1.0%
47	South Dakota	9	0.1%
15	Tennessee	145	2.3%
4	Texas	479	7.6%
27	Utah	68	1.1%
47	Vermont	9	0.1%
11	Virginia	165	2.6%
18	Washington	115	1.8%
36	West Virginia	28	0.4%
26	Wisconsin	80	1.3%
50	Wyoming	3	0.0%

RANK ORDER

RANK	STATE	PHYSICIANS	% of USA
1	California	927	14.7%
2	New York	621	9.8%
3	Florida	501	7.9%
4	Texas	479	7.6%
5	Pennsylvania	247	3.9%
6	Illinois	230	3.6%
7	New Jersey	205	3.2%
8	Ohio	196	3.1%
9	Michigan	190	3.0%
10	Massachusetts	174	2.8%
11	Virginia	165	2.6%
12	North Carolina	159	2.5%
13	Georgia	157	2.5%
14	Maryland	150	2.4%
15	Tennessee	145	2.3%
16	Missouri	128	2.0%
17	Arizona	122	1.9%
18	Washington	115	1.8%
19	Connecticut	96	1.5%
20	Colorado	94	1.5%
21	Kentucky	89	1.4%
22	Indiana	88	1.4%
23	Louisiana	86	1.4%
24	Alabama	84	1.3%
25	Minnesota	82	1.3%
26	Wisconsin	80	1.3%
27	Utah	68	1.1%
28	South Carolina	64	1.0%
29	Oregon	59	0.9%
30	Kansas	53	0.8%
31	Nevada	42	0.7%
31	Oklahoma	42	0.7%
33	Mississippi	39	0.6%
34	Hawaii	33	0.5%
35	Arkansas	31	0.5%
36	West Virginia	28	0.4%
37	Nebraska	27	0.4%
38	Iowa	25	0.4%
39	Rhode Island	24	0.4%
40	Idaho	23	0.4%
41	New Mexico	22	0.3%
42	Delaware	18	0.3%
42	New Hampshire	18	0.3%
44	Montana	17	0.3%
45	Maine	14	0.2%
46	North Dakota	10	0.2%
47	South Dakota	9	0.1%
47	Vermont	9	0.1%
49	Alaska	6	0.1%
50	Wyoming	3	0.0%
	District of Columbia	29	0.5%

Source: American Medical Association (Chicago, Illinois)
"Physician Characteristics and Distribution in the U.S." (2003-2004 Edition)
*As of December 31, 2001. Total does not include 40 physicians in U.S. territories and possessions.

Rate of Nonfederal Physicians in Plastic Surgery in 2001

National Rate = 2.2 Physicians per 100,000 Population*

ALPHA ORDER

RANK	STATE	RATE
22	Alabama	1.9
48	Alaska	0.9
11	Arizona	2.3
43	Arkansas	1.2
6	California	2.7
18	Colorado	2.1
4	Connecticut	2.8
11	Delaware	2.3
2	Florida	3.1
22	Georgia	1.9
6	Hawaii	2.7
30	Idaho	1.7
29	Illinois	1.8
40	Indiana	1.4
48	Iowa	0.9
19	Kansas	2.0
16	Kentucky	2.2
22	Louisiana	1.9
47	Maine	1.1
4	Maryland	2.8
6	Massachusetts	2.7
22	Michigan	1.9
33	Minnesota	1.6
40	Mississippi	1.4
11	Missouri	2.3
22	Montana	1.9
33	Nebraska	1.6
19	Nevada	2.0
40	New Hampshire	1.4
10	New Jersey	2.4
43	New Mexico	1.2
1	New York	3.3
22	North Carolina	1.9
33	North Dakota	1.6
30	Ohio	1.7
43	Oklahoma	1.2
30	Oregon	1.7
19	Pennsylvania	2.0
11	Rhode Island	2.3
33	South Carolina	1.6
43	South Dakota	1.2
9	Tennessee	2.5
16	Texas	2.2
3	Utah	3.0
38	Vermont	1.5
11	Virginia	2.3
22	Washington	1.9
33	West Virginia	1.6
38	Wisconsin	1.5
50	Wyoming	0.6

RANK ORDER

RANK	STATE	RATE
1	New York	3.3
2	Florida	3.1
3	Utah	3.0
4	Connecticut	2.8
4	Maryland	2.8
6	California	2.7
6	Hawaii	2.7
6	Massachusetts	2.7
9	Tennessee	2.5
10	New Jersey	2.4
11	Arizona	2.3
11	Delaware	2.3
11	Missouri	2.3
11	Rhode Island	2.3
11	Virginia	2.3
16	Kentucky	2.2
16	Texas	2.2
18	Colorado	2.1
19	Kansas	2.0
19	Nevada	2.0
19	Pennsylvania	2.0
22	Alabama	1.9
22	Georgia	1.9
22	Louisiana	1.9
22	Michigan	1.9
22	Montana	1.9
22	North Carolina	1.9
22	Washington	1.9
29	Illinois	1.8
30	Idaho	1.7
30	Ohio	1.7
30	Oregon	1.7
33	Minnesota	1.6
33	Nebraska	1.6
33	North Dakota	1.6
33	South Carolina	1.6
33	West Virginia	1.6
38	Vermont	1.5
38	Wisconsin	1.5
40	Indiana	1.4
40	Mississippi	1.4
40	New Hampshire	1.4
43	Arkansas	1.2
43	New Mexico	1.2
43	Oklahoma	1.2
43	South Dakota	1.2
47	Maine	1.1
48	Alaska	0.9
48	Iowa	0.9
50	Wyoming	0.6

	District of Columbia	5.1

Source: Morgan Quitno Press using data from American Medical Association (Chicago, Illinois)
"Physician Characteristics and Distribution in the U.S." (2003-2004 Edition)
*As of December 31, 2001. National rate does not include physicians in U.S. territories and possessions.

Nonfederal Physicians in Other Specialties in 2001

National Total = 193,374 Physicians*

ALPHA ORDER

RANK	STATE	PHYSICIANS	% of USA
28	Alabama	2,127	1.1%
49	Alaska	304	0.2%
23	Arizona	2,934	1.5%
33	Arkansas	1,260	0.7%
1	California	23,629	12.2%
22	Colorado	2,969	1.5%
18	Connecticut	3,429	1.8%
45	Delaware	503	0.3%
45	Idaho	503	0.3%
5	Florida	9,891	5.1%
14	Georgia	4,515	2.3%
39	Hawaii	921	0.5%
45	Idaho	503	0.3%
6	Illinois	8,571	4.4%
19	Indiana	3,382	1.7%
31	Iowa	1,280	0.7%
29	Kansas	1,495	0.8%
27	Kentucky	2,273	1.2%
24	Louisiana	2,865	1.5%
41	Maine	890	0.5%
11	Maryland	5,683	2.9%
7	Massachusetts	7,949	4.1%
10	Michigan	6,168	3.2%
21	Minnesota	3,228	1.7%
34	Mississippi	1,187	0.6%
20	Missouri	3,375	1.7%
44	Montana	518	0.3%
38	Nebraska	947	0.5%
37	Nevada	991	0.5%
42	New Hampshire	884	0.5%
9	New Jersey	6,452	3.3%
35	New Mexico	1,091	0.6%
2	New York	19,689	10.2%
12	North Carolina	5,008	2.6%
48	North Dakota	348	0.2%
8	Ohio	7,156	3.7%
30	Oklahoma	1,492	0.8%
26	Oregon	2,301	1.2%
4	Pennsylvania	10,063	5.2%
40	Rhode Island	901	0.5%
25	South Carolina	2,316	1.2%
47	South Dakota	351	0.2%
17	Tennessee	3,449	1.8%
3	Texas	11,512	6.0%
32	Utah	1,271	0.7%
43	Vermont	591	0.3%
13	Virginia	4,702	2.4%
15	Washington	4,154	2.1%
36	West Virginia	1,010	0.5%
16	Wisconsin	3,498	1.8%
50	Wyoming	224	0.1%

RANK ORDER

RANK	STATE	PHYSICIANS	% of USA
1	California	23,629	12.2%
2	New York	19,689	10.2%
3	Texas	11,512	6.0%
4	Pennsylvania	10,063	5.2%
5	Florida	9,891	5.1%
6	Illinois	8,571	4.4%
7	Massachusetts	7,949	4.1%
8	Ohio	7,156	3.7%
9	New Jersey	6,452	3.3%
10	Michigan	6,168	3.2%
11	Maryland	5,683	2.9%
12	North Carolina	5,008	2.6%
13	Virginia	4,702	2.4%
14	Georgia	4,515	2.3%
15	Washington	4,154	2.1%
16	Wisconsin	3,498	1.8%
17	Tennessee	3,449	1.8%
18	Connecticut	3,429	1.8%
19	Indiana	3,382	1.7%
20	Missouri	3,375	1.7%
21	Minnesota	3,228	1.7%
22	Colorado	2,969	1.5%
23	Arizona	2,934	1.5%
24	Louisiana	2,865	1.5%
25	South Carolina	2,316	1.2%
26	Oregon	2,301	1.2%
27	Kentucky	2,273	1.2%
28	Alabama	2,127	1.1%
29	Kansas	1,495	0.8%
30	Oklahoma	1,492	0.8%
31	Iowa	1,280	0.7%
32	Utah	1,271	0.7%
33	Arkansas	1,260	0.7%
34	Mississippi	1,187	0.6%
35	New Mexico	1,091	0.6%
36	West Virginia	1,010	0.5%
37	Nevada	991	0.5%
38	Nebraska	947	0.5%
39	Hawaii	921	0.5%
40	Rhode Island	901	0.5%
41	Maine	890	0.5%
42	New Hampshire	884	0.5%
43	Vermont	591	0.3%
44	Montana	518	0.3%
45	Delaware	503	0.3%
45	Idaho	503	0.3%
47	South Dakota	351	0.2%
48	North Dakota	348	0.2%
49	Alaska	304	0.2%
50	Wyoming	224	0.1%
	District of Columbia	1,124	0.6%

Source: American Medical Association (Chicago, Illinois)
"Physician Characteristics and Distribution in the U.S." (2003-2004 Edition)
*As of December 31, 2001. Total does not include 2,375 physicians in U.S. territories and possessions. Other Specialties include Aerospace Medicine, Anesthesiology, Child Psychiatry, Diagnostic Radiology, Emergency Medicine, Forensic Pathology, Nuclear Medicine, Occupational Medicine, Neurology, Psychiatry, Public Health, Anatomic/Clinical Pathology, Radiology, Radiation Oncology and other specialties.

Rate of Nonfederal Physicians in Other Specialties in 2001

National Rate = 68 Physicians per 100,000 Population*

ALPHA ORDER

RANK	STATE	RATE
41	Alabama	48
41	Alaska	48
34	Arizona	55
43	Arkansas	47
13	California	68
15	Colorado	67
4	Connecticut	100
21	Delaware	63
25	Florida	60
39	Georgia	54
9	Hawaii	75
50	Idaho	38
13	Illinois	68
34	Indiana	55
47	Iowa	44
34	Kansas	55
31	Kentucky	56
20	Louisiana	64
11	Maine	69
2	Maryland	106
1	Massachusetts	124
23	Michigan	62
17	Minnesota	65
49	Mississippi	42
25	Missouri	60
29	Montana	57
34	Nebraska	55
43	Nevada	47
10	New Hampshire	70
8	New Jersey	76
25	New Mexico	60
3	New York	103
24	North Carolina	61
34	North Dakota	55
21	Ohio	63
48	Oklahoma	43
16	Oregon	66
7	Pennsylvania	82
6	Rhode Island	85
29	South Carolina	57
45	South Dakota	46
25	Tennessee	60
39	Texas	54
31	Utah	56
5	Vermont	96
17	Virginia	65
11	Washington	69
31	West Virginia	56
17	Wisconsin	65
46	Wyoming	45

RANK ORDER

RANK	STATE	RATE
1	Massachusetts	124
2	Maryland	106
3	New York	103
4	Connecticut	100
5	Vermont	96
6	Rhode Island	85
7	Pennsylvania	82
8	New Jersey	76
9	Hawaii	75
10	New Hampshire	70
11	Maine	69
11	Washington	69
13	California	68
13	Illinois	68
15	Colorado	67
16	Oregon	66
17	Minnesota	65
17	Virginia	65
17	Wisconsin	65
20	Louisiana	64
21	Delaware	63
21	Ohio	63
23	Michigan	62
24	North Carolina	61
25	Florida	60
25	Missouri	60
25	New Mexico	60
25	Tennessee	60
29	Montana	57
29	South Carolina	57
31	Kentucky	56
31	Utah	56
31	West Virginia	56
34	Arizona	55
34	Indiana	55
34	Kansas	55
34	Nebraska	55
34	North Dakota	55
39	Georgia	54
39	Texas	54
41	Alabama	48
41	Alaska	48
43	Arkansas	47
43	Nevada	47
45	South Dakota	46
46	Wyoming	45
47	Iowa	44
48	Oklahoma	43
49	Mississippi	42
50	Idaho	38

District of Columbia	196

Source: Morgan Quitno Press using data from American Medical Association (Chicago, Illinois)
"Physician Characteristics and Distribution in the U.S." (2003-2004 Edition)
*As of December 31, 2001. National rate does not include physicians in U.S. territories and possessions. Other Specialties include Aerospace Medicine, Anesthesiology, Child Psychiatry, Diagnostic Radiology, Emergency Medicine, Forensic Pathology, Nuclear Medicine, Occupational Medicine, Neurology, Psychiatry, Public Health, Anatomic/Clinical Pathology, Radiology, Radiation Oncology and other specialties.

Nonfederal Physicians in Anesthesiology in 2001

National Total = 35,826 Physicians*

ALPHA ORDER

RANK	STATE	PHYSICIANS	% of USA
27	Alabama	427	1.2%
47	Alaska	64	0.2%
19	Arizona	658	1.8%
34	Arkansas	248	0.7%
1	California	4,442	12.4%
21	Colorado	579	1.6%
22	Connecticut	524	1.5%
46	Delaware	71	0.2%
4	Florida	2,165	6.0%
13	Georgia	843	2.4%
41	Hawaii	134	0.4%
44	Idaho	88	0.2%
5	Illinois	1,689	4.7%
14	Indiana	820	2.3%
31	Iowa	279	0.8%
31	Kansas	279	0.8%
26	Kentucky	436	1.2%
24	Louisiana	478	1.3%
40	Maine	149	0.4%
10	Maryland	930	2.6%
9	Massachusetts	1,260	3.5%
12	Michigan	873	2.4%
23	Minnesota	505	1.4%
35	Mississippi	247	0.7%
20	Missouri	604	1.7%
42	Montana	117	0.3%
36	Nebraska	194	0.5%
33	Nevada	271	0.8%
38	New Hampshire	157	0.4%
7	New Jersey	1,318	3.7%
37	New Mexico	191	0.5%
2	New York	3,163	8.8%
15	North Carolina	808	2.3%
49	North Dakota	49	0.1%
8	Ohio	1,313	3.7%
29	Oklahoma	315	0.9%
25	Oregon	465	1.3%
6	Pennsylvania	1,656	4.6%
43	Rhode Island	101	0.3%
28	South Carolina	410	1.1%
48	South Dakota	53	0.1%
18	Tennessee	708	2.0%
3	Texas	2,674	7.5%
30	Utah	290	0.8%
45	Vermont	74	0.2%
16	Virginia	775	2.2%
11	Washington	890	2.5%
39	West Virginia	154	0.4%
17	Wisconsin	726	2.0%
50	Wyoming	48	0.1%

RANK ORDER

RANK	STATE	PHYSICIANS	% of USA
1	California	4,442	12.4%
2	New York	3,163	8.8%
3	Texas	2,674	7.5%
4	Florida	2,165	6.0%
5	Illinois	1,689	4.7%
6	Pennsylvania	1,656	4.6%
7	New Jersey	1,318	3.7%
8	Ohio	1,313	3.7%
9	Massachusetts	1,260	3.5%
10	Maryland	930	2.6%
11	Washington	890	2.5%
12	Michigan	873	2.4%
13	Georgia	843	2.4%
14	Indiana	820	2.3%
15	North Carolina	808	2.3%
16	Virginia	775	2.2%
17	Wisconsin	726	2.0%
18	Tennessee	708	2.0%
19	Arizona	658	1.8%
20	Missouri	604	1.7%
21	Colorado	579	1.6%
22	Connecticut	524	1.5%
23	Minnesota	505	1.4%
24	Louisiana	478	1.3%
25	Oregon	465	1.3%
26	Kentucky	436	1.2%
27	Alabama	427	1.2%
28	South Carolina	410	1.1%
29	Oklahoma	315	0.9%
30	Utah	290	0.8%
31	Iowa	279	0.8%
31	Kansas	279	0.8%
33	Nevada	271	0.8%
34	Arkansas	248	0.7%
35	Mississippi	247	0.7%
36	Nebraska	194	0.5%
37	New Mexico	191	0.5%
38	New Hampshire	157	0.4%
39	West Virginia	154	0.4%
40	Maine	149	0.4%
41	Hawaii	134	0.4%
42	Montana	117	0.3%
43	Rhode Island	101	0.3%
44	Idaho	88	0.2%
45	Vermont	74	0.2%
46	Delaware	71	0.2%
47	Alaska	64	0.2%
48	South Dakota	53	0.1%
49	North Dakota	49	0.1%
50	Wyoming	48	0.1%
	District of Columbia	114	0.3%

Source: American Medical Association (Chicago, Illinois)
"Physician Characteristics and Distribution in the U.S." (2003-2004 Edition)
*As of December 31, 2001. Total does not include 241 physicians in U.S. territories and possessions.

Rate of Nonfederal Physicians in Anesthesiology in 2001

National Rate = 12.6 Physicians per 100,000 Population*

ALPHA ORDER

RANK	STATE	RATE
39	Alabama	9.6
33	Alaska	10.1
20	Arizona	12.4
42	Arkansas	9.2
16	California	12.8
13	Colorado	13.1
5	Connecticut	15.3
44	Delaware	8.9
12	Florida	13.2
36	Georgia	10.0
26	Hawaii	10.9
50	Idaho	6.7
7	Illinois	13.5
9	Indiana	13.4
40	Iowa	9.5
32	Kansas	10.3
28	Kentucky	10.7
28	Louisiana	10.7
23	Maine	11.6
2	Maryland	17.3
1	Massachusetts	19.7
45	Michigan	8.7
33	Minnesota	10.1
46	Mississippi	8.6
28	Missouri	10.7
14	Montana	12.9
25	Nebraska	11.3
14	Nevada	12.9
18	New Hampshire	12.5
4	New Jersey	15.5
31	New Mexico	10.4
3	New York	16.6
37	North Carolina	9.8
48	North Dakota	7.7
24	Ohio	11.5
43	Oklahoma	9.1
9	Oregon	13.4
7	Pennsylvania	13.5
40	Rhode Island	9.5
33	South Carolina	10.1
49	South Dakota	7.0
21	Tennessee	12.3
18	Texas	12.5
17	Utah	12.7
22	Vermont	12.1
27	Virginia	10.8
6	Washington	14.8
46	West Virginia	8.6
9	Wisconsin	13.4
38	Wyoming	9.7

RANK ORDER

RANK	STATE	RATE
1	Massachusetts	19.7
2	Maryland	17.3
3	New York	16.6
4	New Jersey	15.5
5	Connecticut	15.3
6	Washington	14.8
7	Illinois	13.5
7	Pennsylvania	13.5
9	Indiana	13.4
9	Oregon	13.4
9	Wisconsin	13.4
12	Florida	13.2
13	Colorado	13.1
14	Montana	12.9
14	Nevada	12.9
16	California	12.8
17	Utah	12.7
18	New Hampshire	12.5
18	Texas	12.5
20	Arizona	12.4
21	Tennessee	12.3
22	Vermont	12.1
23	Maine	11.6
24	Ohio	11.5
25	Nebraska	11.3
26	Hawaii	10.9
27	Virginia	10.8
28	Kentucky	10.7
28	Louisiana	10.7
28	Missouri	10.7
31	New Mexico	10.4
32	Kansas	10.3
33	Alaska	10.1
33	Minnesota	10.1
33	South Carolina	10.1
36	Georgia	10.0
37	North Carolina	9.8
38	Wyoming	9.7
39	Alabama	9.6
40	Iowa	9.5
40	Rhode Island	9.5
42	Arkansas	9.2
43	Oklahoma	9.1
44	Delaware	8.9
45	Michigan	8.7
46	Mississippi	8.6
46	West Virginia	8.6
48	North Dakota	7.7
49	South Dakota	7.0
50	Idaho	6.7

District of Columbia   19.9

Source: Morgan Quitno Press using data from American Medical Association (Chicago, Illinois)
"Physician Characteristics and Distribution in the U.S." (2003-2004 Edition)
*As of December 31, 2001. National rate does not include physicians in U.S. territories and possessions.

Nonfederal Physicians in Psychiatry in 2001

National Total = 37,616 Physicians*

ALPHA ORDER

RANK	STATE	PHYSICIANS	% of USA
28	Alabama	303	0.8%
47	Alaska	62	0.2%
23	Arizona	481	1.3%
37	Arkansas	185	0.5%
2	California	5,089	13.5%
18	Colorado	538	1.4%
14	Connecticut	877	2.3%
44	Delaware	86	0.2%
6	Florida	1,569	4.2%
15	Georgia	818	2.2%
34	Hawaii	208	0.6%
48	Idaho	61	0.2%
7	Illinois	1,526	4.1%
24	Indiana	469	1.2%
36	Iowa	188	0.5%
29	Kansas	298	0.8%
27	Kentucky	369	1.0%
21	Louisiana	510	1.4%
33	Maine	209	0.6%
9	Maryland	1,248	3.3%
3	Massachusetts	2,017	5.4%
11	Michigan	1,051	2.8%
22	Minnesota	485	1.3%
38	Mississippi	173	0.5%
19	Missouri	532	1.4%
45	Montana	74	0.2%
41	Nebraska	152	0.4%
43	Nevada	132	0.4%
35	New Hampshire	190	0.5%
8	New Jersey	1,368	3.6%
31	New Mexico	234	0.6%
1	New York	5,439	14.5%
13	North Carolina	939	2.5%
48	North Dakota	61	0.2%
10	Ohio	1,147	3.0%
30	Oklahoma	261	0.7%
26	Oregon	399	1.1%
4	Pennsylvania	1,918	5.1%
32	Rhode Island	227	0.6%
25	South Carolina	430	1.1%
46	South Dakota	63	0.2%
20	Tennessee	511	1.4%
5	Texas	1,691	4.5%
38	Utah	173	0.5%
40	Vermont	157	0.4%
12	Virginia	949	2.5%
16	Washington	701	1.9%
42	West Virginia	150	0.4%
17	Wisconsin	558	1.5%
50	Wyoming	30	0.1%

RANK ORDER

RANK	STATE	PHYSICIANS	% of USA
1	New York	5,439	14.5%
2	California	5,089	13.5%
3	Massachusetts	2,017	5.4%
4	Pennsylvania	1,918	5.1%
5	Texas	1,691	4.5%
6	Florida	1,569	4.2%
7	Illinois	1,526	4.1%
8	New Jersey	1,368	3.6%
9	Maryland	1,248	3.3%
10	Ohio	1,147	3.0%
11	Michigan	1,051	2.8%
12	Virginia	949	2.5%
13	North Carolina	939	2.5%
14	Connecticut	877	2.3%
15	Georgia	818	2.2%
16	Washington	701	1.9%
17	Wisconsin	558	1.5%
18	Colorado	538	1.4%
19	Missouri	532	1.4%
20	Tennessee	511	1.4%
21	Louisiana	510	1.4%
22	Minnesota	485	1.3%
23	Arizona	481	1.3%
24	Indiana	469	1.2%
25	South Carolina	430	1.1%
26	Oregon	399	1.1%
27	Kentucky	369	1.0%
28	Alabama	303	0.8%
29	Kansas	298	0.8%
30	Oklahoma	261	0.7%
31	New Mexico	234	0.6%
32	Rhode Island	227	0.6%
33	Maine	209	0.6%
34	Hawaii	208	0.6%
35	New Hampshire	190	0.5%
36	Iowa	188	0.5%
37	Arkansas	185	0.5%
38	Mississippi	173	0.5%
38	Utah	173	0.5%
40	Vermont	157	0.4%
41	Nebraska	152	0.4%
42	West Virginia	150	0.4%
43	Nevada	132	0.4%
44	Delaware	86	0.2%
45	Montana	74	0.2%
46	South Dakota	63	0.2%
47	Alaska	62	0.2%
48	Idaho	61	0.2%
48	North Dakota	61	0.2%
50	Wyoming	30	0.1%
	District of Columbia	310	0.8%

Source: American Medical Association (Chicago, Illinois)
    "Physician Characteristics and Distribution in the U.S." (2003-2004 Edition)
*As of December 31, 2001. Total does not include 417 physicians in U.S. territories and possessions. Psychiatry includes psychoanalysis.

Rate of Nonfederal Physicians in Psychiatry in 2001

National Rate = 13.2 Physicians per 100,000 Population*

ALPHA ORDER

RANK	STATE	RATE
45	Alabama	6.8
27	Alaska	9.8
33	Arizona	9.1
44	Arkansas	6.9
12	California	14.7
16	Colorado	12.1
4	Connecticut	25.5
22	Delaware	10.8
30	Florida	9.6
28	Georgia	9.7
7	Hawaii	17.0
50	Idaho	4.6
15	Illinois	12.2
41	Indiana	7.7
46	Iowa	6.4
21	Kansas	11.0
33	Kentucky	9.1
19	Louisiana	11.4
8	Maine	16.3
5	Maryland	23.2
1	Massachusetts	31.5
24	Michigan	10.5
28	Minnesota	9.7
49	Mississippi	6.0
32	Missouri	9.4
39	Montana	8.2
36	Nebraska	8.8
47	Nevada	6.3
11	New Hampshire	15.1
9	New Jersey	16.1
14	New Mexico	12.8
2	New York	28.5
19	North Carolina	11.4
30	North Dakota	9.6
26	Ohio	10.1
43	Oklahoma	7.5
18	Oregon	11.5
10	Pennsylvania	15.6
6	Rhode Island	21.4
23	South Carolina	10.6
37	South Dakota	8.3
35	Tennessee	8.9
40	Texas	7.9
42	Utah	7.6
3	Vermont	25.6
13	Virginia	13.2
17	Washington	11.7
37	West Virginia	8.3
25	Wisconsin	10.3
48	Wyoming	6.1

RANK ORDER

RANK	STATE	RATE
1	Massachusetts	31.5
2	New York	28.5
3	Vermont	25.6
4	Connecticut	25.5
5	Maryland	23.2
6	Rhode Island	21.4
7	Hawaii	17.0
8	Maine	16.3
9	New Jersey	16.1
10	Pennsylvania	15.6
11	New Hampshire	15.1
12	California	14.7
13	Virginia	13.2
14	New Mexico	12.8
15	Illinois	12.2
16	Colorado	12.1
17	Washington	11.7
18	Oregon	11.5
19	Louisiana	11.4
19	North Carolina	11.4
21	Kansas	11.0
22	Delaware	10.8
23	South Carolina	10.6
24	Michigan	10.5
25	Wisconsin	10.3
26	Ohio	10.1
27	Alaska	9.8
28	Georgia	9.7
28	Minnesota	9.7
30	Florida	9.6
30	North Dakota	9.6
32	Missouri	9.4
33	Arizona	9.1
33	Kentucky	9.1
35	Tennessee	8.9
36	Nebraska	8.8
37	South Dakota	8.3
37	West Virginia	8.3
39	Montana	8.2
40	Texas	7.9
41	Indiana	7.7
42	Utah	7.6
43	Oklahoma	7.5
44	Arkansas	6.9
45	Alabama	6.8
46	Iowa	6.4
47	Nevada	6.3
48	Wyoming	6.1
49	Mississippi	6.0
50	Idaho	4.6

District of Columbia	54.0

Source: Morgan Quitno Press using data from American Medical Association (Chicago, Illinois)
"Physician Characteristics and Distribution in the U.S." (2003-2004 Edition)
*As of December 31, 2001. National rate does not include physicians in U.S. territories and possessions.
Psychiatry includes psychoanalysis.

Percent of Population Lacking Access to Mental Health Care in 2002

National Percent = 13.3% of Population*

ALPHA ORDER

RANK	STATE	PERCENT
2	Alabama	46.6
13	Alaska	32.5
30	Arizona	10.5
4	Arkansas	42.7
38	California	7.0
43	Colorado	2.7
49	Connecticut	0.7
50	Delaware	0.0
39	Florida	6.9
21	Georgia	17.6
36	Hawaii	8.1
3	Idaho	44.0
26	Illinois	15.0
42	Indiana	5.3
9	Iowa	36.4
14	Kansas	32.0
17	Kentucky	21.9
45	Louisiana	2.2
34	Maine	9.0
47	Maryland	1.9
48	Massachusetts	1.2
22	Michigan	17.4
24	Minnesota	16.1
19	Mississippi	19.1
20	Missouri	18.9
5	Montana	41.9
12	Nebraska	33.5
32	Nevada	9.1
40	New Hampshire	5.8
46	New Jersey	2.1
7	New Mexico	38.1
40	New York	5.8
31	North Carolina	9.8
10	North Dakota	35.9
35	Ohio	8.3
8	Oklahoma	36.9
18	Oregon	19.9
32	Pennsylvania	9.1
29	Rhode Island	10.8
11	South Carolina	34.2
6	South Dakota	39.9
23	Tennessee	16.7
16	Texas	22.0
15	Utah	23.9
28	Vermont	12.6
44	Virginia	2.5
27	Washington	13.4
37	West Virginia	7.8
25	Wisconsin	15.2
1	Wyoming	67.3

RANK ORDER

RANK	STATE	PERCENT
1	Wyoming	67.3
2	Alabama	46.6
3	Idaho	44.0
4	Arkansas	42.7
5	Montana	41.9
6	South Dakota	39.9
7	New Mexico	38.1
8	Oklahoma	36.9
9	Iowa	36.4
10	North Dakota	35.9
11	South Carolina	34.2
12	Nebraska	33.5
13	Alaska	32.5
14	Kansas	32.0
15	Utah	23.9
16	Texas	22.0
17	Kentucky	21.9
18	Oregon	19.9
19	Mississippi	19.1
20	Missouri	18.9
21	Georgia	17.6
22	Michigan	17.4
23	Tennessee	16.7
24	Minnesota	16.1
25	Wisconsin	15.2
26	Illinois	15.0
27	Washington	13.4
28	Vermont	12.6
29	Rhode Island	10.8
30	Arizona	10.5
31	North Carolina	9.8
32	Nevada	9.1
32	Pennsylvania	9.1
34	Maine	9.0
35	Ohio	8.3
36	Hawaii	8.1
37	West Virginia	7.8
38	California	7.0
39	Florida	6.9
40	New Hampshire	5.8
40	New York	5.8
42	Indiana	5.3
43	Colorado	2.7
44	Virginia	2.5
45	Louisiana	2.2
46	New Jersey	2.1
47	Maryland	1.9
48	Massachusetts	1.2
49	Connecticut	0.7
50	Delaware	0.0

District of Columbia 0.7

Source: Morgan Quitno Press using data from U.S. Dept. of Health and Human Services, Div. of Shortage Designation
"Selected Statistics on Health Professional Shortage Areas, As of December 31, 2002"
*Percent of population considered under-served by mental health practitioners. An under-served population does
not have primary medical care within reasonable economic and geographic bounds.

International Medical School Graduates Practicing in the U.S. in 2001

National Total = 193,910 Nonfederal Physicians*

ALPHA ORDER

RANK	STATE	PHYSICIANS	% of USA
26	Alabama	1,419	0.7%
47	Alaska	92	0.0%
20	Arizona	2,098	1.1%
34	Arkansas	713	0.4%
2	California	21,474	11.1%
33	Colorado	735	0.4%
13	Connecticut	3,735	1.9%
37	Delaware	612	0.3%
3	Florida	15,958	8.2%
14	Georgia	3,269	1.7%
38	Hawaii	583	0.3%
49	Idaho	58	0.0%
5	Illinois	12,383	6.4%
16	Indiana	2,568	1.3%
32	Iowa	966	0.5%
27	Kansas	1,076	0.6%
23	Kentucky	1,855	1.0%
21	Louisiana	2,033	1.0%
42	Maine	419	0.2%
10	Maryland	6,176	3.2%
11	Massachusetts	5,972	3.1%
9	Michigan	8,132	4.2%
22	Minnesota	1,876	1.0%
39	Mississippi	575	0.3%
15	Missouri	2,974	1.5%
47	Montana	92	0.0%
40	Nebraska	496	0.3%
31	Nevada	985	0.5%
41	New Hampshire	462	0.2%
4	New Jersey	12,401	6.4%
36	New Mexico	616	0.3%
1	New York	33,028	17.0%
17	North Carolina	2,385	1.2%
43	North Dakota	345	0.2%
8	Ohio	8,137	4.2%
28	Oklahoma	1,071	0.6%
35	Oregon	711	0.4%
7	Pennsylvania	9,336	4.8%
30	Rhode Island	1,005	0.5%
29	South Carolina	1,066	0.5%
45	South Dakota	206	0.1%
19	Tennessee	2,199	1.1%
6	Texas	10,604	5.5%
44	Utah	328	0.2%
46	Vermont	190	0.1%
12	Virginia	4,096	2.1%
24	Washington	1,701	0.9%
25	West Virginia	1,485	0.8%
18	Wisconsin	2,360	1.2%
50	Wyoming	55	0.0%

RANK ORDER

RANK	STATE	PHYSICIANS	% of USA
1	New York	33,028	17.0%
2	California	21,474	11.1%
3	Florida	15,958	8.2%
4	New Jersey	12,401	6.4%
5	Illinois	12,383	6.4%
6	Texas	10,604	5.5%
7	Pennsylvania	9,336	4.8%
8	Ohio	8,137	4.2%
9	Michigan	8,132	4.2%
10	Maryland	6,176	3.2%
11	Massachusetts	5,972	3.1%
12	Virginia	4,096	2.1%
13	Connecticut	3,735	1.9%
14	Georgia	3,269	1.7%
15	Missouri	2,974	1.5%
16	Indiana	2,568	1.3%
17	North Carolina	2,385	1.2%
18	Wisconsin	2,360	1.2%
19	Tennessee	2,199	1.1%
20	Arizona	2,098	1.1%
21	Louisiana	2,033	1.0%
22	Minnesota	1,876	1.0%
23	Kentucky	1,855	1.0%
24	Washington	1,701	0.9%
25	West Virginia	1,485	0.8%
26	Alabama	1,419	0.7%
27	Kansas	1,076	0.6%
28	Oklahoma	1,071	0.6%
29	South Carolina	1,066	0.5%
30	Rhode Island	1,005	0.5%
31	Nevada	985	0.5%
32	Iowa	966	0.5%
33	Colorado	735	0.4%
34	Arkansas	713	0.4%
35	Oregon	711	0.4%
36	New Mexico	616	0.3%
37	Delaware	612	0.3%
38	Hawaii	583	0.3%
39	Mississippi	575	0.3%
40	Nebraska	496	0.3%
41	New Hampshire	462	0.2%
42	Maine	419	0.2%
43	North Dakota	345	0.2%
44	Utah	328	0.2%
45	South Dakota	206	0.1%
46	Vermont	190	0.1%
47	Alaska	92	0.0%
47	Montana	92	0.0%
49	Idaho	58	0.0%
50	Wyoming	55	0.0%
	District of Columbia	799	0.4%

Source: American Medical Association (Chicago, Illinois)
    "Physician Characteristics and Distribution in the U.S." (2003-2004 Edition)
*Nonfederal physicians as of December 31, 2001. Total does not include 5,594 physicians in U.S. territories and possessions.

Rate of International Medical School Graduates Practicing in the U.S. in 2001

National Rate = 68 Nonfederal Physicians per 100,000 Population*

ALPHA ORDER

RANK	STATE	RATE
34	Alabama	32
46	Alaska	15
25	Arizona	40
41	Arkansas	26
14	California	62
45	Colorado	17
4	Connecticut	109
11	Delaware	77
6	Florida	97
27	Georgia	39
19	Hawaii	48
50	Idaho	4
5	Illinois	99
24	Indiana	42
32	Iowa	33
25	Kansas	40
21	Kentucky	46
22	Louisiana	45
32	Maine	33
3	Maryland	115
8	Massachusetts	93
10	Michigan	81
28	Minnesota	38
43	Mississippi	20
17	Missouri	53
49	Montana	10
37	Nebraska	29
20	Nevada	47
30	New Hampshire	37
2	New Jersey	146
31	New Mexico	34
1	New York	173
37	North Carolina	29
16	North Dakota	54
13	Ohio	71
35	Oklahoma	31
43	Oregon	20
12	Pennsylvania	76
7	Rhode Island	95
41	South Carolina	26
40	South Dakota	27
28	Tennessee	38
18	Texas	50
47	Utah	14
35	Vermont	31
15	Virginia	57
39	Washington	28
9	West Virginia	82
23	Wisconsin	44
48	Wyoming	11

RANK ORDER

RANK	STATE	RATE
1	New York	173
2	New Jersey	146
3	Maryland	115
4	Connecticut	109
5	Illinois	99
6	Florida	97
7	Rhode Island	95
8	Massachusetts	93
9	West Virginia	82
10	Michigan	81
11	Delaware	77
12	Pennsylvania	76
13	Ohio	71
14	California	62
15	Virginia	57
16	North Dakota	54
17	Missouri	53
18	Texas	50
19	Hawaii	48
20	Nevada	47
21	Kentucky	46
22	Louisiana	45
23	Wisconsin	44
24	Indiana	42
25	Arizona	40
25	Kansas	40
27	Georgia	39
28	Minnesota	38
28	Tennessee	38
30	New Hampshire	37
31	New Mexico	34
32	Iowa	33
32	Maine	33
34	Alabama	32
35	Oklahoma	31
35	Vermont	31
37	Nebraska	29
37	North Carolina	29
39	Washington	28
40	South Dakota	27
41	Arkansas	26
41	South Carolina	26
43	Mississippi	20
43	Oregon	20
45	Colorado	17
46	Alaska	15
47	Utah	14
48	Wyoming	11
49	Montana	10
50	Idaho	4

District of Columbia 139

Source: Morgan Quitno Press using data from American Medical Association (Chicago, Illinois)
"Physician Characteristics and Distribution in the U.S." (2003-2004 Edition)
*As of December 31, 2001. National rate does not include physicians in U.S. territories and possessions.

International Medical School Graduates
As a Percent of Nonfederal Physicians in 2001
National Percent = 24.2% of Nonfederal Physicians*

ALPHA ORDER

RANK	STATE	PERCENT
30	Alabama	14.5
45	Alaska	7.3
22	Arizona	17.2
35	Arkansas	12.5
15	California	22.1
47	Colorado	6.3
9	Connecticut	27.7
7	Delaware	29.1
3	Florida	34.6
22	Georgia	17.2
29	Hawaii	15.4
50	Idaho	2.5
3	Illinois	34.6
21	Indiana	18.7
28	Iowa	16.3
24	Kansas	16.9
20	Kentucky	19.5
26	Louisiana	16.7
37	Maine	11.5
8	Maryland	28.1
18	Massachusetts	20.7
6	Michigan	32.0
34	Minnesota	13.0
41	Mississippi	10.9
17	Missouri	21.2
49	Montana	4.1
37	Nebraska	11.5
12	Nevada	23.7
33	New Hampshire	13.1
1	New Jersey	44.5
32	New Mexico	13.9
2	New York	42.0
39	North Carolina	11.2
15	North Dakota	22.1
10	Ohio	26.8
25	Oklahoma	16.8
44	Oregon	7.5
13	Pennsylvania	23.6
11	Rhode Island	26.0
40	South Carolina	11.0
36	South Dakota	12.4
31	Tennessee	14.4
14	Texas	22.7
46	Utah	6.5
43	Vermont	8.0
18	Virginia	20.7
42	Washington	10.1
5	West Virginia	34.1
27	Wisconsin	16.6
48	Wyoming	5.6

RANK ORDER

RANK	STATE	PERCENT
1	New Jersey	44.5
2	New York	42.0
3	Florida	34.6
3	Illinois	34.6
5	West Virginia	34.1
6	Michigan	32.0
7	Delaware	29.1
8	Maryland	28.1
9	Connecticut	27.7
10	Ohio	26.8
11	Rhode Island	26.0
12	Nevada	23.7
13	Pennsylvania	23.6
14	Texas	22.7
15	California	22.1
15	North Dakota	22.1
17	Missouri	21.2
18	Massachusetts	20.7
18	Virginia	20.7
20	Kentucky	19.5
21	Indiana	18.7
22	Arizona	17.2
22	Georgia	17.2
24	Kansas	16.9
25	Oklahoma	16.8
26	Louisiana	16.7
27	Wisconsin	16.6
28	Iowa	16.3
29	Hawaii	15.4
30	Alabama	14.5
31	Tennessee	14.4
32	New Mexico	13.9
33	New Hampshire	13.1
34	Minnesota	13.0
35	Arkansas	12.5
36	South Dakota	12.4
37	Maine	11.5
37	Nebraska	11.5
39	North Carolina	11.2
40	South Carolina	11.0
41	Mississippi	10.9
42	Washington	10.1
43	Vermont	8.0
44	Oregon	7.5
45	Alaska	7.3
46	Utah	6.5
47	Colorado	6.3
48	Wyoming	5.6
49	Montana	4.1
50	Idaho	2.5

District of Columbia   19.3

Source: Morgan Quitno Press using data from American Medical Association (Chicago, Illinois)
   "Physician Characteristics and Distribution in the U.S." (2003-2004 Edition)
*As of December 31, 2001. National percent does not include physicians in U.S. territories and possessions.

Osteopathic Physicians in 2002

National Total = 43,910 Osteopathic Physicians*

<u>ALPHA ORDER</u>

RANK	STATE	OSTEOPATHS	% of USA
29	Alabama	304	0.7%
44	Alaska	92	0.2%
12	Arizona	1,143	2.6%
38	Arkansas	173	0.4%
7	California	2,532	5.8%
14	Colorado	690	1.6%
33	Connecticut	261	0.6%
36	Delaware	194	0.4%
4	Florida	2,865	6.5%
16	Georgia	590	1.3%
40	Hawaii	137	0.3%
42	Idaho	132	0.3%
9	Illinois	1,908	4.3%
15	Indiana	631	1.4%
13	Iowa	930	2.1%
18	Kansas	523	1.2%
32	Kentucky	266	0.6%
46	Louisiana	84	0.2%
22	Maine	498	1.1%
23	Maryland	475	1.1%
24	Massachusetts	405	0.9%
2	Michigan	4,443	10.1%
31	Minnesota	274	0.6%
35	Mississippi	246	0.6%
10	Missouri	1,650	3.8%
45	Montana	88	0.2%
43	Nebraska	112	0.3%
30	Nevada	279	0.6%
41	New Hampshire	135	0.3%
8	New Jersey	2,509	5.7%
28	New Mexico	308	0.7%
5	New York	2,817	6.4%
26	North Carolina	400	0.9%
48	North Dakota	57	0.1%
3	Ohio	3,197	7.3%
11	Oklahoma	1,266	2.9%
25	Oregon	403	0.9%
1	Pennsylvania	4,900	11.2%
37	Rhode Island	176	0.4%
34	South Carolina	256	0.6%
47	South Dakota	64	0.1%
27	Tennessee	355	0.8%
6	Texas	2,691	6.1%
39	Utah	160	0.4%
49	Vermont	48	0.1%
20	Virginia	517	1.2%
17	Washington	536	1.2%
19	West Virginia	522	1.2%
21	Wisconsin	501	1.1%
50	Wyoming	45	0.1%

<u>RANK ORDER</u>

RANK	STATE	OSTEOPATHS	% of USA
1	Pennsylvania	4,900	11.2%
2	Michigan	4,443	10.1%
3	Ohio	3,197	7.3%
4	Florida	2,865	6.5%
5	New York	2,817	6.4%
6	Texas	2,691	6.1%
7	California	2,532	5.8%
8	New Jersey	2,509	5.7%
9	Illinois	1,908	4.3%
10	Missouri	1,650	3.8%
11	Oklahoma	1,266	2.9%
12	Arizona	1,143	2.6%
13	Iowa	930	2.1%
14	Colorado	690	1.6%
15	Indiana	631	1.4%
16	Georgia	590	1.3%
17	Washington	536	1.2%
18	Kansas	523	1.2%
19	West Virginia	522	1.2%
20	Virginia	517	1.2%
21	Wisconsin	501	1.1%
22	Maine	498	1.1%
23	Maryland	475	1.1%
24	Massachusetts	405	0.9%
25	Oregon	403	0.9%
26	North Carolina	400	0.9%
27	Tennessee	355	0.8%
28	New Mexico	308	0.7%
29	Alabama	304	0.7%
30	Nevada	279	0.6%
31	Minnesota	274	0.6%
32	Kentucky	266	0.6%
33	Connecticut	261	0.6%
34	South Carolina	256	0.6%
35	Mississippi	246	0.6%
36	Delaware	194	0.4%
37	Rhode Island	176	0.4%
38	Arkansas	173	0.4%
39	Utah	160	0.4%
40	Hawaii	137	0.3%
41	New Hampshire	135	0.3%
42	Idaho	132	0.3%
43	Nebraska	112	0.3%
44	Alaska	92	0.2%
45	Montana	88	0.2%
46	Louisiana	84	0.2%
47	South Dakota	64	0.1%
48	North Dakota	57	0.1%
49	Vermont	48	0.1%
50	Wyoming	45	0.1%
	District of Columbia	34	0.1%

Source: American Osteopathic Association
   "Fact Sheet: Active D.O.'s by State" (November 2002, http://www.aoa.net/AOAGeneral/AOAFactsnov02.pdf)
*Excludes retired, disabled, foreign and federal osteopaths. Osteopaths practice a system of medicine based on the theory that disturbances in the musculoskeletal system affect other body parts, causing many disorders that can be corrected by various manipulative techniques in conjunction with conventional medical, surgical, pharmacological, and other therapeutic procedures.

Rate of Osteopathic Physicians in 2002

National Rate = 15 Osteopaths per 100,000 Population*

ALPHA ORDER

RANK	STATE	RATE
37	Alabama	7
19	Alaska	14
11	Arizona	21
42	Arkansas	6
37	California	7
16	Colorado	15
34	Connecticut	8
10	Delaware	24
13	Florida	17
37	Georgia	7
22	Hawaii	11
25	Idaho	10
16	Illinois	15
25	Indiana	10
5	Iowa	32
12	Kansas	19
42	Kentucky	6
50	Louisiana	2
3	Maine	38
28	Maryland	9
42	Massachusetts	6
1	Michigan	44
48	Minnesota	5
28	Mississippi	9
6	Missouri	29
25	Montana	10
42	Nebraska	6
20	Nevada	13
22	New Hampshire	11
6	New Jersey	29
13	New Mexico	17
16	New York	15
48	North Carolina	5
28	North Dakota	9
9	Ohio	28
4	Oklahoma	36
22	Oregon	11
2	Pennsylvania	40
15	Rhode Island	16
42	South Carolina	6
34	South Dakota	8
42	Tennessee	6
21	Texas	12
37	Utah	7
34	Vermont	8
37	Virginia	7
28	Washington	9
6	West Virginia	29
28	Wisconsin	9
28	Wyoming	9

RANK ORDER

RANK	STATE	RATE
1	Michigan	44
2	Pennsylvania	40
3	Maine	38
4	Oklahoma	36
5	Iowa	32
6	Missouri	29
6	New Jersey	29
6	West Virginia	29
9	Ohio	28
10	Delaware	24
11	Arizona	21
12	Kansas	19
13	Florida	17
13	New Mexico	17
15	Rhode Island	16
16	Colorado	15
16	Illinois	15
16	New York	15
19	Alaska	14
20	Nevada	13
21	Texas	12
22	Hawaii	11
22	New Hampshire	11
22	Oregon	11
25	Idaho	10
25	Indiana	10
25	Montana	10
28	Maryland	9
28	Mississippi	9
28	North Dakota	9
28	Washington	9
28	Wisconsin	9
28	Wyoming	9
34	Connecticut	8
34	South Dakota	8
34	Vermont	8
37	Alabama	7
37	California	7
37	Georgia	7
37	Utah	7
37	Virginia	7
42	Arkansas	6
42	Kentucky	6
42	Massachusetts	6
42	Nebraska	6
42	South Carolina	6
42	Tennessee	6
48	Minnesota	5
48	North Carolina	5
50	Louisiana	2
	District of Columbia	6

Source: Morgan Quitno Press using data from American Osteopathic Association
    "Fact Sheet: Active D.O.'s by State" (November 2002, http://www.aoa.net/AOAGeneral/AOAFactsnov02.pdf)
*Calculated using 2002 population estimates. Excludes retired, disabled, foreign and federal osteopaths.
Osteopaths practice a system of medicine based on the theory that disturbances in the musculoskeletal system
affect other body parts, causing many disorders that can be corrected by various manipulative techniques in
conjunction with conventional medical, surgical, pharmacological, and other therapeutic procedures.

Podiatric Physicians in 2002

National Total = 14,850 Podiatric Physicians*

<u>ALPHA ORDER</u>

RANK	STATE	PODIATRISTS	% of USA
25	Alabama	128	0.9%
49	Alaska	15	0.1%
18	Arizona	230	1.5%
36	Arkansas	68	0.5%
2	California	1,545	10.4%
23	Colorado	148	1.0%
14	Connecticut	248	1.7%
41	Delaware	49	0.3%
3	Florida	1,152	7.8%
13	Georgia	287	1.9%
50	Hawaii	8	0.1%
44	Idaho	41	0.3%
5	Illinois	882	5.9%
15	Indiana	240	1.6%
20	Iowa	174	1.2%
31	Kansas	93	0.6%
29	Kentucky	104	0.7%
27	Louisiana	120	0.8%
35	Maine	73	0.5%
11	Maryland	357	2.4%
10	Massachusetts	403	2.7%
9	Michigan	612	4.1%
24	Minnesota	140	0.9%
41	Mississippi	49	0.3%
21	Missouri	172	1.2%
43	Montana	42	0.3%
40	Nebraska	55	0.4%
34	Nevada	83	0.6%
39	New Hampshire	61	0.4%
6	New Jersey	823	5.5%
37	New Mexico	64	0.4%
1	New York	1,941	13.1%
16	North Carolina	238	1.6%
47	North Dakota	21	0.1%
7	Ohio	805	5.4%
32	Oklahoma	92	0.6%
26	Oregon	126	0.8%
4	Pennsylvania	1,069	7.2%
33	Rhode Island	84	0.6%
30	South Carolina	97	0.7%
45	South Dakota	33	0.2%
22	Tennessee	170	1.1%
8	Texas	695	4.7%
28	Utah	105	0.7%
46	Vermont	23	0.2%
12	Virginia	322	2.2%
17	Washington	233	1.6%
37	West Virginia	64	0.4%
19	Wisconsin	202	1.4%
48	Wyoming	16	0.1%

<u>RANK ORDER</u>

RANK	STATE	PODIATRISTS	% of USA
1	New York	1,941	13.1%
2	California	1,545	10.4%
3	Florida	1,152	7.8%
4	Pennsylvania	1,069	7.2%
5	Illinois	882	5.9%
6	New Jersey	823	5.5%
7	Ohio	805	5.4%
8	Texas	695	4.7%
9	Michigan	612	4.1%
10	Massachusetts	403	2.7%
11	Maryland	357	2.4%
12	Virginia	322	2.2%
13	Georgia	287	1.9%
14	Connecticut	248	1.7%
15	Indiana	240	1.6%
16	North Carolina	238	1.6%
17	Washington	233	1.6%
18	Arizona	230	1.5%
19	Wisconsin	202	1.4%
20	Iowa	174	1.2%
21	Missouri	172	1.2%
22	Tennessee	170	1.1%
23	Colorado	148	1.0%
24	Minnesota	140	0.9%
25	Alabama	128	0.9%
26	Oregon	126	0.8%
27	Louisiana	120	0.8%
28	Utah	105	0.7%
29	Kentucky	104	0.7%
30	South Carolina	97	0.7%
31	Kansas	93	0.6%
32	Oklahoma	92	0.6%
33	Rhode Island	84	0.6%
34	Nevada	83	0.6%
35	Maine	73	0.5%
36	Arkansas	68	0.5%
37	New Mexico	64	0.4%
37	West Virginia	64	0.4%
39	New Hampshire	61	0.4%
40	Nebraska	55	0.4%
41	Delaware	49	0.3%
41	Mississippi	49	0.3%
43	Montana	42	0.3%
44	Idaho	41	0.3%
45	South Dakota	33	0.2%
46	Vermont	23	0.2%
47	North Dakota	21	0.1%
48	Wyoming	16	0.1%
49	Alaska	15	0.1%
50	Hawaii	8	0.1%
	District of Columbia	48	0.3%

Source: American Podiatric Medical Association, Inc.
  "Podiatric Physicians in Active Practice"
*Podiatry deals with the diagnosis, treatment, and prevention of diseases of the human foot. National total does not include 49 podiatrists in Puerto Rico, Virgin Islands and U.S. Armed Services.

Rate of Podiatric Physicians in 2002

National Rate = 5.1 Podiatrists per 100,000 Population*

RANK	STATE	RATE
39	Alabama	2.9
48	Alaska	2.3
21	Arizona	4.2
45	Arkansas	2.5
18	California	4.4
32	Colorado	3.3
5	Connecticut	7.2
11	Delaware	6.1
8	Florida	6.9
30	Georgia	3.4
50	Hawaii	0.6
37	Idaho	3.1
6	Illinois	7.0
22	Indiana	3.9
13	Iowa	5.9
30	Kansas	3.4
45	Kentucky	2.5
43	Louisiana	2.7
14	Maine	5.6
9	Maryland	6.5
10	Massachusetts	6.3
11	Michigan	6.1
42	Minnesota	2.8
49	Mississippi	1.7
38	Missouri	3.0
16	Montana	4.6
34	Nebraska	3.2
23	Nevada	3.8
15	New Hampshire	4.8
2	New Jersey	9.6
29	New Mexico	3.5
1	New York	10.1
39	North Carolina	2.9
32	North Dakota	3.3
6	Ohio	7.0
44	Oklahoma	2.6
27	Oregon	3.6
3	Pennsylvania	8.7
4	Rhode Island	7.9
47	South Carolina	2.4
20	South Dakota	4.3
39	Tennessee	2.9
34	Texas	3.2
17	Utah	4.5
25	Vermont	3.7
18	Virginia	4.4
23	Washington	3.8
27	West Virginia	3.6
25	Wisconsin	3.7
34	Wyoming	3.2

RANK	STATE	RATE
1	New York	10.1
2	New Jersey	9.6
3	Pennsylvania	8.7
4	Rhode Island	7.9
5	Connecticut	7.2
6	Illinois	7.0
6	Ohio	7.0
8	Florida	6.9
9	Maryland	6.5
10	Massachusetts	6.3
11	Delaware	6.1
11	Michigan	6.1
13	Iowa	5.9
14	Maine	5.6
15	New Hampshire	4.8
16	Montana	4.6
17	Utah	4.5
18	California	4.4
18	Virginia	4.4
20	South Dakota	4.3
21	Arizona	4.2
22	Indiana	3.9
23	Nevada	3.8
23	Washington	3.8
25	Vermont	3.7
25	Wisconsin	3.7
27	Oregon	3.6
27	West Virginia	3.6
29	New Mexico	3.5
30	Georgia	3.4
30	Kansas	3.4
32	Colorado	3.3
32	North Dakota	3.3
34	Nebraska	3.2
34	Texas	3.2
34	Wyoming	3.2
37	Idaho	3.1
38	Missouri	3.0
39	Alabama	2.9
39	North Carolina	2.9
39	Tennessee	2.9
42	Minnesota	2.8
43	Louisiana	2.7
44	Oklahoma	2.6
45	Arkansas	2.5
45	Kentucky	2.5
47	South Carolina	2.4
48	Alaska	2.3
49	Mississippi	1.7
50	Hawaii	0.6

District of Columbia 8.4

Source: Morgan Quitno Press using data from American Podiatric Medical Association, Inc.
    "Podiatric Physicians in Active Practice"
*Podiatry deals with the diagnosis, treatment, and prevention of diseases of the human foot. National rate does not include podiatrists in Puerto Rico, Virgin Islands and U.S. Armed Services.

Doctors of Chiropractic in 2000

National Total = 81,011 Chiropractors*

ALPHA ORDER

RANK	STATE	CHIROPRACTOR	% of USA
30	Alabama	759	0.9%
48	Alaska	175	0.2%
10	Arizona	2,488	3.1%
33	Arkansas	557	0.7%
1	California	12,600	15.6%
11	Colorado	2,063	2.5%
27	Connecticut	893	1.1%
45	Delaware	242	0.3%
3	Florida	4,335	5.4%
6	Georgia	3,552	4.4%
34	Hawaii	521	0.6%
38	Idaho	363	0.4%
8	Illinois	2,925	3.6%
25	Indiana	964	1.2%
21	Iowa	1,309	1.6%
26	Kansas	932	1.2%
24	Kentucky	1,121	1.4%
22	Louisiana	1,289	1.6%
39	Maine	355	0.4%
32	Maryland	587	0.7%
15	Massachusetts	1,934	2.4%
9	Michigan	2,755	3.4%
13	Minnesota	1,960	2.4%
41	Mississippi	339	0.4%
16	Missouri	1,917	2.4%
43	Montana	302	0.4%
42	Nebraska	324	0.4%
37	Nevada	427	0.5%
36	New Hampshire	449	0.6%
7	New Jersey	3,383	4.2%
35	New Mexico	493	0.6%
2	New York	5,885	7.3%
17	North Carolina	1,628	2.0%
46	North Dakota	240	0.3%
12	Ohio	2,015	2.5%
28	Oklahoma	867	1.1%
19	Oregon	1,396	1.7%
5	Pennsylvania	3,704	4.6%
NA	Rhode Island**	NA	NA
23	South Carolina	1,263	1.6%
40	South Dakota	346	0.4%
29	Tennessee	802	1.0%
4	Texas	4,268	5.3%
31	Utah	754	0.9%
47	Vermont	215	0.3%
20	Virginia	1,311	1.6%
14	Washington	1,938	2.4%
44	West Virginia	276	0.3%
18	Wisconsin	1,584	2.0%
49	Wyoming	171	0.2%

RANK ORDER

RANK	STATE	CHIROPRACTOR	% of USA
1	California	12,600	15.6%
2	New York	5,885	7.3%
3	Florida	4,335	5.4%
4	Texas	4,268	5.3%
5	Pennsylvania	3,704	4.6%
6	Georgia	3,552	4.4%
7	New Jersey	3,383	4.2%
8	Illinois	2,925	3.6%
9	Michigan	2,755	3.4%
10	Arizona	2,488	3.1%
11	Colorado	2,063	2.5%
12	Ohio	2,015	2.5%
13	Minnesota	1,960	2.4%
14	Washington	1,938	2.4%
15	Massachusetts	1,934	2.4%
16	Missouri	1,917	2.4%
17	North Carolina	1,628	2.0%
18	Wisconsin	1,584	2.0%
19	Oregon	1,396	1.7%
20	Virginia	1,311	1.6%
21	Iowa	1,309	1.6%
22	Louisiana	1,289	1.6%
23	South Carolina	1,263	1.6%
24	Kentucky	1,121	1.4%
25	Indiana	964	1.2%
26	Kansas	932	1.2%
27	Connecticut	893	1.1%
28	Oklahoma	867	1.1%
29	Tennessee	802	1.0%
30	Alabama	759	0.9%
31	Utah	754	0.9%
32	Maryland	587	0.7%
33	Arkansas	557	0.7%
34	Hawaii	521	0.6%
35	New Mexico	493	0.6%
36	New Hampshire	449	0.6%
37	Nevada	427	0.5%
38	Idaho	363	0.4%
39	Maine	355	0.4%
40	South Dakota	346	0.4%
41	Mississippi	339	0.4%
42	Nebraska	324	0.4%
43	Montana	302	0.4%
44	West Virginia	276	0.3%
45	Delaware	242	0.3%
46	North Dakota	240	0.3%
47	Vermont	215	0.3%
48	Alaska	175	0.2%
49	Wyoming	171	0.2%
NA	Rhode Island**	NA	NA
	District of Columbia	35	0.0%

Source: Federation of Chiropractic Licensing Boards
"Official Directory" (http://www.fclb.org/directory/index.htm)

As of December 2000. Licensed active doctors. There is some duplication as some doctors are licensed in more than one state.
***Not available.*

Rate of Doctors of Chiropractic in 2000

National Rate = 29 Chiropractors per 100,000 Population*

ALPHA ORDER

RANK	STATE	RATE
44	Alabama	17
27	Alaska	28
1	Arizona	48
37	Arkansas	21
10	California	37
1	Colorado	48
34	Connecticut	26
20	Delaware	31
32	Florida	27
5	Georgia	43
5	Hawaii	43
27	Idaho	28
36	Illinois	24
45	Indiana	16
4	Iowa	45
13	Kansas	35
27	Kentucky	28
25	Louisiana	29
27	Maine	28
49	Maryland	11
23	Massachusetts	30
27	Michigan	28
8	Minnesota	40
48	Mississippi	12
16	Missouri	34
18	Montana	33
41	Nebraska	19
37	Nevada	21
12	New Hampshire	36
8	New Jersey	40
32	New Mexico	27
20	New York	31
39	North Carolina	20
10	North Dakota	37
42	Ohio	18
35	Oklahoma	25
7	Oregon	41
23	Pennsylvania	30
NA	Rhode Island**	NA
20	South Carolina	31
3	South Dakota	46
47	Tennessee	14
39	Texas	20
16	Utah	34
13	Vermont	35
42	Virginia	18
18	Washington	33
46	West Virginia	15
25	Wisconsin	29
13	Wyoming	35

RANK ORDER

RANK	STATE	RATE
1	Arizona	48
1	Colorado	48
3	South Dakota	46
4	Iowa	45
5	Georgia	43
5	Hawaii	43
7	Oregon	41
8	Minnesota	40
8	New Jersey	40
10	California	37
10	North Dakota	37
12	New Hampshire	36
13	Kansas	35
13	Vermont	35
13	Wyoming	35
16	Missouri	34
16	Utah	34
18	Montana	33
18	Washington	33
20	Delaware	31
20	New York	31
20	South Carolina	31
23	Massachusetts	30
23	Pennsylvania	30
25	Louisiana	29
25	Wisconsin	29
27	Alaska	28
27	Idaho	28
27	Kentucky	28
27	Maine	28
27	Michigan	28
32	Florida	27
32	New Mexico	27
34	Connecticut	26
35	Oklahoma	25
36	Illinois	24
37	Arkansas	21
37	Nevada	21
39	North Carolina	20
39	Texas	20
41	Nebraska	19
42	Ohio	18
42	Virginia	18
44	Alabama	17
45	Indiana	16
46	West Virginia	15
47	Tennessee	14
48	Mississippi	12
49	Maryland	11
NA	Rhode Island**	NA
	District of Columbia	6

Source: Morgan Quitno Press using data from Federation of Chiropractic Licensing Boards
"Official Directory" (http://www.fclb.org/directory/index.htm)
*As of December 2000. Licensed active doctors. There is some duplication as some doctors are licensed in more than one state.
**Not available.

Physician Assistants in Clinical Practice in 2003

National Total = 45,765 Physician Assistants*

ALPHA ORDER

RANK	STATE	PA'S	% of USA
41	Alabama	242	0.5%
37	Alaska	278	0.6%
16	Arizona	894	2.0%
49	Arkansas	55	0.1%
2	California	4,561	10.0%
13	Colorado	1,083	2.4%
17	Connecticut	884	1.9%
47	Delaware	125	0.3%
5	Florida	2,548	5.6%
8	Georgia	1,537	3.4%
48	Hawaii	109	0.2%
38	Idaho	275	0.6%
12	Illinois	1,152	2.5%
32	Indiana	382	0.8%
26	Iowa	530	1.2%
23	Kansas	572	1.2%
24	Kentucky	562	1.2%
35	Louisiana	319	0.7%
29	Maine	436	1.0%
11	Maryland	1,300	2.8%
14	Massachusetts	971	2.1%
7	Michigan	1,928	4.2%
19	Minnesota	706	1.5%
50	Mississippi	30	0.1%
34	Missouri	330	0.7%
42	Montana	212	0.5%
25	Nebraska	537	1.2%
39	Nevada	265	0.6%
40	New Hampshire	255	0.6%
21	New Jersey	654	1.4%
33	New Mexico	363	0.8%
1	New York	5,371	11.7%
6	North Carolina	2,285	5.0%
43	North Dakota	200	0.4%
9	Ohio	1,348	2.9%
20	Oklahoma	667	1.5%
28	Oregon	461	1.0%
4	Pennsylvania	2,629	5.7%
44	Rhode Island	154	0.3%
31	South Carolina	398	0.9%
36	South Dakota	298	0.7%
22	Tennessee	580	1.3%
3	Texas	2,827	6.2%
30	Utah	411	0.9%
45	Vermont	151	0.3%
18	Virginia	771	1.7%
10	Washington	1,347	2.9%
27	West Virginia	511	1.1%
15	Wisconsin	950	2.1%
46	Wyoming	131	0.3%

RANK ORDER

RANK	STATE	PA'S	% of USA
1	New York	5,371	11.7%
2	California	4,561	10.0%
3	Texas	2,827	6.2%
4	Pennsylvania	2,629	5.7%
5	Florida	2,548	5.6%
6	North Carolina	2,285	5.0%
7	Michigan	1,928	4.2%
8	Georgia	1,537	3.4%
9	Ohio	1,348	2.9%
10	Washington	1,347	2.9%
11	Maryland	1,300	2.8%
12	Illinois	1,152	2.5%
13	Colorado	1,083	2.4%
14	Massachusetts	971	2.1%
15	Wisconsin	950	2.1%
16	Arizona	894	2.0%
17	Connecticut	884	1.9%
18	Virginia	771	1.7%
19	Minnesota	706	1.5%
20	Oklahoma	667	1.5%
21	New Jersey	654	1.4%
22	Tennessee	580	1.3%
23	Kansas	572	1.2%
24	Kentucky	562	1.2%
25	Nebraska	537	1.2%
26	Iowa	530	1.2%
27	West Virginia	511	1.1%
28	Oregon	461	1.0%
29	Maine	436	1.0%
30	Utah	411	0.9%
31	South Carolina	398	0.9%
32	Indiana	382	0.8%
33	New Mexico	363	0.8%
34	Missouri	330	0.7%
35	Louisiana	319	0.7%
36	South Dakota	298	0.7%
37	Alaska	278	0.6%
38	Idaho	275	0.6%
39	Nevada	265	0.6%
40	New Hampshire	255	0.6%
41	Alabama	242	0.5%
42	Montana	212	0.5%
43	North Dakota	200	0.4%
44	Rhode Island	154	0.3%
45	Vermont	151	0.3%
46	Wyoming	131	0.3%
47	Delaware	125	0.3%
48	Hawaii	109	0.2%
49	Arkansas	55	0.1%
50	Mississippi	30	0.1%
	District of Columbia	180	0.4%

Source: The American Academy of Physician Assistants
"Projected Number of PAs in Clinical Practice as of January 1, 2003"
(http://www.aapa.org/research/03projClinPracPAs.html)
*Projected. National total does not include 237 physician assistants who work outside the United States or whose location is unknown.

Rate of Physician Assistants in Clinical Practice in 2003

National Rate = 15.9 PA's per 100,000 Population*

ALPHA ORDER

RANK	STATE	RATE
48	Alabama	5.4
1	Alaska	43.2
27	Arizona	16.4
49	Arkansas	2.0
35	California	13.0
12	Colorado	24.0
10	Connecticut	25.5
28	Delaware	15.5
29	Florida	15.2
23	Georgia	18.0
43	Hawaii	8.8
18	Idaho	20.5
42	Illinois	9.1
46	Indiana	6.2
23	Iowa	18.0
17	Kansas	21.1
33	Kentucky	13.7
45	Louisiana	7.1
3	Maine	33.7
13	Maryland	23.8
30	Massachusetts	15.1
21	Michigan	19.2
32	Minnesota	14.1
50	Mississippi	1.0
47	Missouri	5.8
14	Montana	23.3
5	Nebraska	31.1
37	Nevada	12.2
19	New Hampshire	20.0
44	New Jersey	7.6
20	New Mexico	19.6
7	New York	28.0
8	North Carolina	27.5
4	North Dakota	31.5
38	Ohio	11.8
22	Oklahoma	19.1
34	Oregon	13.1
16	Pennsylvania	21.3
31	Rhode Island	14.4
41	South Carolina	9.7
2	South Dakota	39.2
40	Tennessee	10.0
35	Texas	13.0
25	Utah	17.7
11	Vermont	24.5
39	Virginia	10.6
15	Washington	22.2
6	West Virginia	28.4
26	Wisconsin	17.5
9	Wyoming	26.3

RANK ORDER

RANK	STATE	RATE
1	Alaska	43.2
2	South Dakota	39.2
3	Maine	33.7
4	North Dakota	31.5
5	Nebraska	31.1
6	West Virginia	28.4
7	New York	28.0
8	North Carolina	27.5
9	Wyoming	26.3
10	Connecticut	25.5
11	Vermont	24.5
12	Colorado	24.0
13	Maryland	23.8
14	Montana	23.3
15	Washington	22.2
16	Pennsylvania	21.3
17	Kansas	21.1
18	Idaho	20.5
19	New Hampshire	20.0
20	New Mexico	19.6
21	Michigan	19.2
22	Oklahoma	19.1
23	Georgia	18.0
23	Iowa	18.0
25	Utah	17.7
26	Wisconsin	17.5
27	Arizona	16.4
28	Delaware	15.5
29	Florida	15.2
30	Massachusetts	15.1
31	Rhode Island	14.4
32	Minnesota	14.1
33	Kentucky	13.7
34	Oregon	13.1
35	California	13.0
35	Texas	13.0
37	Nevada	12.2
38	Ohio	11.8
39	Virginia	10.6
40	Tennessee	10.0
41	South Carolina	9.7
42	Illinois	9.1
43	Hawaii	8.8
44	New Jersey	7.6
45	Louisiana	7.1
46	Indiana	6.2
47	Missouri	5.8
48	Alabama	5.4
49	Arkansas	2.0
50	Mississippi	1.0

District of Columbia 31.5

Source: Morgan Quitno Press using data from The American Academy of Physician Assistants
"Projected Number of PAs in Clinical Practice as of January 1, 2003"
(http://www.aapa.org/research/03projClinPracPAs.html)
*Projected. Rates calculated using 2002 Census population figures.

Registered Nurses in 2000

National Total = 2,201,813 Registered Nurses*

ALPHA ORDER			
RANK	STATE	NURSES	% of USA
22	Alabama	34,073	1.5%
49	Alaska	4,914	0.2%
24	Arizona	32,222	1.5%
33	Arkansas	18,752	0.9%
1	California	184,329	8.4%
26	Colorado	31,695	1.4%
25	Connecticut	32,073	1.5%
45	Delaware	7,337	0.3%
4	Florida	125,439	5.7%
12	Georgia	55,881	2.5%
42	Hawaii	8,518	0.4%
44	Idaho	8,230	0.4%
6	Illinois	101,660	4.6%
18	Indiana	46,244	2.1%
27	Iowa	31,020	1.4%
30	Kansas	23,779	1.1%
23	Kentucky	33,655	1.5%
21	Louisiana	37,275	1.7%
37	Maine	13,072	0.6%
19	Maryland	45,323	2.1%
9	Massachusetts	75,795	3.4%
8	Michigan	79,353	3.6%
17	Minnesota	47,102	2.1%
32	Mississippi	21,338	1.0%
13	Missouri	53,730	2.4%
46	Montana	7,327	0.3%
34	Nebraska	16,399	0.7%
41	Nevada	10,384	0.5%
40	New Hampshire	11,321	0.5%
11	New Jersey	67,280	3.1%
38	New Mexico	11,932	0.5%
2	New York	160,009	7.3%
10	North Carolina	69,057	3.1%
47	North Dakota	7,039	0.3%
7	Ohio	100,144	4.5%
31	Oklahoma	21,905	1.0%
29	Oregon	27,121	1.2%
5	Pennsylvania	123,997	5.6%
39	Rhode Island	11,542	0.5%
28	South Carolina	29,226	1.3%
43	South Dakota	8,511	0.4%
15	Tennessee	49,626	2.3%
3	Texas	126,436	5.7%
36	Utah	13,229	0.6%
48	Vermont	5,829	0.3%
14	Virginia	50,359	2.3%
20	Washington	43,482	2.0%
35	West Virginia	15,523	0.7%
16	Wisconsin	47,895	2.2%
50	Wyoming	3,849	0.2%

RANK ORDER			
RANK	STATE	NURSES	% of USA
1	California	184,329	8.4%
2	New York	160,009	7.3%
3	Texas	126,436	5.7%
4	Florida	125,439	5.7%
5	Pennsylvania	123,997	5.6%
6	Illinois	101,660	4.6%
7	Ohio	100,144	4.5%
8	Michigan	79,353	3.6%
9	Massachusetts	75,795	3.4%
10	North Carolina	69,057	3.1%
11	New Jersey	67,280	3.1%
12	Georgia	55,881	2.5%
13	Missouri	53,730	2.4%
14	Virginia	50,359	2.3%
15	Tennessee	49,626	2.3%
16	Wisconsin	47,895	2.2%
17	Minnesota	47,102	2.1%
18	Indiana	46,244	2.1%
19	Maryland	45,323	2.1%
20	Washington	43,482	2.0%
21	Louisiana	37,275	1.7%
22	Alabama	34,073	1.5%
23	Kentucky	33,655	1.5%
24	Arizona	32,222	1.5%
25	Connecticut	32,073	1.5%
26	Colorado	31,695	1.4%
27	Iowa	31,020	1.4%
28	South Carolina	29,226	1.3%
29	Oregon	27,121	1.2%
30	Kansas	23,779	1.1%
31	Oklahoma	21,905	1.0%
32	Mississippi	21,338	1.0%
33	Arkansas	18,752	0.9%
34	Nebraska	16,399	0.7%
35	West Virginia	15,523	0.7%
36	Utah	13,229	0.6%
37	Maine	13,072	0.6%
38	New Mexico	11,932	0.5%
39	Rhode Island	11,542	0.5%
40	New Hampshire	11,321	0.5%
41	Nevada	10,384	0.5%
42	Hawaii	8,518	0.4%
43	South Dakota	8,511	0.4%
44	Idaho	8,230	0.4%
45	Delaware	7,337	0.3%
46	Montana	7,327	0.3%
47	North Dakota	7,039	0.3%
48	Vermont	5,829	0.3%
49	Alaska	4,914	0.2%
50	Wyoming	3,849	0.2%
	District of Columbia	9,583	0.4%

*Source: U.S. Department of Health and Human Services, Health Resources and Services Administration
"The Registered Nurse Population" (February 2001)*
Preliminary as of March 2000. Does not include 494,727 registered nurses not employed in nursing.

Rate of Registered Nurses in 2000

National Rate = 782 Nurses per 100,000 Population*

ALPHA ORDER

RANK ORDER

RANK	STATE	RATE	RANK	STATE	RATE
33	Alabama	766	1	Massachusetts	1,194
31	Alaska	784	2	South Dakota	1,128
46	Arizona	628	3	Rhode Island	1,101
41	Arkansas	701	4	North Dakota	1,096
49	California	544	5	Iowa	1,060
37	Colorado	737	6	Maine	1,025
12	Connecticut	942	7	Pennsylvania	1,010
13	Delaware	936	8	Missouri	960
30	Florida	785	9	Nebraska	958
42	Georgia	683	10	Minnesota	957
40	Hawaii	703	10	Vermont	957
44	Idaho	636	12	Connecticut	942
25	Illinois	819	13	Delaware	936
34	Indiana	761	14	New Hampshire	916
5	Iowa	1,060	15	Wisconsin	893
16	Kansas	885	16	Kansas	885
24	Kentucky	833	17	Ohio	882
23	Louisiana	834	18	Tennessee	872
6	Maine	1,025	19	North Carolina	858
21	Maryland	856	19	West Virginia	858
1	Massachusetts	1,194	21	Maryland	856
28	Michigan	798	22	New York	843
10	Minnesota	957	23	Louisiana	834
35	Mississippi	750	24	Kentucky	833
8	Missouri	960	25	Illinois	819
26	Montana	812	26	Montana	812
9	Nebraska	958	27	New Jersey	800
50	Nevada	520	28	Michigan	798
14	New Hampshire	916	29	Oregon	793
27	New Jersey	800	30	Florida	785
43	New Mexico	656	31	Alaska	784
22	New York	843	32	Wyoming	780
19	North Carolina	858	33	Alabama	766
4	North Dakota	1,096	34	Indiana	761
17	Ohio	882	35	Mississippi	750
45	Oklahoma	635	36	Washington	738
29	Oregon	793	37	Colorado	737
7	Pennsylvania	1,010	38	South Carolina	728
3	Rhode Island	1,101	39	Virginia	711
38	South Carolina	728	40	Hawaii	703
2	South Dakota	1,128	41	Arkansas	701
18	Tennessee	872	42	Georgia	683
47	Texas	606	43	New Mexico	656
48	Utah	592	44	Idaho	636
10	Vermont	957	45	Oklahoma	635
39	Virginia	711	46	Arizona	628
36	Washington	738	47	Texas	606
19	West Virginia	858	48	Utah	592
15	Wisconsin	893	49	California	544
32	Wyoming	780	50	Nevada	520
				District of Columbia	1,675

Source: U.S. Department of Health and Human Services, Health Resources and Services Administration
"The Registered Nurse Population" (February 2001)
*Preliminary as of March 2000. Rates do not include registered nurses not employed in nursing.

Dentists in 2000

National Total = 166,383 Dentists*

ALPHA ORDER

RANK	STATE	DENTISTS	% of USA
27	Alabama	1,912	1.1%
45	Alaska	467	0.3%
23	Arizona	2,322	1.4%
35	Arkansas	1,080	0.6%
1	California	22,963	13.8%
20	Colorado	2,818	1.7%
22	Connecticut	2,636	1.6%
47	Delaware	357	0.2%
5	Florida	8,170	4.9%
14	Georgia	3,611	2.2%
36	Hawaii	992	0.6%
41	Idaho	678	0.4%
4	Illinois	8,205	4.9%
19	Indiana	2,867	1.7%
30	Iowa	1,564	0.9%
32	Kansas	1,329	0.8%
25	Kentucky	2,258	1.4%
26	Louisiana	2,086	1.3%
42	Maine	601	0.4%
12	Maryland	3,986	2.4%
10	Massachusetts	5,137	3.1%
9	Michigan	5,913	3.6%
18	Minnesota	2,960	1.8%
33	Mississippi	1,115	0.7%
21	Missouri	2,680	1.6%
44	Montana	485	0.3%
34	Nebraska	1,087	0.7%
39	Nevada	763	0.5%
40	New Hampshire	707	0.4%
7	New Jersey	6,607	4.0%
38	New Mexico	809	0.5%
2	New York	15,159	9.1%
15	North Carolina	3,394	2.0%
49	North Dakota	300	0.2%
8	Ohio	6,108	3.7%
29	Oklahoma	1,683	1.0%
24	Oregon	2,273	1.4%
6	Pennsylvania	8,031	4.8%
43	Rhode Island	589	0.4%
28	South Carolina	1,803	1.1%
46	South Dakota	359	0.2%
17	Tennessee	2,993	1.8%
3	Texas	9,873	5.9%
31	Utah	1,398	0.8%
48	Vermont	353	0.2%
11	Virginia	4,036	2.4%
13	Washington	3,860	2.3%
37	West Virginia	828	0.5%
16	Wisconsin	3,119	1.9%
50	Wyoming	267	0.2%

RANK ORDER

RANK	STATE	DENTISTS	% of USA
1	California	22,963	13.8%
2	New York	15,159	9.1%
3	Texas	9,873	5.9%
4	Illinois	8,205	4.9%
5	Florida	8,170	4.9%
6	Pennsylvania	8,031	4.8%
7	New Jersey	6,607	4.0%
8	Ohio	6,108	3.7%
9	Michigan	5,913	3.6%
10	Massachusetts	5,137	3.1%
11	Virginia	4,036	2.4%
12	Maryland	3,986	2.4%
13	Washington	3,860	2.3%
14	Georgia	3,611	2.2%
15	North Carolina	3,394	2.0%
16	Wisconsin	3,119	1.9%
17	Tennessee	2,993	1.8%
18	Minnesota	2,960	1.8%
19	Indiana	2,867	1.7%
20	Colorado	2,818	1.7%
21	Missouri	2,680	1.6%
22	Connecticut	2,636	1.6%
23	Arizona	2,322	1.4%
24	Oregon	2,273	1.4%
25	Kentucky	2,258	1.4%
26	Louisiana	2,086	1.3%
27	Alabama	1,912	1.1%
28	South Carolina	1,803	1.1%
29	Oklahoma	1,683	1.0%
30	Iowa	1,564	0.9%
31	Utah	1,398	0.8%
32	Kansas	1,329	0.8%
33	Mississippi	1,115	0.7%
34	Nebraska	1,087	0.7%
35	Arkansas	1,080	0.6%
36	Hawaii	992	0.6%
37	West Virginia	828	0.5%
38	New Mexico	809	0.5%
39	Nevada	763	0.5%
40	New Hampshire	707	0.4%
41	Idaho	678	0.4%
42	Maine	601	0.4%
43	Rhode Island	589	0.4%
44	Montana	485	0.3%
45	Alaska	467	0.3%
46	South Dakota	359	0.2%
47	Delaware	357	0.2%
48	Vermont	353	0.2%
49	North Dakota	300	0.2%
50	Wyoming	267	0.2%
	District of Columbia	728	0.4%

Source: American Dental Association
   "Distribution of Dentists, by Region and State, 2000"
Professionally active dentists. Total includes 64 dentists for whom state is no known. Total does not include 2,366 dentists in territories nor dentists in the Armed Forces stationed overseas.

Rate of Dentists in 2000

National Rate = 59 Dentists per 100,000 Population*

ALPHA ORDER

RANK	STATE	RATE
46	Alabama	43
7	Alaska	74
41	Arizona	45
48	Arkansas	40
8	California	68
11	Colorado	65
5	Connecticut	77
41	Delaware	45
30	Florida	51
44	Georgia	44
1	Hawaii	82
28	Idaho	52
9	Illinois	66
35	Indiana	47
27	Iowa	53
31	Kansas	49
22	Kentucky	56
35	Louisiana	47
35	Maine	47
6	Maryland	75
2	Massachusetts	81
17	Michigan	59
16	Minnesota	60
49	Mississippi	39
33	Missouri	48
24	Montana	54
14	Nebraska	63
50	Nevada	38
20	New Hampshire	57
4	New Jersey	78
44	New Mexico	44
3	New York	80
47	North Carolina	42
35	North Dakota	47
24	Ohio	54
31	Oklahoma	49
9	Oregon	66
11	Pennsylvania	65
22	Rhode Island	56
41	South Carolina	45
33	South Dakota	48
28	Tennessee	52
35	Texas	47
15	Utah	62
18	Vermont	58
20	Virginia	57
11	Washington	65
40	West Virginia	46
18	Wisconsin	58
24	Wyoming	54

RANK ORDER

RANK	STATE	RATE
1	Hawaii	82
2	Massachusetts	81
3	New York	80
4	New Jersey	78
5	Connecticut	77
6	Maryland	75
7	Alaska	74
8	California	68
9	Illinois	66
9	Oregon	66
11	Colorado	65
11	Pennsylvania	65
11	Washington	65
14	Nebraska	63
15	Utah	62
16	Minnesota	60
17	Michigan	59
18	Vermont	58
18	Wisconsin	58
20	New Hampshire	57
20	Virginia	57
22	Kentucky	56
22	Rhode Island	56
24	Montana	54
24	Ohio	54
24	Wyoming	54
27	Iowa	53
28	Idaho	52
28	Tennessee	52
30	Florida	51
31	Kansas	49
31	Oklahoma	49
33	Missouri	48
33	South Dakota	48
35	Indiana	47
35	Louisiana	47
35	Maine	47
35	North Dakota	47
35	Texas	47
40	West Virginia	46
41	Arizona	45
41	Delaware	45
41	South Carolina	45
44	Georgia	44
44	New Mexico	44
46	Alabama	43
47	North Carolina	42
48	Arkansas	40
49	Mississippi	39
50	Nevada	38

District of Columbia	127

Source: Morgan Quitno Press using data from American Dental Association
   "Distribution of Dentists, by Region and State, 2000"
Professionally active dentists. National rate includes dentists for whom state is no known. National rate does not include dentists in territories nor dentists in the Armed Forces stationed overseas.

Percent of Population Lacking Access to Dental Care in 2002

National Percent = 9.1% of Population*

ALPHA ORDER

RANK	STATE	PERCENT
1	Alabama	32.6
14	Alaska	13.9
28	Arizona	8.4
41	Arkansas	4.6
47	California	2.4
44	Colorado	3.9
40	Connecticut	4.9
11	Delaware	16.2
23	Florida	9.8
25	Georgia	9.4
27	Hawaii	8.7
12	Idaho	16.0
28	Illinois	8.4
42	Indiana	4.2
10	Iowa	17.0
8	Kansas	19.5
35	Kentucky	6.3
34	Louisiana	6.4
5	Maine	21.3
39	Maryland	5.1
43	Massachusetts	4.0
18	Michigan	11.4
45	Minnesota	3.5
20	Mississippi	10.6
4	Missouri	22.4
6	Montana	20.9
49	Nebraska	1.2
15	Nevada	12.7
36	New Hampshire	5.4
48	New Jersey	1.8
2	New Mexico	24.4
38	New York	5.2
15	North Carolina	12.7
31	North Dakota	7.1
30	Ohio	7.4
37	Oklahoma	5.3
13	Oregon	14.9
21	Pennsylvania	10.5
26	Rhode Island	8.8
3	South Carolina	24.1
24	South Dakota	9.6
7	Tennessee	20.1
17	Texas	11.7
9	Utah	17.5
46	Vermont	3.3
32	Virginia	6.9
22	Washington	10.2
33	West Virginia	6.6
19	Wisconsin	10.8
50	Wyoming	0.5

RANK ORDER

RANK	STATE	PERCENT
1	Alabama	32.6
2	New Mexico	24.4
3	South Carolina	24.1
4	Missouri	22.4
5	Maine	21.3
6	Montana	20.9
7	Tennessee	20.1
8	Kansas	19.5
9	Utah	17.5
10	Iowa	17.0
11	Delaware	16.2
12	Idaho	16.0
13	Oregon	14.9
14	Alaska	13.9
15	Nevada	12.7
15	North Carolina	12.7
17	Texas	11.7
18	Michigan	11.4
19	Wisconsin	10.8
20	Mississippi	10.6
21	Pennsylvania	10.5
22	Washington	10.2
23	Florida	9.8
24	South Dakota	9.6
25	Georgia	9.4
26	Rhode Island	8.8
27	Hawaii	8.7
28	Arizona	8.4
28	Illinois	8.4
30	Ohio	7.4
31	North Dakota	7.1
32	Virginia	6.9
33	West Virginia	6.6
34	Louisiana	6.4
35	Kentucky	6.3
36	New Hampshire	5.4
37	Oklahoma	5.3
38	New York	5.2
39	Maryland	5.1
40	Connecticut	4.9
41	Arkansas	4.6
42	Indiana	4.2
43	Massachusetts	4.0
44	Colorado	3.9
45	Minnesota	3.5
46	Vermont	3.3
47	California	2.4
48	New Jersey	1.8
49	Nebraska	1.2
50	Wyoming	0.5

| | District of Columbia | 7.6 |

Source: Morgan Quitno Press using data from U.S. Dept. of Health and Human Services, Div. of Shortage Designation "Selected Statistics on Health Professional Shortage Areas, As of December 31, 2002"

*Percent of population considered under-served by dental practitioners. An under-served population does not have primary medical care within reasonable economic and geographic bounds.

Employment in Health Care in 2000

National Total = 12,172,956 Employees*

ALPHA ORDER

RANK	STATE	EMPLOYEES	% of USA
23	Alabama	180,369	1.5%
49	Alaska	23,340	0.2%
25	Arizona	170,829	1.4%
32	Arkansas	113,531	0.9%
1	California	1,133,256	9.3%
26	Colorado	162,113	1.3%
22	Connecticut	181,533	1.5%
47	Delaware	35,478	0.3%
4	Florida	654,046	5.4%
12	Georgia	295,414	2.4%
44	Hawaii	42,355	0.3%
42	Idaho	46,428	0.4%
7	Illinois	539,203	4.4%
14	Indiana	279,301	2.3%
27	Iowa	161,581	1.3%
30	Kansas	132,964	1.1%
24	Kentucky	179,803	1.5%
21	Louisiana	203,383	1.7%
37	Maine	71,854	0.6%
20	Maryland	220,469	1.8%
9	Massachusetts	379,275	3.1%
8	Michigan	429,085	3.5%
15	Minnesota	273,671	2.2%
33	Mississippi	109,819	0.9%
13	Missouri	280,341	2.3%
45	Montana	40,793	0.3%
34	Nebraska	88,603	0.7%
40	Nevada	57,628	0.5%
41	New Hampshire	56,175	0.5%
10	New Jersey	363,043	3.0%
38	New Mexico	63,360	0.5%
2	New York	1,003,828	8.2%
11	North Carolina	345,082	2.8%
46	North Dakota	39,613	0.3%
6	Ohio	565,860	4.6%
29	Oklahoma	145,225	1.2%
31	Oregon	131,439	1.1%
5	Pennsylvania	644,112	5.3%
39	Rhode Island	58,027	0.5%
28	South Carolina	151,329	1.2%
43	South Dakota	43,869	0.4%
18	Tennessee	254,525	2.1%
3	Texas	813,680	6.7%
36	Utah	74,672	0.6%
48	Vermont	28,488	0.2%
16	Virginia	260,209	2.1%
19	Washington	237,666	2.0%
35	West Virginia	87,227	0.7%
17	Wisconsin	255,687	2.1%
50	Wyoming	17,898	0.1%

RANK ORDER

RANK	STATE	EMPLOYEES	% of USA
1	California	1,133,256	9.3%
2	New York	1,003,828	8.2%
3	Texas	813,680	6.7%
4	Florida	654,046	5.4%
5	Pennsylvania	644,112	5.3%
6	Ohio	565,860	4.6%
7	Illinois	539,203	4.4%
8	Michigan	429,085	3.5%
9	Massachusetts	379,275	3.1%
10	New Jersey	363,043	3.0%
11	North Carolina	345,082	2.8%
12	Georgia	295,414	2.4%
13	Missouri	280,341	2.3%
14	Indiana	279,301	2.3%
15	Minnesota	273,671	2.2%
16	Virginia	260,209	2.1%
17	Wisconsin	255,687	2.1%
18	Tennessee	254,525	2.1%
19	Washington	237,666	2.0%
20	Maryland	220,469	1.8%
21	Louisiana	203,383	1.7%
22	Connecticut	181,533	1.5%
23	Alabama	180,369	1.5%
24	Kentucky	179,803	1.5%
25	Arizona	170,829	1.4%
26	Colorado	162,113	1.3%
27	Iowa	161,581	1.3%
28	South Carolina	151,329	1.2%
29	Oklahoma	145,225	1.2%
30	Kansas	132,964	1.1%
31	Oregon	131,439	1.1%
32	Arkansas	113,531	0.9%
33	Mississippi	109,819	0.9%
34	Nebraska	88,603	0.7%
35	West Virginia	87,227	0.7%
36	Utah	74,672	0.6%
37	Maine	71,854	0.6%
38	New Mexico	63,360	0.5%
39	Rhode Island	58,027	0.5%
40	Nevada	57,628	0.5%
41	New Hampshire	56,175	0.5%
42	Idaho	46,428	0.4%
43	South Dakota	43,869	0.4%
44	Hawaii	42,355	0.3%
45	Montana	40,793	0.3%
46	North Dakota	39,613	0.3%
47	Delaware	35,478	0.3%
48	Vermont	28,488	0.2%
49	Alaska	23,340	0.2%
50	Wyoming	17,898	0.1%
	District of Columbia	47,192	0.4%

Source: U.S. Bureau of the Census
"County Business Patterns 2000 (NAICS)" (http://censtats.census.gov/cbpnaic/cbpnaic.shtml)
*Includes employees at establishments exempt from as well as subject to the federal income tax. Includes employees at those establishments within the North American Industry Classification System (NAICS) classifications 621 (ambulatory health care services), 622 (hospitals) and 623 (nursing and residential care facilities). See Facilities Chapter for establishments.

VII. PHYSICAL FITNESS

Users of Exercise Equipment in 2001

National Total = 43,028,000 Users

ALPHA ORDER

RANK	STATE	USERS	% of USA
23	Alabama	690,000	1.6%
NA	Alaska*	NA	NA
17	Arizona	865,000	2.0%
37	Arkansas	215,000	0.5%
1	California	5,645,000	13.1%
22	Colorado	727,000	1.7%
21	Connecticut	789,000	1.8%
41	Delaware	138,000	0.3%
4	Florida	2,579,000	6.0%
10	Georgia	1,323,000	3.1%
NA	Hawaii*	NA	NA
38	Idaho	181,000	0.4%
5	Illinois	2,190,000	5.1%
13	Indiana	1,020,000	2.4%
33	Iowa	362,000	0.8%
32	Kansas	427,000	1.0%
26	Kentucky	566,000	1.3%
30	Louisiana	449,000	1.0%
40	Maine	140,000	0.3%
20	Maryland	806,000	1.9%
14	Massachusetts	1,012,000	2.4%
7	Michigan	1,707,000	4.0%
18	Minnesota	847,000	2.0%
31	Mississippi	436,000	1.0%
12	Missouri	1,091,000	2.5%
44	Montana	111,000	0.3%
35	Nebraska	265,000	0.6%
28	Nevada	474,000	1.1%
42	New Hampshire	132,000	0.3%
9	New Jersey	1,497,000	3.5%
39	New Mexico	153,000	0.4%
2	New York	2,783,000	6.5%
19	North Carolina	836,000	1.9%
44	North Dakota	111,000	0.3%
6	Ohio	1,814,000	4.2%
34	Oklahoma	347,000	0.8%
25	Oregon	592,000	1.4%
8	Pennsylvania	1,519,000	3.5%
36	Rhode Island	243,000	0.6%
27	South Carolina	493,000	1.1%
43	South Dakota	123,000	0.3%
24	Tennessee	642,000	1.5%
3	Texas	2,670,000	6.2%
29	Utah	456,000	1.1%
47	Vermont	101,000	0.2%
11	Virginia	1,217,000	2.8%
16	Washington	951,000	2.2%
46	West Virginia	107,000	0.2%
15	Wisconsin	973,000	2.3%
48	Wyoming	77,000	0.2%

RANK ORDER

RANK	STATE	USERS	% of USA
1	California	5,645,000	13.1%
2	New York	2,783,000	6.5%
3	Texas	2,670,000	6.2%
4	Florida	2,579,000	6.0%
5	Illinois	2,190,000	5.1%
6	Ohio	1,814,000	4.2%
7	Michigan	1,707,000	4.0%
8	Pennsylvania	1,519,000	3.5%
9	New Jersey	1,497,000	3.5%
10	Georgia	1,323,000	3.1%
11	Virginia	1,217,000	2.8%
12	Missouri	1,091,000	2.5%
13	Indiana	1,020,000	2.4%
14	Massachusetts	1,012,000	2.4%
15	Wisconsin	973,000	2.3%
16	Washington	951,000	2.2%
17	Arizona	865,000	2.0%
18	Minnesota	847,000	2.0%
19	North Carolina	836,000	1.9%
20	Maryland	806,000	1.9%
21	Connecticut	789,000	1.8%
22	Colorado	727,000	1.7%
23	Alabama	690,000	1.6%
24	Tennessee	642,000	1.5%
25	Oregon	592,000	1.4%
26	Kentucky	566,000	1.3%
27	South Carolina	493,000	1.1%
28	Nevada	474,000	1.1%
29	Utah	456,000	1.1%
30	Louisiana	449,000	1.0%
31	Mississippi	436,000	1.0%
32	Kansas	427,000	1.0%
33	Iowa	362,000	0.8%
34	Oklahoma	347,000	0.8%
35	Nebraska	265,000	0.6%
36	Rhode Island	243,000	0.6%
37	Arkansas	215,000	0.5%
38	Idaho	181,000	0.4%
39	New Mexico	153,000	0.4%
40	Maine	140,000	0.3%
41	Delaware	138,000	0.3%
42	New Hampshire	132,000	0.3%
43	South Dakota	123,000	0.3%
44	Montana	111,000	0.3%
44	North Dakota	111,000	0.3%
46	West Virginia	107,000	0.2%
47	Vermont	101,000	0.2%
48	Wyoming	77,000	0.2%
NA	Alaska*	NA	NA
NA	Hawaii*	NA	NA
	District of Columbia*	NA	NA

Source: The National Sporting Goods Association
"NSGA Sports Participation Survey, January-December 2001 (Copyright 2002, reprinted with permission)
*Not available.

Participants in Golf in 2001

National Total = 26,637,000 Golfers

RANK	STATE	GOLFERS	% of USA
20	Alabama	445,000	1.7%
NA	Alaska*	NA	NA
22	Arizona	432,000	1.6%
38	Arkansas	153,000	0.6%
1	California	2,894,000	10.9%
26	Colorado	316,000	1.2%
27	Connecticut	313,000	1.2%
36	Delaware	179,000	0.7%
3	Florida	1,747,000	6.6%
16	Georgia	543,000	2.0%
NA	Hawaii*	NA	NA
33	Idaho	217,000	0.8%
4	Illinois	1,619,000	6.1%
11	Indiana	711,000	2.7%
21	Iowa	437,000	1.6%
24	Kansas	324,000	1.2%
19	Kentucky	507,000	1.9%
37	Louisiana	174,000	0.7%
39	Maine	123,000	0.5%
28	Maryland	303,000	1.1%
9	Massachusetts	800,000	3.0%
5	Michigan	1,575,000	5.9%
12	Minnesota	665,000	2.5%
35	Mississippi	201,000	0.8%
18	Missouri	513,000	1.9%
42	Montana	85,000	0.3%
31	Nebraska	260,000	1.0%
29	Nevada	302,000	1.1%
46	New Hampshire	54,000	0.2%
15	New Jersey	570,000	2.1%
44	New Mexico	70,000	0.3%
2	New York	1,819,000	6.8%
13	North Carolina	645,000	2.4%
41	North Dakota	88,000	0.3%
6	Ohio	1,572,000	5.9%
34	Oklahoma	210,000	0.8%
30	Oregon	264,000	1.0%
8	Pennsylvania	943,000	3.5%
45	Rhode Island	63,000	0.2%
32	South Carolina	251,000	0.9%
40	South Dakota	104,000	0.4%
23	Tennessee	361,000	1.4%
7	Texas	1,346,000	5.1%
25	Utah	323,000	1.2%
48	Vermont	33,000	0.1%
17	Virginia	518,000	1.9%
14	Washington	600,000	2.3%
42	West Virginia	85,000	0.3%
10	Wisconsin	780,000	2.9%
47	Wyoming	43,000	0.2%

RANK	STATE	GOLFERS	% of USA
1	California	2,894,000	10.9%
2	New York	1,819,000	6.8%
3	Florida	1,747,000	6.6%
4	Illinois	1,619,000	6.1%
5	Michigan	1,575,000	5.9%
6	Ohio	1,572,000	5.9%
7	Texas	1,346,000	5.1%
8	Pennsylvania	943,000	3.5%
9	Massachusetts	800,000	3.0%
10	Wisconsin	780,000	2.9%
11	Indiana	711,000	2.7%
12	Minnesota	665,000	2.5%
13	North Carolina	645,000	2.4%
14	Washington	600,000	2.3%
15	New Jersey	570,000	2.1%
16	Georgia	543,000	2.0%
17	Virginia	518,000	1.9%
18	Missouri	513,000	1.9%
19	Kentucky	507,000	1.9%
20	Alabama	445,000	1.7%
21	Iowa	437,000	1.6%
22	Arizona	432,000	1.6%
23	Tennessee	361,000	1.4%
24	Kansas	324,000	1.2%
25	Utah	323,000	1.2%
26	Colorado	316,000	1.2%
27	Connecticut	313,000	1.2%
28	Maryland	303,000	1.1%
29	Nevada	302,000	1.1%
30	Oregon	264,000	1.0%
31	Nebraska	260,000	1.0%
32	South Carolina	251,000	0.9%
33	Idaho	217,000	0.8%
34	Oklahoma	210,000	0.8%
35	Mississippi	201,000	0.8%
36	Delaware	179,000	0.7%
37	Louisiana	174,000	0.7%
38	Arkansas	153,000	0.6%
39	Maine	123,000	0.5%
40	South Dakota	104,000	0.4%
41	North Dakota	88,000	0.3%
42	Montana	85,000	0.3%
42	West Virginia	85,000	0.3%
44	New Mexico	70,000	0.3%
45	Rhode Island	63,000	0.2%
46	New Hampshire	54,000	0.2%
47	Wyoming	43,000	0.2%
48	Vermont	33,000	0.1%
NA	Alaska*	NA	NA
NA	Hawaii*	NA	NA
	District of Columbia*	NA	NA

Source: The National Sporting Goods Association
    "NSGA Sports Participation Survey, January-December 2001 (Copyright 2002, reprinted with permission)
*Not available.

Participants in Running/Jogging in 2001

National Total = 24,537,000 Runners/Joggers

ALPHA ORDER

RANK	STATE	RUNNERS	% of USA
28	Alabama	263,000	1.1%
NA	Alaska*	NA	NA
18	Arizona	451,000	1.8%
40	Arkansas	105,000	0.4%
1	California	3,498,000	14.3%
20	Colorado	413,000	1.7%
27	Connecticut	276,000	1.1%
NA	Delaware*	NA	NA
4	Florida	1,383,000	5.6%
8	Georgia	803,000	3.3%
NA	Hawaii*	NA	NA
33	Idaho	162,000	0.7%
11	Illinois	668,000	2.7%
21	Indiana	409,000	1.7%
29	Iowa	258,000	1.1%
37	Kansas	138,000	0.6%
23	Kentucky	371,000	1.5%
31	Louisiana	249,000	1.0%
38	Maine	113,000	0.5%
19	Maryland	429,000	1.7%
14	Massachusetts	605,000	2.5%
6	Michigan	929,000	3.8%
17	Minnesota	471,000	1.9%
32	Mississippi	167,000	0.7%
9	Missouri	791,000	3.2%
42	Montana	96,000	0.4%
39	Nebraska	108,000	0.4%
30	Nevada	257,000	1.0%
44	New Hampshire	63,000	0.3%
5	New Jersey	1,046,000	4.3%
34	New Mexico	161,000	0.7%
3	New York	1,760,000	7.2%
13	North Carolina	616,000	2.5%
47	North Dakota	25,000	0.1%
7	Ohio	905,000	3.7%
35	Oklahoma	159,000	0.6%
26	Oregon	278,000	1.1%
12	Pennsylvania	620,000	2.5%
41	Rhode Island	104,000	0.4%
25	South Carolina	308,000	1.3%
46	South Dakota	41,000	0.2%
24	Tennessee	368,000	1.5%
2	Texas	2,173,000	8.9%
22	Utah	374,000	1.5%
45	Vermont	49,000	0.2%
10	Virginia	705,000	2.9%
16	Washington	503,000	2.0%
36	West Virginia	148,000	0.6%
15	Wisconsin	513,000	2.1%
43	Wyoming	68,000	0.3%

RANK ORDER

RANK	STATE	RUNNERS	% of USA
1	California	3,498,000	14.3%
2	Texas	2,173,000	8.9%
3	New York	1,760,000	7.2%
4	Florida	1,383,000	5.6%
5	New Jersey	1,046,000	4.3%
6	Michigan	929,000	3.8%
7	Ohio	905,000	3.7%
8	Georgia	803,000	3.3%
9	Missouri	791,000	3.2%
10	Virginia	705,000	2.9%
11	Illinois	668,000	2.7%
12	Pennsylvania	620,000	2.5%
13	North Carolina	616,000	2.5%
14	Massachusetts	605,000	2.5%
15	Wisconsin	513,000	2.1%
16	Washington	503,000	2.0%
17	Minnesota	471,000	1.9%
18	Arizona	451,000	1.8%
19	Maryland	429,000	1.7%
20	Colorado	413,000	1.7%
21	Indiana	409,000	1.7%
22	Utah	374,000	1.5%
23	Kentucky	371,000	1.5%
24	Tennessee	368,000	1.5%
25	South Carolina	308,000	1.3%
26	Oregon	278,000	1.1%
27	Connecticut	276,000	1.1%
28	Alabama	263,000	1.1%
29	Iowa	258,000	1.1%
30	Nevada	257,000	1.0%
31	Louisiana	249,000	1.0%
32	Mississippi	167,000	0.7%
33	Idaho	162,000	0.7%
34	New Mexico	161,000	0.7%
35	Oklahoma	159,000	0.6%
36	West Virginia	148,000	0.6%
37	Kansas	138,000	0.6%
38	Maine	113,000	0.5%
39	Nebraska	108,000	0.4%
40	Arkansas	105,000	0.4%
41	Rhode Island	104,000	0.4%
42	Montana	96,000	0.4%
43	Wyoming	68,000	0.3%
44	New Hampshire	63,000	0.3%
45	Vermont	49,000	0.2%
46	South Dakota	41,000	0.2%
47	North Dakota	25,000	0.1%
NA	Alaska*	NA	NA
NA	Delaware*	NA	NA
NA	Hawaii*	NA	NA
	District of Columbia*	NA	NA

Source: The National Sporting Goods Association
"NSGA Sports Participation Survey, January-December 2001 (Copyright 2002, reprinted with permission)
*Not available.

Participants in Swimming in 2001

National Total = 54,788,000 Swimmers

ALPHA ORDER

RANK	STATE	SWIMMERS	% of USA
27	Alabama	724,000	1.3%
NA	Alaska*	NA	NA
11	Arizona	1,526,000	2.8%
28	Arkansas	666,000	1.2%
1	California	5,815,000	10.6%
19	Colorado	1,075,000	2.0%
31	Connecticut	613,000	1.1%
39	Delaware	306,000	0.6%
3	Florida	3,735,000	6.8%
10	Georgia	1,645,000	3.0%
NA	Hawaii*	NA	NA
38	Idaho	312,000	0.6%
7	Illinois	2,322,000	4.2%
16	Indiana	1,196,000	2.2%
35	Iowa	377,000	0.7%
29	Kansas	641,000	1.2%
24	Kentucky	789,000	1.4%
22	Louisiana	833,000	1.5%
36	Maine	362,000	0.7%
21	Maryland	865,000	1.6%
17	Massachusetts	1,179,000	2.2%
9	Michigan	1,961,000	3.6%
20	Minnesota	1,006,000	1.8%
30	Mississippi	615,000	1.1%
13	Missouri	1,295,000	2.4%
45	Montana	95,000	0.2%
42	Nebraska	224,000	0.4%
26	Nevada	744,000	1.4%
40	New Hampshire	255,000	0.5%
5	New Jersey	2,420,000	4.4%
44	New Mexico	151,000	0.3%
2	New York	4,059,000	7.4%
14	North Carolina	1,276,000	2.3%
47	North Dakota	40,000	0.1%
6	Ohio	2,416,000	4.4%
34	Oklahoma	489,000	0.9%
32	Oregon	589,000	1.1%
8	Pennsylvania	2,170,000	4.0%
43	Rhode Island	195,000	0.4%
25	South Carolina	770,000	1.4%
46	South Dakota	75,000	0.1%
23	Tennessee	828,000	1.5%
4	Texas	3,224,000	5.9%
33	Utah	513,000	0.9%
41	Vermont	225,000	0.4%
12	Virginia	1,442,000	2.6%
18	Washington	1,079,000	2.0%
37	West Virginia	313,000	0.6%
15	Wisconsin	1,219,000	2.2%
48	Wyoming	39,000	0.1%

RANK ORDER

RANK	STATE	SWIMMERS	% of USA
1	California	5,815,000	10.6%
2	New York	4,059,000	7.4%
3	Florida	3,735,000	6.8%
4	Texas	3,224,000	5.9%
5	New Jersey	2,420,000	4.4%
6	Ohio	2,416,000	4.4%
7	Illinois	2,322,000	4.2%
8	Pennsylvania	2,170,000	4.0%
9	Michigan	1,961,000	3.6%
10	Georgia	1,645,000	3.0%
11	Arizona	1,526,000	2.8%
12	Virginia	1,442,000	2.6%
13	Missouri	1,295,000	2.4%
14	North Carolina	1,276,000	2.3%
15	Wisconsin	1,219,000	2.2%
16	Indiana	1,196,000	2.2%
17	Massachusetts	1,179,000	2.2%
18	Washington	1,079,000	2.0%
19	Colorado	1,075,000	2.0%
20	Minnesota	1,006,000	1.8%
21	Maryland	865,000	1.6%
22	Louisiana	833,000	1.5%
23	Tennessee	828,000	1.5%
24	Kentucky	789,000	1.4%
25	South Carolina	770,000	1.4%
26	Nevada	744,000	1.4%
27	Alabama	724,000	1.3%
28	Arkansas	666,000	1.2%
29	Kansas	641,000	1.2%
30	Mississippi	615,000	1.1%
31	Connecticut	613,000	1.1%
32	Oregon	589,000	1.1%
33	Utah	513,000	0.9%
34	Oklahoma	489,000	0.9%
35	Iowa	377,000	0.7%
36	Maine	362,000	0.7%
37	West Virginia	313,000	0.6%
38	Idaho	312,000	0.6%
39	Delaware	306,000	0.6%
40	New Hampshire	255,000	0.5%
41	Vermont	225,000	0.4%
42	Nebraska	224,000	0.4%
43	Rhode Island	195,000	0.4%
44	New Mexico	151,000	0.3%
45	Montana	95,000	0.2%
46	South Dakota	75,000	0.1%
47	North Dakota	40,000	0.1%
48	Wyoming	39,000	0.1%
NA	Alaska*	NA	NA
NA	Hawaii*	NA	NA
	District of Columbia*	NA	NA

Source: The National Sporting Goods Association
"NSGA Sports Participation Survey, January-December 2001 (Copyright 2002, reprinted with permission)
*Not available.

Participants in Tennis in 2001

National Total = 10,911,000 Tennis Players

ALPHA ORDER

RANK	STATE	PLAYERS	% of USA
26	Alabama	96,000	0.9%
NA	Alaska*	NA	NA
25	Arizona	98,000	0.9%
35	Arkansas	29,000	0.3%
1	California	1,427,000	13.1%
19	Colorado	172,000	1.6%
21	Connecticut	142,000	1.3%
43	Delaware	12,000	0.1%
2	Florida	877,000	8.0%
8	Georgia	562,000	5.2%
NA	Hawaii*	NA	NA
46	Idaho	9,000	0.1%
9	Illinois	405,000	3.7%
24	Indiana	112,000	1.0%
32	Iowa	54,000	0.5%
45	Kansas	10,000	0.1%
17	Kentucky	194,000	1.8%
12	Louisiana	325,000	3.0%
42	Maine	13,000	0.1%
20	Maryland	168,000	1.5%
31	Massachusetts	61,000	0.6%
10	Michigan	388,000	3.6%
14	Minnesota	281,000	2.6%
40	Mississippi	18,000	0.2%
11	Missouri	331,000	3.0%
34	Montana	37,000	0.3%
29	Nebraska	78,000	0.7%
27	Nevada	94,000	0.9%
35	New Hampshire	29,000	0.3%
5	New Jersey	611,000	5.6%
30	New Mexico	72,000	0.7%
3	New York	862,000	7.9%
23	North Carolina	121,000	1.1%
43	North Dakota	12,000	0.1%
6	Ohio	592,000	5.4%
22	Oklahoma	136,000	1.2%
28	Oregon	86,000	0.8%
15	Pennsylvania	275,000	2.5%
39	Rhode Island	25,000	0.2%
33	South Carolina	43,000	0.4%
35	South Dakota	29,000	0.3%
35	Tennessee	29,000	0.3%
4	Texas	657,000	6.0%
18	Utah	177,000	1.6%
47	Vermont	6,000	0.1%
7	Virginia	567,000	5.2%
16	Washington	254,000	2.3%
NA	West Virginia*	NA	NA
13	Wisconsin	300,000	2.7%
40	Wyoming	18,000	0.2%

RANK ORDER

RANK	STATE	PLAYERS	% of USA
1	California	1,427,000	13.1%
2	Florida	877,000	8.0%
3	New York	862,000	7.9%
4	Texas	657,000	6.0%
5	New Jersey	611,000	5.6%
6	Ohio	592,000	5.4%
7	Virginia	567,000	5.2%
8	Georgia	562,000	5.2%
9	Illinois	405,000	3.7%
10	Michigan	388,000	3.6%
11	Missouri	331,000	3.0%
12	Louisiana	325,000	3.0%
13	Wisconsin	300,000	2.7%
14	Minnesota	281,000	2.6%
15	Pennsylvania	275,000	2.5%
16	Washington	254,000	2.3%
17	Kentucky	194,000	1.8%
18	Utah	177,000	1.6%
19	Colorado	172,000	1.6%
20	Maryland	168,000	1.5%
21	Connecticut	142,000	1.3%
22	Oklahoma	136,000	1.2%
23	North Carolina	121,000	1.1%
24	Indiana	112,000	1.0%
25	Arizona	98,000	0.9%
26	Alabama	96,000	0.9%
27	Nevada	94,000	0.9%
28	Oregon	86,000	0.8%
29	Nebraska	78,000	0.7%
30	New Mexico	72,000	0.7%
31	Massachusetts	61,000	0.6%
32	Iowa	54,000	0.5%
33	South Carolina	43,000	0.4%
34	Montana	37,000	0.3%
35	Arkansas	29,000	0.3%
35	New Hampshire	29,000	0.3%
35	South Dakota	29,000	0.3%
35	Tennessee	29,000	0.3%
39	Rhode Island	25,000	0.2%
40	Mississippi	18,000	0.2%
40	Wyoming	18,000	0.2%
42	Maine	13,000	0.1%
43	Delaware	12,000	0.1%
43	North Dakota	12,000	0.1%
45	Kansas	10,000	0.1%
46	Idaho	9,000	0.1%
47	Vermont	6,000	0.1%
NA	Alaska*	NA	NA
NA	Hawaii*	NA	NA
NA	West Virginia*	NA	NA
	District of Columbia*	NA	NA

Source: The National Sporting Goods Association
"NSGA Sports Participation Survey, January-December 2001 (Copyright 2002, reprinted with permission)
*Not available.

Alcohol Consumption in 1999

National Total = 482,678,000 Gallons*

ALPHA ORDER

RANK	STATE	GALLONS	% of USA
25	Alabama	6,656,000	1.4%
47	Alaska	1,346,000	0.3%
15	Arizona	9,971,000	2.1%
35	Arkansas	3,725,000	0.8%
1	California	57,195,000	11.8%
23	Colorado	8,305,000	1.7%
27	Connecticut	5,953,000	1.2%
45	Delaware	1,812,000	0.4%
3	Florida	32,773,000	6.8%
10	Georgia	14,019,000	2.9%
41	Hawaii	2,212,000	0.5%
39	Idaho	2,355,000	0.5%
5	Illinois	22,337,000	4.6%
18	Indiana	9,371,000	1.9%
32	Iowa	4,601,000	1.0%
34	Kansas	3,925,000	0.8%
29	Kentucky	5,662,000	1.2%
21	Louisiana	8,678,000	1.8%
40	Maine	2,348,000	0.5%
20	Maryland	8,740,000	1.8%
11	Massachusetts	12,290,000	2.5%
8	Michigan	16,625,000	3.4%
19	Minnesota	9,189,000	1.9%
30	Mississippi	4,801,000	1.0%
16	Missouri	9,962,000	2.1%
44	Montana	1,828,000	0.4%
37	Nebraska	2,979,000	0.6%
28	Nevada	5,765,000	1.2%
33	New Hampshire	3,943,000	0.8%
9	New Jersey	14,416,000	3.0%
36	New Mexico	3,308,000	0.7%
4	New York	28,187,000	5.8%
12	North Carolina	12,241,000	2.5%
48	North Dakota	1,264,000	0.3%
7	Ohio	18,203,000	3.8%
31	Oklahoma	4,624,000	1.0%
26	Oregon	6,239,000	1.3%
6	Pennsylvania	18,723,000	3.9%
43	Rhode Island	1,936,000	0.4%
24	South Carolina	7,590,000	1.6%
46	South Dakota	1,354,000	0.3%
22	Tennessee	8,468,000	1.8%
2	Texas	35,677,000	7.4%
42	Utah	2,105,000	0.4%
49	Vermont	1,144,000	0.2%
14	Virginia	11,107,000	2.3%
16	Washington	9,962,000	2.1%
38	West Virginia	2,492,000	0.5%
13	Wisconsin	11,664,000	2.4%
50	Wyoming	961,000	0.2%

RANK ORDER

RANK	STATE	GALLONS	% of USA
1	California	57,195,000	11.8%
2	Texas	35,677,000	7.4%
3	Florida	32,773,000	6.8%
4	New York	28,187,000	5.8%
5	Illinois	22,337,000	4.6%
6	Pennsylvania	18,723,000	3.9%
7	Ohio	18,203,000	3.8%
8	Michigan	16,625,000	3.4%
9	New Jersey	14,416,000	3.0%
10	Georgia	14,019,000	2.9%
11	Massachusetts	12,290,000	2.5%
12	North Carolina	12,241,000	2.5%
13	Wisconsin	11,664,000	2.4%
14	Virginia	11,107,000	2.3%
15	Arizona	9,971,000	2.1%
16	Missouri	9,962,000	2.1%
16	Washington	9,962,000	2.1%
18	Indiana	9,371,000	1.9%
19	Minnesota	9,189,000	1.9%
20	Maryland	8,740,000	1.8%
21	Louisiana	8,678,000	1.8%
22	Tennessee	8,468,000	1.8%
23	Colorado	8,305,000	1.7%
24	South Carolina	7,590,000	1.6%
25	Alabama	6,656,000	1.4%
26	Oregon	6,239,000	1.3%
27	Connecticut	5,953,000	1.2%
28	Nevada	5,765,000	1.2%
29	Kentucky	5,662,000	1.2%
30	Mississippi	4,801,000	1.0%
31	Oklahoma	4,624,000	1.0%
32	Iowa	4,601,000	1.0%
33	New Hampshire	3,943,000	0.8%
34	Kansas	3,925,000	0.8%
35	Arkansas	3,725,000	0.8%
36	New Mexico	3,308,000	0.7%
37	Nebraska	2,979,000	0.6%
38	West Virginia	2,492,000	0.5%
39	Idaho	2,355,000	0.5%
40	Maine	2,348,000	0.5%
41	Hawaii	2,212,000	0.5%
42	Utah	2,105,000	0.4%
43	Rhode Island	1,936,000	0.4%
44	Montana	1,828,000	0.4%
45	Delaware	1,812,000	0.4%
46	South Dakota	1,354,000	0.3%
47	Alaska	1,346,000	0.3%
48	North Dakota	1,264,000	0.3%
49	Vermont	1,144,000	0.2%
50	Wyoming	961,000	0.2%
	District of Columbia	1,647,000	0.3%

*Source: U.S. Department of Health and Human Services, National Institute on Alcohol Abuse and Alcoholism
"Volume Beverage and Ethanol Consumption for States" (http://www.niaaa.nih.gov/databases/consum02.txt)
This is apparent consumption of actual alcohol, not entire volume of an alcoholic beverage (e.g. wine is roughly 11% absolute alcohol content). Apparent consumption is based on several sources which together approximate sales but do not actually measure consumption. Accordingly, figures for some states may be skewed by purchases by nonresidents.

Adult Per Capita Alcohol Consumption in 1999

National Per Capita = 2.5 Gallons Consumed per Adult Age 21 & Older*

ALPHA ORDER

RANK	STATE	PER CAPITA
44	Alabama	2.1
3	Alaska	3.5
6	Arizona	3.1
44	Arkansas	2.1
30	California	2.5
7	Colorado	3.0
30	Connecticut	2.5
4	Delaware	3.4
7	Florida	3.0
24	Georgia	2.6
24	Hawaii	2.6
14	Idaho	2.8
17	Illinois	2.7
36	Indiana	2.3
36	Iowa	2.3
44	Kansas	2.1
47	Kentucky	2.0
10	Louisiana	2.9
24	Maine	2.6
34	Maryland	2.4
17	Massachusetts	2.7
34	Michigan	2.4
14	Minnesota	2.8
24	Mississippi	2.6
24	Missouri	2.6
7	Montana	3.0
24	Nebraska	2.6
1	Nevada	4.6
1	New Hampshire	4.6
30	New Jersey	2.5
10	New Mexico	2.9
41	New York	2.2
36	North Carolina	2.3
10	North Dakota	2.9
36	Ohio	2.3
47	Oklahoma	2.0
17	Oregon	2.7
41	Pennsylvania	2.2
17	Rhode Island	2.7
14	South Carolina	2.8
17	South Dakota	2.7
41	Tennessee	2.2
17	Texas	2.7
50	Utah	1.6
17	Vermont	2.7
36	Virginia	2.3
30	Washington	2.5
49	West Virginia	1.9
5	Wisconsin	3.2
10	Wyoming	2.9

RANK ORDER

RANK	STATE	PER CAPITA
1	Nevada	4.6
1	New Hampshire	4.6
3	Alaska	3.5
4	Delaware	3.4
5	Wisconsin	3.2
6	Arizona	3.1
7	Colorado	3.0
7	Florida	3.0
7	Montana	3.0
10	Louisiana	2.9
10	New Mexico	2.9
10	North Dakota	2.9
10	Wyoming	2.9
14	Idaho	2.8
14	Minnesota	2.8
14	South Carolina	2.8
17	Illinois	2.7
17	Massachusetts	2.7
17	Oregon	2.7
17	Rhode Island	2.7
17	South Dakota	2.7
17	Texas	2.7
17	Vermont	2.7
24	Georgia	2.6
24	Hawaii	2.6
24	Maine	2.6
24	Mississippi	2.6
24	Missouri	2.6
24	Nebraska	2.6
30	California	2.5
30	Connecticut	2.5
30	New Jersey	2.5
30	Washington	2.5
34	Maryland	2.4
34	Michigan	2.4
36	Indiana	2.3
36	Iowa	2.3
36	North Carolina	2.3
36	Ohio	2.3
36	Virginia	2.3
41	New York	2.2
41	Pennsylvania	2.2
41	Tennessee	2.2
44	Alabama	2.1
44	Arkansas	2.1
44	Kansas	2.1
47	Kentucky	2.0
47	Oklahoma	2.0
49	West Virginia	1.9
50	Utah	1.6

District of Columbia   4.1

Source: Morgan Quitno Press using data from U.S. Dept. of HHS, National Institute on Alcohol Abuse and Alcoholism
"Volume Beverage and Ethanol Consumption for States" (http://www.niaaa.nih.gov/databases/consum02.txt)
*This is apparent consumption of actual alcohol, not entire volume of an alcoholic beverage (e.g. wine is roughly 11% absolute alcohol content). Apparent consumption is based on several sources which together approximate sales but do not actually measure consumption. Accordingly, figures for some states may be skewed by purchases by nonresidents.

Apparent Beer Consumption in 1999

National Total = 6,076,042,000 Gallons of Beer Consumed*

ALPHA ORDER

RANK	STATE	GALLONS	% of USA
25	Alabama	93,828,000	1.5%
48	Alaska	15,334,000	0.3%
15	Arizona	130,093,000	2.1%
34	Arkansas	51,627,000	0.8%
1	California	638,017,000	10.5%
23	Colorado	100,219,000	1.6%
32	Connecticut	57,183,000	0.9%
45	Delaware	19,379,000	0.3%
3	Florida	383,187,000	6.3%
9	Georgia	174,292,000	2.9%
40	Hawaii	28,405,000	0.5%
42	Idaho	25,885,000	0.4%
5	Illinois	281,042,000	4.6%
17	Indiana	124,425,000	2.0%
29	Iowa	70,297,000	1.2%
33	Kansas	53,926,000	0.9%
26	Kentucky	77,257,000	1.3%
19	Louisiana	120,389,000	2.0%
41	Maine	26,745,000	0.4%
24	Maryland	97,210,000	1.6%
16	Massachusetts	124,764,000	2.1%
8	Michigan	208,268,000	3.4%
21	Minnesota	106,645,000	1.8%
28	Mississippi	71,842,000	1.2%
14	Missouri	133,462,000	2.2%
43	Montana	25,067,000	0.4%
36	Nebraska	43,009,000	0.7%
31	Nevada	62,261,000	1.0%
38	New Hampshire	38,265,000	0.6%
13	New Jersey	144,382,000	2.4%
35	New Mexico	47,563,000	0.8%
4	New York	314,368,000	5.2%
10	North Carolina	165,398,000	2.7%
47	North Dakota	17,338,000	0.3%
7	Ohio	266,374,000	4.4%
30	Oklahoma	68,060,000	1.1%
27	Oregon	73,905,000	1.2%
6	Pennsylvania	267,927,000	4.4%
44	Rhode Island	21,501,000	0.4%
22	South Carolina	101,782,000	1.7%
46	South Dakota	18,955,000	0.3%
18	Tennessee	122,535,000	2.0%
2	Texas	546,353,000	9.0%
39	Utah	29,072,000	0.5%
49	Vermont	13,496,000	0.2%
11	Virginia	147,953,000	2.4%
20	Washington	114,135,000	1.9%
37	West Virginia	39,547,000	0.7%
12	Wisconsin	146,162,000	2.4%
50	Wyoming	12,423,000	0.2%

RANK ORDER

RANK	STATE	GALLONS	% of USA
1	California	638,017,000	10.5%
2	Texas	546,353,000	9.0%
3	Florida	383,187,000	6.3%
4	New York	314,368,000	5.2%
5	Illinois	281,042,000	4.6%
6	Pennsylvania	267,927,000	4.4%
7	Ohio	266,374,000	4.4%
8	Michigan	208,268,000	3.4%
9	Georgia	174,292,000	2.9%
10	North Carolina	165,398,000	2.7%
11	Virginia	147,953,000	2.4%
12	Wisconsin	146,162,000	2.4%
13	New Jersey	144,382,000	2.4%
14	Missouri	133,462,000	2.2%
15	Arizona	130,093,000	2.1%
16	Massachusetts	124,764,000	2.1%
17	Indiana	124,425,000	2.0%
18	Tennessee	122,535,000	2.0%
19	Louisiana	120,389,000	2.0%
20	Washington	114,135,000	1.9%
21	Minnesota	106,645,000	1.8%
22	South Carolina	101,782,000	1.7%
23	Colorado	100,219,000	1.6%
24	Maryland	97,210,000	1.6%
25	Alabama	93,828,000	1.5%
26	Kentucky	77,257,000	1.3%
27	Oregon	73,905,000	1.2%
28	Mississippi	71,842,000	1.2%
29	Iowa	70,297,000	1.2%
30	Oklahoma	68,060,000	1.1%
31	Nevada	62,261,000	1.0%
32	Connecticut	57,183,000	0.9%
33	Kansas	53,926,000	0.9%
34	Arkansas	51,627,000	0.8%
35	New Mexico	47,563,000	0.8%
36	Nebraska	43,009,000	0.7%
37	West Virginia	39,547,000	0.7%
38	New Hampshire	38,265,000	0.6%
39	Utah	29,072,000	0.5%
40	Hawaii	28,405,000	0.5%
41	Maine	26,745,000	0.4%
42	Idaho	25,885,000	0.4%
43	Montana	25,067,000	0.4%
44	Rhode Island	21,501,000	0.4%
45	Delaware	19,379,000	0.3%
46	South Dakota	18,955,000	0.3%
47	North Dakota	17,338,000	0.3%
48	Alaska	15,334,000	0.3%
49	Vermont	13,496,000	0.2%
50	Wyoming	12,423,000	0.2%
	District of Columbia	14,491,000	0.2%

Source: U.S. Department of Health and Human Services, National Institute on Alcohol Abuse and Alcoholism "Volume Beverage and Ethanol Consumption for States" (http://www.niaaa.nih.gov/databases/consum02.txt)
This is apparent consumption and is based on several sources which together approximate sales but do not actually measure consumption. Reported state volumes reflect only in-state purchases. Accordingly, figures for some states may be skewed by purchases by nonresidents.

Adult Per Capita Beer Consumption in 1999

National Per Capita = 31.9 Gallons Consumed per Adult 21 Years and Older*

ALPHA ORDER

RANK	STATE	PER CAPITA
33	Alabama	30.2
9	Alaska	39.4
7	Arizona	40.2
41	Arkansas	29.1
43	California	28.1
17	Colorado	35.7
48	Connecticut	24.5
16	Delaware	35.9
18	Florida	34.9
24	Georgia	32.4
21	Hawaii	33.7
29	Idaho	31.1
23	Illinois	33.4
36	Indiana	30.0
18	Iowa	34.9
38	Kansas	29.5
45	Kentucky	27.5
5	Louisiana	40.7
39	Maine	29.4
46	Maryland	26.6
44	Massachusetts	27.9
32	Michigan	30.3
24	Minnesota	32.4
11	Mississippi	38.3
18	Missouri	34.9
5	Montana	40.7
14	Nebraska	37.7
1	Nevada	49.9
2	New Hampshire	45.0
47	New Jersey	24.7
3	New Mexico	41.0
49	New York	24.1
31	North Carolina	30.7
10	North Dakota	39.3
22	Ohio	33.6
39	Oklahoma	29.4
26	Oregon	31.5
30	Pennsylvania	30.9
33	Rhode Island	30.2
15	South Carolina	37.0
12	South Dakota	38.1
28	Tennessee	31.4
4	Texas	40.9
50	Utah	22.6
26	Vermont	31.5
35	Virginia	30.1
42	Washington	28.4
37	West Virginia	29.9
8	Wisconsin	39.9
13	Wyoming	38.0

RANK ORDER

RANK	STATE	PER CAPITA
1	Nevada	49.9
2	New Hampshire	45.0
3	New Mexico	41.0
4	Texas	40.9
5	Louisiana	40.7
5	Montana	40.7
7	Arizona	40.2
8	Wisconsin	39.9
9	Alaska	39.4
10	North Dakota	39.3
11	Mississippi	38.3
12	South Dakota	38.1
13	Wyoming	38.0
14	Nebraska	37.7
15	South Carolina	37.0
16	Delaware	35.9
17	Colorado	35.7
18	Florida	34.9
18	Iowa	34.9
18	Missouri	34.9
21	Hawaii	33.7
22	Ohio	33.6
23	Illinois	33.4
24	Georgia	32.4
24	Minnesota	32.4
26	Oregon	31.5
26	Vermont	31.5
28	Tennessee	31.4
29	Idaho	31.1
30	Pennsylvania	30.9
31	North Carolina	30.7
32	Michigan	30.3
33	Alabama	30.2
33	Rhode Island	30.2
35	Virginia	30.1
36	Indiana	30.0
37	West Virginia	29.9
38	Kansas	29.5
39	Maine	29.4
39	Oklahoma	29.4
41	Arkansas	29.1
42	Washington	28.4
43	California	28.1
44	Massachusetts	27.9
45	Kentucky	27.5
46	Maryland	26.6
47	New Jersey	24.7
48	Connecticut	24.5
49	New York	24.1
50	Utah	22.6
	District of Columbia	35.8

Source: Morgan Quitno Press using data from U.S. Dept. of HHS, National Institute on Alcohol Abuse and Alcoholism
"Volume Beverage and Ethanol Consumption for States" (http://www.niaaa.nih.gov/databases/consum02.txt)
*This is apparent consumption and is based on several sources which together approximate sales but do not
actually measure consumption. Reported state volumes reflect only in-state purchases. Accordingly, figures for
some states may be skewed by purchases by nonresidents.

Wine Consumption in 1999

National Total = 533,709,000 Gallons of Wine Consumed*

ALPHA ORDER

RANK	STATE	GALLONS	% of USA
29	Alabama	4,694,000	0.9%
45	Alaska	1,463,000	0.3%
15	Arizona	10,619,000	2.0%
40	Arkansas	1,996,000	0.4%
1	California	94,262,000	17.7%
18	Colorado	9,778,000	1.8%
16	Connecticut	10,421,000	2.0%
38	Delaware	2,312,000	0.4%
3	Florida	39,783,000	7.5%
13	Georgia	13,544,000	2.5%
34	Hawaii	2,975,000	0.6%
28	Idaho	5,230,000	1.0%
5	Illinois	24,834,000	4.7%
24	Indiana	7,276,000	1.4%
39	Iowa	2,309,000	0.4%
35	Kansas	2,725,000	0.5%
31	Kentucky	3,398,000	0.6%
25	Louisiana	6,438,000	1.2%
32	Maine	2,984,000	0.6%
17	Maryland	9,880,000	1.9%
7	Massachusetts	20,194,000	3.8%
9	Michigan	14,582,000	2.7%
21	Minnesota	8,083,000	1.5%
43	Mississippi	1,656,000	0.3%
22	Missouri	7,933,000	1.5%
43	Montana	1,656,000	0.3%
42	Nebraska	1,786,000	0.3%
23	Nevada	7,507,000	1.4%
30	New Hampshire	4,231,000	0.8%
6	New Jersey	24,204,000	4.5%
37	New Mexico	2,655,000	0.5%
2	New York	43,254,000	8.1%
14	North Carolina	11,717,000	2.2%
49	North Dakota	598,000	0.1%
11	Ohio	14,432,000	2.7%
36	Oklahoma	2,656,000	0.5%
19	Oregon	9,205,000	1.7%
8	Pennsylvania	15,914,000	3.0%
32	Rhode Island	2,984,000	0.6%
26	South Carolina	5,483,000	1.0%
48	South Dakota	641,000	0.1%
27	Tennessee	5,417,000	1.0%
4	Texas	25,386,000	4.8%
46	Utah	1,313,000	0.2%
41	Vermont	1,788,000	0.3%
12	Virginia	13,876,000	2.6%
10	Washington	14,532,000	2.7%
47	West Virginia	1,151,000	0.2%
20	Wisconsin	8,709,000	1.6%
50	Wyoming	538,000	0.1%

RANK ORDER

RANK	STATE	GALLONS	% of USA
1	California	94,262,000	17.7%
2	New York	43,254,000	8.1%
3	Florida	39,783,000	7.5%
4	Texas	25,386,000	4.8%
5	Illinois	24,834,000	4.7%
6	New Jersey	24,204,000	4.5%
7	Massachusetts	20,194,000	3.8%
8	Pennsylvania	15,914,000	3.0%
9	Michigan	14,582,000	2.7%
10	Washington	14,532,000	2.7%
11	Ohio	14,432,000	2.7%
12	Virginia	13,876,000	2.6%
13	Georgia	13,544,000	2.5%
14	North Carolina	11,717,000	2.2%
15	Arizona	10,619,000	2.0%
16	Connecticut	10,421,000	2.0%
17	Maryland	9,880,000	1.9%
18	Colorado	9,778,000	1.8%
19	Oregon	9,205,000	1.7%
20	Wisconsin	8,709,000	1.6%
21	Minnesota	8,083,000	1.5%
22	Missouri	7,933,000	1.5%
23	Nevada	7,507,000	1.4%
24	Indiana	7,276,000	1.4%
25	Louisiana	6,438,000	1.2%
26	South Carolina	5,483,000	1.0%
27	Tennessee	5,417,000	1.0%
28	Idaho	5,230,000	1.0%
29	Alabama	4,694,000	0.9%
30	New Hampshire	4,231,000	0.8%
31	Kentucky	3,398,000	0.6%
32	Maine	2,984,000	0.6%
32	Rhode Island	2,984,000	0.6%
34	Hawaii	2,975,000	0.6%
35	Kansas	2,725,000	0.5%
36	Oklahoma	2,656,000	0.5%
37	New Mexico	2,655,000	0.5%
38	Delaware	2,312,000	0.4%
39	Iowa	2,309,000	0.4%
40	Arkansas	1,996,000	0.4%
41	Vermont	1,788,000	0.3%
42	Nebraska	1,786,000	0.3%
43	Mississippi	1,656,000	0.3%
43	Montana	1,656,000	0.3%
45	Alaska	1,463,000	0.3%
46	Utah	1,313,000	0.2%
47	West Virginia	1,151,000	0.2%
48	South Dakota	641,000	0.1%
49	North Dakota	598,000	0.1%
50	Wyoming	538,000	0.1%
	District of Columbia	2,707,000	0.5%

Source: U.S. Department of Health and Human Services, National Institute on Alcohol Abuse and Alcoholism
"Volume Beverage and Ethanol Consumption for States" (http://www.niaaa.nih.gov/databases/consum02.txt)
*This is apparent consumption and is based on several sources which together approximate sales but do not actually measure consumption. Reported state volumes reflect only in-state purchases. Accordingly, figures for some states may be skewed by purchases by nonresidents.

Adult Per Capita Wine Consumption in 1999

National Per Capita = 2.8 Gallons Consumed per Adult 21 Years and Older

ALPHA ORDER

RANK	STATE	PER CAPITA
39	Alabama	1.5
12	Alaska	3.8
17	Arizona	3.3
45	Arkansas	1.1
9	California	4.1
15	Colorado	3.5
4	Connecticut	4.5
6	Delaware	4.3
13	Florida	3.6
24	Georgia	2.5
15	Hawaii	3.5
1	Idaho	6.3
20	Illinois	2.9
34	Indiana	1.8
45	Iowa	1.1
39	Kansas	1.5
44	Kentucky	1.2
28	Louisiana	2.2
17	Maine	3.3
22	Maryland	2.7
4	Massachusetts	4.5
30	Michigan	2.1
24	Minnesota	2.5
49	Mississippi	0.9
30	Missouri	2.1
22	Montana	2.7
37	Nebraska	1.6
2	Nevada	6.0
3	New Hampshire	5.0
9	New Jersey	4.1
27	New Mexico	2.3
17	New York	3.3
28	North Carolina	2.2
41	North Dakota	1.4
34	Ohio	1.8
45	Oklahoma	1.1
11	Oregon	3.9
34	Pennsylvania	1.8
7	Rhode Island	4.2
32	South Carolina	2.0
43	South Dakota	1.3
41	Tennessee	1.4
33	Texas	1.9
48	Utah	1.0
7	Vermont	4.2
21	Virginia	2.8
13	Washington	3.6
49	West Virginia	0.9
26	Wisconsin	2.4
37	Wyoming	1.6

RANK ORDER

RANK	STATE	PER CAPITA
1	Idaho	6.3
2	Nevada	6.0
3	New Hampshire	5.0
4	Connecticut	4.5
4	Massachusetts	4.5
6	Delaware	4.3
7	Rhode Island	4.2
7	Vermont	4.2
9	California	4.1
9	New Jersey	4.1
11	Oregon	3.9
12	Alaska	3.8
13	Florida	3.6
13	Washington	3.6
15	Colorado	3.5
15	Hawaii	3.5
17	Arizona	3.3
17	Maine	3.3
17	New York	3.3
20	Illinois	2.9
21	Virginia	2.8
22	Maryland	2.7
22	Montana	2.7
24	Georgia	2.5
24	Minnesota	2.5
26	Wisconsin	2.4
27	New Mexico	2.3
28	Louisiana	2.2
28	North Carolina	2.2
30	Michigan	2.1
30	Missouri	2.1
32	South Carolina	2.0
33	Texas	1.9
34	Indiana	1.8
34	Ohio	1.8
34	Pennsylvania	1.8
37	Nebraska	1.6
37	Wyoming	1.6
39	Alabama	1.5
39	Kansas	1.5
41	North Dakota	1.4
41	Tennessee	1.4
43	South Dakota	1.3
44	Kentucky	1.2
45	Arkansas	1.1
45	Iowa	1.1
45	Oklahoma	1.1
48	Utah	1.0
49	Mississippi	0.9
49	West Virginia	0.9
	District of Columbia	6.7

Source: Morgan Quitno Press using data from U.S. Dept. of HHS, National Institute on Alcohol Abuse and Alcoholism "Volume Beverage and Ethanol Consumption for States" (http://www.niaaa.nih.gov/databases/consum02.txt)
*This is apparent consumption and is based on several sources which together approximate sales but do not actually measure consumption. Reported state volumes reflect only in-state purchases. Accordingly, figures for some states may be skewed by purchases by nonresidents.

Distilled Spirits Consumption in 1999

National Total = 341,625,000 Gallons of Distilled Spirits Consumed*

RANK	STATE	GALLONS	% of USA
27	Alabama	4,449,000	1.3%
46	Alaska	1,138,000	0.3%
19	Arizona	6,683,000	2.0%
34	Arkansas	2,783,000	0.8%
1	California	39,718,000	11.6%
21	Colorado	6,164,000	1.8%
25	Connecticut	4,952,000	1.4%
39	Delaware	1,561,000	0.5%
2	Florida	25,299,000	7.4%
9	Georgia	10,777,000	3.2%
43	Hawaii	1,338,000	0.4%
44	Idaho	1,255,000	0.4%
5	Illinois	15,782,000	4.6%
18	Indiana	6,894,000	2.0%
35	Iowa	2,774,000	0.8%
33	Kansas	2,790,000	0.8%
28	Kentucky	4,250,000	1.2%
22	Louisiana	5,913,000	1.7%
38	Maine	1,847,000	0.5%
15	Maryland	7,522,000	2.2%
11	Massachusetts	9,905,000	2.9%
6	Michigan	13,069,000	3.8%
13	Minnesota	8,143,000	2.4%
31	Mississippi	3,295,000	1.0%
17	Missouri	7,136,000	2.1%
45	Montana	1,183,000	0.3%
37	Nebraska	1,979,000	0.6%
26	Nevada	4,853,000	1.4%
30	New Hampshire	4,076,000	1.2%
7	New Jersey	11,671,000	3.4%
36	New Mexico	2,007,000	0.6%
3	New York	20,585,000	6.0%
14	North Carolina	7,997,000	2.3%
48	North Dakota	989,000	0.3%
10	Ohio	10,594,000	3.1%
32	Oklahoma	2,964,000	0.9%
29	Oregon	4,199,000	1.2%
8	Pennsylvania	11,225,000	3.3%
41	Rhode Island	1,420,000	0.4%
23	South Carolina	5,602,000	1.6%
47	South Dakota	1,019,000	0.3%
24	Tennessee	5,486,000	1.6%
4	Texas	19,018,000	5.6%
40	Utah	1,526,000	0.4%
50	Vermont	746,000	0.2%
20	Virginia	6,469,000	1.9%
16	Washington	7,181,000	2.1%
42	West Virginia	1,373,000	0.4%
12	Wisconsin	9,644,000	2.8%
49	Wyoming	810,000	0.2%

RANK	STATE	GALLONS	% of USA
1	California	39,718,000	11.6%
2	Florida	25,299,000	7.4%
3	New York	20,585,000	6.0%
4	Texas	19,018,000	5.6%
5	Illinois	15,782,000	4.6%
6	Michigan	13,069,000	3.8%
7	New Jersey	11,671,000	3.4%
8	Pennsylvania	11,225,000	3.3%
9	Georgia	10,777,000	3.2%
10	Ohio	10,594,000	3.1%
11	Massachusetts	9,905,000	2.9%
12	Wisconsin	9,644,000	2.8%
13	Minnesota	8,143,000	2.4%
14	North Carolina	7,997,000	2.3%
15	Maryland	7,522,000	2.2%
16	Washington	7,181,000	2.1%
17	Missouri	7,136,000	2.1%
18	Indiana	6,894,000	2.0%
19	Arizona	6,683,000	2.0%
20	Virginia	6,469,000	1.9%
21	Colorado	6,164,000	1.8%
22	Louisiana	5,913,000	1.7%
23	South Carolina	5,602,000	1.6%
24	Tennessee	5,486,000	1.6%
25	Connecticut	4,952,000	1.4%
26	Nevada	4,853,000	1.4%
27	Alabama	4,449,000	1.3%
28	Kentucky	4,250,000	1.2%
29	Oregon	4,199,000	1.2%
30	New Hampshire	4,076,000	1.2%
31	Mississippi	3,295,000	1.0%
32	Oklahoma	2,964,000	0.9%
33	Kansas	2,790,000	0.8%
34	Arkansas	2,783,000	0.8%
35	Iowa	2,774,000	0.8%
36	New Mexico	2,007,000	0.6%
37	Nebraska	1,979,000	0.6%
38	Maine	1,847,000	0.5%
39	Delaware	1,561,000	0.5%
40	Utah	1,526,000	0.4%
41	Rhode Island	1,420,000	0.4%
42	West Virginia	1,373,000	0.4%
43	Hawaii	1,338,000	0.4%
44	Idaho	1,255,000	0.4%
45	Montana	1,183,000	0.3%
46	Alaska	1,138,000	0.3%
47	South Dakota	1,019,000	0.3%
48	North Dakota	989,000	0.3%
49	Wyoming	810,000	0.2%
50	Vermont	746,000	0.2%
	District of Columbia	1,572,000	0.5%

Source: U.S. Department of Health and Human Services, National Institute on Alcohol Abuse and Alcoholism "Volume Beverage and Ethanol Consumption for States" (http://www.niaaa.nih.gov/databases/consum02.txt)
This is apparent consumption and is based on several sources which together approximate sales but do not actually measure consumption. Reported state volumes reflect only in-state purchases. Accordingly, figures for some states may be skewed by purchases by nonresidents.

Adult Per Capita Distilled Spirits Consumption in 1999

National Per Capita = 1.8 Gallons Consumed per Adult 21 Years and Older*

ALPHA ORDER

RANK	STATE	PER CAPITA
41	Alabama	1.4
3	Alaska	2.9
12	Arizona	2.1
34	Arkansas	1.6
29	California	1.7
9	Colorado	2.2
12	Connecticut	2.1
3	Delaware	2.9
8	Florida	2.3
15	Georgia	2.0
34	Hawaii	1.6
37	Idaho	1.5
22	Illinois	1.9
29	Indiana	1.7
41	Iowa	1.4
37	Kansas	1.5
37	Kentucky	1.5
15	Louisiana	2.0
15	Maine	2.0
12	Maryland	2.1
9	Massachusetts	2.2
22	Michigan	1.9
6	Minnesota	2.5
26	Mississippi	1.8
22	Missouri	1.9
22	Montana	1.9
29	Nebraska	1.7
2	Nevada	3.9
1	New Hampshire	4.8
15	New Jersey	2.0
29	New Mexico	1.7
34	New York	1.6
37	North Carolina	1.5
9	North Dakota	2.2
45	Ohio	1.3
45	Oklahoma	1.3
26	Oregon	1.8
45	Pennsylvania	1.3
15	Rhode Island	2.0
15	South Carolina	2.0
15	South Dakota	2.0
41	Tennessee	1.4
41	Texas	1.4
49	Utah	1.2
29	Vermont	1.7
45	Virginia	1.3
26	Washington	1.8
50	West Virginia	1.0
5	Wisconsin	2.6
6	Wyoming	2.5

RANK ORDER

RANK	STATE	PER CAPITA
1	New Hampshire	4.8
2	Nevada	3.9
3	Alaska	2.9
3	Delaware	2.9
5	Wisconsin	2.6
6	Minnesota	2.5
6	Wyoming	2.5
8	Florida	2.3
9	Colorado	2.2
9	Massachusetts	2.2
9	North Dakota	2.2
12	Arizona	2.1
12	Connecticut	2.1
12	Maryland	2.1
15	Georgia	2.0
15	Louisiana	2.0
15	Maine	2.0
15	New Jersey	2.0
15	Rhode Island	2.0
15	South Carolina	2.0
15	South Dakota	2.0
22	Illinois	1.9
22	Michigan	1.9
22	Missouri	1.9
22	Montana	1.9
26	Mississippi	1.8
26	Oregon	1.8
26	Washington	1.8
29	California	1.7
29	Indiana	1.7
29	Nebraska	1.7
29	New Mexico	1.7
29	Vermont	1.7
34	Arkansas	1.6
34	Hawaii	1.6
34	New York	1.6
37	Idaho	1.5
37	Kansas	1.5
37	Kentucky	1.5
37	North Carolina	1.5
41	Alabama	1.4
41	Iowa	1.4
41	Tennessee	1.4
41	Texas	1.4
45	Ohio	1.3
45	Oklahoma	1.3
45	Pennsylvania	1.3
45	Virginia	1.3
49	Utah	1.2
50	West Virginia	1.0

District of Columbia 3.9

Source: Morgan Quitno Press using data from U.S. Dept. of HHS, National Institute on Alcohol Abuse and Alcoholism
"Volume Beverage and Ethanol Consumption for States" (http://www.niaaa.nih.gov/databases/consum02.txt)
*This is apparent consumption and is based on several sources which together approximate sales but do not actually measure consumption. Reported state volumes reflect only in-state purchases. Accordingly, figures for some states may be skewed by purchases by nonresidents.

Average Alcohol Consumption per Drinker in 1999

National Average = 4.21 Gallons*

ALPHA ORDER

RANK	STATE	GALLONS
19	Alabama	4.74
10	Alaska	5.06
1	Arizona	7.76
17	Arkansas	4.75
46	California	3.64
33	Colorado	4.00
40	Connecticut	3.81
12	Delaware	4.94
14	Florida	4.82
16	Georgia	4.76
17	Hawaii	4.75
13	Idaho	4.88
32	Illinois	4.04
47	Indiana	3.62
48	Iowa	3.59
35	Kansas	3.95
11	Kentucky	5.03
8	Louisiana	5.51
41	Maine	3.79
44	Maryland	3.65
34	Massachusetts	3.98
49	Michigan	3.56
20	Minnesota	4.72
7	Mississippi	5.67
28	Missouri	4.24
23	Montana	4.48
27	Nebraska	4.29
2	Nevada	6.44
4	New Hampshire	6.34
31	New Jersey	4.07
22	New Mexico	4.50
44	New York	3.65
15	North Carolina	4.79
25	North Dakota	4.43
21	Ohio	4.58
5	Oklahoma	6.01
39	Oregon	3.82
42	Pennsylvania	3.71
30	Rhode Island	4.14
6	South Carolina	5.74
35	South Dakota	3.95
3	Tennessee	6.41
29	Texas	4.18
23	Utah	4.48
38	Vermont	3.86
43	Virginia	3.67
49	Washington	3.56
9	West Virginia	5.08
37	Wisconsin	3.87
25	Wyoming	4.43

RANK ORDER

RANK	STATE	GALLONS
1	Arizona	7.76
2	Nevada	6.44
3	Tennessee	6.41
4	New Hampshire	6.34
5	Oklahoma	6.01
6	South Carolina	5.74
7	Mississippi	5.67
8	Louisiana	5.51
9	West Virginia	5.08
10	Alaska	5.06
11	Kentucky	5.03
12	Delaware	4.94
13	Idaho	4.88
14	Florida	4.82
15	North Carolina	4.79
16	Georgia	4.76
17	Arkansas	4.75
17	Hawaii	4.75
19	Alabama	4.74
20	Minnesota	4.72
21	Ohio	4.58
22	New Mexico	4.50
23	Montana	4.48
23	Utah	4.48
25	North Dakota	4.43
25	Wyoming	4.43
27	Nebraska	4.29
28	Missouri	4.24
29	Texas	4.18
30	Rhode Island	4.14
31	New Jersey	4.07
32	Illinois	4.04
33	Colorado	4.00
34	Massachusetts	3.98
35	Kansas	3.95
35	South Dakota	3.95
37	Wisconsin	3.87
38	Vermont	3.86
39	Oregon	3.82
40	Connecticut	3.81
41	Maine	3.79
42	Pennsylvania	3.71
43	Virginia	3.67
44	Maryland	3.65
44	New York	3.65
46	California	3.64
47	Indiana	3.62
48	Iowa	3.59
49	Michigan	3.56
49	Washington	3.56
	District of Columbia	7.43

Source: U.S. Department of Health and Human Services, National Institute on Alcohol Abuse and Alcoholism
"Per Capita and Per Drinker Ethanol Consumption for States" (http://www.niaaa.nih.gov/databases/consum04.txt)
National percent calculated by the editors. This is consumption of actual alcohol, not entire volume of an alcoholic beverage (e.g. wine is roughly 11% absolute alcohol content).

Percent of Adults Who Do Not Drink Alcohol: 1999

National Percent = 47.5% of Population 18 Years and Older*

ALPHA ORDER

RANK	STATE	PERCENT
9	Alabama	60.4
32	Alaska	43.1
5	Arizona	65.5
7	Arkansas	61.7
42	California	39.6
48	Colorado	35.8
39	Connecticut	40.6
41	Delaware	40.0
29	Florida	44.8
16	Georgia	52.3
14	Hawaii	54.1
17	Idaho	51.1
34	Illinois	42.7
25	Indiana	45.7
28	Iowa	45.0
15	Kansas	53.2
6	Kentucky	65.1
13	Louisiana	54.6
40	Maine	40.2
35	Maryland	42.2
46	Massachusetts	38.5
38	Michigan	40.8
18	Minnesota	48.9
8	Mississippi	61.4
22	Missouri	46.6
32	Montana	43.1
20	Nebraska	47.8
47	Nevada	36.9
48	New Hampshire	35.8
23	New Jersey	46.0
24	New Mexico	45.9
21	New York	47.4
10	North Carolina	58.3
30	North Dakota	44.6
12	Ohio	56.2
1	Oklahoma	71.4
45	Oregon	39.1
19	Pennsylvania	48.5
36	Rhode Island	41.7
11	South Carolina	58.0
37	South Dakota	41.4
2	Tennessee	70.3
27	Texas	45.2
2	Utah	70.3
43	Vermont	39.5
25	Virginia	45.7
44	Washington	39.3
4	West Virginia	67.4
50	Wisconsin	28.9
31	Wyoming	43.9

RANK ORDER

RANK	STATE	PERCENT
1	Oklahoma	71.4
2	Tennessee	70.3
2	Utah	70.3
4	West Virginia	67.4
5	Arizona	65.5
6	Kentucky	65.1
7	Arkansas	61.7
8	Mississippi	61.4
9	Alabama	60.4
10	North Carolina	58.3
11	South Carolina	58.0
12	Ohio	56.2
13	Louisiana	54.6
14	Hawaii	54.1
15	Kansas	53.2
16	Georgia	52.3
17	Idaho	51.1
18	Minnesota	48.9
19	Pennsylvania	48.5
20	Nebraska	47.8
21	New York	47.4
22	Missouri	46.6
23	New Jersey	46.0
24	New Mexico	45.9
25	Indiana	45.7
25	Virginia	45.7
27	Texas	45.2
28	Iowa	45.0
29	Florida	44.8
30	North Dakota	44.6
31	Wyoming	43.9
32	Alaska	43.1
32	Montana	43.1
34	Illinois	42.7
35	Maryland	42.2
36	Rhode Island	41.7
37	South Dakota	41.4
38	Michigan	40.8
39	Connecticut	40.6
40	Maine	40.2
41	Delaware	40.0
42	California	39.6
43	Vermont	39.5
44	Washington	39.3
45	Oregon	39.1
46	Massachusetts	38.5
47	Nevada	36.9
48	Colorado	35.8
48	New Hampshire	35.8
50	Wisconsin	28.9
	District of Columbia	49.7

Source: U.S. Department of Health and Human Services, National Institute on Alcohol Abuse and Alcoholism
   "Per Capita and Per Drinker Ethanol Consumption for States" (http://www.niaaa.nih.gov/databases/consum04.txt)
*National percent calculated by the editors.

Percent of Adults Who Are Binge Drinkers: 2001

National Median = 14.8% of Adults*

ALPHA ORDER

RANK	STATE	PERCENT
42	Alabama	11.6
5	Alaska	18.2
9	Arizona	16.8
43	Arkansas	11.3
21	California	15.5
10	Colorado	16.7
32	Connecticut	13.8
18	Delaware	15.7
38	Florida	12.0
39	Georgia	11.9
45	Hawaii	10.4
36	Idaho	12.8
8	Illinois	17.3
32	Indiana	13.8
13	Iowa	16.2
26	Kansas	14.7
49	Kentucky	8.7
32	Louisiana	13.8
22	Maine	15.4
39	Maryland	11.9
6	Massachusetts	18.1
7	Michigan	18.0
3	Minnesota	19.6
41	Mississippi	11.8
31	Missouri	14.1
10	Montana	16.7
28	Nebraska	14.6
10	Nevada	16.7
16	New Hampshire	15.8
35	New Jersey	13.5
16	New Mexico	15.8
29	New York	14.4
46	North Carolina	9.8
2	North Dakota	22.3
13	Ohio	16.2
44	Oklahoma	11.0
26	Oregon	14.7
20	Pennsylvania	15.6
23	Rhode Island	15.1
37	South Carolina	12.3
4	South Dakota	18.5
50	Tennessee	6.8
23	Texas	15.1
47	Utah	9.7
18	Vermont	15.7
30	Virginia	14.3
25	Washington	14.9
48	West Virginia	9.4
1	Wisconsin	25.7
15	Wyoming	16.0

RANK ORDER

RANK	STATE	PERCENT
1	Wisconsin	25.7
2	North Dakota	22.3
3	Minnesota	19.6
4	South Dakota	18.5
5	Alaska	18.2
6	Massachusetts	18.1
7	Michigan	18.0
8	Illinois	17.3
9	Arizona	16.8
10	Colorado	16.7
10	Montana	16.7
10	Nevada	16.7
13	Iowa	16.2
13	Ohio	16.2
15	Wyoming	16.0
16	New Hampshire	15.8
16	New Mexico	15.8
18	Delaware	15.7
18	Vermont	15.7
20	Pennsylvania	15.6
21	California	15.5
22	Maine	15.4
23	Rhode Island	15.1
23	Texas	15.1
25	Washington	14.9
26	Kansas	14.7
26	Oregon	14.7
28	Nebraska	14.6
29	New York	14.4
30	Virginia	14.3
31	Missouri	14.1
32	Connecticut	13.8
32	Indiana	13.8
32	Louisiana	13.8
35	New Jersey	13.5
36	Idaho	12.8
37	South Carolina	12.3
38	Florida	12.0
39	Georgia	11.9
39	Maryland	11.9
41	Mississippi	11.8
42	Alabama	11.6
43	Arkansas	11.3
44	Oklahoma	11.0
45	Hawaii	10.4
46	North Carolina	9.8
47	Utah	9.7
48	West Virginia	9.4
49	Kentucky	8.7
50	Tennessee	6.8
	District of Columbia	14.8

Source: U.S. Department of Health and Human Services, Centers for Disease Control and Prevention
"2001 Behavioral Risk Factor Surveillance Summary Prevalence Report" (August 9, 2002)
*Persons 18 and older reporting consumption of five or more alcoholic drinks on one or more occasions during the previous month.

Percent of Adults Who Smoke: 2001

National Median = 22.9% of Adults*

ALPHA ORDER				RANK ORDER		
RANK	STATE	PERCENT		RANK	STATE	PERCENT
21	Alabama	23.8		1	Kentucky	30.9
7	Alaska	26.2		2	Oklahoma	28.7
40	Arizona	21.5		3	West Virginia	28.2
12	Arkansas	25.5		4	Ohio	27.6
49	California	17.2		5	Indiana	27.4
32	Colorado	22.3		6	Nevada	26.9
43	Connecticut	20.6		7	Alaska	26.2
14	Delaware	25.0		8	South Carolina	26.0
29	Florida	22.4		9	Missouri	25.9
23	Georgia	23.7		10	North Carolina	25.7
44	Hawaii	20.5		11	Michigan	25.6
47	Idaho	19.6		12	Arkansas	25.5
23	Illinois	23.7		13	Mississippi	25.3
5	Indiana	27.4		14	Delaware	25.0
37	Iowa	22.1		15	Louisiana	24.6
34	Kansas	22.2		16	Pennsylvania	24.5
1	Kentucky	30.9		17	Tennessee	24.4
15	Louisiana	24.6		18	New Hampshire	24.1
19	Maine	23.9		19	Maine	23.9
41	Maryland	21.1		19	Rhode Island	23.9
48	Massachusetts	19.5		21	Alabama	23.8
11	Michigan	25.6		21	New Mexico	23.8
34	Minnesota	22.2		23	Georgia	23.7
13	Mississippi	25.3		23	Illinois	23.7
9	Missouri	25.9		25	Wisconsin	23.6
39	Montana	21.9		26	New York	23.2
46	Nebraska	20.2		27	Virginia	22.5
6	Nevada	26.9		27	Washington	22.5
18	New Hampshire	24.1		29	Florida	22.4
41	New Jersey	21.1		29	Texas	22.4
21	New Mexico	23.8		29	Vermont	22.4
26	New York	23.2		32	Colorado	22.3
10	North Carolina	25.7		32	South Dakota	22.3
37	North Dakota	22.1		34	Kansas	22.2
4	Ohio	27.6		34	Minnesota	22.2
2	Oklahoma	28.7		34	Wyoming	22.2
44	Oregon	20.5		37	Iowa	22.1
16	Pennsylvania	24.5		37	North Dakota	22.1
19	Rhode Island	23.9		39	Montana	21.9
8	South Carolina	26.0		40	Arizona	21.5
32	South Dakota	22.3		41	Maryland	21.1
17	Tennessee	24.4		41	New Jersey	21.1
29	Texas	22.4		43	Connecticut	20.6
50	Utah	13.2		44	Hawaii	20.5
29	Vermont	22.4		44	Oregon	20.5
27	Virginia	22.5		46	Nebraska	20.2
27	Washington	22.5		47	Idaho	19.6
3	West Virginia	28.2		48	Massachusetts	19.5
25	Wisconsin	23.6		49	California	17.2
34	Wyoming	22.2		50	Utah	13.2
					District of Columbia	20.8

Source: U.S. Department of Health and Human Services, Centers for Disease Control and Prevention
"2001 Behavioral Risk Factor Surveillance Summary Prevalence Report" (August 9, 2002)
*Persons 18 and older who smoke everyday or some days.

Percent of Males Who Smoke: 2001

National Median = 25.5% of Men*

ALPHA ORDER

RANK	STATE	PERCENT
22	Alabama	25.8
18	Alaska	26.4
39	Arizona	23.1
14	Arkansas	27.2
47	California	20.6
36	Colorado	23.7
45	Connecticut	21.2
9	Delaware	28.2
25	Florida	25.6
24	Georgia	25.7
30	Hawaii	24.7
46	Idaho	21.0
16	Illinois	26.7
3	Indiana	29.7
35	Iowa	24.2
40	Kansas	22.5
1	Kentucky	31.9
7	Louisiana	28.7
15	Maine	27.0
31	Maryland	24.6
49	Massachusetts	20.4
16	Michigan	26.7
29	Minnesota	24.8
4	Mississippi	29.3
13	Missouri	27.6
42	Montana	21.7
47	Nebraska	20.6
12	Nevada	27.8
25	New Hampshire	25.6
43	New Jersey	21.6
10	New Mexico	27.9
20	New York	26.1
8	North Carolina	28.6
31	North Dakota	24.6
5	Ohio	29.1
2	Oklahoma	31.1
44	Oregon	21.4
19	Pennsylvania	26.3
22	Rhode Island	25.8
10	South Carolina	27.9
38	South Dakota	23.2
20	Tennessee	26.1
28	Texas	25.1
50	Utah	14.6
34	Vermont	24.4
37	Virginia	23.5
33	Washington	24.5
6	West Virginia	28.9
27	Wisconsin	25.3
40	Wyoming	22.5

RANK ORDER

RANK	STATE	PERCENT
1	Kentucky	31.9
2	Oklahoma	31.1
3	Indiana	29.7
4	Mississippi	29.3
5	Ohio	29.1
6	West Virginia	28.9
7	Louisiana	28.7
8	North Carolina	28.6
9	Delaware	28.2
10	New Mexico	27.9
10	South Carolina	27.9
12	Nevada	27.8
13	Missouri	27.6
14	Arkansas	27.2
15	Maine	27.0
16	Illinois	26.7
16	Michigan	26.7
18	Alaska	26.4
19	Pennsylvania	26.3
20	New York	26.1
20	Tennessee	26.1
22	Alabama	25.8
22	Rhode Island	25.8
24	Georgia	25.7
25	Florida	25.6
25	New Hampshire	25.6
27	Wisconsin	25.3
28	Texas	25.1
29	Minnesota	24.8
30	Hawaii	24.7
31	Maryland	24.6
31	North Dakota	24.6
33	Washington	24.5
34	Vermont	24.4
35	Iowa	24.2
36	Colorado	23.7
37	Virginia	23.5
38	South Dakota	23.2
39	Arizona	23.1
40	Kansas	22.5
40	Wyoming	22.5
42	Montana	21.7
43	New Jersey	21.6
44	Oregon	21.4
45	Connecticut	21.2
46	Idaho	21.0
47	California	20.6
47	Nebraska	20.6
49	Massachusetts	20.4
50	Utah	14.6

District of Columbia   24.9

Source: U.S. Department of Health and Human Services, Centers for Disease Control and Prevention
"2001 Behavioral Risk Factor Surveillance Summary Prevalence Report" (August 9, 2002)
*Persons 18 and older who smoke everyday or some days.

Percent of Women Who Smoke: 2001

National Percent = 21.3% of Women*

ALPHA ORDER

RANK	STATE	PERCENT
16	Alabama	22.1
6	Alaska	25.9
36	Arizona	20.1
11	Arkansas	24.0
49	California	14.0
29	Colorado	20.9
36	Connecticut	20.1
16	Delaware	22.1
44	Florida	19.4
22	Georgia	21.8
48	Hawaii	16.3
46	Idaho	18.2
29	Illinois	20.9
7	Indiana	25.3
35	Iowa	20.3
20	Kansas	22.0
1	Kentucky	30.0
28	Louisiana	21.0
27	Maine	21.1
47	Maryland	17.9
45	Massachusetts	18.7
8	Michigan	24.5
43	Minnesota	19.6
24	Mississippi	21.7
9	Missouri	24.4
16	Montana	22.1
39	Nebraska	19.8
5	Nevada	26.0
15	New Hampshire	22.7
31	New Jersey	20.7
38	New Mexico	20.0
31	New York	20.7
12	North Carolina	23.1
41	North Dakota	19.7
4	Ohio	26.3
3	Oklahoma	26.4
41	Oregon	19.7
13	Pennsylvania	22.8
16	Rhode Island	22.1
10	South Carolina	24.3
26	South Dakota	21.4
13	Tennessee	22.8
39	Texas	19.8
50	Utah	12.0
33	Vermont	20.5
25	Virginia	21.6
33	Washington	20.5
2	West Virginia	27.6
21	Wisconsin	21.9
22	Wyoming	21.8

RANK ORDER

RANK	STATE	PERCENT
1	Kentucky	30.0
2	West Virginia	27.6
3	Oklahoma	26.4
4	Ohio	26.3
5	Nevada	26.0
6	Alaska	25.9
7	Indiana	25.3
8	Michigan	24.5
9	Missouri	24.4
10	South Carolina	24.3
11	Arkansas	24.0
12	North Carolina	23.1
13	Pennsylvania	22.8
13	Tennessee	22.8
15	New Hampshire	22.7
16	Alabama	22.1
16	Delaware	22.1
16	Montana	22.1
16	Rhode Island	22.1
20	Kansas	22.0
21	Wisconsin	21.9
22	Georgia	21.8
22	Wyoming	21.8
24	Mississippi	21.7
25	Virginia	21.6
26	South Dakota	21.4
27	Maine	21.1
28	Louisiana	21.0
29	Colorado	20.9
29	Illinois	20.9
31	New Jersey	20.7
31	New York	20.7
33	Vermont	20.5
33	Washington	20.5
35	Iowa	20.3
36	Arizona	20.1
36	Connecticut	20.1
38	New Mexico	20.0
39	Nebraska	19.8
39	Texas	19.8
41	North Dakota	19.7
41	Oregon	19.7
43	Minnesota	19.6
44	Florida	19.4
45	Massachusetts	18.7
46	Idaho	18.2
47	Maryland	17.9
48	Hawaii	16.3
49	California	14.0
50	Utah	12.0
	District of Columbia	17.3

Source: U.S. Department of Health and Human Services, Centers for Disease Control and Prevention
"2001 Behavioral Risk Factor Surveillance Summary Prevalence Report" (August 9, 2002)
*Persons 18 and older who smoke everyday or some days.

Percent of Population Who are Illicit Drug Users: 2000

National Percent = 6.3% of Population*

ALPHA ORDER				RANK ORDER		
RANK	STATE	PERCENT		RANK	STATE	PERCENT
35	Alabama	5.4		1	Massachusetts	11.4
3	Alaska	8.8		2	Colorado	8.9
22	Arizona	6.1		3	Alaska	8.8
35	Arkansas	5.4		4	Delaware	8.5
8	California	7.6		4	Vermont	8.5
2	Colorado	8.9		6	Rhode Island	8.1
12	Connecticut	7.3		7	Hawaii	7.7
4	Delaware	8.5		8	California	7.6
26	Florida	5.9		9	Nevada	7.5
19	Georgia	6.3		9	Oregon	7.5
7	Hawaii	7.7		9	Washington	7.5
35	Idaho	5.4		12	Connecticut	7.3
19	Illinois	6.3		13	New Mexico	7.1
26	Indiana	5.9		14	Maine	6.9
49	Iowa	4.3		14	Michigan	6.9
41	Kansas	5.1		16	North Carolina	6.7
26	Kentucky	5.9		16	Wisconsin	6.7
22	Louisiana	6.1		18	New Hampshire	6.6
14	Maine	6.9		19	Georgia	6.3
32	Maryland	5.7		19	Illinois	6.3
1	Massachusetts	11.4		19	Montana	6.3
14	Michigan	6.9		22	Arizona	6.1
25	Minnesota	6.0		22	Louisiana	6.1
39	Mississippi	5.2		22	New Jersey	6.1
38	Missouri	5.3		25	Minnesota	6.0
19	Montana	6.3		26	Florida	5.9
48	Nebraska	4.5		26	Indiana	5.9
9	Nevada	7.5		26	Kentucky	5.9
18	New Hampshire	6.6		26	Pennsylvania	5.9
22	New Jersey	6.1		26	Tennessee	5.9
13	New Mexico	7.1		31	New York	5.8
31	New York	5.8		32	Maryland	5.7
16	North Carolina	6.7		32	Wyoming	5.7
50	North Dakota	4.2		34	Ohio	5.6
34	Ohio	5.6		35	Alabama	5.4
42	Oklahoma	5.0		35	Arkansas	5.4
9	Oregon	7.5		35	Idaho	5.4
26	Pennsylvania	5.9		38	Missouri	5.3
6	Rhode Island	8.1		39	Mississippi	5.2
39	South Carolina	5.2		39	South Carolina	5.2
45	South Dakota	4.8		41	Kansas	5.1
26	Tennessee	5.9		42	Oklahoma	5.0
44	Texas	4.9		42	Utah	5.0
42	Utah	5.0		44	Texas	4.9
4	Vermont	8.5		45	South Dakota	4.8
45	Virginia	4.8		45	Virginia	4.8
9	Washington	7.5		47	West Virginia	4.7
47	West Virginia	4.7		48	Nebraska	4.5
16	Wisconsin	6.7		49	Iowa	4.3
32	Wyoming	5.7		50	North Dakota	4.2
					District of Columbia	7.1

Source: U.S. Department of Health and Human Services, Substance Abuse and Mental Health Services Administration
"2000 National Household Survey on Drug Abuse" (October 2002)
*Population 12 years old and over who used any illicit drug at least once within month of survey.

Percent of Adults Obese: 2001

National Median = 21.1% of Adults*

<table>
<tr><td colspan="3">ALPHA ORDER</td><td colspan="3">RANK ORDER</td></tr>
<tr><td>RANK</td><td>STATE</td><td>PERCENT</td><td>RANK</td><td>STATE</td><td>PERCENT</td></tr>
<tr><td>6</td><td>Alabama</td><td>24.5</td><td>1</td><td>Mississippi</td><td>26.5</td></tr>
<tr><td>19</td><td>Alaska</td><td>22.1</td><td>2</td><td>West Virginia</td><td>25.1</td></tr>
<tr><td>44</td><td>Arizona</td><td>18.5</td><td>3</td><td>Michigan</td><td>25.0</td></tr>
<tr><td>16</td><td>Arkansas</td><td>22.4</td><td>4</td><td>Kentucky</td><td>24.6</td></tr>
<tr><td>21</td><td>California</td><td>21.9</td><td>4</td><td>Texas</td><td>24.6</td></tr>
<tr><td>50</td><td>Colorado</td><td>14.9</td><td>6</td><td>Alabama</td><td>24.5</td></tr>
<tr><td>45</td><td>Connecticut</td><td>17.9</td><td>6</td><td>Indiana</td><td>24.5</td></tr>
<tr><td>27</td><td>Delaware</td><td>20.8</td><td>8</td><td>Louisiana</td><td>24.0</td></tr>
<tr><td>42</td><td>Florida</td><td>18.8</td><td>9</td><td>Tennessee</td><td>23.4</td></tr>
<tr><td>12</td><td>Georgia</td><td>22.7</td><td>10</td><td>Missouri</td><td>23.2</td></tr>
<tr><td>45</td><td>Hawaii</td><td>17.9</td><td>11</td><td>North Carolina</td><td>22.9</td></tr>
<tr><td>29</td><td>Idaho</td><td>20.5</td><td>12</td><td>Georgia</td><td>22.7</td></tr>
<tr><td>25</td><td>Illinois</td><td>21.0</td><td>13</td><td>Oklahoma</td><td>22.6</td></tr>
<tr><td>6</td><td>Indiana</td><td>24.5</td><td>14</td><td>Iowa</td><td>22.5</td></tr>
<tr><td>14</td><td>Iowa</td><td>22.5</td><td>14</td><td>South Carolina</td><td>22.5</td></tr>
<tr><td>22</td><td>Kansas</td><td>21.6</td><td>16</td><td>Arkansas</td><td>22.4</td></tr>
<tr><td>4</td><td>Kentucky</td><td>24.6</td><td>16</td><td>Ohio</td><td>22.4</td></tr>
<tr><td>8</td><td>Louisiana</td><td>24.0</td><td>16</td><td>Wisconsin</td><td>22.4</td></tr>
<tr><td>37</td><td>Maine</td><td>19.5</td><td>19</td><td>Alaska</td><td>22.1</td></tr>
<tr><td>29</td><td>Maryland</td><td>20.5</td><td>19</td><td>Pennsylvania</td><td>22.1</td></tr>
<tr><td>49</td><td>Massachusetts</td><td>16.6</td><td>21</td><td>California</td><td>21.9</td></tr>
<tr><td>3</td><td>Michigan</td><td>25.0</td><td>22</td><td>Kansas</td><td>21.6</td></tr>
<tr><td>33</td><td>Minnesota</td><td>19.9</td><td>23</td><td>South Dakota</td><td>21.2</td></tr>
<tr><td>1</td><td>Mississippi</td><td>26.5</td><td>24</td><td>Oregon</td><td>21.1</td></tr>
<tr><td>10</td><td>Missouri</td><td>23.2</td><td>25</td><td>Illinois</td><td>21.0</td></tr>
<tr><td>42</td><td>Montana</td><td>18.8</td><td>26</td><td>Virginia</td><td>20.9</td></tr>
<tr><td>28</td><td>Nebraska</td><td>20.7</td><td>27</td><td>Delaware</td><td>20.8</td></tr>
<tr><td>37</td><td>Nevada</td><td>19.5</td><td>28</td><td>Nebraska</td><td>20.7</td></tr>
<tr><td>39</td><td>New Hampshire</td><td>19.4</td><td>29</td><td>Idaho</td><td>20.5</td></tr>
<tr><td>36</td><td>New Jersey</td><td>19.6</td><td>29</td><td>Maryland</td><td>20.5</td></tr>
<tr><td>34</td><td>New Mexico</td><td>19.7</td><td>31</td><td>North Dakota</td><td>20.4</td></tr>
<tr><td>32</td><td>New York</td><td>20.3</td><td>32</td><td>New York</td><td>20.3</td></tr>
<tr><td>11</td><td>North Carolina</td><td>22.9</td><td>33</td><td>Minnesota</td><td>19.9</td></tr>
<tr><td>31</td><td>North Dakota</td><td>20.4</td><td>34</td><td>New Mexico</td><td>19.7</td></tr>
<tr><td>16</td><td>Ohio</td><td>22.4</td><td>34</td><td>Wyoming</td><td>19.7</td></tr>
<tr><td>13</td><td>Oklahoma</td><td>22.6</td><td>36</td><td>New Jersey</td><td>19.6</td></tr>
<tr><td>24</td><td>Oregon</td><td>21.1</td><td>37</td><td>Maine</td><td>19.5</td></tr>
<tr><td>19</td><td>Pennsylvania</td><td>22.1</td><td>37</td><td>Nevada</td><td>19.5</td></tr>
<tr><td>47</td><td>Rhode Island</td><td>17.7</td><td>39</td><td>New Hampshire</td><td>19.4</td></tr>
<tr><td>14</td><td>South Carolina</td><td>22.5</td><td>40</td><td>Washington</td><td>19.3</td></tr>
<tr><td>23</td><td>South Dakota</td><td>21.2</td><td>41</td><td>Utah</td><td>19.1</td></tr>
<tr><td>9</td><td>Tennessee</td><td>23.4</td><td>42</td><td>Florida</td><td>18.8</td></tr>
<tr><td>4</td><td>Texas</td><td>24.6</td><td>42</td><td>Montana</td><td>18.8</td></tr>
<tr><td>41</td><td>Utah</td><td>19.1</td><td>44</td><td>Arizona</td><td>18.5</td></tr>
<tr><td>48</td><td>Vermont</td><td>17.6</td><td>45</td><td>Connecticut</td><td>17.9</td></tr>
<tr><td>26</td><td>Virginia</td><td>20.9</td><td>45</td><td>Hawaii</td><td>17.9</td></tr>
<tr><td>40</td><td>Washington</td><td>19.3</td><td>47</td><td>Rhode Island</td><td>17.7</td></tr>
<tr><td>2</td><td>West Virginia</td><td>25.1</td><td>48</td><td>Vermont</td><td>17.6</td></tr>
<tr><td>16</td><td>Wisconsin</td><td>22.4</td><td>49</td><td>Massachusetts</td><td>16.6</td></tr>
<tr><td>34</td><td>Wyoming</td><td>19.7</td><td>50</td><td>Colorado</td><td>14.9</td></tr>
<tr><td></td><td></td><td></td><td></td><td>District of Columbia</td><td>20.0</td></tr>
</table>

Source: U.S. Department of Health and Human Services, Centers for Disease Control and Prevention
"2001 Behavioral Risk Factor Surveillance Summary Prevalence Report" (August 9, 2002)
*Persons 18 and older. Obese is defined as a Body Mass Index (BMI) of 30.0 or more regardless of sex. BMI is a ratio of height to weight. As an example, a person 5' 8" and weighing 197 pounds has a BMI of 30.
See http://www.cdc.gov/nccdphp/dnpa/bmi/bmi-adult.htm.

Percent of Adults Overweight: 2001

National Median = 37.1% of Adults*

ALPHA ORDER

RANK	STATE	PERCENT
26	Alabama	37.1
1	Alaska	41.1
20	Arizona	37.4
26	Arkansas	37.1
17	California	37.5
37	Colorado	36.5
25	Connecticut	37.2
8	Delaware	38.4
28	Florida	37.0
32	Georgia	36.7
50	Hawaii	33.4
6	Idaho	38.8
17	Illinois	37.5
45	Indiana	35.4
22	Iowa	37.3
45	Kansas	35.4
17	Kentucky	37.5
40	Louisiana	36.2
4	Maine	39.2
37	Maryland	36.5
15	Massachusetts	37.8
48	Michigan	35.1
3	Minnesota	40.6
22	Mississippi	37.3
39	Missouri	36.3
14	Montana	37.9
7	Nebraska	38.5
28	Nevada	37.0
32	New Hampshire	36.7
11	New Jersey	38.2
20	New Mexico	37.4
43	New York	35.7
42	North Carolina	35.9
1	North Dakota	41.1
16	Ohio	37.7
5	Oklahoma	39.0
28	Oregon	37.0
11	Pennsylvania	38.2
8	Rhode Island	38.4
22	South Carolina	37.3
10	South Dakota	38.3
45	Tennessee	35.4
35	Texas	36.6
44	Utah	35.6
49	Vermont	34.5
31	Virginia	36.9
32	Washington	36.7
13	West Virginia	38.0
35	Wisconsin	36.6
41	Wyoming	36.0

RANK ORDER

RANK	STATE	PERCENT
1	Alaska	41.1
1	North Dakota	41.1
3	Minnesota	40.6
4	Maine	39.2
5	Oklahoma	39.0
6	Idaho	38.8
7	Nebraska	38.5
8	Delaware	38.4
8	Rhode Island	38.4
10	South Dakota	38.3
11	New Jersey	38.2
11	Pennsylvania	38.2
13	West Virginia	38.0
14	Montana	37.9
15	Massachusetts	37.8
16	Ohio	37.7
17	California	37.5
17	Illinois	37.5
17	Kentucky	37.5
20	Arizona	37.4
20	New Mexico	37.4
22	Iowa	37.3
22	Mississippi	37.3
22	South Carolina	37.3
25	Connecticut	37.2
26	Alabama	37.1
26	Arkansas	37.1
28	Florida	37.0
28	Nevada	37.0
28	Oregon	37.0
31	Virginia	36.9
32	Georgia	36.7
32	New Hampshire	36.7
32	Washington	36.7
35	Texas	36.6
35	Wisconsin	36.6
37	Colorado	36.5
37	Maryland	36.5
39	Missouri	36.3
40	Louisiana	36.2
41	Wyoming	36.0
42	North Carolina	35.9
43	New York	35.7
44	Utah	35.6
45	Indiana	35.4
45	Kansas	35.4
45	Tennessee	35.4
48	Michigan	35.1
49	Vermont	34.5
50	Hawaii	33.4
	District of Columbia	32.0

Source: U.S. Department of Health and Human Services, Centers for Disease Control and Prevention
"2001 Behavioral Risk Factor Surveillance Summary Prevalence Report" (August 9, 2002)
*Persons 18 and older. Overweight is defined as a Body Mass Index (BMI) of 25.0 to 29.9 regardless of sex. BMI
is a ratio of height to weight. As an example, a person 5' 8" and weighing 171 pounds has a BMI of 26.
See http://www.cdc.gov/nccdphp/dnpa/bmi/bmi-adult.htm.

Percent of Adults Who Exercise Vigorously: 2001

National Median = 24.5% of Adults*

ALPHA ORDER

RANK	STATE	PERCENT
38	Alabama	21.3
1	Alaska	33.7
12	Arizona	28.1
31	Arkansas	23.7
18	California	26.1
8	Colorado	28.9
13	Connecticut	27.6
38	Delaware	21.3
36	Florida	22.6
34	Georgia	23.1
17	Hawaii	26.4
6	Idaho	29.7
20	Illinois	25.2
22	Indiana	24.9
45	Iowa	19.5
32	Kansas	23.5
50	Kentucky	10.9
48	Louisiana	17.9
16	Maine	26.6
22	Maryland	24.9
9	Massachusetts	28.7
28	Michigan	24.1
25	Minnesota	24.5
47	Mississippi	18.6
40	Missouri	20.8
28	Montana	24.1
49	Nebraska	16.4
15	Nevada	26.7
11	New Hampshire	28.3
35	New Jersey	22.7
19	New Mexico	25.8
37	New York	22.5
42	North Carolina	20.5
27	North Dakota	24.2
28	Ohio	24.1
46	Oklahoma	18.8
6	Oregon	29.7
25	Pennsylvania	24.5
24	Rhode Island	24.6
21	South Carolina	25.0
40	South Dakota	20.8
43	Tennessee	19.6
33	Texas	23.4
2	Utah	31.9
3	Vermont	30.6
14	Virginia	26.9
5	Washington	29.8
43	West Virginia	19.6
10	Wisconsin	28.4
4	Wyoming	30.5

RANK ORDER

RANK	STATE	PERCENT
1	Alaska	33.7
2	Utah	31.9
3	Vermont	30.6
4	Wyoming	30.5
5	Washington	29.8
6	Idaho	29.7
6	Oregon	29.7
8	Colorado	28.9
9	Massachusetts	28.7
10	Wisconsin	28.4
11	New Hampshire	28.3
12	Arizona	28.1
13	Connecticut	27.6
14	Virginia	26.9
15	Nevada	26.7
16	Maine	26.6
17	Hawaii	26.4
18	California	26.1
19	New Mexico	25.8
20	Illinois	25.2
21	South Carolina	25.0
22	Indiana	24.9
22	Maryland	24.9
24	Rhode Island	24.6
25	Minnesota	24.5
25	Pennsylvania	24.5
27	North Dakota	24.2
28	Michigan	24.1
28	Montana	24.1
28	Ohio	24.1
31	Arkansas	23.7
32	Kansas	23.5
33	Texas	23.4
34	Georgia	23.1
35	New Jersey	22.7
36	Florida	22.6
37	New York	22.5
38	Alabama	21.3
38	Delaware	21.3
40	Missouri	20.8
40	South Dakota	20.8
42	North Carolina	20.5
43	Tennessee	19.6
43	West Virginia	19.6
45	Iowa	19.5
46	Oklahoma	18.8
47	Mississippi	18.6
48	Louisiana	17.9
49	Nebraska	16.4
50	Kentucky	10.9

| | District of Columbia | 27.0 |

Source: U.S. Department of Health and Human Services, Centers for Disease Control and Prevention
  "2001 Behavioral Risk Factor Surveillance Summary Prevalence Report" (August 9, 2002)
*Persons 18 and older.   Activity that caused large increases in breathing or heart rate at least 20 minutes three or
more times per week (such as running, aerobics or heavy yardwork).

Percent of Adults With No Leisure Time Physical Activity: 2001

National Median = 25.8% of Adults*

ALPHA ORDER

RANK	STATE	PERCENT
9	Alabama	31.2
40	Alaska	21.1
37	Arizona	21.9
7	Arkansas	31.5
16	California	26.6
46	Colorado	19.2
30	Connecticut	24.0
25	Delaware	25.7
11	Florida	27.7
13	Georgia	27.3
47	Hawaii	18.9
41	Idaho	21.0
18	Illinois	26.5
21	Indiana	26.2
23	Iowa	25.9
15	Kansas	26.7
3	Kentucky	33.4
1	Louisiana	35.6
32	Maine	23.2
29	Maryland	24.2
35	Massachusetts	22.8
31	Michigan	23.4
48	Minnesota	17.1
3	Mississippi	33.4
12	Missouri	27.5
37	Montana	21.9
8	Nebraska	31.4
36	Nevada	22.6
45	New Hampshire	19.5
16	New Jersey	26.6
24	New Mexico	25.8
10	New York	28.7
19	North Carolina	26.4
32	North Dakota	23.2
21	Ohio	26.2
5	Oklahoma	32.8
42	Oregon	20.8
28	Pennsylvania	24.7
27	Rhode Island	24.9
19	South Carolina	26.4
26	South Dakota	25.4
2	Tennessee	35.1
14	Texas	27.1
50	Utah	16.5
44	Vermont	20.3
32	Virginia	23.2
48	Washington	17.1
6	West Virginia	31.7
43	Wisconsin	20.7
39	Wyoming	21.2

RANK ORDER

RANK	STATE	PERCENT
1	Louisiana	35.6
2	Tennessee	35.1
3	Kentucky	33.4
3	Mississippi	33.4
5	Oklahoma	32.8
6	West Virginia	31.7
7	Arkansas	31.5
8	Nebraska	31.4
9	Alabama	31.2
10	New York	28.7
11	Florida	27.7
12	Missouri	27.5
13	Georgia	27.3
14	Texas	27.1
15	Kansas	26.7
16	California	26.6
16	New Jersey	26.6
18	Illinois	26.5
19	North Carolina	26.4
19	South Carolina	26.4
21	Indiana	26.2
21	Ohio	26.2
23	Iowa	25.9
24	New Mexico	25.8
25	Delaware	25.7
26	South Dakota	25.4
27	Rhode Island	24.9
28	Pennsylvania	24.7
29	Maryland	24.2
30	Connecticut	24.0
31	Michigan	23.4
32	Maine	23.2
32	North Dakota	23.2
32	Virginia	23.2
35	Massachusetts	22.8
36	Nevada	22.6
37	Arizona	21.9
37	Montana	21.9
39	Wyoming	21.2
40	Alaska	21.1
41	Idaho	21.0
42	Oregon	20.8
43	Wisconsin	20.7
44	Vermont	20.3
45	New Hampshire	19.5
46	Colorado	19.2
47	Hawaii	18.9
48	Minnesota	17.1
48	Washington	17.1
50	Utah	16.5

	District of Columbia	24.2

Source: U.S. Department of Health and Human Services, Centers for Disease Control and Prevention
"2001 Behavioral Risk Factor Surveillance Summary Prevalence Report" (August 9, 2002)
*Persons 18 and older reporting no leisure time physical activity in the past month.

Number of Days in Past Month When Physical Health was "Not Good": 2001

National Average = 3.5 Days*

ALPHA ORDER

RANK	STATE	DAYS
3	Alabama	4.2
18	Alaska	3.5
7	Arizona	3.9
2	Arkansas	4.5
18	California	3.5
27	Colorado	3.3
36	Connecticut	3.2
22	Delaware	3.4
18	Florida	3.5
27	Georgia	3.3
50	Hawaii	2.1
27	Idaho	3.3
43	Illinois	3.0
18	Indiana	3.5
43	Iowa	3.0
45	Kansas	2.9
6	Kentucky	4.0
36	Louisiana	3.2
10	Maine	3.7
40	Maryland	3.1
22	Massachusetts	3.4
10	Michigan	3.7
40	Minnesota	3.1
3	Mississippi	4.2
15	Missouri	3.6
22	Montana	3.4
48	Nebraska	2.8
15	Nevada	3.6
45	New Hampshire	2.9
27	New Jersey	3.3
10	New Mexico	3.7
10	New York	3.7
15	North Carolina	3.6
49	North Dakota	2.7
27	Ohio	3.3
5	Oklahoma	4.1
10	Oregon	3.7
22	Pennsylvania	3.4
8	Rhode Island	3.8
8	South Carolina	3.8
45	South Dakota	2.9
27	Tennessee	3.3
36	Texas	3.2
27	Utah	3.3
27	Vermont	3.3
27	Virginia	3.3
22	Washington	3.4
1	West Virginia	5.3
36	Wisconsin	3.2
40	Wyoming	3.1

RANK ORDER

RANK	STATE	DAYS
1	West Virginia	5.3
2	Arkansas	4.5
3	Alabama	4.2
3	Mississippi	4.2
5	Oklahoma	4.1
6	Kentucky	4.0
7	Arizona	3.9
8	Rhode Island	3.8
8	South Carolina	3.8
10	Maine	3.7
10	Michigan	3.7
10	New Mexico	3.7
10	New York	3.7
10	Oregon	3.7
15	Missouri	3.6
15	Nevada	3.6
15	North Carolina	3.6
18	Alaska	3.5
18	California	3.5
18	Florida	3.5
18	Indiana	3.5
22	Delaware	3.4
22	Massachusetts	3.4
22	Montana	3.4
22	Pennsylvania	3.4
22	Washington	3.4
27	Colorado	3.3
27	Georgia	3.3
27	Idaho	3.3
27	New Jersey	3.3
27	Ohio	3.3
27	Tennessee	3.3
27	Utah	3.3
27	Vermont	3.3
27	Virginia	3.3
36	Connecticut	3.2
36	Louisiana	3.2
36	Texas	3.2
36	Wisconsin	3.2
40	Maryland	3.1
40	Minnesota	3.1
40	Wyoming	3.1
43	Illinois	3.0
43	Iowa	3.0
45	Kansas	2.9
45	New Hampshire	2.9
45	South Dakota	2.9
48	Nebraska	2.8
49	North Dakota	2.7
50	Hawaii	2.1
	District of Columbia**	NA

Source: U.S. Department of Health and Human Services, Centers for Disease Control and Prevention
   "2001 Behavioral Risk Factor Surveillance Summary Prevalence Report" (August 9, 2002)
*Persons 18 and older.
**Not available.

Number of Days in Past Month When Mental Health was "Not Good": 2001

National Average = 3.4 Days*

ALPHA ORDER

RANK	STATE	DAYS
3	Alabama	4.3
29	Alaska	3.2
17	Arizona	3.4
4	Arkansas	3.8
14	California	3.5
8	Colorado	3.6
29	Connecticut	3.2
29	Delaware	3.2
34	Florida	3.1
5	Georgia	3.7
50	Hawaii	1.5
14	Idaho	3.5
41	Illinois	2.9
8	Indiana	3.6
44	Iowa	2.7
41	Kansas	2.9
1	Kentucky	4.7
41	Louisiana	2.9
26	Maine	3.3
29	Maryland	3.2
17	Massachusetts	3.4
5	Michigan	3.7
34	Minnesota	3.1
34	Mississippi	3.1
17	Missouri	3.4
48	Montana	2.5
44	Nebraska	2.7
5	Nevada	3.7
40	New Hampshire	3.0
17	New Jersey	3.4
17	New Mexico	3.4
14	New York	3.5
44	North Carolina	2.7
47	North Dakota	2.6
26	Ohio	3.3
17	Oklahoma	3.4
17	Oregon	3.4
8	Pennsylvania	3.6
8	Rhode Island	3.6
17	South Carolina	3.4
48	South Dakota	2.5
34	Tennessee	3.1
17	Texas	3.4
8	Utah	3.6
34	Vermont	3.1
8	Virginia	3.6
26	Washington	3.3
2	West Virginia	4.4
29	Wisconsin	3.2
34	Wyoming	3.1

RANK ORDER

RANK	STATE	DAYS
1	Kentucky	4.7
2	West Virginia	4.4
3	Alabama	4.3
4	Arkansas	3.8
5	Georgia	3.7
5	Michigan	3.7
5	Nevada	3.7
8	Colorado	3.6
8	Indiana	3.6
8	Pennsylvania	3.6
8	Rhode Island	3.6
8	Utah	3.6
8	Virginia	3.6
14	California	3.5
14	Idaho	3.5
14	New York	3.5
17	Arizona	3.4
17	Massachusetts	3.4
17	Missouri	3.4
17	New Jersey	3.4
17	New Mexico	3.4
17	Oklahoma	3.4
17	Oregon	3.4
17	South Carolina	3.4
17	Texas	3.4
26	Maine	3.3
26	Ohio	3.3
26	Washington	3.3
29	Alaska	3.2
29	Connecticut	3.2
29	Delaware	3.2
29	Maryland	3.2
29	Wisconsin	3.2
34	Florida	3.1
34	Minnesota	3.1
34	Mississippi	3.1
34	Tennessee	3.1
34	Vermont	3.1
34	Wyoming	3.1
40	New Hampshire	3.0
41	Illinois	2.9
41	Kansas	2.9
41	Louisiana	2.9
44	Iowa	2.7
44	Nebraska	2.7
44	North Carolina	2.7
47	North Dakota	2.6
48	Montana	2.5
48	South Dakota	2.5
50	Hawaii	1.5

District of Columbia**   NA

Source: U.S. Department of Health and Human Services, Centers for Disease Control and Prevention
"2001 Behavioral Risk Factor Surveillance Summary Prevalence Report" (August 9, 2002)
*Persons 18 and older.
**Not available.

Percent of Population Rating Their Health as Fair or Poor in 2001

National Median = 15.5% of Adults*

ALPHA ORDER

RANK	STATE	PERCENT
4	Alabama	21.2
45	Alaska	11.3
12	Arizona	16.1
7	Arkansas	19.5
13	California	16.0
31	Colorado	13.2
43	Connecticut	11.5
33	Delaware	13.1
13	Florida	16.0
15	Georgia	15.9
40	Hawaii	12.4
34	Idaho	13.0
28	Illinois	13.5
25	Indiana	14.0
42	Iowa	11.9
37	Kansas	12.6
3	Kentucky	21.7
17	Louisiana	15.5
31	Maine	13.2
27	Maryland	13.8
41	Massachusetts	12.1
22	Michigan	14.6
47	Minnesota	11.0
2	Mississippi	22.9
17	Missouri	15.5
23	Montana	14.4
34	Nebraska	13.0
29	Nevada	13.4
50	New Hampshire	9.4
17	New Jersey	15.5
9	New Mexico	16.9
11	New York	16.3
10	North Carolina	16.4
37	North Dakota	12.6
24	Ohio	14.2
6	Oklahoma	19.6
21	Oregon	14.8
25	Pennsylvania	14.0
20	Rhode Island	15.3
16	South Carolina	15.6
37	South Dakota	12.6
5	Tennessee	19.9
8	Texas	19.3
49	Utah	10.0
43	Vermont	11.5
30	Virginia	13.3
36	Washington	12.8
1	West Virginia	24.2
46	Wisconsin	11.1
48	Wyoming	10.9

RANK ORDER

RANK	STATE	PERCENT
1	West Virginia	24.2
2	Mississippi	22.9
3	Kentucky	21.7
4	Alabama	21.2
5	Tennessee	19.9
6	Oklahoma	19.6
7	Arkansas	19.5
8	Texas	19.3
9	New Mexico	16.9
10	North Carolina	16.4
11	New York	16.3
12	Arizona	16.1
13	California	16.0
13	Florida	16.0
15	Georgia	15.9
16	South Carolina	15.6
17	Louisiana	15.5
17	Missouri	15.5
17	New Jersey	15.5
20	Rhode Island	15.3
21	Oregon	14.8
22	Michigan	14.6
23	Montana	14.4
24	Ohio	14.2
25	Indiana	14.0
25	Pennsylvania	14.0
27	Maryland	13.8
28	Illinois	13.5
29	Nevada	13.4
30	Virginia	13.3
31	Colorado	13.2
31	Maine	13.2
33	Delaware	13.1
34	Idaho	13.0
34	Nebraska	13.0
36	Washington	12.8
37	Kansas	12.6
37	North Dakota	12.6
37	South Dakota	12.6
40	Hawaii	12.4
41	Massachusetts	12.1
42	Iowa	11.9
43	Connecticut	11.5
43	Vermont	11.5
45	Alaska	11.3
46	Wisconsin	11.1
47	Minnesota	11.0
48	Wyoming	10.9
49	Utah	10.0
50	New Hampshire	9.4
	District of Columbia**	NA

Source: U.S. Department of Health and Human Services, Centers for Disease Control and Prevention
"2001 Behavioral Risk Factor Surveillance Summary Prevalence Report" (August 9, 2002)
*Persons 18 and older.
**Not available.

Safety Belt Usage Rate in 2001

National Rate = 73.0% Use Safety Belts*

<table>
<tr><td colspan="3">ALPHA ORDER</td><td colspan="3">RANK ORDER</td></tr>
<tr><th>RANK</th><th>STATE</th><th>PERCENT</th><th>RANK</th><th>STATE</th><th>PERCENT</th></tr>
<tr><td>11</td><td>Alabama</td><td>79.4</td><td>1</td><td>California</td><td>91.1</td></tr>
<tr><td>39</td><td>Alaska</td><td>62.6</td><td>2</td><td>New Mexico</td><td>87.8</td></tr>
<tr><td>19</td><td>Arizona</td><td>74.4</td><td>3</td><td>Oregon</td><td>87.5</td></tr>
<tr><td>46</td><td>Arkansas</td><td>54.5</td><td>4</td><td>Maryland</td><td>82.9</td></tr>
<tr><td>1</td><td>California</td><td>91.1</td><td>5</td><td>North Carolina</td><td>82.7</td></tr>
<tr><td>22</td><td>Colorado</td><td>72.1</td><td>6</td><td>Washington</td><td>82.6</td></tr>
<tr><td>13</td><td>Connecticut</td><td>78.0</td><td>7</td><td>Hawaii</td><td>82.5</td></tr>
<tr><td>35</td><td>Delaware</td><td>67.3</td><td>8</td><td>Michigan</td><td>82.3</td></tr>
<tr><td>27</td><td>Florida</td><td>69.5</td><td>9</td><td>Iowa</td><td>80.9</td></tr>
<tr><td>12</td><td>Georgia</td><td>79.0</td><td>10</td><td>New York</td><td>80.3</td></tr>
<tr><td>7</td><td>Hawaii</td><td>82.5</td><td>11</td><td>Alabama</td><td>79.4</td></tr>
<tr><td>43</td><td>Idaho</td><td>60.4</td><td>12</td><td>Georgia</td><td>79.0</td></tr>
<tr><td>23</td><td>Illinois</td><td>71.4</td><td>13</td><td>Connecticut</td><td>78.0</td></tr>
<tr><td>33</td><td>Indiana</td><td>67.4</td><td>14</td><td>Utah</td><td>77.8</td></tr>
<tr><td>9</td><td>Iowa</td><td>80.9</td><td>15</td><td>New Jersey</td><td>77.6</td></tr>
<tr><td>42</td><td>Kansas</td><td>60.8</td><td>16</td><td>Montana</td><td>76.3</td></tr>
<tr><td>40</td><td>Kentucky</td><td>61.9</td><td>17</td><td>Texas</td><td>76.1</td></tr>
<tr><td>30</td><td>Louisiana</td><td>68.1</td><td>18</td><td>Nevada</td><td>74.5</td></tr>
<tr><td>NA</td><td>Maine**</td><td>NA</td><td>19</td><td>Arizona</td><td>74.4</td></tr>
<tr><td>4</td><td>Maryland</td><td>82.9</td><td>20</td><td>Minnesota</td><td>73.9</td></tr>
<tr><td>45</td><td>Massachusetts</td><td>56.0</td><td>21</td><td>Virginia</td><td>72.3</td></tr>
<tr><td>8</td><td>Michigan</td><td>82.3</td><td>22</td><td>Colorado</td><td>72.1</td></tr>
<tr><td>20</td><td>Minnesota</td><td>73.9</td><td>23</td><td>Illinois</td><td>71.4</td></tr>
<tr><td>41</td><td>Mississippi</td><td>61.6</td><td>24</td><td>Pennsylvania</td><td>70.5</td></tr>
<tr><td>31</td><td>Missouri</td><td>67.9</td><td>25</td><td>Nebraska</td><td>70.2</td></tr>
<tr><td>16</td><td>Montana</td><td>76.3</td><td>26</td><td>South Carolina</td><td>69.6</td></tr>
<tr><td>25</td><td>Nebraska</td><td>70.2</td><td>27</td><td>Florida</td><td>69.5</td></tr>
<tr><td>18</td><td>Nevada</td><td>74.5</td><td>28</td><td>Wisconsin</td><td>68.7</td></tr>
<tr><td>NA</td><td>New Hampshire**</td><td>NA</td><td>29</td><td>Tennessee</td><td>68.3</td></tr>
<tr><td>15</td><td>New Jersey</td><td>77.6</td><td>30</td><td>Louisiana</td><td>68.1</td></tr>
<tr><td>2</td><td>New Mexico</td><td>87.8</td><td>31</td><td>Missouri</td><td>67.9</td></tr>
<tr><td>10</td><td>New York</td><td>80.3</td><td>31</td><td>Oklahoma</td><td>67.9</td></tr>
<tr><td>5</td><td>North Carolina</td><td>82.7</td><td>33</td><td>Indiana</td><td>67.4</td></tr>
<tr><td>44</td><td>North Dakota</td><td>57.9</td><td>33</td><td>Vermont</td><td>67.4</td></tr>
<tr><td>36</td><td>Ohio</td><td>66.9</td><td>35</td><td>Delaware</td><td>67.3</td></tr>
<tr><td>31</td><td>Oklahoma</td><td>67.9</td><td>36</td><td>Ohio</td><td>66.9</td></tr>
<tr><td>3</td><td>Oregon</td><td>87.5</td><td>37</td><td>South Dakota</td><td>63.3</td></tr>
<tr><td>24</td><td>Pennsylvania</td><td>70.5</td><td>38</td><td>Rhode Island</td><td>63.2</td></tr>
<tr><td>38</td><td>Rhode Island</td><td>63.2</td><td>39</td><td>Alaska</td><td>62.6</td></tr>
<tr><td>26</td><td>South Carolina</td><td>69.6</td><td>40</td><td>Kentucky</td><td>61.9</td></tr>
<tr><td>37</td><td>South Dakota</td><td>63.3</td><td>41</td><td>Mississippi</td><td>61.6</td></tr>
<tr><td>29</td><td>Tennessee</td><td>68.3</td><td>42</td><td>Kansas</td><td>60.8</td></tr>
<tr><td>17</td><td>Texas</td><td>76.1</td><td>43</td><td>Idaho</td><td>60.4</td></tr>
<tr><td>14</td><td>Utah</td><td>77.8</td><td>44</td><td>North Dakota</td><td>57.9</td></tr>
<tr><td>33</td><td>Vermont</td><td>67.4</td><td>45</td><td>Massachusetts</td><td>56.0</td></tr>
<tr><td>21</td><td>Virginia</td><td>72.3</td><td>46</td><td>Arkansas</td><td>54.5</td></tr>
<tr><td>6</td><td>Washington</td><td>82.6</td><td>47</td><td>West Virginia</td><td>52.3</td></tr>
<tr><td>47</td><td>West Virginia</td><td>52.3</td><td>NA</td><td>Maine**</td><td>NA</td></tr>
<tr><td>28</td><td>Wisconsin</td><td>68.7</td><td>NA</td><td>New Hampshire**</td><td>NA</td></tr>
<tr><td>NA</td><td>Wyoming**</td><td>NA</td><td>NA</td><td>Wyoming**</td><td>NA</td></tr>
<tr><td></td><td></td><td></td><td></td><td>District of Columbia</td><td>83.6</td></tr>
</table>

Source: U.S. Department of Transportation, National Highway Traffic Safety Administration
    "Traffic Safety Facts 2001" (http://www-nrd.nhtsa.dot.gov/pdf/nrd-30/NCSA/TSF2001/2001statedata.pdf)
As of December 2001.
**Not available.*

VIII. APPENDIX

Population Charts

Population in 2002

National Total = 288,368,698*

ALPHA ORDER

RANK	STATE	POPULATION	% of USA
23	Alabama	4,486,508	1.6%
47	Alaska	643,786	0.2%
19	Arizona	5,456,453	1.9%
33	Arkansas	2,710,079	0.9%
1	California	35,116,033	12.2%
22	Colorado	4,506,542	1.6%
29	Connecticut	3,460,503	1.2%
45	Delaware	807,385	0.3%
4	Florida	16,713,149	5.8%
10	Georgia	8,560,310	3.0%
42	Hawaii	1,244,898	0.4%
39	Idaho	1,341,131	0.5%
5	Illinois	12,600,620	4.4%
14	Indiana	6,159,068	2.1%
30	Iowa	2,936,760	1.0%
32	Kansas	2,715,884	0.9%
26	Kentucky	4,092,891	1.4%
24	Louisiana	4,482,646	1.6%
40	Maine	1,294,464	0.4%
18	Maryland	5,458,137	1.9%
13	Massachusetts	6,427,801	2.2%
8	Michigan	10,050,446	3.5%
21	Minnesota	5,019,720	1.7%
31	Mississippi	2,871,782	1.0%
17	Missouri	5,672,579	2.0%
44	Montana	909,453	0.3%
38	Nebraska	1,729,180	0.6%
35	Nevada	2,173,491	0.8%
41	New Hampshire	1,275,056	0.4%
9	New Jersey	8,590,300	3.0%
36	New Mexico	1,855,059	0.6%
3	New York	19,157,532	6.6%
11	North Carolina	8,320,146	2.9%
48	North Dakota	634,110	0.2%
7	Ohio	11,421,267	4.0%
28	Oklahoma	3,493,714	1.2%
27	Oregon	3,521,515	1.2%
6	Pennsylvania	12,335,091	4.3%
43	Rhode Island	1,069,725	0.4%
25	South Carolina	4,107,183	1.4%
46	South Dakota	761,063	0.3%
16	Tennessee	5,797,289	2.0%
2	Texas	21,779,893	7.6%
34	Utah	2,316,256	0.8%
49	Vermont	616,592	0.2%
12	Virginia	7,293,542	2.5%
15	Washington	6,068,996	2.1%
37	West Virginia	1,801,873	0.6%
20	Wisconsin	5,441,196	1.9%
50	Wyoming	498,703	0.2%

RANK ORDER

RANK	STATE	POPULATION	% of USA
1	California	35,116,033	12.2%
2	Texas	21,779,893	7.6%
3	New York	19,157,532	6.6%
4	Florida	16,713,149	5.8%
5	Illinois	12,600,620	4.4%
6	Pennsylvania	12,335,091	4.3%
7	Ohio	11,421,267	4.0%
8	Michigan	10,050,446	3.5%
9	New Jersey	8,590,300	3.0%
10	Georgia	8,560,310	3.0%
11	North Carolina	8,320,146	2.9%
12	Virginia	7,293,542	2.5%
13	Massachusetts	6,427,801	2.2%
14	Indiana	6,159,068	2.1%
15	Washington	6,068,996	2.1%
16	Tennessee	5,797,289	2.0%
17	Missouri	5,672,579	2.0%
18	Maryland	5,458,137	1.9%
19	Arizona	5,456,453	1.9%
20	Wisconsin	5,441,196	1.9%
21	Minnesota	5,019,720	1.7%
22	Colorado	4,506,542	1.6%
23	Alabama	4,486,508	1.6%
24	Louisiana	4,482,646	1.6%
25	South Carolina	4,107,183	1.4%
26	Kentucky	4,092,891	1.4%
27	Oregon	3,521,515	1.2%
28	Oklahoma	3,493,714	1.2%
29	Connecticut	3,460,503	1.2%
30	Iowa	2,936,760	1.0%
31	Mississippi	2,871,782	1.0%
32	Kansas	2,715,884	0.9%
33	Arkansas	2,710,079	0.9%
34	Utah	2,316,256	0.8%
35	Nevada	2,173,491	0.8%
36	New Mexico	1,855,059	0.6%
37	West Virginia	1,801,873	0.6%
38	Nebraska	1,729,180	0.6%
39	Idaho	1,341,131	0.5%
40	Maine	1,294,464	0.4%
41	New Hampshire	1,275,056	0.4%
42	Hawaii	1,244,898	0.4%
43	Rhode Island	1,069,725	0.4%
44	Montana	909,453	0.3%
45	Delaware	807,385	0.3%
46	South Dakota	761,063	0.3%
47	Alaska	643,786	0.2%
48	North Dakota	634,110	0.2%
49	Vermont	616,592	0.2%
50	Wyoming	498,703	0.2%
	District of Columbia	570,898	0.2%

Source: U.S. Bureau of the Census
  "Population Estimates" (December 20, 2002, http://eire.census.gov/popest/estimates.php)
*Resident population.

Population in 2001

National Total = 285,317,559*

ALPHA ORDER

RANK	STATE	POPULATION	% of USA
23	Alabama	4,468,912	1.6%
48	Alaska	633,630	0.2%
20	Arizona	5,306,966	1.9%
33	Arkansas	2,694,698	0.9%
1	California	34,600,463	12.1%
24	Colorado	4,430,989	1.6%
29	Connecticut	3,434,602	1.2%
45	Delaware	796,599	0.3%
4	Florida	16,373,330	5.7%
10	Georgia	8,405,677	2.9%
42	Hawaii	1,227,024	0.4%
39	Idaho	1,320,585	0.5%
5	Illinois	12,520,227	4.4%
14	Indiana	6,126,743	2.1%
30	Iowa	2,931,967	1.0%
32	Kansas	2,702,125	0.9%
25	Kentucky	4,068,816	1.4%
22	Louisiana	4,470,368	1.6%
40	Maine	1,284,470	0.5%
19	Maryland	5,386,079	1.9%
13	Massachusetts	6,401,164	2.2%
8	Michigan	10,006,266	3.5%
21	Minnesota	4,984,535	1.7%
31	Mississippi	2,859,733	1.0%
17	Missouri	5,637,309	2.0%
44	Montana	905,382	0.3%
38	Nebraska	1,720,039	0.6%
35	Nevada	2,097,722	0.7%
41	New Hampshire	1,259,359	0.4%
9	New Jersey	8,511,116	3.0%
36	New Mexico	1,830,935	0.6%
3	New York	19,084,350	6.7%
11	North Carolina	8,206,105	2.9%
47	North Dakota	636,550	0.2%
7	Ohio	11,389,785	4.0%
28	Oklahoma	3,469,577	1.2%
27	Oregon	3,473,441	1.2%
6	Pennsylvania	12,303,104	4.3%
43	Rhode Island	1,059,659	0.4%
26	South Carolina	4,062,125	1.4%
46	South Dakota	758,324	0.3%
16	Tennessee	5,749,398	2.0%
2	Texas	21,370,983	7.5%
34	Utah	2,278,712	0.8%
49	Vermont	612,978	0.2%
12	Virginia	7,196,750	2.5%
15	Washington	5,993,390	2.1%
37	West Virginia	1,800,975	0.6%
18	Wisconsin	5,405,947	1.9%
50	Wyoming	493,754	0.2%

RANK ORDER

RANK	STATE	POPULATION	% of USA
1	California	34,600,463	12.1%
2	Texas	21,370,983	7.5%
3	New York	19,084,350	6.7%
4	Florida	16,373,330	5.7%
5	Illinois	12,520,227	4.4%
6	Pennsylvania	12,303,104	4.3%
7	Ohio	11,389,785	4.0%
8	Michigan	10,006,266	3.5%
9	New Jersey	8,511,116	3.0%
10	Georgia	8,405,677	2.9%
11	North Carolina	8,206,105	2.9%
12	Virginia	7,196,750	2.5%
13	Massachusetts	6,401,164	2.2%
14	Indiana	6,126,743	2.1%
15	Washington	5,993,390	2.1%
16	Tennessee	5,749,398	2.0%
17	Missouri	5,637,309	2.0%
18	Wisconsin	5,405,947	1.9%
19	Maryland	5,386,079	1.9%
20	Arizona	5,306,966	1.9%
21	Minnesota	4,984,535	1.7%
22	Louisiana	4,470,368	1.6%
23	Alabama	4,468,912	1.6%
24	Colorado	4,430,989	1.6%
25	Kentucky	4,068,816	1.4%
26	South Carolina	4,062,125	1.4%
27	Oregon	3,473,441	1.2%
28	Oklahoma	3,469,577	1.2%
29	Connecticut	3,434,602	1.2%
30	Iowa	2,931,967	1.0%
31	Mississippi	2,859,733	1.0%
32	Kansas	2,702,125	0.9%
33	Arkansas	2,694,698	0.9%
34	Utah	2,278,712	0.8%
35	Nevada	2,097,722	0.7%
36	New Mexico	1,830,935	0.6%
37	West Virginia	1,800,975	0.6%
38	Nebraska	1,720,039	0.6%
39	Idaho	1,320,585	0.5%
40	Maine	1,284,470	0.5%
41	New Hampshire	1,259,359	0.4%
42	Hawaii	1,227,024	0.4%
43	Rhode Island	1,059,659	0.4%
44	Montana	905,382	0.3%
45	Delaware	796,599	0.3%
46	South Dakota	758,324	0.3%
47	North Dakota	636,550	0.2%
48	Alaska	633,630	0.2%
49	Vermont	612,978	0.2%
50	Wyoming	493,754	0.2%
	District of Columbia	573,822	0.2%

Source: U.S. Bureau of the Census
  "Population Estimates" (December 20, 2002, http://eire.census.gov/popest/estimates.php)
*Resident population. Revised estimates.

Male Population in 2000

National Total = 138,053,563 Males

ALPHA ORDER

RANK	STATE	MALES	% of USA
24	Alabama	2,146,504	1.6%
47	Alaska	324,112	0.2%
19	Arizona	2,561,057	1.9%
33	Arkansas	1,304,693	0.9%
1	California	16,874,892	12.2%
22	Colorado	2,165,983	1.6%
29	Connecticut	1,649,319	1.2%
45	Delaware	380,541	0.3%
4	Florida	7,797,715	5.6%
10	Georgia	4,027,113	2.9%
41	Hawaii	608,671	0.4%
39	Idaho	648,660	0.5%
5	Illinois	6,080,336	4.4%
14	Indiana	2,982,474	2.2%
30	Iowa	1,435,515	1.0%
32	Kansas	1,328,474	1.0%
25	Kentucky	1,975,368	1.4%
23	Louisiana	2,162,903	1.6%
40	Maine	620,309	0.4%
20	Maryland	2,557,794	1.9%
13	Massachusetts	3,058,816	2.2%
8	Michigan	4,873,095	3.5%
21	Minnesota	2,435,631	1.8%
31	Mississippi	1,373,554	1.0%
17	Missouri	2,720,177	2.0%
44	Montana	449,480	0.3%
38	Nebraska	843,351	0.6%
35	Nevada	1,018,051	0.7%
42	New Hampshire	607,687	0.4%
9	New Jersey	4,082,813	3.0%
36	New Mexico	894,317	0.6%
3	New York	9,146,748	6.6%
11	North Carolina	3,942,695	2.9%
48	North Dakota	320,524	0.2%
7	Ohio	5,512,262	4.0%
28	Oklahoma	1,695,895	1.2%
27	Oregon	1,696,550	1.2%
6	Pennsylvania	5,929,663	4.3%
43	Rhode Island	503,635	0.4%
26	South Carolina	1,948,929	1.4%
46	South Dakota	374,558	0.3%
16	Tennessee	2,770,275	2.0%
2	Texas	10,352,910	7.5%
34	Utah	1,119,031	0.8%
49	Vermont	298,337	0.2%
12	Virginia	3,471,895	2.5%
15	Washington	2,934,300	2.1%
37	West Virginia	879,170	0.6%
18	Wisconsin	2,649,041	1.9%
50	Wyoming	248,374	0.2%

RANK ORDER

RANK	STATE	MALES	% of USA
1	California	16,874,892	12.2%
2	Texas	10,352,910	7.5%
3	New York	9,146,748	6.6%
4	Florida	7,797,715	5.6%
5	Illinois	6,080,336	4.4%
6	Pennsylvania	5,929,663	4.3%
7	Ohio	5,512,262	4.0%
8	Michigan	4,873,095	3.5%
9	New Jersey	4,082,813	3.0%
10	Georgia	4,027,113	2.9%
11	North Carolina	3,942,695	2.9%
12	Virginia	3,471,895	2.5%
13	Massachusetts	3,058,816	2.2%
14	Indiana	2,982,474	2.2%
15	Washington	2,934,300	2.1%
16	Tennessee	2,770,275	2.0%
17	Missouri	2,720,177	2.0%
18	Wisconsin	2,649,041	1.9%
19	Arizona	2,561,057	1.9%
20	Maryland	2,557,794	1.9%
21	Minnesota	2,435,631	1.8%
22	Colorado	2,165,983	1.6%
23	Louisiana	2,162,903	1.6%
24	Alabama	2,146,504	1.6%
25	Kentucky	1,975,368	1.4%
26	South Carolina	1,948,929	1.4%
27	Oregon	1,696,550	1.2%
28	Oklahoma	1,695,895	1.2%
29	Connecticut	1,649,319	1.2%
30	Iowa	1,435,515	1.0%
31	Mississippi	1,373,554	1.0%
32	Kansas	1,328,474	1.0%
33	Arkansas	1,304,693	0.9%
34	Utah	1,119,031	0.8%
35	Nevada	1,018,051	0.7%
36	New Mexico	894,317	0.6%
37	West Virginia	879,170	0.6%
38	Nebraska	843,351	0.6%
39	Idaho	648,660	0.5%
40	Maine	620,309	0.4%
41	Hawaii	608,671	0.4%
42	New Hampshire	607,687	0.4%
43	Rhode Island	503,635	0.4%
44	Montana	449,480	0.3%
45	Delaware	380,541	0.3%
46	South Dakota	374,558	0.3%
47	Alaska	324,112	0.2%
48	North Dakota	320,524	0.2%
49	Vermont	298,337	0.2%
50	Wyoming	248,374	0.2%
	District of Columbia	269,366	0.2%

Source: U.S. Bureau of the Census
"Census 2000 Summary File 1"

Female Population in 2000

National Total = 143,368,343 Females

ALPHA ORDER

ALPHA ORDER

RANK	STATE	FEMALES	% of USA
23	Alabama	2,300,596	1.6%
49	Alaska	302,820	0.2%
20	Arizona	2,569,575	1.8%
32	Arkansas	1,368,707	1.0%
1	California	16,996,756	11.9%
24	Colorado	2,135,278	1.5%
27	Connecticut	1,756,246	1.2%
45	Delaware	403,059	0.3%
4	Florida	8,184,663	5.7%
10	Georgia	4,159,340	2.9%
42	Hawaii	602,866	0.4%
40	Idaho	645,293	0.5%
6	Illinois	6,338,957	4.4%
14	Indiana	3,098,011	2.2%
30	Iowa	1,490,809	1.0%
33	Kansas	1,359,944	0.9%
25	Kentucky	2,066,401	1.4%
22	Louisiana	2,306,073	1.6%
39	Maine	654,614	0.5%
18	Maryland	2,738,692	1.9%
13	Massachusetts	3,290,281	2.3%
8	Michigan	5,065,349	3.5%
21	Minnesota	2,483,848	1.7%
31	Mississippi	1,471,104	1.0%
17	Missouri	2,875,034	2.0%
44	Montana	452,715	0.3%
38	Nebraska	867,912	0.6%
35	Nevada	980,206	0.7%
41	New Hampshire	628,099	0.4%
9	New Jersey	4,331,537	3.0%
37	New Mexico	924,729	0.6%
3	New York	9,829,709	6.9%
11	North Carolina	4,106,618	2.9%
47	North Dakota	321,676	0.2%
7	Ohio	5,840,878	4.1%
28	Oklahoma	1,754,759	1.2%
29	Oregon	1,724,849	1.2%
5	Pennsylvania	6,351,391	4.4%
43	Rhode Island	544,684	0.4%
26	South Carolina	2,063,083	1.4%
46	South Dakota	380,286	0.3%
16	Tennessee	2,919,008	2.0%
2	Texas	10,498,910	7.3%
34	Utah	1,114,138	0.8%
48	Vermont	310,490	0.2%
12	Virginia	3,606,620	2.5%
15	Washington	2,959,821	2.1%
36	West Virginia	929,174	0.6%
19	Wisconsin	2,714,634	1.9%
50	Wyoming	245,408	0.2%

RANK ORDER

RANK	STATE	FEMALES	% of USA
1	California	16,996,756	11.9%
2	Texas	10,498,910	7.3%
3	New York	9,829,709	6.9%
4	Florida	8,184,663	5.7%
5	Pennsylvania	6,351,391	4.4%
6	Illinois	6,338,957	4.4%
7	Ohio	5,840,878	4.1%
8	Michigan	5,065,349	3.5%
9	New Jersey	4,331,537	3.0%
10	Georgia	4,159,340	2.9%
11	North Carolina	4,106,618	2.9%
12	Virginia	3,606,620	2.5%
13	Massachusetts	3,290,281	2.3%
14	Indiana	3,098,011	2.2%
15	Washington	2,959,821	2.1%
16	Tennessee	2,919,008	2.0%
17	Missouri	2,875,034	2.0%
18	Maryland	2,738,692	1.9%
19	Wisconsin	2,714,634	1.9%
20	Arizona	2,569,575	1.8%
21	Minnesota	2,483,848	1.7%
22	Louisiana	2,306,073	1.6%
23	Alabama	2,300,596	1.6%
24	Colorado	2,135,278	1.5%
25	Kentucky	2,066,401	1.4%
26	South Carolina	2,063,083	1.4%
27	Connecticut	1,756,246	1.2%
28	Oklahoma	1,754,759	1.2%
29	Oregon	1,724,849	1.2%
30	Iowa	1,490,809	1.0%
31	Mississippi	1,471,104	1.0%
32	Arkansas	1,368,707	1.0%
33	Kansas	1,359,944	0.9%
34	Utah	1,114,138	0.8%
35	Nevada	980,206	0.7%
36	West Virginia	929,174	0.6%
37	New Mexico	924,729	0.6%
38	Nebraska	867,912	0.6%
39	Maine	654,614	0.5%
40	Idaho	645,293	0.5%
41	New Hampshire	628,099	0.4%
42	Hawaii	602,866	0.4%
43	Rhode Island	544,684	0.4%
44	Montana	452,715	0.3%
45	Delaware	403,059	0.3%
46	South Dakota	380,286	0.3%
47	North Dakota	321,676	0.2%
48	Vermont	310,490	0.2%
49	Alaska	302,820	0.2%
50	Wyoming	245,408	0.2%
	District of Columbia	302,693	0.2%

Source: U.S. Bureau of the Census
"Census 2000 Summary File 1"

Population in 1998

National Total = 270,248,003*

RANK	STATE	POPULATION	% of USA
23	Alabama	4,351,037	1.6%
48	Alaska	615,205	0.2%
21	Arizona	4,667,277	1.7%
33	Arkansas	2,538,202	0.9%
1	California	32,682,794	12.1%
24	Colorado	3,968,967	1.5%
29	Connecticut	3,272,563	1.2%
45	Delaware	744,066	0.3%
4	Florida	14,908,230	5.5%
10	Georgia	7,636,522	2.8%
41	Hawaii	1,190,472	0.4%
40	Idaho	1,230,923	0.5%
5	Illinois	12,069,774	4.5%
14	Indiana	5,907,617	2.2%
30	Iowa	2,861,025	1.1%
32	Kansas	2,638,667	1.0%
25	Kentucky	3,934,310	1.5%
22	Louisiana	4,362,758	1.6%
39	Maine	1,247,554	0.5%
19	Maryland	5,130,072	1.9%
13	Massachusetts	6,144,407	2.3%
8	Michigan	9,820,231	3.6%
20	Minnesota	4,726,411	1.7%
31	Mississippi	2,751,335	1.0%
16	Missouri	5,437,562	2.0%
44	Montana	879,533	0.3%
38	Nebraska	1,660,772	0.6%
36	Nevada	1,743,772	0.6%
42	New Hampshire	1,185,823	0.4%
9	New Jersey	8,095,542	3.0%
37	New Mexico	1,733,535	0.6%
3	New York	18,159,175	6.7%
11	North Carolina	7,545,828	2.8%
47	North Dakota	637,808	0.2%
7	Ohio	11,237,752	4.2%
27	Oklahoma	3,339,478	1.2%
28	Oregon	3,282,055	1.2%
6	Pennsylvania	12,002,329	4.4%
43	Rhode Island	987,704	0.4%
26	South Carolina	3,839,578	1.4%
46	South Dakota	730,789	0.3%
17	Tennessee	5,432,679	2.0%
2	Texas	19,712,389	7.3%
34	Utah	2,100,562	0.8%
49	Vermont	590,579	0.2%
12	Virginia	6,789,225	2.5%
15	Washington	5,687,832	2.1%
35	West Virginia	1,811,688	0.7%
18	Wisconsin	5,222,124	1.9%
50	Wyoming	480,045	0.2%

RANK	STATE	POPULATION	% of USA
1	California	32,682,794	12.1%
2	Texas	19,712,389	7.3%
3	New York	18,159,175	6.7%
4	Florida	14,908,230	5.5%
5	Illinois	12,069,774	4.5%
6	Pennsylvania	12,002,329	4.4%
7	Ohio	11,237,752	4.2%
8	Michigan	9,820,231	3.6%
9	New Jersey	8,095,542	3.0%
10	Georgia	7,636,522	2.8%
11	North Carolina	7,545,828	2.8%
12	Virginia	6,789,225	2.5%
13	Massachusetts	6,144,407	2.3%
14	Indiana	5,907,617	2.2%
15	Washington	5,687,832	2.1%
16	Missouri	5,437,562	2.0%
17	Tennessee	5,432,679	2.0%
18	Wisconsin	5,222,124	1.9%
19	Maryland	5,130,072	1.9%
20	Minnesota	4,726,411	1.7%
21	Arizona	4,667,277	1.7%
22	Louisiana	4,362,758	1.6%
23	Alabama	4,351,037	1.6%
24	Colorado	3,968,967	1.5%
25	Kentucky	3,934,310	1.5%
26	South Carolina	3,839,578	1.4%
27	Oklahoma	3,339,478	1.2%
28	Oregon	3,282,055	1.2%
29	Connecticut	3,272,563	1.2%
30	Iowa	2,861,025	1.1%
31	Mississippi	2,751,335	1.0%
32	Kansas	2,638,667	1.0%
33	Arkansas	2,538,202	0.9%
34	Utah	2,100,562	0.8%
35	West Virginia	1,811,688	0.7%
36	Nevada	1,743,772	0.6%
37	New Mexico	1,733,535	0.6%
38	Nebraska	1,660,772	0.6%
39	Maine	1,247,554	0.5%
40	Idaho	1,230,923	0.5%
41	Hawaii	1,190,472	0.4%
42	New Hampshire	1,185,823	0.4%
43	Rhode Island	987,704	0.4%
44	Montana	879,533	0.3%
45	Delaware	744,066	0.3%
46	South Dakota	730,789	0.3%
47	North Dakota	637,808	0.2%
48	Alaska	615,205	0.2%
49	Vermont	590,579	0.2%
50	Wyoming	480,045	0.2%
	District of Columbia	521,426	0.2%

Source: U.S. Bureau of the Census
"State Population Estimates" (December 29, 1999, http://www.census.gov/population/estimates/state/st-99-3.txt)
*Includes armed forces residing in each state. This updates earlier 1998 population estimates.

IX. SOURCES

American Academy of Physicians Assistants
950 North Washington Street
Alexandria, VA 22314-1552
703-836-2272
Internet: www.aapa.org

American Cancer Society, Inc.
1599 Clifton Road, NE.
Atlanta, GA 30329-4251
800-227-2345
Internet: http://www.cancer.org

American Dental Association
211 E. Chicago Ave.
Chicago, IL 60611
312-440-2500
Internet: www.ada.org

American Hospital Association
One North Franklin
Chicago, IL 60606-3421
312-422-3000
Internet: www.aha.org

American Medical Association
515 North State Street
Chicago, IL 60610
312-464-5000
Internet: http://www.ama-assn.org

American Osteopathic Association
142 East Ontario Street
Chicago, IL 60611
800-621-1773
Internet: www.aoa-net.org

American Podiatric Medical Association
9312 Old Georgetown Road
Bethesda, MD 20814-1698
301-581-9221
Internet: www.apma.org

Bureau of Labor Statistics
Census of Fatal Occupational Injuries
2 Massachusetts Ave., NE
Washington, DC 20212
202-691-6175
Internet: http://stats.bls.gov/oshhome.htm

Census Bureau
4700 Silver Hill Road
Suitland, MD 20746
301-457-2800
Internet: http://www.census.gov

Centers for Disease Control and Prevention
1600 Clifton Road, NE.
Atlanta, GA 30333
404-639-3534 (Public Affairs)
800-458-5231 (AIDS Clearinghouse)
Internet: http://www.cdc.gov

Centers for Medicare and Medicaid Services
(Formerly Health Care Financing Administration)
7500 Security Boulevard
Baltimore, MD 21244
410-786-3000
Internet: http://www.cms.gov

Federation of Chiropractic Licensing Boards
901 54th Ave., Ste. 101
Greeley, CO 80634-4400
970-356-3500
Internet: www.fclb.org

Health Care Financing Administration
See Centers for Medicare and Medicaid Services

InterStudy
P.O. Box 4366
St. Paul, MN 55104
800-844-3351
Internet: www.hmodata.com

National Center for Health Statistics
U.S. Department of Health and Human Services
3311 Toledo Road
Hyattsville, MD 20782-2003
301-458-4636
Internet: http://www.cdc.gov/nchs/

National Institute on Alcohol Abuse
and Alcoholism
National Institutes of Health
6000 Executive Boulevard
Bethesda, MD 20892-7003
301-443-9970
Internet: www.niaaa.nih.gov/

National Highway Traffic Safety Admin.
400 Seventh Street, SW
Washington, DC 20590
202-366-9550
Internet: www.nhtsa.dot.gov

National Sporting Goods Association
1601 Feehanville Drive, Ste 300
Mt. Prospect, IL 60056-6035
847-296-6742
Internet: www.nsga.org

Smoking and Health Office
Centers for Disease Control and Prevention
4770 Buford Hwy, NE., Mail Stop K-50
Atlanta, GA 30341-3724
770-488-5701
www.cdc.gov/tobacco/

X. INDEX

X. INDEX (continued)

X. INDEX (continued)

Births and Reproductive Health

Deaths

Facilities

Finance

Incidence of Disease

Providers

Physical Fitness

CHAPTER INDEX

HOW TO USE THIS INDEX

Place left thumb on the outer edge of this page. To locate the desired entry, fold back the remaining page edges and align the index edge mark with the appropriate page edge mark.